D0138223

Lumbar

accessory process	
inferior articular process	inferior apophyseal process
mammillary process	
superior articular process	superior apophyseal process

Sacrum and Coccyx

base	body
coccygeal horn	coccygeal cornu
lumbosacral junction	sacrovertebral junction
median sacral crest	medial sacral crest
pelvic sacral foramina	anterior sacral foramina
sacral horn	sacral cornu
superior articular process	articular process
vertebral canal	spinal canal

Chapter 9 Bony Thorax

body of sternum	gladiolus
jugular notch	manubrial notch
xiphoid process	ensiform cartilage

Chapter 10 Thoracic Viscera

cardiac impression	cardiac fossa
costodiaphragmatic recess	costophrenic, or phrenicostal sinus
hilum	hilus
impression	fossa
inferior lobe	lower lobe
jugular notch	manubrial notch
main bronchus	primary bronchus
pulmonary pleura	visceral
superior lobe	upper lobe
superior thoracic aperture	thoracic inlet

Chapter 11 Long Bone Measurement

limb	extremity

Chapter 12 Contrast Arthrography

limb	extremity

Chapter 13 Foreign Body Localization and Trauma Radiography Guidelines

limb	extremity

Chapter 14 Mouth and Salivary Glands

Mouth

frenulum of tongue	frenulum linguae
soft palate	velum
sublingual fold	plica sublingualis

Salivary Glands

parotid duct	Stensen's duct
sublingual caruncle	
sublingual ducts	ducts of Rivinus, or Bartholin's duct
submandibular duct	submaxillary, or Wharton's duct
submandibular gland	submaxillary gland

Chapter 15 Anterior Part of Neck

auditory tubes	eustachian tubes
choanae	
cricothyroid ligament	cricothyroid interval
inferior constrictor muscle	cricopharyngeus muscle
laryngeal inlet	laryngeal orifice
laryngeal pharynx	hypopharynx
lymphoid	lymphadenoid
piriformis recess	piriformis sinus
rima vestibuli	vestibular slit
valleculae epiglottica	epiglottic valleculae
vestibula folds	false vocal cords

Chapter 16 Digestive System
Abdomen, Liver, Spleen, Biliary Tract

Liver

hilum	hilus
porta	porta hepatis
visceral surface of liver	posterior surface of liver

Pancreas and Spleen

accessory pancreatic duct	duct of Santorini
pancreatic duct	duct of Wirsung
pancreatic islets	islets of Langerhans

Biliary Tract

gall bladder	gallbladder
hepatopancreatic ampulla	ampulla of Vater
sphincter of the hepatopancreatic ampulla	sphincter of Oddi

Chapter 17 Digestive System
Alimentary Tract

Stomach

angular notch	incisura angularis
cardia	
cardiac notch	cardiac incisura
esophagogastric junction	esophageal orifice
gastric folds	rugae
pyloric antrum	pyloric vestibule
pyloric canal	
pyloric orifice	

Small Intestine

first portion	superior portion
second portion	descending portion
third portion	horizontal portion
fourth portion	ascending portion
common hepatic duct	hepatic duct
duodenojejunal flexure	angle of Treitz

Large Intestine

left colic flexure	splenic flexure
right colic flexure	hepatic flexure

Chapter 18 Urinary System

glomerular capsule	capsule of Bowman
hilum	hilus
major calyces	infundibula
renal papilla	apex
spongy portion [of male urethra]	cavernous portion
straight tubule	descending and ascending limbs of the loop of Henle
suprarenal glands	adrenal glands
uriniferous tubules	

Chapter 19 Reproductive System

Male Reproductive System

ductus deferens	vas deferens
spongy portion [of male urethra]	cavernous portion

Female Reproductive System

cervix	neck
intestinal surface	posterior surface [of uterus]
isthmus	superior cervix, internal os
lateral angles	cornua
ovarian vesicular follicles	ovisac
perineal body	
uterine ostium	external os, or external orifice of cervix
uterine tube	fallopian tube [oviduct deleted]
vesical surface	anterior surface of uterus

Continued on inside back cover.

MERRILL'S ATLAS OF

RADIOGRAPHIC POSITIONS and RADIOLOGIC PROCEDURES

VOLUME ONE

MERRILL'S ATLAS OF

RADIOGRAPHIC POSITIONS and RADIOLOGIC PROCEDURES

Philip W. Ballinger, M.S., R.T.(R)

Director and Assistant Professor, Radiologic Technology Division
School of Allied Medical Professions
The Ohio State University
Columbus, Ohio

EIGHTH EDITION

with **2863** illustrations, including **9** in full color

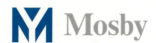 Mosby

St. Louis Baltimore Boston Carlsbad Chicago Naples New York Philadelphia Portland
London Madrid Mexico City Singapore Sydney Tokyo Toronto Wiesbaden

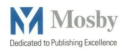

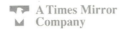

Editor: Jeanne Rowland
Developmental Editor: Linda Wendling
Project Manager: Gayle May Morris
Production Editors: Deborah Vogel, Karen Allman
Manufacturing Manager: Theresa Fuchs
Design Manager: Susan Lane

EIGHTH EDITION

Copyright © 1995 by Mosby–Year Book, Inc.

Previous editions copyrighted 1949, 1959, 1967, 1975, 1982, 1986, 1991

All rights reserved. No part of this publication may be reproduced,
stored in a retrieval system, or transmitted, in any form or by any
means, electronic, mechanical, photocopying, recording, or otherwise,
without prior written permission from the publisher.

Permission to photocopy or reproduce solely for internal or personal
use is permitted for libraries or other users registered with the Copyright
Clearance Center, provided that the base fee of $4.00 per chapter plus $.10
per page is paid directly to the Copyright Clearance Center, 27 Congress
Street, Salem, MA 01970. This consent does not extend to other kinds
of copying, such as copying for general distribution, for advertising or
promotional purposes, for creating new collected works, or for resale.

Printed in the United States of America
Composition by The Clarinda Company
Printing/binding by R.R. Donnelley

Mosby–Year Book, Inc.
11830 Westline Industrial Drive
St. Louis, Missouri 63146

International Standard Book Number 0-8016-7936-2

95 96 97 98 99 / 9 8 7 6 5 4 3 2

CONTRIBUTOR

STEWART C. BUSHONG, Sc.D.,
FACR, FACMP
Professor of Radiologic Science
Department of Radiology
Baylor College of Medicine
Houston, Texas

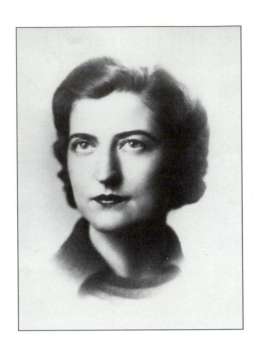

VINITA MERRILL

1905-1977

Miss Vinita Merrill had the foresight,
talent, and knowledge to author the
first edition of this atlas in 1949.
The eighth edition was published
in 1995, the centennial year
of the discovery of x-radiation.

PREFACE

With the 1995 centennial of the discovery of x-radiation, radiography students and practitioners throughout the world are reflecting on our history, celebrating our profession's contributions, and speculating about our future in the changing health care environment. *Merrill's Atlas of Radiographic Positions and Radiologic Procedures* has quite a history of its own. It has been recognized as a classic text in the field for almost half a century. In the eighth edition we believe we have successfully built on the pioneering work begun forty-six years ago by Vinita Merrill in the first edition of the atlas. Readers familiar with the atlas will find many improvements. For those using the atlas for the first time, our hope is that you will find it a highly reliable, comprehensive resource that will serve you well for many years to come.

The planning process for the new edition included soliciting input from *Merrill's Atlas* users and from many educators, who were teaching anatomy and positioning. In response to their insightful suggestions, we have made some significant improvements.

Standardization of terminology

The use of the important radiography terms, projection and position, has been standardized throughout the atlas. In particular, the comments of Eugene D. Frank, Radiography Program Director at Mayo Clinic/Foundation, provided the catalyst for these terminology changes. After many hours of discussion with Gene, who served as a special consultant on the revision, as well as Curt Serbus, who contributed greatly to our efforts, we worked out terminology we believe will be easier for students, radiographers and physicians to understand and use. The terminology continues to be in agreement with the American Registry of Radiologic Technologists and the Canadian Association of Medical Radiation Technologists. Chapter 3 provides a complete explanation of the modified terminology, and headers throughout the text reflect the improvements.

Essential projections

As a result of surveying all radiography programs in the United States and Canada, we identified 181 essential competency projections. These projections are the ones most frequently performed and are deemed necessary for competency of entry-level practitioners.

We have designated these with a special icon to alert students and instructors that these positioning skills are essential knowledge for the beginning radiographer. Instructors may, of course, modify the list of essential competency projections as appropriate to their specific geographic locations.

Bulleted positioning descriptions

Descriptions of positioning of patient and body part have been reformatted in bulleted lists for ease of reading and understanding.

Second color

Readers will notice that headings are set in color for emphasis. The second color has been incorporated in anatomic illustrations and is also used for demonstration of central ray angle and cassette positioning.

New and modified illustrations

The new edition has hundreds of new illustrations. Of particular note are the new photographs for cranium positioning. Also important is the inclusion of degree angulation information on most illustrations involving angulation of the x-ray tube to assist the reader in quickly identifying the degree of central ray angulation or the degree of body rotation.

Historical photographs

In recognition of the 1995 centennial of the discovery of x-radiation, we have included historical photographs on the opening page of each chapter. Many are from the first edition of the atlas published in 1949, some were taken during a visit to the Röntgen Museum and birthplace of Dr. Röntgen in Lennep, Germany, and a few are from other credited sources. These photographs provide a historical perspective on the evolution of radiography and help us appreciate its significance.

Ancillaries

For the first time, the atlas has a comprehensive set of ancillaries. In addition to the third edition of *Pocket Guide to Radiography,* also available are an anatomy and positioning instructional program in slide/audiotape or CD-ROM format, student workbooks, instructor's manuals, and a 1000-question test bank on floppy disk and in bound form.

Anatomic terminology

With each new edition, anatomic terminology is updated to reflect the latest information from the International Congress of Anatomists. As in previous editions, this information is printed on the inside covers of the atlas for easy reference.

We hope you find this new edition the very best ever. Your comments and suggestions are always welcome. We are constantly striving to improve the atlas and are dependent on your input to help us in that process.

Philip W. Ballinger

ACKNOWLEDGMENTS

Sincere appreciation to the following individuals for having reviewed three or more chapters for the new edition:

Lana Andrews-Havron, B.S.R.T., R.T.(R)(T)
Baylor University Medical Center, Dallas, Texas

Michael Fugate, M.Ed., R.T.(R)
Santa Fe Community College, Gainesville, Florida

Linda Cox, M.S., R.T.(R)
Indiana University, Indianapolis, Indiana

Diane M. Kawamura, Ph.D., R.T.(R), RDMS
Weber State University, Ogden, Utah

Debra S. McMahan, B.S., PA-C, R.T.(R)
Daniel Freeman Memorial Hospital, Inglewood, California

Betty L. Palmer, A.A.S., R.T.(R)
Portland Community College, Portland, Oregon

Helen Marie Peters, ACR
Northern Alberta Institute of Technology, Edmonton, Alberta, Canada

Janet K. Scherer, DCR, RT(R), ACR
McMaster University Medical Centre, Hamilton, Ontario, Canada

Curt Serbus, M.Ed., R.T.(R)
University of Southern Indiana, Evansville, Indiana

Donald C. Shoaf, M.Ed., R.T.(R)
Forsyth Technical Community College, Winston-Salem, North Carolina

O. Scott Staley, M.S., R.T.(R)
Boise State University, Boise, Idaho

James Temme M.P.A., R.T.(R)
University of Nebraska Medical Center, Omaha, Nebraska

I am grateful to the following professionals for their constructive comments on selected chapters:

Allan C. Beebe, M.D.

Scott A. Berg, B.S., R.T.(R)

Donald R. Bernier, CNMT

Janice M. Blanchard, R.T.(R)

Steven J. Bollin Sr., B.S, R.T.(R)

Dianna Childs, R.T.(R)

Joan Clark, M.S., R.T.(R)

Kathryn S. Durand, A.S., R.T.(R)

Kevin D. Evans, B.S., R.T.(R), RDMS

Sharyn Gibson, M.H.S., R.T.(R)

Ruth M. Hackworth, B.S., R.T.(R)(T)

Steven G. Hayes, B.S.R.T., R.T.(R)

Keith R. Johnson, R.T.(R)(CV)

John Raphael Kenney, R.T.(R)

Michael E. Madden, Ph.D., R.T.(R)

Elaine M. Markon, M.S., R.T.(N), CNMT

Darrell E. McKay, Ph.D., R.T.(R), FASRT

Rita M. Oswald, B.S., R.T.(R)(CV)

Robert Reid, M.S., R.T.(N)

Ken Roszel, M.S., R.T.(R)

Cheryl K. Sanders, M.P.A., R.T.(R)(T), FAERS

Nancy S. Sawyer, B.S., CNMT, R.T.(N)

Rees Stuteville, M.Ed., R.T.(R)

Tom F. Torres, B.S., R.T.(R)

Beverly J. Tupper, B.S., R.T.(R)(CV)

Melinda S. Vasila, B.S., R.T.(R)(N)

Users of the atlas will notice hundreds of new illustrations. Perhaps the most noticeable additions are the new photographic illustrations for the positioning involving the cranium. **James Temme MPA, R.T.(R),** Radiography Program Director at the University of Nebraska served as patient model and demonstrated his dedication to the profession by devoting several long, grueling, and uncomfortable days and nights of being positioned. Thank you, Jim. Thanks are also extended to the photographer, **Mr. Brent Turner** of BLT Productions, Inc. for his dedication and concern for producing high quality photographic images. Numerous photographic illustrations have also had degree angulation symbols placed on the illustration along with the degrees of angulation to assist the reader in quickly identifying the degree of central ray angulation or the degree of body part rotation.

Special thanks go to **Eugene D. Frank, M.A., R.T.(R), FASRT,** who provided invaluable help standardizing the projection and position terminology and for reviewing galleys and pages for this edition. Thanks, Gene, for devoting generous amounts of time, effort and talent during the production process and for helping to bring consistency to the atlas.

To the professional staff of the medical illustrators, medical photographers and staff of the Biomedical Communications Division in the School of Allied Medical Professions at The Ohio State University. Thanks to you the quality of the illustrations in the atlas remains high. To **Harry Condry** and **Janet Nelms** who kept track of my many orders, thank you. Thanks also to medical illustrators **Dave Schumick** and **Robert Hummel** for their competent work. To **Theron Ellinger,** thank you for printing the illustrations to demonstrate the anatomy and positioning, and to **Jenny Torbett,** senior medical photographer, thanks for your photography of numerous atlas illustrations.

To **Eileen Buckholz,** I admire your ability to manage the Radiologic Technology Division at The Ohio State University. Your skills in keeping track of student schedules, clinical and academic records, faculty, due dates and my schedule continue to amaze me. You were always there when something was needed and you always pleasantly responded to my many requests like "Eileen I can't find my copy of . . ." You would retrieve the missing item and keep all of us on schedule in your own special, caring and gentle way. A sincere thank you is not enough, but thank you again.

For more than a decade I have had the pleasure of working with **Don Ladig** of the Mosby–Year Book family. Thanks, Don. Your support and encouragement have been a constant positive driving force. During the last few years I have had the rewarding experience of working with **Jeanne Rowland,** Editor at Mosby–Year Book. Jeanne, I enjoy your honest and straight-forward manner of communicating, have found you to be readily available, and always striving to improve the atlas. Thank you, Jeanne, I have enjoyed working with you. Thanks to **Linda Wendling** for superb copyediting. You have really learned to talk like a radiographer in the last eighteen months. To **Debbie Vogel,** Project Manager, we have all appreciated your patience and calm demeanor in dealing with looming deadlines and revisions that just kept coming.

To **Terri Bruckner, M.A., R.T.(R),** where do I begin to say thank you. To keep current with the advancing profession of radiology, literally thousands of recent journal articles have been reviewed. Terri, while competently serving as my production assistant, you did an outstanding job in searching, screening, organizing and compiling the updated bibliographies for all three volumes. During the revision process, your ability to write, compile and critically evaluate new material was truly appreciated. During the production stages, your eye for consistency and detail was evident. It has indeed been a pleasure working with you, Terri.

The love and support provided by my family permitted my total involvement in this revision project. To my in-laws, **L. Neil** and **Ruth Hathaway,** thank you for accepting my absence too many times. I plan to improve upon the time available to spend with you as I accept early retirement from The Ohio State University. To my parents, **Dwight W. and Mildred Ballinger,** this work would not have been possible had you not supported me after I initially made the decision to enter radiology. You were always there whenever I needed something, and your love and affection truly made the project easier.

To my son and daughter, **Eric and Monica Ballinger,** now that you are in college I hope you find professions that you will enjoy as much as I do radiology. There were many times I was not available to spend time with you because "I was working on the book." I hope you understand that in spite of my sometimes absence, I do love you.

To my wife of twenty-five years, **Nancy Ballinger,** thanks for always being there when I wasn't. And thanks for saying yes when I called "Hey Nanc, got a minute?" For all the times you dropped what you were doing to proofread, check, and double check a revised manuscript, thank you. For over half of our married life you have juggled the family schedule to accommodate my involvement with the atlas. Thank you, Nancy, for your tolerance, support and love. I do love you and appreciate your active involvement in my publishing efforts.

P.W.B.

CONTENTS

VOLUME ONE

VOLUME TWO

VOLUME THREE

MERRILL'S ATLAS OF

RADIOGRAPHIC POSITIONS and RADIOLOGIC PROCEDURES

Chapter 1

PRELIMINARY STEPS IN RADIOGRAPHY

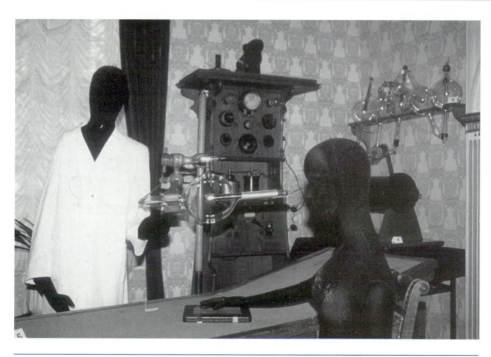

A radiographic room from 1901 displayed in the Roentgen Museum in Lennep, Germany.

Fig. 1-1. Sufficient radiographic density is needed to make a diagnosis. **A,** Insufficient density. **B,** Proper density, **C,** Too dense.

(Courtesy Frank J. Brewster, R.T.)

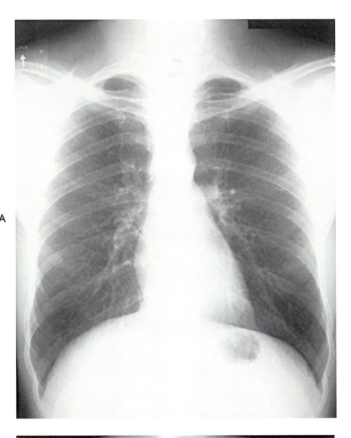

A

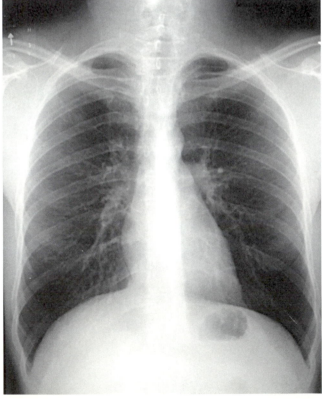

B

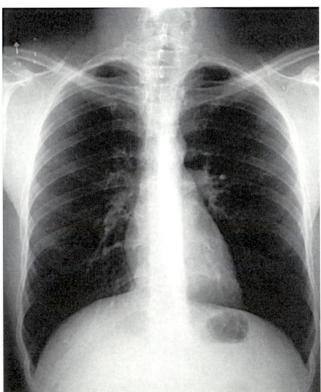

C

Radiograph

Each step in performing a radiographic procedure must be accurately completed to ensure that the maximum amount of information is recorded on the image receptor (film). The information gained as a result of performing the radiographic examination generally demonstrates the presence, or absence, of pathology or trauma. This information assists in the diagnosis and treatment of the patient. There is no examination in radiology in which accuracy and attention to detail are not essential.

The radiographer should be thoroughly familiar with the radiographic images cast by normal structures. To develop the ability to properly analyze radiographs and to correct or prevent errors in technique, the radiographer should study radiographs from the following standpoints:

1. The relationship of the structural superimpositions as to size, shape, position, and angulation must be reviewed.
2. Each anatomic structure must be compared with that of adjacent structures, such as the head of the humerus compared with the glenoid cavity and acromion process.

3. The optical density of the radiograph (the degree of film blackening) must be within a diagnostic range. If a radiograph is too light or too dark, an accurate diagnosis becomes difficult or impossible. Fig. 1-1 illustrates radiographs of proper and improper densities. If a change in technique is necessary, each of the following factors controlling density must be taken into account: milliamperage (mA); time (in seconds); or a combination of milliamperage and time (mAs); and source-to-image receptor distance (SID).

4. The contrast (the difference in density, or blackness, of any two areas on a radiograph) must be sufficient to allow radiographic distinction of adjacent structures with different tissue densities. Fig. 1-2 demonstrates three different scales of contrast. The primary controlling factor of radiographic contrast is kilovoltage peak (kVp).

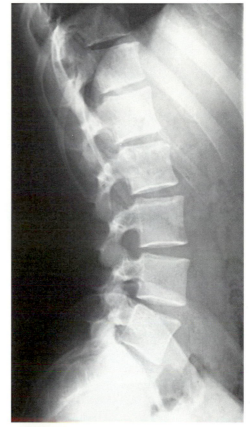

A

Fig. 1-2. Three different scales of contrast. **A,** Long scale (low contrast). **B,** Moderate scale (moderate contrast). **C,** Short scale (high contrast).

(Courtesy John Syring, R.T.)

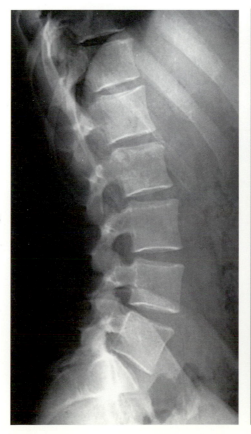

B

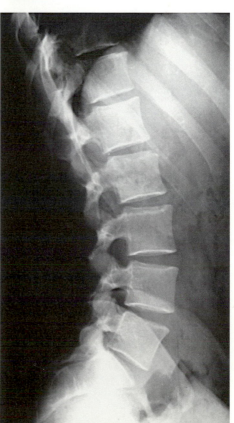

C

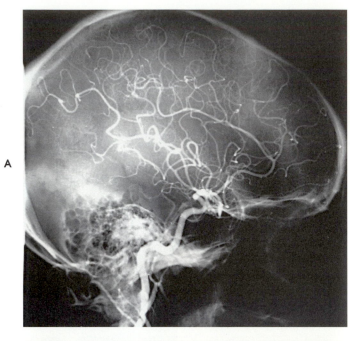

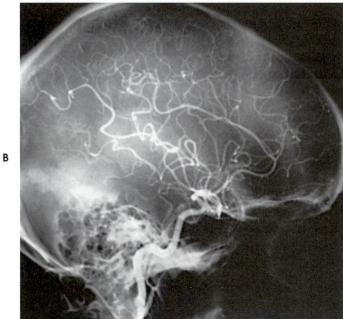

Fig. 1-3. Different levels of recorded detail. **A,** Sharp image. **B,** Unsharp image.

(Courtesy Joyce Tarzewski, R.T.)

5. The recorded detail (ability to visualize small structures) must be sufficient to clearly demonstrate the desired anatomic part. Recorded detail is controlled by several factors, categorized as geometric factors, motion, and structural material. The importance of recorded detail is illustrated in Fig. 1-3.

6. The *magnification* of the body part must be evaluated, taking into account the controlling factors of object-to-image receptor distance (OID) and source-to-image receptor distance (SID). All radiographs yield some degree of magnification, because all body parts are three dimensional.

7. The shape *distortion* of the body part must be analyzed, and the following controlling factors must be studied: direction of the central ray, central ray–film alignment, and part-film alignment. Shape distortion is often used to an advantage in radiography. An example of shape distortion is the axial image of the cranium. This image offers a distortion which more clearly demonstrates the occipital bone.

A sound knowledge of anatomy and the ability to analyze radiographs correctly are of particular importance—especially to radiographers who work without a physician in constant attendance. Under this condition the physician must be able to depend on the radiographer to perform the technical phase of the examinations without aid.

DISPLAYING RADIOGRAPHS

Radiographs are generally displayed according to the preference of the interpreting physician. Because such methods of displaying radiographic images have developed largely through custom, no fixed rules have been established. Therefore the following guidelines are presented to assist in the placement of radiographs on a viewbox.

Radiographs are usually placed on the viewbox, or viewing device, and oriented so the person viewing the radiographic image can envision the patient standing in the anatomical position, face-to-face with the viewer. (*Anatomical position* is assumed when the patient stands erect, face and eyes directed forward, arms extended by the sides with the palms of the hands facing forward, heels together, the toes pointing anteriorly with the great toes touching.) When the radiograph is displayed, the patient's left side is on the viewer's right side and vice versa.

Whereas Fig. 1-4 illustrates the patient's anterior (front) closest to the image receptor, other positions place the posterior (back) body surface closest. Regardless of which body surface is closest to the image receptor, the radiographs in this text are displayed in the anterior-posterior orientation. (Positioning terminology is fully described in Chapter 3.) A properly displayed PA chest radiograph is shown in Fig. 1-5. Exceptions to these global guidelines often include the hand, wrists, feet, and toes. Hand and wrist radiographs are routinely displayed with the digits (fingers) pointed toward the ceiling. In addition, foot and toe radiographs are generally placed on the viewbox so the toes also point toward the ceiling. Instead of hanging the radiographs with respect to the anatomical position, the radiographs are often hung just the opposite; they are hung from the perspective of the x-ray tube. "From the perspective of the x-ray tube" means one "views" the x-ray image with the eyes being in the same orientation as the body surface that the x-rays first enter.

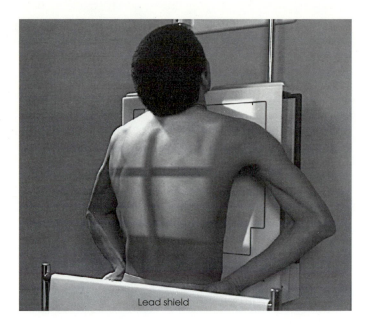

Fig. 1-4. Positioning to obtain a PA chest radiograph.

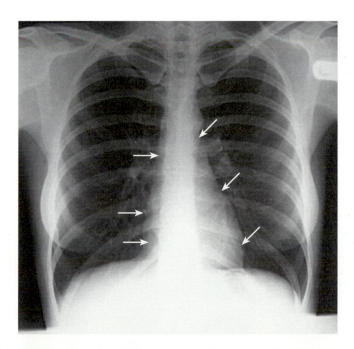

Fig. 1-5. Normal PA chest radiograph as displayed AP on viewbox (as though the patient were in the anatomical position). Note the large area of decreased density *(arrows)* on the patient's midline and left side (the reader's right) representing the patient's spine, heart, and blood vessels.

(Courtesy Elizabeth Zuffuto, R.T.)

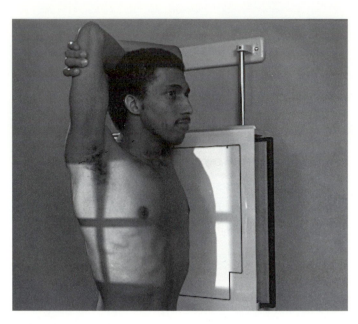

Fig. 1-6. Proper positioning to obtain a left lateral chest radiograph.

Lateral radiographic images are generally placed on the viewbox in the same orientation as if the viewer were looking at the patient from the perspective of the x-ray tube from the side where the x-radiation first *enters* the patient. Another way to describe this is to display the radiograph so that the side of the patient *closest* to the cassette during the procedure is also the side in the image closest to the viewbox. For example, a patient positioned for a left lateral chest radiograph is depicted in Fig. 1-6. The resulting left lateral chest radiograph is usually placed on the viewbox as printed in Fig. 1-7.

Another *possible* exception relates to how decubitus images of the abdomen are displayed. (Terminology for decubitus positions is described in Chapter 3, and multiple decubitus radiographs are contained in Chapters 16 and 17.) While a consensus in radiology regarding how decubitus radiographs are displayed does not exist, the two most common ways of displaying decubitus radiographs are: (1) in accordance with the anatomical position described above, or (2) in the manner in which the x-ray film cassette was positioned when the radiograph was exposed (i.e., the radiograph is displayed so it appears the patient is lying on one side). Decubitus radiographs in this text are displayed using the latter orientation.

Collimator borders

Lung apex

Esophagus

Trachea

Sternum

Posterior ribs (superimposed)

A

Heart shadow

Diaphragm

Costophrenic angle

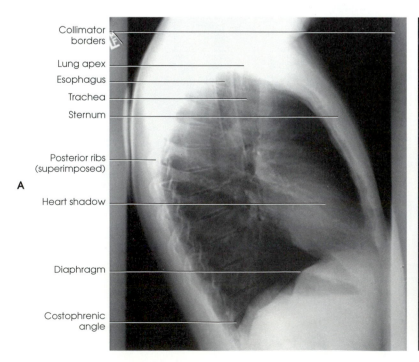

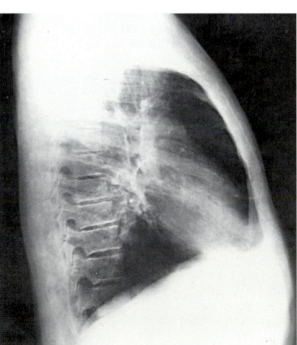

B

Fig. 1-7. Usual display of a left lateral chest radiograph.

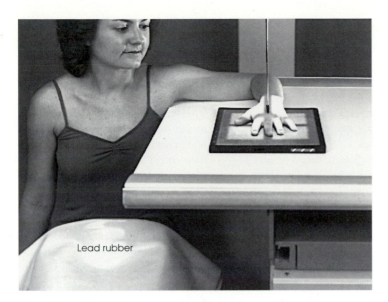

Lead rubber

Fig. 1-8. Positioning for a PA projection of the left hand.

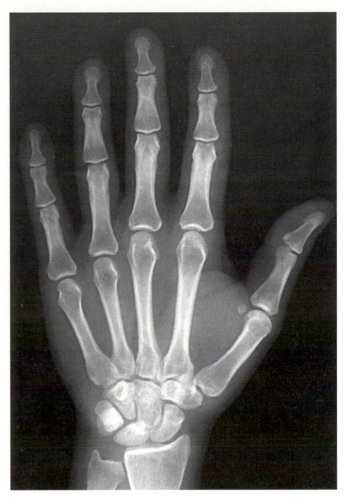

Fig. 1-9. Usual display of the PA left hand radiograph.

Clinical History Needed by Radiographer

All radiographs in this text are displayed from the perspective of the x-ray tube. For example, to obtain a PA radiograph of the patient's left hand, the patient is positioned as shown in Fig. 1-8. The PA radiograph of the left hand is printed in this text as if it were displayed on the viewbox (Fig. 1-9).

These are, of course, only guidelines. For example, some physicians prefer to view radiographs of the spine as if he or she were viewing the patient from the posterior body surface. (If the physician is a surgeon, for example, the posterior body surface is the site most often entered during surgery involving the spine.) Other physicians prefer to display radiographic images differently than any method described above. Since no universal fixed rules exist for displaying radiographs, flexibility is essential.

The radiographer is responsible for performing radiographic examinations according to the standard procedure, except when contraindicated because of the patient's condition. As the demands for physicians' time increase, less time is available to devote to the technical phase of radiology. This makes the physician more dependent on the radiographer to carry out this phase of patient care. This additional responsibility makes it necessary that the radiographer know (1) normal anatomy and normal anatomic variations so the patient can be accurately positioned, and (2) the radiographic characteristics of numerous pathologic conditions, that is, their effect on the normal radiopacity of structures (their penetrability by roentgen rays), so the exposure factors can be accurately selected. Although the

radiographer is not responsible for explaining the cause, diagnosis, or treatment of disease, it is the radiographer's responsibility to produce an image to demonstrate the conditions.

When the physician does not see the patient, the radiographer is responsible for obtaining the necessary history and observing any apparent abnormality that might affect the radiographic result. Examples include jaundice in gall bladder examinations and surface masses that might cast shadows that could be mistaken for internal changes. When the radiographer assumes this responsibility, the physician should give specific instructions as to the information desired.

The requisition received by the radiographer should clearly identify the exact region to be radiographed and the suspected or existing patient diagnosis. The patient must be positioned and the exposure factors selected according to the region involved and the radiographic characteristics of the existent abnormality. The radiographer must understand the rationale behind the examination; otherwise he or she cannot produce radiographs of the greatest possible diagnostic value. Having the information in advance saves the delay and expense of reexamination, not to mention the inconvenience and, much more important, the unnecessary radiation exposure to the patient.

Initial Examination

The radiographs obtained for the initial examination of each body part are based on the anatomy and/or function of the part and the nature of the abnormality indicated by the clinical history. The radiographs obtained for the initial examination are usually held to the minimum required to detect any demonstrable abnormality in the region. Supplemental studies for further investigation are then made as indicated. This method saves time, eliminates unnecessary radiographs, and reduces patient exposure to radiation.

Diagnosis and the Radiographer

It is quite natural for a patient to be anxious about examination results and to ask questions. The radiographer should tactfully advise the patient that the referring physician will receive the report as soon as the radiographs have been interpreted. Referring physicians also ask questions of the radiographer; they should be asked to contact the interpreting physician.

Ethics in Radiologic Technology

Ethics is the term applied to the science of duty and right conduct toward others. The nature of the work in the medical profession requires that the rules of conduct be strict. The physician, being responsible for the welfare of the patient, must be able to depend on the absolute honesty of all health professionals in carrying out orders and in reporting any mistakes.

The "Code of Ethics" initially developed and adopted by The American Society of Radiologic Technologists (ASRT) identified 10 ethical principles[1]. The ASRT's "Code of Ethics" in its present form[2] was also adopted by the American Registry of Radiologic Technologists and is reprinted by permission.[3] The Canadian Association of Medical Radiation Technologists (C.A.M.R.T.) similarly has an approved "Code of Ethics." The C.A.M.R.T. "Code of Ethics" is reprinted by permission.[4]

CODE OF ETHICS (U.S.)

1. The Radiologic Technologist conducts himself/herself in a professional manner, responds to patient needs and supports colleagues and associates in providing quality patient care.
2. The Radiologic Technologist acts to advance the principal objective of the profession to provide services to humanity with full respect for the dignity of mankind.
3. The Radiologic Technologist delivers patient care and service unrestricted by concerns of personal attributes or the nature of the disease or illness, and without discrimination, regardless of sex, race, creed, religion, or socioeconomic status.
4. The Radiologic Technologist practices technology founded upon theoretical knowledge and concepts, utilizes equipment and accessories consistent with the purposes for which they have been designed, and employs procedures and techniques appropriately.

5. The Radiologic Technologist assesses situations, exercises care, discretion and judgment, assumes responsibility for professional decisions, and acts in the best interest of the patient.
6. The Radiologic Technologist acts as an agent through observation and communication to obtain pertinent information for the physician to aid in the diagnosis and treatment management of the patient, and recognizes that interpretation and diagnosis are outside the scope of practice for the profession.
7. The Radiologic Technologist utilizes equipment and accessories, employs techniques and procedures, performs services in accordance with an accepted standard of practice, and demonstrates expertise in limiting the radiation exposure to the patient, self and other members of the health care team.
8. The Radiologic Technologist practices ethical conduct appropriate to the profession, and protects the patient's right to quality radiologic technology care.
9. The Radiologic Technologist respects confidences entrusted in the course of professional practice, protects the patient's right to privacy, and reveals confidential information only as required by law or to protect the welfare of the individual or the community.
10. The Radiologic Technologist continually strives to improve knowledge and skills by participating in educational and professional activities, sharing knowledge with colleagues and investigating new and innovative aspects of professional practice. One means available to improve knowledge and skills is through professional continuing education.

CANADIAN ASSOCIATION OF MEDICAL RADIATION TECHNOLOGISTS CODE OF ETHICS

The Canadian Association of Medical Radiation Technologists recognizes its obligation to identify and promote professional standards of conduct and performance. The execution of such standards is the personal responsibility of each member.

---

[1]"Code of Ethics," Radiol Technol 54:48, 1982.
[2]"Code of Ethics," Radiol Technol 61(5):362, 1990.
[3]ARRT, Personal communication (support and adoption), July 1993.
[4]C.A.M.R.T., Personal communication and permission, July 1992.

The C.A.M.R.T. Code of Ethics requires that every member shall:

1. Provide service with dignity and respect to all people regardless of race, national or ethnic origin, colour, sex, religion, age, type of illness, mental or physical challenges.
2. Encourage the trust and confidence of the public through high standards of professional competence, conduct, and appearance.
3. Conduct all technical procedures with due regard to current radiation safety standards.
4. Practice only those procedures for which the necessary qualifications are held unless such procedures have been properly delegated by an appropriate medical authority and for which the technologist has received adequate training to an acceptable level of competence.
5. Practice only those disciplines of medical radiation technology for which he or she has been certified by the C.A.M.R.T. and is currently competent.
6. Be mindful that patients must seek diagnostic information from their treating physician. In those instances where a discreet comment to the appropriate authority may assist diagnosis or treatment, the technologist may feel morally obliged to provide one.
7. Preserve and protect the confidentiality of any information, either medical or personal, acquired through professional contact with the patient. An exception may be appropriate when the disclosure of such information is necessary to the treatment of the patient, the safety of other patients or health care providers, or is a legal requirement.
8. Cooperate with other health care providers.
9. Advance the art and science of medical radiation technology through ongoing professional development.
10. Recognize that participation and support of our association is a professional responsibility.

June 1991

Care of Radiographic Examining Room

The radiographic examining room should be as scrupulously clean as any other room used for medical purposes. The mechanical parts of the x-ray machine, such as the table, x-ray tube and its supporting structure, and the collimator, should be wiped with a clean, damp (not wet) cloth every day. The metal parts should be periodically cleaned with a disinfectant. The overhead system, x-ray tube, and other parts that conduct electricity should be cleaned with alcohol or a clean, dry cloth. Water is never used to clean electrical parts.

Cones, collimators, compression devices, gonad shields, and other accessories should be cleaned daily and after any contact with a patient. Adhesive tape residue left on cassettes and cassette stands should be removed and the cassette disinfected. Cassettes should be protected from patients with bleeding, ulcerated, or other exudative lesions by the use of disposable protective covers. Use of stained and damaged cassettes is inexcusable and does not represent a professional atmosphere.

The radiographic room should be prepared for the examination before the patient is brought into the room. Fresh linen should be put on the table and pillow. Everything should be in place so that the room looks clean and fresh, not disarranged from the previous examination. Accessories to be used during the examination should be placed nearby. These pre-examination steps require only a few minutes but create a lasting impression on the patient. Not performing these beforehand will also leave a lasting impression.

Aseptic Technique

Radiographers are engaged in caring for sick people and therefore should be thoroughly familiar with *aseptic technique*. They should know how to handle patients who are on precaution or isolation without contaminating their hands, clothing, or apparatus, and they must know how to disinfect these things when they do become contaminated. As one of the first steps in aseptic technique, the radiographer's hands should be kept smooth and free from roughness or chapping by the frequent use of soothing lotions. Any abrasion should be protected by a bandage to prevent the entrance of bacteria. The hands should be washed before and after each patient and should be kept away from the face and head.

For the protection of the radiographer's health, as well as that of the patient, the laws of asepsis and prophylaxis must be obeyed. Scrupulous cleanliness should be used in handling all patients, whether they are known to have an infectious disease or not. If the patient's head, face, or teeth are to be examined, the patient should see the radiographer wash his or her hands. If this is not possible, the radiographer should wash his or her hands and then enter the room drying the hands with a fresh towel. If the patient's face is to come in contact with the cassette front, or table, the patient should see the radiographer clean the device with a disinfectant or cover it with a clean drape.

A sufficient supply of gowns and disposable gloves should be kept in the radiology department to care for infectious patients. After examining any patient, the radiographer must wash his hands in warm running water and soap-suds, rinse them, and dry them thoroughly. If the sink is not equipped with a knee control for the water supply, the valve of the faucet should be opened with a paper towel when the hands are contaminated. After proper hand washing, the valve of the faucet should be closed with a paper towel.

Before bringing isolation unit patients to the radiology department, the transporter should drape the stretcher or wheelchair with a clean sheet to prevent contamination of anything the patient might touch. When it is necessary to transfer these patients to the radiographic table, it should first be draped with a sheet. The edges of the sheet may then be folded back over the patient so the radiographer can position him or her through the clean side of the sheet without becoming contaminated.

For the protection of cassettes when a non-Bucky technique is used, a folded sheet should be placed over the end of the stretcher or table. The cassette is then placed between the clean fold of the sheet, and, with the hands between the clean fold, the radiographer can position the patient through the sheet. If the radiographer must handle the patient directly, an assistant should position the tube and operate the equipment to prevent contamination.

When the examination is finished, the contaminated linen should be folded with the clean side out and returned to the unit with the patient. There it will receive the special attention given to linen used for these patients or be disposed of according to the established policy of the institution.

In an effort to protect health care workers, the Centers for Disease Control (CDC) issued recommendations for handling blood and other body fluids in 1987. According to the CDC, all human blood and certain body fluids should be treated as if they contain pathogenic microorganisms. In addition to human blood, the identified fluids include: amniotic, pericardial, pleural, synovial, cerebrospinal, semen, vaginal secretions, or any fluid visibly contaminated with human blood. These precautions should apply to all contacts involving patients. Health care workers should wear gloves whenever they may come into contact with blood, mucous membranes, wounds, or any surface or body fluid containing blood. In any procedure in which blood or other body fluids may be sprayed or splashed, the radiographer should wear masks, protective eyewear (sold as eye shields and goggles), and a gown.

Health care workers must be cautious to prevent needle stick injuries. Needles should never be recapped, bent, broken, or clipped. Instead, they should be placed in a puncture-proof container and properly discarded.

Disinfectants and Antiseptics

Chemical substances that kill pathogenic bacteria are classified as *germicides* or *disinfectants.* Chemical substances that inhibit the growth of, without necessarily killing, pathogenic microorganisms are called *antiseptics. Sterilization,* which is usually performed by means of heat or chemicals, is the destruction of all microorganisms. Thus sterilization is the killing of all microorganisms, whereas *disinfection* is the process of killing only those which are pathogenic. The objection to many chemical disinfectants is that to be effective they must be used in solutions so strong that they damage the material being disinfected.

Because alcohol is commonly used for medical or practical asepsis in medical facilities, it should be noted that alcohol has antiseptic but not disinfectant properties. Dilute bleach is sometimes used as a disinfectant. No matter what is being done involving a patient, washing the hands with warm, soapy water is always appropriate.

Isolation Unit

Two types of patients are often cared for in isolation units: patients containing infectious microorganisms causing their disease, and patients needing protection from potentially lethal microorganisms carried by health care givers or visitors. A radiographer entering an isolation room must be aware of the patient's disease, how it is transmitted, and how to properly clean and disinfect the equipment both before and after use in the isolation unit.

When performing portable, or bedside, procedures in an isolation unit, the radiographer should obtain the required protective apparel—a gown, cap, mask, and/or gloves. Again the hands should *always* be washed prior to putting on gloves or touching the patient. If more than one radiograph is to be taken, the radiographer should stand any additional cassettes on paper towels outside the patient's room. The machine is taken into the room and manipulated into position. Care is taken not to let the machine touch the bed. The cassette is put in a clean protective cover (a clean cover for each cassette used), and an assistant performs the contamination work of adjusting the cassette and patient. If it is not possible to have an experienced radiography assistant, necessary adjustments can be made on the control panel and tube, and the machine operated through a clean cloth. Care must be taken not to let the contaminated side of the cloth come in contact with the equipment.

When the exposures have been finished, the mask, cap, and gown are removed and placed in the precaution hamper. The radiographer washes his or her hands before leaving the room. Again, all equipment that touched the patient or the patient's bed must be wiped with a disinfectant (following appropriate aseptic procedures), including the cable of the x-ray machine, which has of necessity been on the floor.

Venipuncture

The job responsibilities of radiographers are constantly changing. The ASRT include in their "Scope of Practice" responsibility for understanding and performing the methods for venipuncture. Another listed responsibility is to prepare, identify, and/or administer contrast media and/or medications as prescribed by a licensed practitioner.[1] These tasks are dependent on state statutes, institutional policy, and physician support.

Because the venipuncture technique is beyond the scope of this text, radiographers should be aware of four considerations before performing venipuncture. These are as follows:

1. The laws and/or statutes of the state must permit such.[2]
2. Injections are only permitted when authorized by a licensed physician.
3. Instruction must be received (and documented) in venipuncture and related aseptic technique and medication administration.
4. Instruction must be provided and documented regarding the appropriate response in case of an adverse reaction to the contrast medium.

General patient care textbooks provide information on performing venipuncture.

[1]The Scopes of Practice for Health Care Professionals in the Radiologic Sciences, The American Society of Radiologic Technologists, Albuquerque, 1992, p. 27.
[2]Tortorici M and MacDonald J: RTs performing venipuncture: a survey of state regulations, Radiol Technol 64:368-372, 1993.

Operating Room

Radiographers who have not had extensive patient care education must exercise constant watchfulness to avoid doing anything that will contaminate sterile objects in the operating room. After washing the hands and putting on scrub clothing, cap, and mask, the radiographer should step into the operating room to survey the particular setup before taking in the x-ray equipment. By taking this precaution the radiographer can ensure that sufficient room is available to do the work without the danger of contaminating anything. If necessary the radiographer asks the circulating nurse to move any sterile items. Because of the danger of contamination of the sterile field, sterile supplies, or persons scrubbed for the procedure, the radiographer should never approach the operative side of the surgical table.

After checking the room setup, the x-ray equipment should be thoroughly wiped with a damp (not wet) cloth before it is taken into the operating room. The x-ray machine or C-arm unit is taken to the free side of the operating table, that is, the side opposite the surgeon, scrub nurse, and sterile layout. The machine should be maneuvered into a general position that will make the final adjustments easy when the surgeon is ready to proceed with the examination.

The cassette is placed in a sterile covering, depending on the type of examination to be performed. The surgeon or one of the assistants holds the sterile case open while the radiographer gently drops the cassette into it, being careful not to touch the sterile case. The radiographer may then give directions for positioning and securing the cassette for the exposure.

The radiographer should make the necessary arrangements with the operating room supervisor when performing work that requires the use of a tunnel or other special equipment. Any cassette tunnel or grid should be placed on the table when it is being prepared for the patient, with the tray opening to the side of the table opposite the sterile field. With the cooperation of the surgeon and operating room supervisor, a system can be developed for performing radiographic examinations accurately and quickly, without moving the patient or endangering the sterile field.

Minor Surgical Procedures in the Radiology Department

Many procedures that require a rigid aseptic technique, such as cystography, intravenous urography, spinal punctures, angiography, and angiocardiography, are often carried out in the radiology department (Fig. 1-10). Although the physician needs the assistance of a nurse in certain procedures, the radiographer can make the necessary preparations and provide assistance in many procedures.

For procedures that do not require a nurse, the radiographer should know what surgical instruments and supplies are needed and how to prepare and sterilize such. Radiographers may make arrangements with the surgical supervisor for the education necessary to carry out these procedures.

Procedure Book

There should be a procedure, or protocol, book covering each examination performed in the radiology department. Under the appropriate heading, each procedure should be outlined and state the staff required and the duties of each member of the team. There should be a listing of the sterile and nonsterile items. A copy of the sterile instrument requirement should be given to the supervisor of the central sterile supply (CSS) department to facilitate preparation of the trays for each procedure.

Bowel Preparation

Radiologic examinations involving the abdomen often require that the entire colon be cleansed before the examination to obtain diagnostic quality radiographs. The patient's colon may be cleansed by one or any combination of the following: limited diet, laxatives, and enemas. The technique used to cleanse the patient's colon is generally selected by the medical facility or physician. Before beginning an abdominal procedure, it is prudent to question the patient about any bowel preparation that may have been completed. For additional information on bowel preparation, see Chapter 17, Volume Two, of this atlas

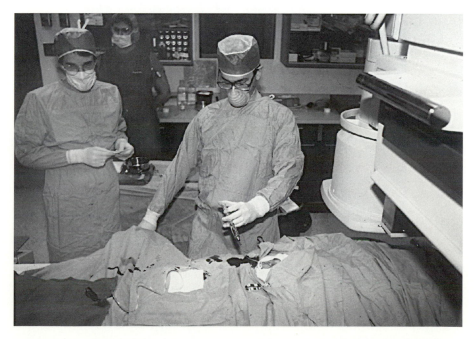

Fig. 1-10. Many radiologic procedures require that strict aseptic technique be followed, as seen in this procedure involving passing a catheter into the patient's femoral artery.

Motion and Its Control

Patient motion plays a large role in radiography (Fig. 1-11). Because motion is the result of muscle action it is important to know something of the function of muscles to eliminate or control motion for the period of time necessary for a satisfactory examination. There are three types of muscular tissue: smooth, cardiac, and striated. The first two types are classified as involuntary muscles and the third as voluntary.

INVOLUNTARY MUSCLES

The visceral (organ) muscles are composed of *smooth* muscular tissue and are controlled partially by their inherent characteristic of rhythmic contractility and partially by the autonomic nervous system. By their rhythmic contraction and relaxation these muscles perform the movements of the internal organs. The rhythmic action of the muscular tissue of the alimentary tract, called *peristalsis,* is normally more active in the stomach (about three or four waves per minute) and gradually diminishes along the intestine. The specialized *cardiac* muscular tissue functions by contracting the heart to pump blood into the arteries and by expanding or relaxing to permit the heart to receive blood from the veins. The normal rhythmic actions of cardiac muscular tissue are independent of nerve stimulus and thus are said to be myogenic in origin or to be an inherent characteristic of the muscle tissue. The phase of contraction is termed *systole,* and the phase of relaxation is termed *diastole.* One phase of contraction and one phase of relaxation, that is, a systole and a diastole, are called a complete cardiac cycle. The pulse rate of the heart varies with emotions, exercise, and food, as well as with size, age, and sex.

Involuntary motion is caused by the following:

Heart pulsation	Chills
Peristalsis	Tremor
Spasm	Pain

Involuntary muscle control

Length of exposure time is the only recourse against involuntary motion; the shorter the exposure time, the better.

VOLUNTARY MUSCLES

The voluntary, or skeletal, muscles are composed of *striated* muscular tissue and are controlled by the central nervous system. These muscles perform the movements of the body initiated by the will. Each striated (skeletal) muscle has a name derived from its position, shape, structure, action, direction, or points of attachment. Each muscle consists of a *body,* or *belly,* and two tendinous extremities for attachment.

The body of the muscle is made up of cylindrical fibers covered with a thin membrane and bound together into primary bundles called *fasciculi.* The covering sheaths of the individual fibers, the fasciculi, and that of the muscle are prolonged into round, fibrous cords called *tendons* or into flattened tendons called *aponeuroses.* The tendons attach the muscles to bone. When the muscle contracts, one end is moved toward the other. Although most of the striated muscles can be made to act from either limb (extremity), the less movable attachment is called the *origin* of the muscle, and the more movable is called the *insertion.* The contraction acts in the direction of the tendinous attachments.

The striated (skeletal) muscles never work singly. A combination of muscles is brought into play in any movement. One set acts as the *prime movers;* one set, called *synergists,* acts to assist or complement movements not required; one set acts as fixation muscles in steadying the point from which the force is being applied; and one set, the antagonists of the prime movers, relaxes to remove resistance to the action.

In radiography the patient's body must be positioned in such a way that the synergetic, antagonistic, and fixation muscles can perform their part of the work; otherwise the action of the prime movers will be hampered. The patient's comfort is a good index to the success of the position.

Voluntary motion resulting from lack of control is caused by the following:

Nervousness	Discomfort
Excitability	Mental illness
Fear	Age (child)

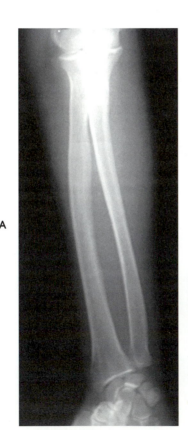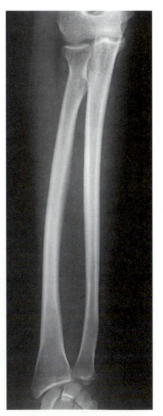

Fig. 1-11. A, Forearm radiograph on patient who moved during the exposure. **B,** Radiograph of patient without motion. Note the fuzzy appearance of the edges of the bones on the patient who moved.

(Courtesy Delores Goodwin, R.T.)

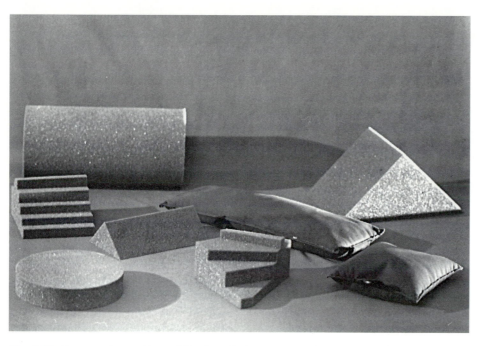

Fig. 1-12. Commonly used immobilization devices are positioning sponges and sandbags.

Voluntary muscle control

The radiographer can control voluntary patient motion by giving clear instructions, providing for the patient's comfort, and correctly applying and adjusting support and immobilization. Voluntary motion as a result of mental illness and age can best be controlled by decreasing the length of the exposure. Immobilization for limb (extremity) work can often be obtained for the duration of the exposure by having the patient phonate an "m—m—m" sound with the mouth closed or an "ah—h—h" sound with the mouth open. Selected immobilization devices of positioning sponges and sandbags are shown in Fig. 1-12.

Structural Relationship in Positioning

The position and relationship of the organs of the trunk vary considerably with the position of the body. Naturally, the radiographer must know not only the size, shape, position, and relationship of the organs when the body is in the anatomic position. But just as important is a thorough knowledge of the change in these relationships when the body is moved from the erect to recumbent and sitting positions.

For example, when the body is erect, the diaphragm lies in an oblique plane on a level with the sixth costal cartilage anteriorly and with the tenth rib posteriorly. With the body in the dorsal recumbent, or supine, position, the diaphragm is situated from 2 to 4 inches higher than when erect. The exact elevation depends on the curvature of the spine and the pressure of the abdominal viscera and muscles. The elevation will be less in thin patients. When the body is in the ventral recumbent, or prone, position, the diaphragm will be from 2 to 4 inches lower than in the erect position. This is because of the relaxation of pressure from the abdominal viscera and muscles and removal of the tilting of the spinal curvature. The depression of the diaphragm will be greater in thin patients.

When the body is in a seated position, the diaphragm assumes its lowest position because of lung pressure, relaxation of the abdominal muscles, and relaxation of pressure from the abdominal viscera. When the body is in a lateral recumbent position (lying on one's side), the upper half of the diaphragm assumes a position lower than when seated, and the lower half assumes a position higher than when supine because of unequal pressure from the abdominal viscera. Here the two

halves of the diaphragm cease to function in unison with breathing; the lower half has a greater excursion than the upper half. The original height of the diaphragm varies constantly during respiration. Its excursion between deep inspiration and deep expiration is approximately 1 inch, the right side of the diaphragm having a slightly greater excursion than the left.

The thoracic and abdominal viscera vary in location along with the diaphragm through all its movements. Likewise the anterior bony structures of the trunk vary in their relation to posterior structures as the position of the body is changed. For this reason the surface landmark for any given body position cannot be relied on when the body is in any position other than the one specified. Nor can surface landmarks be depended on to hold for one position on all patients. Landmarks are based on the *average,* and although they are applicable to a majority of patients, they cannot be used when a patient's form varies considerably from the normal.

If all patients were average in size and shape, the radiographer would have few problems. Because this is not the case, the radiographer must study anatomy from the standpoint of relationship and mechanics. With a reasonable knowledge of normal anatomy, the mechanics of body movement, and the usual deviations from the normal, the element of error in positioning is reduced to a minimum.

Patient Instructions

When the examination requires preparation, as in kidney and gastrointestinal examinations, the radiographer must instruct the patient carefully. Although the particular examination or procedure may be an "old story" to us, it is new to the patient. Frequently, what a radiographer sees as stupidity results from lack of sufficiently explicit directions. The radiographer must be sure that the patient understands not only what to do but also why it is to be done. Patients are more likely to follow instructions correctly if they see the reason for them. If the instructions are complicated, they should be written out. For example, because few patients know how to take an enema correctly, it is advisable to question the patient and, when necessary, take the time to explain the correct procedure. This will often save film, radiation exposure to the patient, and time.

Patient's Attire, Ornaments, and Surgical Dressings

The patient should be dressed in a gown that, with the use of a sheet where necessary, allows exposure of the region under examination. *Never expose a patient unnecessarily.* Only the area under examination should be uncovered, and the rest of the patient's body should be covered well enough for warmth. For examining parts that must be covered, disposable patient gowns or cotton is the preferred gowning material. If washable gowns are used, they should not be starched; starch is somewhat radiopaque—that is, it cannot be easily penetrated by x-rays. Any folds in the cloth should be straightened out to prevent confusing shadows. It is important to remember that a material that will not cast a shadow on a heavy exposure, such as that used on an adult abdomen, may show clearly on a light exposure, such as that used on a child's abdomen.

Any radiopaque object should be removed from the region to be radiographed. Zippers, snaps, thick elastic, or buttons should be removed when radiographs of the chest and abdomen are produced (Fig. 1-13). When radiographing the skull, the radiographer must make sure that dentures, removable bridgework, earrings, necklaces, and all hairpins are removed.

When radiographing the abdomen, pelvis, or hips of an infant, the diaper should be removed. Some diaper rash ointments are somewhat radiopaque and may need to be removed prior to the procedure.

Surgical dressings should be examined for radiopaque substances, such as metallic salves and adhesive tape. If permission to remove the dressings has not been obtained or the radiographer does not know how and the radiology department physician is not present, the surgeon or nurse should be asked to accompany the patient to the radiology department to remove the dressings. When dressings are removed, the radiographer should always make sure that open wounds are adequately protected by a cover of sterile gauze.

Lifting and Handling Patients

Any patient who is coherent and capable of understanding deserves an explanation of the procedure to be performed. The patient should understand just what is expected and be made comfortable. If the patient is apprehensive about the examination, his or her fears should be alleviated. However, if the procedure is one that will cause discomfort or be unpleasant, as in cystoscopy and intravenous injections, the patient should not be told otherwise. The procedure is explained calmly. The patient is told that it will cause some discomfort or be unpleasant, as the case may be but, since it is a necessary part of the examination, that full cooperation is needed. If patients see that everything is being done for their comfort, they will usually respond favorably.

Because the whole procedure is new to the patient, he or she usually works in reverse when given more than one order at a time. For example, when instructed to get up on the table and lie on his or her abdomen, the patient will usually get onto the table in the most awkward possible manner and lie down on the back. Instead of asking the patient to get onto the table in a specific position, the radiographer should first have the patient sit on the table and then instruct him or her to assume the desired position. If the patient sits on the table first, the position can be assumed with less strain and fewer awkward movements. *Never rush a patient.* If a patient feels hurried, he or she will be under a nervous strain and therefore unable to relax and cooperate. In moving and adjusting a patient into position, the radiographer should handle him or her gently but firmly. A too light touch can be as irritating as one that is too firm. The patient should be instructed and allowed to do as much of the moving as possible.

X-ray grids move under the radiographic table, and with the introduction of floating, or moving, tabletops, patients may injure their fingers. To reduce the possibility of injury, ask patients to keep their fingers on top of the table at all times. Regardless of what part is being examined, the entire body must be adjusted to avoid muscle pull against the part being examined, with resultant motion or rotation. When the patient is in an oblique position, the radiographer should apply support and adjust it to relieve the patient of strain while holding the position. Immobilization devices and compression bands are used whenever necessary, but not to a point of discomfort to the patient. Care is taken in releasing a compression band

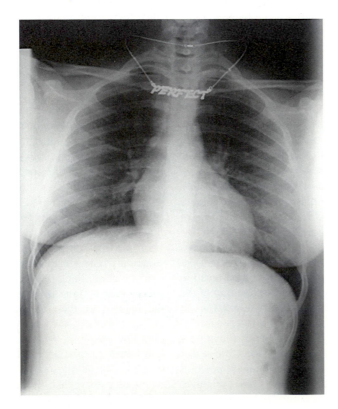

Fig. 1-13. Failure to remove the necklace required that this less than "perfect" radiograph be repeated.

over the abdomen; this should be done slowly.

In making the final adjustments on a position, the radiographer should stand with the eyes in line with the position of the focal spot, visualize the internal structures, and adjust the part accordingly. The rules of positioning are few, and many repeat examinations can be eliminated by following the rules.

Great care must be exercised in handling trauma patients, particularly those with skull, spinal, and long bone injuries. Because of the possibility of fragment displacement, any necessary manipulation should be performed by a physician. The positioning technique should be adapted to the patient to move him or her as little as possible. If the tube-part-film relationship is maintained, the resultant projection will be the same regardless of the patient's position.

When it is necessary to move a patient who is too sick to move on his or her own, the following considerations must be kept in mind:

1. To protect the patient, move him or her as little as possible.
2. Never try to lift a helpless patient alone.
3. To avoid straining the muscles of the back when lifting a heavy patient, flex the knees, straighten the back, and bend from the hips.
4. When a patient's shoulders are lifted, the head should be supported. While the head is held with one hand, the opposite arm is slid under the shoulders and the axilla grasped in such a way that the head can rest on the bend of the elbow when the patient is raised.
5. When it is necessary to move the patient's hips, the knees are flexed first. In this position patients may be able to raise themselves. If not, it is easier to lift the body when the knees are bent.
6. When helpless patients must be transferred to the radiographic table from a stretcher or bed, they should be moved on a sheet by at least four, preferably six, people. The stretcher is placed parallel to and touching the table. Two people should be stationed on the side of the stretcher and two on the far side of the radiographic table to grasp the sheet at the shoulder and hip levels. One person should support the patient's

head and another his feet. When the signal is given, all six should lift and move the patient in unison.

Many hospitals now have a specially equipped radiographic room adjoining the emergency department. These units often have special radiographic equipment and stretchers with radiolucent tops, so that severely injured patients can be examined in the position in which they arrive. Where this ideal setup does not exist, trauma patients are often conveyed to the main radiology department. There they must be given precedence over nonemergency patients.

Preexposure Instructions

The radiographer instructs the patient in breathing, practicing until the patient understands exactly what to do. After the patient is in position and before leaving to make the exposure, the radiographer should have the patient practice the breathing once more. This requires a few minutes, but it saves much time and radiation and many repeats. There are definite reasons for the phase of breathing used in trunk examinations. The correct *respiration phase* is printed under the positioning instructions in this atlas.

Inspiration depresses the diaphragm and abdominal viscera, lengthens and expands the lung fields, elevates the sternum and pushes it anteriorly, and elevates the ribs and reduces their angle near the spine. *Expiration* elevates the diaphragm and abdominal viscera, shortens the lung fields, depresses the sternum, and lowers the ribs and increases their angle near the spine.

When exposures are to be made during quiet breathing, the patient should practice slow, even breathing, so that only the structures above the one being examined will move. When lung motion, but not rib motion, is desired, the patient should practice slow, deep breathing after the compression band has been applied across the chest.

Foundation Exposure Technique

Specific exposure techniques are not included in this text. Too many variable factors are involved, not only from one department to another but from one unit to another within the same department. Only by familiarity with the characteristics of the particular equipment and accessories

employed and a knowledge of the physician's preference in image quality can a satisfactory technique be established. In establishing the correct foundation technique for each unit, *all* of the following must be taken into account: the electrical current applied to the x-ray tube (three phase, single phase, or high frequency); the kilowatt rating of the generator and tube; the radiation characteristics (wavelength); the filtration used; the type and speed of both film and intensification screens; the grid; and the type of processor and processing solutions. With this information available, the exposure factors can be selected for each region of the body and balanced in such a way to produce radiographs of the greatest possible radiographic quality.

Adaptation of Exposure Technique to Patient

It is the radiographer's responsibility to select the combination of exposure factors that produces the desired quality of radiograph for each region of the body and to standardize this quality. Once the standard quality is established, there should be as little deviation as possible. The foundation factors should be adjusted to the individual patient to maintain uniform quality throughout the range of patients. However, correctly balanced factors cannot be expected to produce the same definition on all subjects any more than one combination of exposure factors can be expected to produce the same contrast standard on all subjects. Just as people have different colors of hair, some patients have fine, distinct bony trabecular markings and others do not. Congenital and developmental changes from the normal, age changes, and pathologic changes must all be considered when the quality of the radiograph is judged.

Certain pathologic conditions require the radiographer to compensate when establishing an exposure technique. Selected conditions requiring a decrease in patient radiation exposure include age (infants, children, and the elderly), emphysema, degenerative arthritis, atrophy, multiple myeloma, active osteomyelitis, and sarcoma. Other conditions require increased radiation exposure to penetrate the part: selected conditions include atelectasis, advanced carcinoma, edema, pleural effusion, pneumoconiosis, and osteopetrosis.

Identification of Radiographs

All radiographs should be identified to include at least the following information: (1) the patient's name and/or identification or case number, (2) the date, (3) the side marker, right or left, and (4) institutional identity. See Fig. 1-14 for an example. The importance of correct identification bears stressing and restressing. There is no instance in which it is not important, but it becomes vital in comparison studies, on follow-up examinations, and in medicolegal and compensation cases. It is advisable to develop the habit of rechecking the identification marker just before placing it on the film.

Other patient identification markings may include such items as patient age/birthday, time of day, and name of the radiographer and/or attending physician. For certain examinations, the radiograph should include such markings as cumulative time following introduction of contrast medium (e.g., 5 min postinjection) and, in tomography, the level of the fulcrum (e.g., 9 cm). Other radiographs are marked to indicate the position of the patient (upright or decubitus) or other markings specified by the institution.

Numerous methods of marking films for identification are available. They range from the direct method of radiographing it along with the part, to "flashing" it onto the film in the darkroom or examination room before development, to writing it on the film after it has been processed, to perforating the information on the film, to specialty cassette-marking systems designed for accurate and efficient operation.

Film Placement

The part of interest is usually centered to the center point of the cassette or to where the angulation of the central ray will project it to the center. The cassette should be adjusted in such a way that its long axis will lie parallel with the long axis of the part being examined. Although having a long bone angled across the radiograph does not impair its diagnostic value, such an arrangement can be aesthetically distracting.

Even though the lesion may be known to be at the midshaft area of a long bone, a film large enough to include at least one joint should be used on all long bone studies. This is the only means of determining the position of the part and localizing the lesion. Many institutions require that both joints be demonstrated when a long bone is initially radiographed. For tall patients, this can necessitate two exposures; one for the long bone and joint closest to the area of concern and a second to demonstrate the joint at the opposite end.

A film large enough to cover the region under examination, but not larger, should always be used. In addition to being extravagant, large films include extraneous parts that detract from the appearance of the radiograph and, more important, cause unnecessary radiation exposure to the patient.

The rule of "place the object as close to the film as possible" might better read "place the object as close to the film as possible for an accurate anatomic image." Although there is greater magnification, less distortion is obtained by increasing the object-to-image receptor distance (OID) in such examinations as lateral images of the middle and ring fingers so that the part will lie parallel with the film. There is also less structural distortion and superimposition if oblique images of the ribs are made with the injured side elevated. Magnification can be reduced in these examinations by increasing the source-to-image receptor distance (SID) to compensate for the increase in OID. In certain instances intentional magnification is desirable, and it is obtained by positioning and supporting the object between the film and the focal spot of the tube. The procedure is known as enlargement or magnification technique.

For ease of comparison, bilateral examinations of small body parts may be placed on one film. However, exact duplication of the location of the images on the film is difficult if the cassette is not accurately marked. Many cassettes have permanent markings on the edges to assist the radiographer in equally spacing multiple images on one film. Depending on the size and shape of the body part being radiographed, the cassette can be divided in half either transversely or longitudinally (see Fig. 1-15, A and B). For smaller body parts, the cassette may be divided into thirds or fourths, as illustrated in Fig. 1-15, C and D.

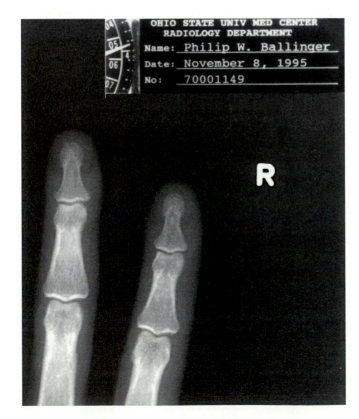

OHIO STATE UNIV MED CENTER
RADIOLOGY DEPARTMENT
Name: Philip W. Ballinger
Date: November 8, 1995
No: 70001149

R

Fig. 1-14. All radiographs must be permanently identified and should contain the minimum four identification markings.

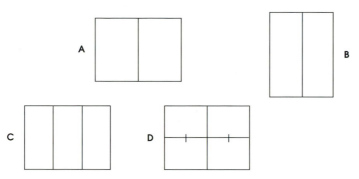

Fig. 1-15. Examples of multiple exposures on one film. **A,** and **B,** Two exposures. **C,** Three exposures. **D,** Four exposures.

It is essential, however, to ensure that the parts are always identified by side and placed on the film in the same manner, either facing or backing each other, according to established routines. Plan the exposures so that the film identification marker will not interfere with the part of interest.

English-Metric Conversion

Measures are the standards used to determine the size of things. People in the United States and a few other countries use standards that belong to the customary, or English, system of measurement. Although this system was developed in England, people in nearly all other countries—including England—now use the metric system of measurement.

In the past couple of decades, efforts have been made to convert all English measurements to the world standard metric system. These efforts have not been particularly effective. Nevertheless, in the future, total conversion to the metric system most likely will occur.

The following information is provided to assist the radiographer in converting measurements from the U.S. customary to the metric system and vice versa:

  1 inch = 2.54 centimeters (cm)
  1 centimeter (cm) = 0.3937 inch
  40 inches SID (source-to-image receptor distance) = 1 meter (m) (approximately)

Cassettes and film are manufactured in both U.S. customary and metric sizes. All U.S. customary and metric film sizes can be evaluated according to the International Standards Organization (ISO) nomenclature. The most common U.S. customary and metric film sizes fall into one of three classifications. Sizes falling within established limitations are listed as *considered equal;* those which are close but not judged equal are classified by the ISO as *slightly different;* some have *no close equivalent.* The most common U.S. customary and metric film sizes are compared in Table 1-1. Also included is a comparison between the U.S. customary and metric film sizes.

In the procedures described in this text, the U.S. customary measurement is listed first, followed by the closest metric film size available printed in parentheses.

Direction of Central Ray

The central or principal beam of rays, simply referred to as the *central ray,* is always centered to the film unless film displacement is being used to include an adjacent area. The central ray is angled through the part of interest under the following conditions:

1. When it is necessary to avoid the superimposition of overlying or underlying structures
2. When it is necessary to avoid stacking a curved structure on itself, such as the sacrum and coccyx
3. When it is necessary to project through angled joints such as the knee joint and lumbosacral junction
4. When it is necessary to project through angled structures without foreshortening or elongation, such as a lateral image of the neck of the femur

The general goal is to place the central ray at right angles to the structure. Accurate positioning of the part and accurate centering of the central ray are of equal importance in securing a true structural projection.

Table 1-1. Comparison of the U.S. customary and metric film sizes

U.S. customary inches (metric cm)	Metric Metric cm (inches)	Size comparison
5 × 7 (12.7 × 17.8)	13 × 18 (5.1 × 7.1)	Slightly different
8 × 10 (20.3 × 25.4)		No close equivalent
	18 × 24 (7.1 × 9.4)	No close equivalent
10 × 12 (25.4 × 30.5)		No close equivalent
	24 × 30 (9.4 × 11.8)	No close equivalent
11 × 14 (27.9 × 35.6)		No close equivalent
	30 × 35 (11.8 × 14.0)	No close equivalent
	30 × 40 (11.8 × 15.7)	No close equivalent
14 × 14 (35.6 × 35.6)	35 × 35 (13.8 × 13.8)	Considered equal
14 × 17 (35.6 × 43.2)	35 × 43 (13.8 × 16.9)	Considered equal
7 × 17 (17.8 × 43.2)	18 × 43 (7.1 × 16.9)	Slightly different
9½ × 9½ (24.1 × 24.1)	24 × 24 (9.4 × 9.4)	Slightly different

Source-to-Image Receptor Distance (SID)

The rule, "use the greatest distance possible consistent with the electrical energy required," does not apply in all examinations. For example, in certain skull examinations, such as that of the paranasal sinuses, it is desirable to use a distance short enough to magnify the opposite side of the skull to make the recorded detail of the side being examined more visible. A more accurate and inclusive rule to follow, therefore, might be, "Consistent with the electrical energy required, use the distance that will give the sharpest recorded detail of the structure examined."

It must be noted that the radiographer is not permitted to use a technique that places the source of the radiation (x-ray tube) closer than 12 inches (30.5 cm) from the nearest patient body surface. The recommended source-to-object distance (SOD) is 15 or more inches (38 cm).

A general rule for placement of the tube might be, "Adjust the tube so that the central ray is at right angles to the structure and the focal spot is at a distance that will project the best recorded detail of the structure."

Collimation of X-Ray Beam

The beam of radiation must be narrow enough to irradiate only the area under examination. This restriction of the x-ray beam serves a twofold purpose. First, it minimizes the amount of radiation to the patient and reduces the amount of in-room scatter radiation that can reach the film. Second, it allows radiographs that show clear structural delineation and increased contrast by (1) reducing scatter radiation, thereby producing a shorter scale of contrast, and (2) preventing secondary radiation from unnecessarily exposing surrounding tissues, with resultant film fogging (Fig. 1-16).

The area of the beam of radiation is reduced to the required size by use of collimators or appropriately apertured sheet diaphragms or shutters constructed of lead or other metal with high radiation absorption power. By this confinement of the beam, the peripheral radiation strikes and is absorbed by the intervening metal, while only the rays in line with the exit aperture are transmitted to the exposure field. Cones or diaphragms can be attached to the collimator, and their effectiveness depends on their proximity to the x-ray source.

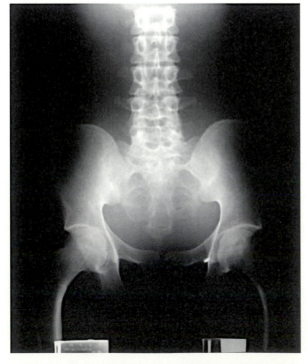

A

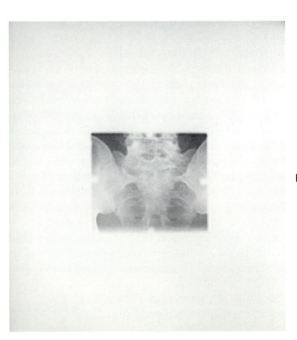

B

Fig. 1-16. Comparison radiographs of a body phantom. **A,** Radiograph with radiation field opened to 14 × 17 inches. **B,** Same technique as **A** with radiation field limited to 6 × 6 inches. Image **B** is less dense but demonstrates a shorter scale of contrast (more black and white) than image **A.**

Gonad Shielding

The patient's gonads may be irradiated when radiologic examinations of the abdomen, pelvis, and hip areas are performed. When practical, gonad shielding should be used to protect the patient as demonstrated in Fig. 1-17. The Center for Devices of Radiological Health (formerly the Bureau of Radiological Health) has developed guidelines recommending gonad shielding in three instances[1]: (1) when the gonads lie within the primary x-ray field or in close proximity (about 5 cm), despite proper beam limitation; (2) if the clinical objective of the examination is not compromised; and (3) if the patient has a reasonable reproductive potential. In addition, gonad shielding is often appropriate when limbs (extremities) are radiographed with the patient seated at the end of the radiographic table, as demonstrated in Fig. 1-8 shown earlier in this chapter. Finally, gonad shielding must be thoroughly considered and used, if indicated, when requested by the patient.

Gonad shielding is included in selected illustrations in this text. For additional information on the rationale of gonad shielding, see Chapter 2.

[1]Gonad shielding in diagnostic radiology, Pub. No. (FDA) 75-8024, Rockville, Md., 1975, Bureau of Radiological Health.

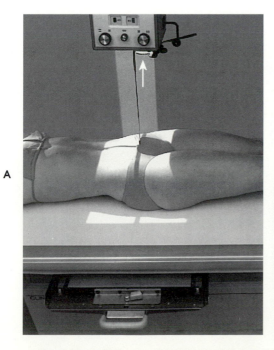
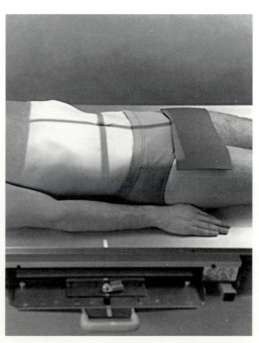

Fig. 1-17. A, Patient positioned for radiographic examination showing proper collimation and the use of gonad (shadow) shield. Lead shielding material placed under the collimator (*arrow*) greatly reduces the exposure to the gonads. **B,** Contact shield (lead rubber) placed between x-ray source and patient's gonads stops radiation from directly striking gonads.

Chapter 2

RADIATION PROTECTION

STEWART C. BUSHONG

Introduction
Radiation units
Radiation sources and levels
Radiation protection guides
Medical radiation dose and
   exposure
Protection of patient
Protection of radiographer

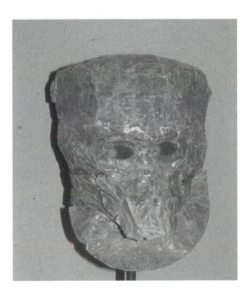

The "latest" in radiation protection:
a lead mask from around 1900.

Introduction

EARLY INJURIES

Perhaps no other event in our technologic history caused as much feverish scientific activity by so many as the accidental discovery of x rays by Wilhelm Roentgen in November of 1895. Because Roentgen was so thorough in his investigations, within a few short weeks he was able to characterize the nature of x rays to nearly the same level of understanding as we have today. This early work earned him the first Nobel prize for physics in 1901. Roentgen immediately recognized the potential diagnostic medical applications of his new "X-light." He produced the first radiograph, that of his wife's hand.

Throughout 1896, the first year after Roentgen's discovery, the world's scientific literature was flooded with reports of experiments with x rays. Very soon thereafter reports appeared relating cases of radiodermatitis, in some instances severe enough to require surgery. These reports had two immediate effects: (1) to speed the experimentation and application of x rays in radiation therapy and (2) to suggest that radiation protection methods were necessary during diagnostic procedures to ensure the safety of both the operator and the patient. However, it took more than 30 years for even moderately consistent radiation protection measures to be universally applied.

By 1910 several hundred cases of severe x-ray burns, many leading to death, had been reported. To illustrate this tragedy in radiation pioneering, consider the case of Clarence Daley, Thomas Edison's friend and principal assistant. Within a couple of days after the cable announcement of the discovery of x rays, Edison was already deeply involved in his own investigations, using an operative x-ray apparatus. Within months several of his assistants experienced a radiodermatitis. Clarence Daley's condition was mild at first but, because of continued exposure, progressed rapidly and resulted in several amputations. He died in 1904 and is considered the first radiation fatality in the United States. When Daley died, Edison discontinued his work with x rays. He had already discovered calcium tungstate as an intensifying phosphor and developed the fluoroscope. Who knows what additional contributions Edison might have made to radiology had he continued his investigations.

PRESENT SUSPECTED RADIATION RESPONSES

In the 1930s a consensus was reached on the need for radiation protection devices and procedures. These radiation protection activities were principally in response to the reported radiation injuries to early radiologists. In the 1950s, scientific reports began to appear that suggested even the low levels of radiation exposure experienced in diagnostic radiology could be responsible for late radiation responses and injury to patients. Current radiation protection practices are prompted by concern for late effects in patients and radiation workers.

After high doses of radiation exposure, a number of acute early responses may appear. Whole body radiation in excess of 200,000 mrads (2000 mGy) can result in death within weeks. Partial body irradiation to any organ or tissue can cause atrophy (shrinking) and dysfunction (improper metabolism). Whole body exposure as low as 25,000 mrads (250 mGy) can produce a measurable hematologic depression (reduction in the number of circulating blood cells) that may require months for recovery. These early effects result from high doses of radiation and therefore are of no concern in diagnostic radiology.

Concern today is for the late effects of radiation exposure. Such effects follow low exposures and may not occur for years. They fall into two natural categories—genetic and somatic effects. Late genetic effects of radiation exposure are suspected; they have not been measured in humans. However, data from a considerable number of animal studies indicate that such effects may occur.

Somatic effects refer to the response to radiation by all cells of the body except the germ (genetic) cells. The principal late somatic effects after low-dose irradiation have only been measured in humans by the use of rather sophisticated epidemiologic and statistical methods. No individual has ever been identified as a radiation victim after low-dose exposure. A low dose is generally considered to be a whole body dose less than about 25,000 mrads (250 mGy). The low dose for partial body irradiation is somewhat higher. Such effects are detectable only when observations are made on thousands and even hundreds of thousands of irradiated individuals.

The shortening of life resulting from nonspecific premature aging was observed many years ago in American pioneer radiologists. This effect does not exist today due to improved radiation protection practices. Local tissues can also experience late radiation effects of a nonmalignant nature. The most prominent late effect, and one that has some significance in diagnostic radiology, is radiation-induced cataracts. However, this effect does not follow low-dose irradiation; it requires at least 200,000 mrads (2000 mGy) of exposure to the lens of the eye.

Radiation-induced malignant disease is the delayed somatic effect of primary concern. Leukemia, solid tumor neoplasia, and cancers of nearly every type involving nearly every organ have been implicated by animal investigations and large-scale observations of humans.

Leukemia is more readily observed in a heavily irradiated population than is cancer. The BEIR (Biologic Effects of Ionizing Radiation) committee estimate for the induction of leukemia by irradiation suggests that if 1 million persons received 1000 mrads (10 mGy), up to 55 additional cases of leukemia would be produced during the 25 years after irradiation. This equals approximately 2 cases/million persons/rad/yr. Without irradiation the incidence of leukemia is approximately 80 cases/million persons/yr.

Cancer is not uncommon, and therefore radiation-induced cancer is difficult to detect, even statistically. The 1990 report of the National Academy of Sciences entitled "The Biologic Effects of Low Doses of Ionizing Radiation"—known as the BEIR-V Report—provides the most authoritative estimate of this radiation response. Although this is an exceedingly thorough report, it can be summarized briefly by the data in Table 2-1. The BEIR

Table 2-1. BEIR committee estimated excess mortality from malignant disease in 100,000 persons

	Male	Female
Normal expectation	20,560	16,680
Excess cases		
Continuous exposure to 1000 mrad/yr	2,880	3,070
Single exposure to 10,000 mrad/yr	770	810
Continuous exposure to 100 mrad/yr	520	600

committee postulated two scenarios. The first assumes an annual 1000 mrad (10 mGy) dose—appropriate to occupational exposure. The second assumes a once-in-a-lifetime 10,000 mrad (100 mGy) dose—simulating an accidental exposure. Of every 100,000 persons, nearly 20,000 will die of malignant disease. After the first assumed exposure, an additional 3000 may die of malignant disease. After a single 10,000 mrad (100 mGy) dose an additional 800 malignant deaths might occur. The range of possible deaths shown in Table 2-1 results from adoption of a relative risk model of radiation response.

These estimates result from extrapolations from high dose data and do not reflect a high degree of certainty. The BEIR committee further concludes that doses "less than 1000 mrads/yr (10 mGy/yr) may not be harmful."

NEED FOR RADIATION PROTECTION

Radiographers receive approximately 70 mrads/yr (0.7 mGy/yr), nearly all during fluoroscopy and portable radiography, during which protective apparel is worn. Consequently, exposures, although identified as whole body on the exposure report, are actually partial body exposures. Although exposure levels are low and the possibility of a late effect is remote, it is prudent to keep radiation exposure to radiographers and patients ALARA (as low as reasonably achievable).

A recent survey of 143,000 radiographers by The American Registry of Radiologic Technologists resulted in much statistical data about dose, demographics, and biologic effects. There was no indication that occupational radiation exposure caused any effects. In fact, in all cases in which radiographers have been studied, no late effects have been observed. Nevertheless, despite the absence of significant data, late genetic and somatic effects of importance are considered possible. There is no dose threshold for such effects. Should a dose threshold exist, all doses below the threshold would be absolutely safe. Even though the occupational exposures that radiographers experience result in a very small and indeterminate probability of producing such effects, an effective radiation protection program is required.

Table 2-2. Conventional radiation units, SI radiation units, and conversion factors

Quantity	Conventional unit	SI unit	Conversion factor
Exposure	roentgen(R)	C/kg	2.58×10^{-4} C/kg/R
Absorbed dose	rad	gray (Gy)	10^{-2} Gy/rad
Dose equivalent	rem	seivert (Sv)	10^{-2} Sv/rem
Activity	curie (Ci)	becquerel (Bq)	3.7×10^{10} Bq/Ci

Radiation Units

A special set of units is used to express the quantity of ionizing radiation. These units, the *roentgen,* the *rad,* and the *rem,* have been developed and defined over many years and are familiar to radiologic workers. However, those in educational programs and in professional practice must become familiar with a second set of radiation units derived from the international system of weights and measures (SI). The SI units associated with classical radiation units and the appropriate conversions are shown in Table 2-2. Although they are only referred to superficially in this chapter, radiographers should be aware that they exist and should be prepared to implement them. At this time the United States is the only developed country that has yet to fully adopt SI radiation units as a system of measure.

UNIT OF EXPOSURE

When an x-ray tube is energized, x rays are emitted in a collimated beam in the same way light is emitted from a flashlight. This useful beam of x rays ionizes the air through which it passes. This is called exposure, and the unit of exposure is the *roentgen* (R). An exposure of 1 R will produce 2.08×10^9 ionizations in a cubic centimeter of air at standard temperature and pressure. The official definition of the roentgen is 2.58×10^{-4} coulombs per kilogram (C/kg) of air, and this is equivalent to the previous quantity. The SI unit of radiation exposure has no special name; it is simply the C/kg.

UNIT OF RADIATION DOSE

When a radiation exposure occurs, the resulting ionizations deposit energy in the air. If an object such as a patient is present at the point of exposure, energy will be deposited by ionization in the patient. This deposition of energy by radiation exposure is called *radiation absorbed dose,* or simply absorbed dose, and it is measured in *rads.* One rad is equivalent to depositing 100 ergs of energy in each gram of the irradiated object. The SI unit of absorbed dose is the *gray* (Gy), and 1 Gy = 100 rads = 1 joule/kg. The *erg* and *joule* are units of energy.

UNIT OF DOSE EQUIVALENT

If the irradiated object is a radiographer or other radiation worker, then the radiation dose resulting from an occupational radiation exposure is said to result in a radiation dose equivalent. The dose equivalent is measured in *rems (radiation equivalent man),* and 1 rem = 100 ergs/g. The SI unit of dose equivalent is the *seivert (Sv),* and 1 Sv = 1 joule/kg. Note that the rad and rem (gray and seivert) are expressed in similar units. The basic difference between the rem and other radiation units is that the rem is used only for radiation protection purposes; it is the unit of occupational exposure.

In diagnostic radiology 1 R can be considered equal to 1 rad and to 1 rem. This simplifying assumption is accurate to within about 15% and therefore is sufficiently precise for nearly all considerations of exposure and dose in diagnostic radiology. Radiation workers in the nuclear power industry and in some other industrial and research activities may be exposed to different kinds of radiation, in which case this simplifying assumption does not apply.

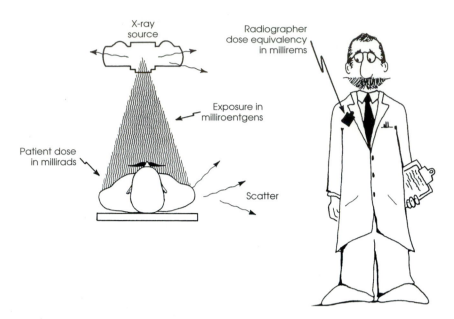

Fig. 2-1. The useful x-ray beam is measured in milliroentgens, the patient dose in millirads, and occupational exposure in millirems.

APPLICATION OF RADIATION UNITS

Although all three units (the roentgen, rad, and rem) are used interchangeably in diagnostic radiology, such use is incorrect, because each unit has a precise application. One roentgen, 1 rad, and 1 rem are all rather large quantities. In practice, quantities that are 1000 times smaller, the milliroentgen (mR), the millirad (mrad), and the millirem (mrem), are used. When a medical physicist calibrates or surveys a radiographic or fluoroscopic x-ray tube, the radiation intensity is expressed in milliroentgens. The radiation intensity will be measured by any one of the various types of radiation detectors; output will be expressed in milliroentgens or sometimes as milliroentgens per milliampere-seconds (mR/mAs) at some given kilovolt peak (kVp). When a patient is irradiated during an examination and the amount of radiation received by the patient is of concern, it is expressed in millirads. If a pregnant patient is irradiated, the fetal dose is also expressed in millirads. The radiation dose to any of the patient's organs would likewise be expressed in millirads. Often, however, the skin dose will be expressed as an exposure in milliroentgens and called an entrance skin exposure (ESE).

Exposure received by radiographers is measured with a personnel radiation monitor. The source of their occupational exposure is nearly always scattered radiation from the patient (Fig. 2-1). The radiation monitor measures exposure; the radiation report indicates the dose equivalent in millirems. The millirem is reserved exclusively for use in radiation protection and therefore is a unit not only of occupational exposure but also sometimes used to express the dose received by populations as the consequence of medical, industrial, and research applications of radiation.

Radiation Sources and Levels

We are exposed to ionizing radiation in our daily lives from multiple sources. The largest source is natural background radiation, something over which we have no control. Other sources are medical diagnostic and therapeutic procedures and radiation applications associated with industry, research, and consumer products. To place in perspective the radiation exposures and risks associated with being a radiographer, one should know something about the radiation levels associated with these other sources (Table 2-3).

NATURAL BACKGROUND

Human beings have inhabited Earth for perhaps 300,000 years and have evolved in the presence of a constant radiation exposure called *natural background radiation*. Natural background radiation comes from three principal sources: (1) terrestrial radiation resulting from naturally occurring radionuclides in the earth, (2) cosmic radiation resulting from sources outside Earth, principally the sun but also sources outside our solar system and galaxy, and (3) internal exposure from radionuclides naturally deposited in the human body, principally potassium 40 (^{40}K). In the United States these sources produce a whole body dose of 50 to 300 mrads/yr (0.5 to 3 mGy/yr), depending on location and diet. Table 2-3 includes these components of the natural background radiation and their quantities.

Table 2-3. Estimated average annual whole-body radiation dose (mrad) in the United States from natural and man-made sources

Radiation source	Annual dose (mrad)	
Man-made		
Diagnostic x-rays	40	
Nuclear medicine	14	
Consumer products	10	
Other	1	
Subtotal		65
Natural		
Internal radionuclides, principally ^{40}K	40	
Terrestrial radionuclides, principally ^{220,222}R, ^{226,228}Ra, ^{14}C	29	
Cosmic rays	29	
Subtotal		98
Radon (dose to lung only)		<u>197</u>
TOTAL		360

Terrestrial radiation

At the time of Earth's formation, some radioactive elements (principally uranium and thorium) were created, having a radioactive half-life of billions of years. As these radionuclides decay, they emit radiation, and this source contributes to the total natural background radiation level. The *terrestrial radiation* level is very dependent on geographic location and particularly the type of soil or rock present. Along the Atlantic and Gulf coasts the terrestrial doses range from 15 to 35 mrads (0.15 to 0.35 mGy). In the northeastern, central, and far western portions of the United States the terrestrial radiation ranges from 35 to 75 mrads (0.35 to 0.75 mGy). In the Colorado plateau area the range is from 75 to 140 mrads (0.75 to 1.4 mGy). By applying the appropriate terrestrial radiation dose rate to the resident population, the average U.S. rate is estimated to be 29 mrads/yr (0.29 mGy/yr). This does not include radon, a radioactive gas that comes from the earth and the earthlike building materials such as concrete and bricks. As a gas, radon contributes only to the dose to the lungs-an estimated 197 mrads/yr (1.9 mGy/yr).

Cosmic radiation

The sources of *cosmic radiation* are many. Photons and particles are emitted by the sun and by sources outside of our solar system—even outside of our galaxy. Because this radiation is incident on the earth, its intensity is influenced by the shielding of the overlying atmosphere and by the geomagnetic latitude. In general, radiation intensity increases with latitude toward the north pole because of the deflection of particles by the earth's magnetic field. The intensity also increases with increasing altitude, so that 1 mile above the earth's surface the cosmic intensity is approximately twice that at sea level. When all of these influences are considered, the U.S. population receives an estimated 29 mrad/yr (0.29 mGy/yr) of cosmic radiation.

Internally deposited radionuclides

The air we breathe, the water we drink, and the food we eat all contain small quantities of naturally occurring radionuclides. Some of these radionuclides are metabolized and incorporated permanently into the tissues of the body. The radionuclides of principal importance are ^3H, ^{14}C, ^{40}K, ^{226}Ra, and ^{210}Po. Collectively, these internally deposited radionuclides result in an average estimated annual dose of 40 mrads (0.40 mGy).

MEDICAL DIAGNOSTIC AND THERAPEUTIC RADIATION

Patients receive radiation exposure from radiographic examinations, fluoroscopic procedures, dental diagnostic procedures, radioisotope procedures, and radiation therapy. By far, most artificial radiation exposure is received from medical radiographic procedures. It is difficult to assign precise dose values to such procedures because of the many associated complications. Approximately 65% of the U.S. population is exposed to radiation each year for medical or dental purposes. Medical applications of radiation represent the second-most intense source of radiation exposure.

Two measures of patient dose are important in assessing the extent of medical radiation exposure on the population: the *genetically significant dose* (GSD) and the *mean marrow dose* (MMD). The GSD is a genetic dose index. It is the gonad dose that, if received by every member of the population, would be expected to produce the sum total effect on the population as the sum of the individual doses actually received. In the United States at this time the GSD is estimated to be 20 mrads (0.2 mGy) per year. The GSD indicates nothing about possible or probable genetic effects. It is only an attempt to estimate the dose received by the population gene pool.

There is a similar index for somatic effects—the MMD; it too is expressed in mrads/yr. The MMD to the U.S. population is currently estimated to be 77 mrads (0.77 mGy). Like the GSD, the MMD is a weighted average over the entire population, including those who are and those who are not irradiated. It takes into account the fraction of anatomic bone marrow irradiated as a function of each type of examination and averages this by the total active bone marrow. Because bone marrow irradiation is considered to be responsible for radiation-induced leukemia, the MMD is a somatic dose index for leukemia. The mean marrow dose is a measure of radiation dose and not of late radiation effect.

INDUSTRIAL APPLICATIONS

Industrial applications of ionizing radiation result in average occupational exposures of up to several hundred millirems per year in some groups such as nuclear power plant workers. In addition to these workers, others employed in the mining, refining, and fabrication of nuclear fuel, in industrial radiography, and in the handling of radioisotopes for a large number of industrial applications receive occupational exposure. Included in these industrial applications is the transportation of radioactive material, particularly as it pertains to the air freight of nuclear medicine radiopharmaceuticals. When prorated over the entire U.S. population these industrial activities add approximately 0.2 mrad/yr (2 μGy/yr) to the population dose.

RESEARCH APPLICATIONS

Research applications of ionizing radiation include particle accelerators, other radiation-producing machines, and radionuclides. Particle accelerators, such as cyclotrons, synchrocyclotrons, Van de Graaff generators, and linear accelerators, are employed in university and industrial research laboratories. Although they can generate intense fields of radiation, these machines are always shielded and protected. X-ray diffraction units and electron microscopes are common research tools employed to investigate the structure of matter. The x-ray diffraction unit generates an intense field of highly collimated and very soft radiation. It does not normally represent a whole body hazard but rather a danger to hands if they are accidentally placed in the useful beam. Electron microscopes likewise produce low-energy x rays, but these are well shielded and do not represent a significant occupational radiation hazard nor a radiation hazard to the population. Many research activities employ radionuclides, mostly low-energy beta-emitting radionuclides such as ^3H and ^{14}C. Although there is a small occupational hazard from these activities, the population exposures are nil. Collectively, these research activities contribute no more than 0.1 mrad/yr (1 μGy/yr) to the population dose.

CONSUMER PRODUCTS

Surprisingly, many consumer products incorporate x-ray devices or radioactive material. Television receivers, video display terminals, and airport surveillance systems are three devices that produce x rays. The first two produce x rays of a very low energy and intensity and pose no hazard to the consumer because these low energy x rays are absorbed completely by the glass envelope at the video tube. Surveillance systems likewise emit low levels of x radiation, and these units are well shielded and are provided with safety interlocks. Radioactive material is incorporated into various luminous products, such as instrument gauges, clocks, and exit signs. Radioactive material is also incorporated into such devices as check sources, static eliminators, and smoke detectors. Collectively, these devices may contribute an additional 4 mrads/yr (40 μGy/yr) to the population dose. Natural radioactive materials are present in many consumer products, such as tobacco, building materials, highway and road construction materials, combustible fuels, glass, and ceramics. Under some circumstances use of these naturally occurring materials can enhance the existing natural background radiation dose by as much as 5 mrads/yr (50 μGy/yr).

Radiation Protection Guides

Most radiation biology research, dealing with experimental animals or observations on humans, has been devoted to describing the quantitative relationship between the radiation dose and biologic effect. Such dose-response relationships have been described with great precision for the early effects of radiation following high doses. Most early effects, such as skin erythema, hematologic depression, and lethality, exhibit a threshold type of dose-response relationship. Such a dose threshold indicates that there is a dose level below which no response will occur.

This is not true for the late effects of low-level radiation exposure. Late effects are considered to have no dose threshold and to increase in incidence with increasing dose (Fig. 2-2). This type of dose-response relationship suggests that no radiation dose, regardless of how small, is considered absolutely safe. At zero dose a small but measurable response may be observed. This represents the natural incidence of effect under observation.

BASIS FOR RADIATION PROTECTION STANDARDS

This linear, nonthreshold type of dose-response relationship is the basis for current radiation protection standards. The late effects of principal concern are leukemia, cancer, and genetic effects, and they have been shown with reasonable accuracy to follow this dose-response model. Some

scientific studies dealing with low doses of x rays have shown that the linear quadratic dose-response model may better represent the actual experience of these effects. This is particularly true for leukemia. Nevertheless, it is conservative and prudent to hold to the linear dose-response model as the basis for radiation protection guides.

This basis for radiation protection guidance in the United States was first enunciated in 1931 when the National Council for Radiation Protection and Measurements (NCRP) recommended a whole body dose-limiting recommendation of 50,000 mrems/yr (500 mSv/yr). Since that time there have been numerous revisions of the dose-limiting recommendation down to the present level of 5000 mrems/yr (50 mSv/yr). Thousands of occupationally exposed persons have been observed, and very few have been exposed to a dose that exceeded the present dose-limiting recommendation. For instance, in diagnostic radiology 88% of radiographers receive less than 100 mrem/yr (1 mSv/yr). Only 3% are exposed to dose levels greater than 1000 mrem/yr (10 mSv/yr). These observations of occupationally exposed radiographers have not resulted in a single observed case of radiation effect.

It should be clear that any attempt to establish a dose-limiting recommendation is highly subjective and requires value assessments beyond the realm of science. The present dose-limiting recommendation has been in effect for more than 20 years and remains a prudent and safe level.

The development of the dose-limiting recommendation and other radiation protection guidelines acknowledges that some risk is involved in all radiation exposure. The task is to set these standards at a level of radiation exposure associated with an acceptable risk. This means recognizing, of course, that what may be an acceptable risk for one individual is unacceptable for another. The dose-limiting recommendation is considered to be an acceptable exposure for all radiation workers. Therefore it is that dose which, if received each year for a 50-year working lifetime, would not be expected to produce any significant effect. The dose-limiting recommendation for the population at large is one tenth of that for occupationally exposed persons, or 500 mrem/yr.

The phrase *dose-limiting recommendation* succeeds earlier phrases such as maximum permissible dose, *tolerance*

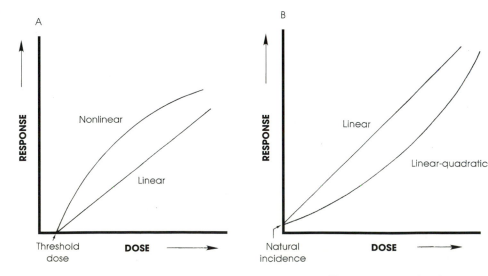

Fig. 2-2. Radiation dose-response relationships appear as either, **A,** threshold, or **B,** nonthreshold in shape.

dose, or *allowable dose.* In addition, radiation protection programs must be consistent with the ALARA concept, as previously defined.

SPECIFIC RADIATION PROTECTION CONCEPTS

In addition to the specification of a whole body dose-limiting recommendation for occupationally exposed persons and the population at large, several tissues and organs of the body are considered for their individual radiosensitivity. Specific individuals in the population are likewise accorded attention in specifying the dose-limiting recommendation. Table 2-4 is a summary of all of these and other dose-limiting recommendations.

In 1987 the NCRP revised the long-standing recommendations in Table 2-4. The new recommendations are slowly being adopted by state and federal regulatory agencies and soon will become law in all states. These newer recommendations are summarized in Table 2-5. It is noted that only SI units are used and the units relate to limits of *dose equivalent.*

The effective dose equivalent for the whole body remains the same—50 mSv/yr. This is the prospective annual effective dose equivalent. The cumulative effective dose equivalent is now 10 mSv × *n,* where *n* is the age of the worker. This is a considerable reduction from the previous level.

Effective dose equivalent is defined as "the sum of the weighted dose equivalents for irradiated tissues or organs. It takes into account the different mortality risks from cancer and the risk of severe hereditary effects in the first two generations associated with irradiation of different organs and tissues."

Effective dose equivalent is expressed symbolically as:

$$H_E = \Sigma w_T\, H_T$$

where:

w_T = the weighting factor representing the proportionate risk of tissue T.
H_T = the average dose equivalent received by tissue T.

The weighting factor, w_T, accounts for the relative radiosensitivity of various tissues and organs. Values for w_T are given in Table 2-6.

Table 2-4. Dose-limiting recommendations (NCRP Report No. 39, 1971)

Subject exposed	Dose
Occupationally exposed persons	
Whole body	
Prospective annual limit	5 rem in any 1 year
Long-term accumulation to age *n* years	*n* × rem
Skin	50 rem in any 1 year
Hands	75 rem in any 1 year (25 rem/3 mo)
Forearms	30 rem in any 1 year (10 rem/3 mo)
Other organs, tissue, and organ systems	15 rem in any 1 year (5 rem/3 mo)
Pregnant women (with respect to fetus)	0.5 rem in gestation period
General population	
Individual or occasional exposed persons	0.5 rem in any 1 year
Students	0.1 rem in any 1 year
Population dose limit	0.17 rem per year (average)

Table 2-5. Current radiation protection guides (NCRP Report No. 91, 1987)

A. *Occupational exposures (annual)*	
1. Effective dose equivalent limit (stochastic effects)	50 mSv
2. Dose equivalent limits for tissues and organs	
a. lens of eye	150 mSv
b. all others (e.g., red bone marrow, breast, lung, gonads, skin and extremities)	500 mSv
3. Cumulative dose equivalent	10 mSv × age
B. *Public exposures (annual)*	1 mSv
C. *Education and training exposures (annual)*	1 mSv
D. *Embryo-fetus exposures*	
1. Total dose equivalent limit	5 mSv
2. Dose equivalent limit in a month	0.5 mSv

Table 2-6. Recommended values of the weighting factors, w^T, for calculating effective dose equivalent

Tissue (T)	Risk coefficient	w_t
Gonads	40×10^{-4} Sv^{-1}	0.25
Breast	25×10^{-4} Sv^{-1}	0.15
Red bone marrow	20×10^{-4} Sv^{-1}	0.12
Lung	20×10^{-4} Sv^{-1}	0.12
Thyroid	5×10^{-4} Sv^{-1}	0.03
Bone surfaces	5×10^{-4} Sv^{-1}	0.03
Remainder	50×10^{-4} Sv^{-1}	0.30
Total	165×10^{-4} Sv^{-1}	1.00

A good radiation protection program must recognize not only the prospective effective dose equivalent but also the long-term cumulative effective dose equivalent. The cumulative figure restricts an individual's lifetime exposure to not more than ten times the worker's age in mSv. This dictates that no one under age 18 be employed as a radiation worker. Students may be under age 18, but a different effective dose equivalent applies to them. Use of the terms *prospective* and *cumulative dose equivalent* serves to emphasize that these are guides only and that exceeding a numerical dose-limiting recommendation may be acceptable under some circumstances.

Other regions of the body have different dose-limiting recommendations. That for the skin is 500 mSv/yr. This dose limitation applies to exposure to nonpenetrating radiation such as electrons and low-energy photons. In diagnostic radiology, mammography is the only type of procedure in which exposure of the radiographer's skin can reach its limit before the whole body limit becomes applicable.

During fluoroscopy it is often necessary for the hands or forearms to be in the useful beam. Usually these parts are protected by lead gloves. However, during certain procedures the use of such protective apparel is not possible. The dose limit for the hands and limbs is 500 mSv/yr. The recommended dose limit for the lens of the eye is now 150 mSv/yr, a threefold increase over the previous level.

The unborn child is known to be particularly sensitive to the effects of ionizing radiation; consequently, a dose limit of 5 mSv/9 mo is applied—the same as the previous recommendations. This presents a special problem in diagnostic radiology. In the case of the pregnant radiographer, it is unlikely that this recommended dose limit for the fetus would ever be approached, much less exceeded, because of the use of protective apparel during fluoroscopy and portable radiography. Nevertheless, rigorous radiation protection methods may be required during pregnancy. In recognizing this special concern, the NCRP has added the additional dose limit of 0.5 mSv/mo once the pregnancy is confirmed.

Under some circumstances students under age 18 may be exposed to radiation during educational experiences. In such cases they are given a separate dose limit of 1 mSv/yr. This dose limit is directed particularly to high school and college students of any age but also to radiography students under age 18.

Although many of the current NCRP recommendations represent an increase in dose limits, that for the general public is a fivefold reduction to 1 mSv/yr. If applied without modification, this means that future radiologic suites will require considerably more shielding than ever before!

Even more changes in recommended dose limits are on the way. The changes are not made because of fear that current limits are dangerous or even harmful; they are made in keeping with ALARA. The changes also acknowledge that we can function efficiently, even with these more restrictive dose-limiting recommendations. In 1991 the International Commission on Radiation Protection (ICRP) issued a number of recommendations, including an annual prospective effective dose equivalent of 20 mSv. Such a reduction is currently under consideration in the United States. Fig. 2-3 summarizes the history of radiation protection guides over the past 90 years.

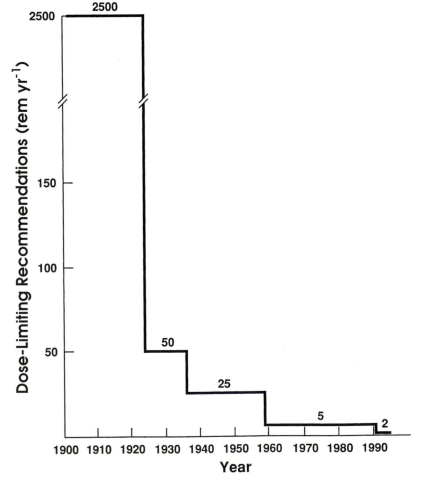

Fig. 2-3. Recommended effective dose equivalent values of the past.

Medical Radiation Dose and Exposure

The output intensity of an x-ray beam from any given radiographic or fluoroscopic unit can vary widely depending on the type of equipment and techniques employed. There may even be a sizable variation among x-ray units of the same manufacture and model when identical techniques are employed. The output intensity of any x-ray unit of course determines the radiation dose not only to the patient but also to the radiographer. Consequently, several methods are used to determine x-ray output to estimate doses to patient and radiographer.

The tabletop output intensity during fluoroscopy is difficult to estimate by computation with even moderate precision; it must be measured. Modern fluoroscopes have beam intensities limited to 10 R/min (2.58×10^{-3} C/kg-min) at the tabletop. Experience has shown that, when operated at a technique of about 100 kVp/1 mA, most fluoroscopes will produce an approximate tabletop exposure of 2 to 3 R/min (5 to 8×10^{-4} C/kg-min). Exposure rates of 4 to 7 R/min (10 to 18×10^{-14} C/kg-min) are common during clinical procedures.

Radiographic output intensities are also difficult to estimate by computation unless at least a single measurement is available. For a properly calibrated radiographic system the output intensity will vary directly with the milliampere-seconds and the square of the kVp. It will also vary inversely as the square of the distance from the target. Mathematically this is represented as follows:

$$\text{Output intensity} = k(mAs)(kVp)^2/d^2$$

where:

k = empirically determined constant
mAs = x-ray tube current multiplied by the exposure time
kVp = tube potential
d = distance from the source to the entrance surface of the patient (SSD)

Using this formulation and one measurement of k, a reasonably accurate estimate of radiographic output intensity can be made for any technique. Usually this one measurement is made at 70 kVp and expressed in milliroentgens per milliampere-seconds at a source-to-image receptor distance (SID) of 100 cm. Experience shows this value to range from about 2 to 8 mR/mAs (5 to 20×10^{-7} C/kg-mAs) depending on the age, manufacture, and adequacy of calibration of the radiographic unit. With this measured value, the output intensity at any other radiographic technique can be computed by using the following expression:

Output intensity (mR) =
   $k(mR/mAs)(mAs^1)(kVp^1/70)^2 (100 \text{ cm}/d')^2$

where:

k = measured value at 70 kVp/100 cm SID
mAs^1 and kVp^1 = the desired technique
d' = SSD

EXAMPLE: The medical physicist's report shows the radiographic output to be 4.8 mR/mAs at 70 kVp/100 cm SID. The technique chart calls for 76 kVp/80 mAs for a KUB examination. If the SSD is 80 cm, the skin exposure will be as follows:

Skin exposure
= $(4.8 \text{ mR/mAs})(80 \text{ mAs})(76/70)^2 (100/80)^2$
= 707 mR

Some investigators have produced nomograms for ease in estimating radiographic output intensity (Fig. 2-4).

PATIENT DOSE

The dose received by patients during diagnostic radiologic examinations is usually expressed in one of three ways: *entrance skin exposure (ESE), organ dose,* or *fetal dose.* Each has a specific application in assessing the risk to the patient, but ESE is the easiest to estimate.

Entrance skin exposure (ESE)

The exposure to the entrance surface of the patient during any radiographic examination can be measured directly or estimated by using the techniques previously described. ESE during fluoroscopy usually must be measured, although it too can be estimated from a tabletop exposure measurement at the technique under investigation.

Two methods generally are employed to measure ESE. Small ion chambers or solid state diodes can be placed on the entrance surface of the patient and exposed during any clinical procedure. Ion chambers and solid state diodes have a sufficiently wide range and are sensitive and accurate. However, they are difficult to position and use, and therefore their application is very limited. Most current estimates of ESE are made with *thermoluminescent dosimeters (TLDs).* TLDs are equally sensitive and precise, and they have a much wider range of response. Furthermore, they are very easy to use and because of their small size can easily be positioned on the skin. TLDs are nearly tissue equivalent and therefore will not be imaged except at a very low kVp.

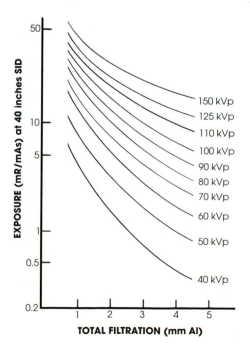

Fig. 2-4. A graphic relationship of radiographic output intensity (mR/mAs) as a function of kVp and added filtration at a source-to-image receptor distance (SID) of 100 cm

Table 2-7. Range of acceptable entrance skin exposures for several commonly performed examinations

Examination	Entrance skin exposure (mR per projection)
Chest (PA)	12-26
Skull (lateral)	105-240
Abdomen (AP)	375-698
Retrograde pyelogram	475-829
Cervical spine (AP)	35-165
Thoracic spine (AP)	295-485
Limb	8-327
Dental (bite-wing and periapical)	227-425

Table 2-8. Representative entrance skin exposure and tissue glandular dose for mammography

Examination	Skin exposure per projection (mR)	Approximate glandular dose per projection (mrad)
Xeromammography	500-1500	400
Screen/film	200-1000	75

Table 2-9. Representative bone marrow doses for selected radiographic examinations

X-ray examination	Mean marrow dose (mrads)
Skull	10
Cervical spine	20
Chest	2
Stomach and upper gastrointestinal	100
Gall bladder	80
Lumbar spine	60
Intravenous urography	25
Abdomen	30
Pelvis	20
Limb	2

Table 2-10. Approximate gonad doses resulting from various radiographic examinations

X-ray examination	Gonad dose (mrad)	
	Male	Female
Skull	<1	<1
Cervical spine	<1	<1
Full-mouth dental	<1	<1
Chest	<1	<1
Stomach and upper gastrointestinal	2	40
Gall bladder	1	20
Lumbar spine	175	400
Intraveneous urography	150	300
Abdomen	100	200
Pelvis	300	150
Upper limb	<1	<1
Lower limb	<1	<1

In recent years some government agencies have attempted to restrict the radiation exposure to patients during commonly performed radiographic examinations. It is also recognized that too low a radiation exposure can be equally hazardous by producing an inadequate image. Table 2-7 shows acceptable ranges for several radiographic examinations. These ranges are rather generous, reflecting the techniques and image receptors currently employed.

Organ dose

Sometimes the radiation dose received by a specific organ or tissue is of primary importance. Of course, organ doses for the most part cannot be measured directly but must be estimated. The breast, for example, is a tissue of primary concern because of the high utilization of x-ray mammography and the potential for radiation-induced breast cancer. Table 2-8 shows the approximate entrance skin exposures and glandular doses received by the breast as a function of the type of image receptor employed. The glandular dose is that which is used to evaluate radiation carcinogenesis.

Another organ of particular concern is the bone marrow. Bone marrow dose is used to estimate the population *mean marrow dose (MMD)* as an index of the somatic effect of radiation exposure. Table 2-9 relates some average bone marrow doses associated with various radiographic exposures. Each of these doses results from partial body exposure and is averaged over the entire body.

The gonads are other organs of concern in diagnostic radiology because of the possible genetic effects of ionizing radiation. Table 2-10 indicates average gonad doses received during various procedures. The large difference between males and females results from the shielding of the ovaries by overlying tissue. The weighted average gonad dose to the general population is used to estimate the *genetically significant dose (GSD)*.

Table 2-11. Approximate fetal dose (mrads) as a function of entrance exposure (1000 mR)

X-ray examination	Fetal dose (mrad/R)
Skull	<0.01
Cervical spine	<0.01
Full-mouth dental	<0.01
Chest	2
Stomach and upper gastrointestinal	25
Gall bladder	3
Lumbar spine	250
Intraveneous urography	265
Abdomen	265
Pelvis	295
Limb	<0.01

Fetal dose

Like most organ doses, fetal dose cannot be measured; it must be estimated. Such estimates are usually obtained from phantom measurements or computer-generated calculations. Table 2-11 shows the results of an analysis by the U.S. Center for Devices and Radiological Health and reports fetal dose as a function of the normalized skin exposure. To use this table, first the ESE for the type of examination in question must be measured. The fetal dose is given in millirads per 1000 milliroentgens ESE. Obviously the fetal dose is highest when the uterus is in the useful beam, such as during abdominal and pelvic examinations. During examination of distal parts of the body, the fetal dose will be very low, often not exceeding 1 mrad.

RADIOGRAPHER EXPOSURE

During the course of normal x-ray examinations, the radiographer receives at least 95% of occupational exposure during fluoroscopy and portable radiography. However, during fluoroscopy and portable radiography the radiographer wears protective apparel, so that only part of the body is exposed.

Adjacent to the examination table exposure rates may approach 500 mR/hr (1.3×10^{-4}C/kg-hr). The protective curtain draping the image intensifier tower will usually reduce the exposure to less than 5 mR/hr (1.3×10^{-6}C/kg-hr). The radiographer exposure can be estimated by assuming a position near the table and determining the x-ray beam on-time. For example, if a barium enema requires 3 minutes of x-ray tube on-time and the radiographer is positioned in a 100 mR/hr (2.58×10^{-5}C/kg-hr) field, then the occupational exposure to the unshielded part of the radiographer would be as follows:

$$100 \text{ mR/hr} \times 3/60 \text{ hr} = 5 \text{ mR}$$

Protective apparel usually provides an exposure reduction factor of at least one tenth, so that in the above example the exposure to the trunk of the body of the radiographer would be less than 1 mR (2.58×10^{-7}C/kg).

During fixed conventional radiography, the radiographer is positioned behind a protective barrier, which often may be a secondary barrier. In such cases the useful beam is never directed at the radiographer. A useful way to estimate exposure to the radiographer during radiography is to apply the rule of thumb that the exposure 1 meter laterally from the patient is approximately 0.1% of the ESE. For example, in Fig. 2-1 on p. 24, the radiographer is positioned 2 m from the patient. If the examination were of the chest, the ESE would be approximately 20 mR (5×10^{-6}C/kg). The scatter radiation 1 m laterally would be 0.1% of the ESE or 0.02 mR (5×10^{-9}C/kg). According to the inverse square law, at 2 m the scatter radiation intensity would be 0.005 mR or 4 µR (2×10^{-9}C/kg).

Protection of Patient

The patient is protected from unnecessary radiation during diagnostic x-ray examinations by certain design features of x-ray equipment and specially fabricated auxiliary apparatus. Special administrative procedures will also help to avoid unnecessary patient dose.

EQUIPMENT AND APPARATUS DESIGN

Usually those features of radiographic and fluoroscopic equipment which are designed to reduce patient dose will also reduce exposure to the radiographer. This aspect of radiation control should be kept in mind when patient protection is considered.

Filtration

A minimum of 2.5 mm Al equivalent total filtration is required on all fluoroscopic tubes and for radiographic tubes operating above 70 kVp. The purpose of filtration is to reduce the amount of low-energy radiation reaching the patient. Because only higher energy x rays are useful in producing an image, low energy x rays are absorbed in the patient and contribute only to patient dose, primarily to the skin, and not to the radiographic or fluoroscopic image. In general, the higher the total filtration, the lower the patient dose.

Collimation

Collimation is, as we have observed in Chapter 1, the restriction of the useful x-ray beam to the body part being examined, thereby sparing adjacent tissue from unnecessary exposure. This is extremely important in patient protection. The x-ray beam should always be collimated to the region of anatomic interest. The larger the useful x-ray beam the higher the patient dose. Restricting the x-ray beam by collimation reduces not only the volume of tissue irradiated but also the absolute dose at any point because of the accompanying reduction in scatter radiation. Reduction of scatter radiation also increases image quality by increasing radiographic contrast.

Specific area shielding

In specific area shielding part of the primary beam is absorbed during the examination by shielding a specific area of the body. Gonad shielding is a good example of specific area shielding and can be applied in two ways—with shadow shields and contact shields. Shadow shields are attached to the radiographic tube head and positioned with the aid of the light localizer between the tube and the patient. Contact shields are usually fabricated of vinyl lead cut into various shapes and are simply laid on the patient. Gonad shielding should be used under the following conditions: (1) on all patients of reproductive age, (2) when the gonads lie in or near the useful beam, and (3) when the use of such shielding will not compromise the required diagnostic information. Gonad shielding will reduce the gonad dose to near zero.

Image receptors

The speed of an image receptor can greatly influence patient dose. Rare earth screens developed in conjunction with matched photographic emulsions show relative speeds of up to twelve times those of a conventional calcium tungstate screen-film combination. Rare earth screen-film combinations that will reduce patient dose to one fourth can be used with no loss of diagnostic information. Higher patient dose reductions are possible, but the quality of the image may be compromised somewhat by radiographic noise. Today's fluoroscopic image intensifier tubes also incorporate more efficient input phosphors that can reduce patient dose by 25% to 50%. Use of these newer imaging modalities has been responsible for the very significant reduction in patient dose in recent years.

Radiographic technique

Radiographic technique not only is important in the production of a quality image but also greatly influences patient dose. Ideally, the higher the kVp the lower the patient dose, because a large reduction in mAs must accompany an increase in kVp. However, as kVp is raised, image contrast is reduced, and for some examinations this reduction in contrast may be unacceptable. For example, mammography could be done at far lower patient doses if the operating kVp were increased. However, the radiographic contrast would be very poor and the image would contain less diagnostic information. In general, the highest practicable kVp with an appropriate low mAs should be employed in all examinations.

ADMINISTRATIVE PROCEDURES

Patient and examination selection are two areas in which radiographers can provide procedures for reducing unnecessary patient dose.

Pregnancy

Safeguards against accidental fetal irradiation early in pregnancy are particularly critical during the first 2 months of pregnancy. In those early weeks, a pregnancy may not be suspected; if exposed unknowingly, the first-trimester fetus is particularly sensitive to radiation exposure. After a couple of months the risk of irradiating an undetected fetus becomes small because the patient is generally aware of her condition.

The radiographer should never knowingly conduct a radiologic examination on a pregnant individual unless a documented decision to do so has been made. When such an examination does proceed, it should be conducted with all of the previously discussed techniques for minimizing patient dose.

For many years, radiologists subscribed to the *10-day rule*. This rule was first stated in 1970 by the ICRP. It recommended that all x-ray examinations of the abdomen or pelvis of a fertile woman be performed only during the 10 days following the onset of menstruation. Over the past 10 years, however, both the American College of Radiology and the ICRP have published thoughtful documents showing why the 10-day rule should be abandoned. The 1983 statement of the ICRP reads:

In the first 10 days following the onset of a menstrual period, there can be no risk to any conceptus, since no conception will have occurred. The risk to a child who had previously been irradiated in utero during the remainder of the 4-week period following the onset of menstruation is likely to be so small that there need be no special limitation on exposures required within these 4 weeks.

The risk of injury following irradiation in utero is small, and the usual benefit so great that if the examination is clinically indicated it should be performed. Many studies have shown that the delay in scheduling such an examination is more harmful to the patient than the x-ray exposure. Fetal doses during radiographic exposure rarely exceed a few hundred millirad. However, if the examination is a high-dose procedure of the pelvis, such as a CT scan or a fluoroscopic examination, special attention may be appropriate if the patient suspects pregnancy. If such an examination can be delayed for a few weeks without compromising the management of the patient, it should. If the examination is necessary at that time, it should be conducted.

When a pregnant patient must be examined, the examination should be done with precisely collimated beams and carefully positioned protective shields. Use of high kVp technique is most appropriate in such situations. The administrative protocols that can be employed to ensure that we do not irradiate pregnant patients vary from simple to complex, with the degree of success proportionally observed.

We meet our responsibility to the potentially pregnant patient by posting in the waiting room and each examining room caution signs warning the patient of the importance of informing the radiographer if pregnancy is a possibility. Fig. 2-5 shows a helpful poster available from the National Center for Devices and Radiological Health.

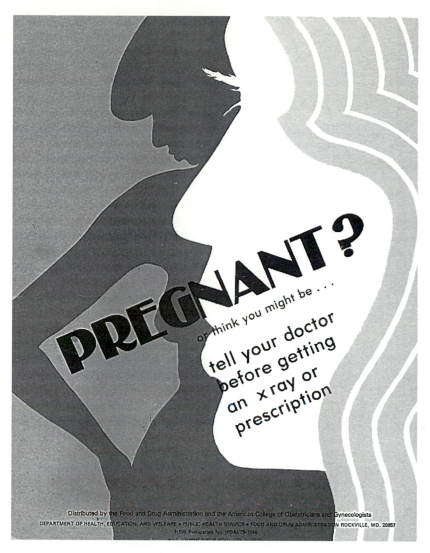

Fig. 2-5. One of many signs available to alert patient to possibility of irradiating an unknown pregnancy.

Patient and examination selection

Certain precautions against unnecessary patient dose are generally the responsibility of the radiologist, not the radiographer. Patient and examination selection are two such situations. Patients selected for x-ray examination fall into two categories: those who have symptoms and those who do not. Patients with symptoms usually require x-ray examinations to evaluate any previous clinical management and to provide the physician with information to plan the patient's future clinical management. Patients without symptoms usually are referred for x-ray examination to provide baseline information for possible future problems or to satisfy certain legal, insurance, or employment requirements.

When accepting a patient with symptoms for x-ray examination, the radiologist must be certain that the type of examination prescribed can provide the information necessary for proper medical management of the patient's condition. Furthermore, even if the findings of the examination are negative or normal, the performance of the examination should be beneficial and should significantly influence the course of management. For example, a skull series following trauma should be carefully evaluated by the radiologist and clinician. Several investigational series have reported that skull examinations are helpful in influencing the medical management of less than 10% of patients. Investigations of other types of examinations, intravenous urography, pelvimetry,

and barium enema, for example, have likewise shown a low yield of significant diagnostic information affecting patients' medical management.

Selection of patients without symptoms for an x-ray examination involves mass screening and selected routine procedures, many of which may not be medically justified. Routine x-ray examinations should not be performed when there is no precise medical indication. Substantial evidence shows that such examinations are of little benefit and are not medically justified because they are not cost effective and the disease detection rate is very low. Examples of such cases follow:

1. Mass screening for tuberculosis. General screening has not been found effective, and better methods of tuberculosis testing are now available. Some x-ray screening in high-risk groups (e.g., medical and paramedical personnel) and in personnel posing a potential community hazard (e.g., miners and workers having contact with beryllium, asbestos, glass, or silica) may be appropriate.
2. Hospital admissions. Chest x-ray examinations for routine hospital admission when there is no clinical indication of chest disease should not be performed. Among patients who would be candidates for such examinations are those admitted to the pulmonary or surgical service or elderly patients.
3. Preemployment physicals. Chest and lower back x-ray examinations are not justified because knowledge gained about previous injury or disease is nil.
4. Periodic health examinations. Many physicians now question the utility of the annual executive physical examination. Certainly, when such an examination is conducted on an asymptomatic patient, it should not include x-ray examination, especially fluoroscopic examination.

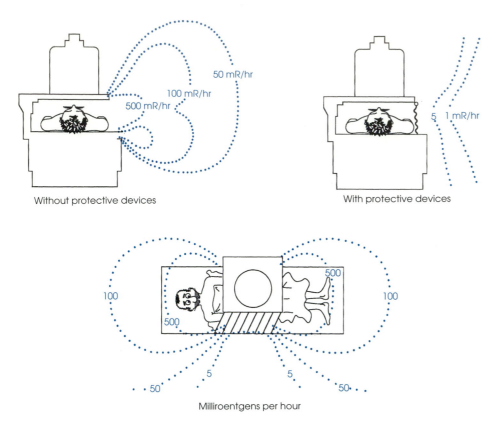

Fig. 2-6. Approximate isoexposure contours during fluoroscopy.

Protection of Radiographer

EQUIPMENT AND APPARATUS DESIGN

The principal source of radiation exposure to the radiographer occurs during fluoroscopy (Fig. 2-6) and portable radiography. Consequently, particular care and attention should be exercised during such situations.

Protective apparel

Protective apparel is used for both fluoroscopic and portable procedures and should be used faithfully. Table 2-12 shows the degree of protection provided by the principal sizes of protective lead (Pb) aprons available. Most find the 0.5 mm Pb apron perfectly adequate. Aprons of 1.0 mm Pb are too heavy for radiographers engaged in a heavy fluoroscopy schedule. Each portable x-ray unit should have assigned to it a protective apron, and the apron should remain with the unit at all times.

Protective barriers

During conventional radiography the radiographer is positioned behind the control booth barrier or other fixed protective barrier. Mobile protective screens should be avoided whenever possible. Although most protective barriers consist of a certain thickness of lead, not all do; nor is it necessary that all contain lead. Table 2-13 shows the British, metric equivalencies, and construction equivalencies of common thicknesses of lead employed in diagnostic radiology. Rarely is it necessary to exceed 1.6 mm thickness of lead.

Newer x-ray equipment and faster image receptors are significantly reducing the intensity of radiation during diagnostic x-ray procedures; therefore the amount of shielding required today is not what it was in years past. Although it is unnecessary for the radiographer to know how to compute the barrier thickness, some of the considerations that enter into that computation should be understood.

Primary versus secondary barriers

A *primary barrier* is any barrier that intercepts the useful, or primary, x-ray beam. A *secondary barrier* is one that intercepts only leakage and scatter radiation. The floor is nearly always considered a primary barrier, and anywhere from one to four walls may also be primary barriers. The ceiling is always considered a secondary barrier. In addition, the control booth barrier is usually considered a secondary barrier. During fluoroscopy all fixed barriers are considered secondary, because the image intensifier tower is designed as a built-in primary barrier.

Dose-limiting recommendations

The effective dose equivalent expressed as a weekly intensity is determined for each barrier on the basis of the use of the area being protected. If the adjacent area, such as another x-ray examination room or the darkroom, is to be occupied only by radiation workers and patients, it is identified as a controlled area. The dose limit for a controlled area is 20 mSv/wk. If the adjacent area is a laboratory, office, or area occupied by persons in the general population, it is called an uncontrolled area, and the dose limit is 1 mSv/wk.

Table 2-12. X-ray attenuation values for the common lead (Pb) equivalent thicknesses of protective aprons

Equivalent thickness (mm Pb)	Percent of x-ray attenuation		
	50 kVp	75 kVp	100 kVp
0.25	97	66	51
0.5	99	88	75
1.0	99	99	94

Modified from Bushong, S.C.: Radiologic science for technologists: physics, biology, and protection, ed 5, St. Louis, 1993, Mosby.

Table 2-13. British, metric, and construction equivalencies of common thicknesses of lead employed in diagnostic radiology*

British (inches)	Metric (mm)	Construction (pounds/square foot)
1/64	0.4	1
1/32	0.8	2
3/64	1.2	3
1/16	1.6	4
5/64	2.0	5
3/32	2.4	6

*Protective lead shielding is usually computed in British or metric units, but it is given to the builder in pounds per square foot.

Distance

The distance from the x-ray tube to the area being protected is important because the radiation intensity decreases rapidly with an increase in distance. If the barrier is designated as a primary barrier, then the distance can hardly be less than 1 m and is usually much more. The distance to a secondary barrier is often shorter. Obviously, for larger examination rooms, the respective distances will be larger and the required shielding will be less.

Workload

Workload is an expression of the total intensity of radiation employed during any week. It is described in units of milliampere-minutes (mA-min) per week and takes into account the number of patients examined, the number of images per patient, and the average mAs per projection. Rarely will the radiographic workload of a busy room exceed 500 mA-min/wk. Special-purpose radiographic units such as chest, head, and pediatric units may have considerably lower workloads. Less shielding is required for low-workload facilities.

Use factor

Under normal conditions, during most of the time that a general-purpose radiographic tube is energized it is pointed toward the floor. During some fraction of its beam on-time it may be pointed toward any vertical barrier. The fraction or percent of time that the useful, energized beam is directed to a barrier is the use factor. The floor is generally assigned a use factor of 1 and each wall a use factor of 0.05 to 0.25. The use factor is 1 for all secondary barriers, because at all times the tube is energized, scatter and leakage radiation are generated.

Occupancy factor

The occupancy factor is an expression of the extent to which the area being protected is occupied. Obviously an area that is always occupied will require more shielding than one that is rarely occupied. The recommended occupancy factors range from full occupancy for an adjacent office or laboratory to partial occupancy for a hallway or restroom to occasional occupancy for outside areas, elevators, and stairwells.

These factors are all considered when the required protective barrier thickness is computed. Although lead is the usual

shielding material for most diagnostic x-ray applications, other types of building material may be acceptable, particularly for secondary barriers. Clay brick, concrete block, gypsum board, and conventional plate glass are sometimes suitable. Frequently, multiple thicknesses of gypsum board may be used instead of lead-lined wallboard. Plate glass that is ½ to 1 inch thick may sometimes be substituted for leaded glass, as in the viewing window of a control booth console. A block, brick, or concrete wall will often satisfy the requirements for a primary barrier. A 4-inch concrete slab floor will likewise usually provide adequate protection as a primary barrier. If the slab is thin, it is sometimes permissible to position additional protective lead under the examination table with an appropriate overhang. If the x-ray room is located on ground level, the earth serves as a primary barrier and no additional shielding is necessary.

ADMINISTRATIVE PROCEDURES

Every radiographer should be familiar with the cardinal principles of radiation protection—time, distance, and shielding: (1) The *time* of exposure to a radiation source should be kept to a minimum; (2) The *distance* between the radiation source and the radiographer should be as great as possible; and (3) When appropriate and practicable, *protective shielding* material should be positioned between the source and the radiographer. A prime example of these cardinal principles occurs in fluoroscopy. During fluoroscopy the maximum exposure rate exists adjacent to the table, as shown in Fig. 2-6. Because the primary beam is emitted by the undertable tube and intercepts the patient, the patient becomes the radiation source because of scatter radiation. The radiologist must minimize the exposure time by activating the foot or hand control *intermittently* for minimum beam on-time. The radiographer can help by making certain that the 5-minute fluoroscopic reset timer is functioning and is used properly. The radiographer can minimize occupational exposure by taking one step back from the edge of the fluoroscopic table when it is not absolutely essential to remain there. Both the radiologist and radiographer wear protective lead apparel during fluoroscopy, which is perhaps the most effective method for reduction of occupational exposure.

Personnel monitoring

Perhaps the single most important aspect of a radiation control program in diagnostic radiology is a properly designed personnel radiation monitoring program. Three types of radiation measuring devices are used as personnel monitors— pocket ionization chambers, film badges, and thermoluminescent dosimetry badges.

Pocket ionization chambers can be used for personnel monitoring, although they seldom are in diagnostic radiology. The singular advantage to these devices is that they can be evaluated daily. However, pocket chamber dosimeters require a great deal of record keeping; thus their use in diagnostic radiology is generally restricted to monitoring occasional visitors.

Photographic film has been successfully used for half a century as a personnel radiation monitor. The design of the *film badge* has undergone many refinements such as integral metal filters that have enabled it to measure not only the quantity of radiation but also the type of radiation, approximate energy, and direction. Consequently it is very important that such a monitor be properly handled and worn.

Thermoluminescent dosimetry (TLD) has been used for approximately 30 years as a personnel radiation monitor. TLD badges have many of the same performance characteristics of film badges. The TLD sensitive material is reusable, and although the initial cost is high, the long-term expense is comparable to that of film badges. Because of the nature of this detector, it can be used for lengths of time exceeding the monthly interval limits placed on film badges. Under some circumstances it is not only permissible but advisable to monitor x-ray workers for calendar quarter intervals rather than for monthly or biweekly intervals. The principal advantage to this mode of radiation monitoring is the reduced record keeping that is required.

Regardless of the type of monitor employed there are certain important aspects to the conduct of a successful personnel radiation monitoring program. Each shipment of personnel monitors will be accompanied by a *control badge*. The control badge should normally be stored in some location distant from any radiation source, such as the office of the director of radiology. Individual radiation monitors should not leave the hospital. A rack or other holding device should be available on which radiographers can store their badges at the hospital at the end of the day. This will help to ensure that the monitors are not inadvertently damaged or exposed to environmental elements outside the hospital. Of course, the holding rack should be positioned distant from any radiation source.

Because radiographers receive most of their occupational exposure during fluoroscopy and portable radiography during which protective apparel is worn, the anatomic position of the personnel monitor is important. It should be worn outside the protective apron, unshielded, at the collar region. This region of the body will receive at least 10 times the radiation exposure of the protected trunk of the body. Therefore it is prudent to monitor the collar region, because it provides a wealth of measures, including the following: a way to estimate thyroid and eye lens dose; a means to estimate effective dose equivalency; and the most realistic means of monitoring the radiation environment. Furthermore, most state regulations require the monitor to be worn at this position. Regardless of the position of the personnel radiation monitor, a notation of where it is worn should be a part of each radiation monitoring report and of department rules and regulations.

The orientation of the monitor is also important. Be sure the front of the monitor faces the radiation source. If the orientation of the monitor is reversed, the filters in the monitor will not be in the correct position and the readings may be false.

A personnel monitoring program is not complete unless proper documentation is provided. Most commercial vendors of personnel radiation monitors will provide the user with a periodic computer-generated report containing all of the required information. For this report to be complete, all of the requested information on each individual must be supplied. This includes name, social security number, birthdate, sex, and previous radiation exposure. The last quantity may sometimes be difficult to obtain. Documentation of efforts initiated to obtain this information must be generated and filed.

Pregnant radiographers

Special administrative procedures are required for pregnant radiographers. It is the responsibility of each radiographer to inform her supervisor when she discovers or suspects that she is pregnant. A supervisor should then consult with the radiographer and review completely the ongoing radiation control program of the department. Under normal circumstances a radiographer will receive less than 5 mSv annually, as recorded by the personnel monitor. Consequently, the exposure under the protective apron should not exceed 0.5 mSv annually, and the resulting fetal dose should not exceed 0.25 mSv. This compares with the dose limitation to the fetus of 5 mSv for the gestation period. Consequently, under most circumstances additional radiation protective measures may not be necessary.

In order to comply with current NCRP recommendations, management must deliberately review each radiation monitoring report to ensure that the occupational fetal dose does not exceed 0.5 mSv in any month. Two measures can aid this compliance. First, if possible, the pregnant radiographer should avoid fluoroscopy or portable radiography. The second measure is to use the collar-positioned monitor to estimate fetal dose. In addition, a second monitor may be positioned at waist level under the protective apron.

When a second monitor is provided, do not let them get mixed up. Label the second one "baby badge" or "fetal monitor" and color it "baby" *blue* or *yellow* "belly." The exposure reported on the baby badge should be maintained on a separate record and identified as exposure to the mother's pelvis. The fetal dose will be 25% to 50% of this value depending on the time and nature of the pregnancy.

Chapter 3

GENERAL ANATOMY AND RADIOGRAPHIC POSITIONING TERMINOLOGY

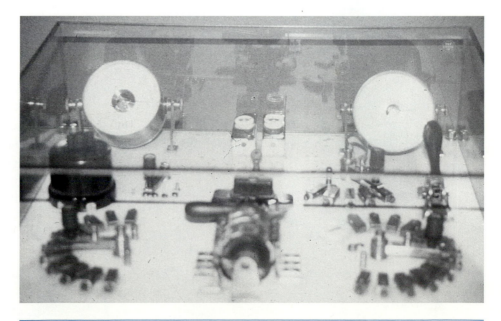

A radiographic control panel (photographed through a protective cover) from 1901. Note the bare electrical contacts on the front left and right corners, which were very hazardous to the operator.

General Anatomy

Radiographers must possess a thorough knowledge of anatomy, physiology, and osteology to obtain radiographs that demonstrate the desired body part. *Anatomy* is the term applied to the science of the structure of the body. *Physiology* is the study of the function of the body organs. *Osteology* is the detailed study of the body of knowledge relating to the bones of the body.

The radiographer must have a general understanding of all body systems and the function of each. Particular emphasis must be devoted to obtaining a thorough understanding of the skeletal system and the surface landmarks used to locate different body parts. It is crucial that the radiographer be able to mentally visualize the internal structures to be radiographed. By using external landmarks, the radiographer can properly position the body part to obtain the best possible diagnostic radiograph.

BODY PLANES AND POSITIONS

The well-established *anatomic position* of the body is defined with the body standing erect, face and eyes directed forward, arms extended by the sides with the palms of the hands facing forward, heels together, the toes pointing anteriorly with the great toes touching. Many of the terms established to describe location or position of parts are based on this body position. Additionally, radiographs are routinely placed on the illuminator for viewing as if the patient were standing before the viewer in this manner (see Displaying Radiographs, Chapter 1).

There are four fundamental planes of the body (Fig. 3-1):

1. The *median sagittal* (midsagittal) *plane* passes vertically through the midline of the body from front to back, dividing it into equal right and left portions. Any plane passing through the body parallel with the median sagittal plane is termed a *sagittal* plane.

2. The *median coronal* (midcoronal, midaxillary or midfrontal) *plane* passes vertically through the coronal suture of the cranium and extends inferiorly through the trunk and limbs at right angles to the median sagittal plane. This plane divides the body into anterior (ventral) and posterior (dorsal) portions. Any plane passing vertically through the body from side to side is called a *coronal* plane.

3. The *horizontal* (transverse or axial) *plane* passes crosswise through the body at right angles to its longitudinal axis and to the median sagittal and coronal planes, dividing it into superior and inferior portions. Any plane passing through the body at right angles to its longitudinal axis is called a horizontal (transverse or axial) plane.

4. An *oblique plane* is any plane that does not conform to the above three descriptions. Oblique planes may be located anywhere in the body, such as those used to pass through the heart in magnetic resonance imaging.

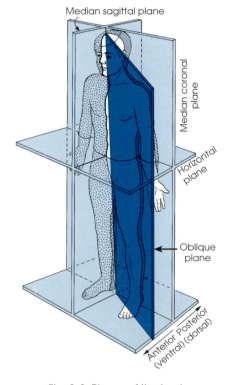

Fig. 3-1. Planes of the body.

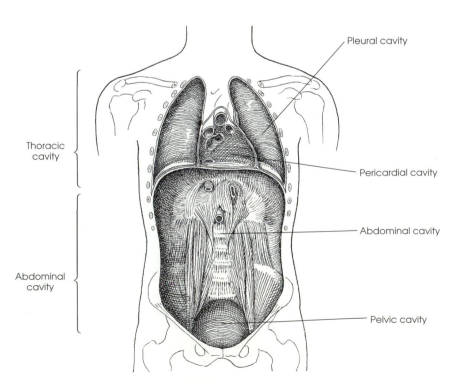

Fig. 3-2. Anterior view of the torso.

BODY CAVITIES

The two great cavities of the torso are the thoracic and abdominal cavities. The thoracic cavity is divided into a *pericardial* and two *pleural* portions as seen in Fig. 3-2. Although the abdominal cavity has no intervening partition, the lower portion is called the pelvic cavity.

The principal structures located in the *thoracic cavity* are the pleural membranes, lungs, trachea, esophagus, pericardium, and heart and great vessels.

The principal structures of the *abdominal cavity* are the peritoneum, liver, gall bladder, pancreas, spleen, stomach, intestines, kidneys, ureters, and major blood vessels.

The *pelvic cavity* contains the rectum, urinary bladder, and parts of the reproductive system.

DIVISIONS OF THE ABDOMEN

The abdomen is the portion of the trunk bordered superiorly by the diaphragm and inferiorly by the superior pelvic aperture (pelvic inlet). To describe the location of organs or an area, the abdomen may be divided either into four quadrants or nine regions.

The abdomen is divided into four *quadrants* (Fig. 3-3) by the median sagittal and a horizontal plane that intersect at the umbilicus. The quadrants are named the *right upper quadrant (RUQ), right lower quadrant (RLQ), left upper quadrant (LUQ),* and *left lower quadrant (LLQ)*. Dividing the abdomen into four quadrants is useful in describing the location of the various abdominal organs. For example, the spleen can be described as being located within the left upper quadrant.

Although this method is seldom used in clinical medicine, some anatomists still divide the abdomen into *nine regions* (Fig. 3-4) by using four planes: two horizontal (transverse) and two vertical (sagittal). The two horizontal planes are drawn at the levels of (1) the tip of the ninth costal cartilage (inferior border of the first lumbar vertebra) and (2) the superior mar-

gin of the crest of the ilium (middle of the fourth lumbar vertebra). Two sagittal planes are drawn, each midway between the anterior superior iliac spines of the pelvis and the median sagittal plane of the body. These planes were described by Addison and may occasionally be called Addison's planes. The nine regions of the body are named as follows:

Superior
Right hypochondrium
Epigastrium
Left hypochondrium
Middle
Right lateral (lumbar)
Umbilical
Left lateral (lumbar)
Inferior
Right inguinal (iliac)
Hypogastrium
Left inguinal (iliac)

In the clinical setting, the patient can be described as having, for example, epigastric pain. With the exception of the epigastric region, health professionals more commonly describe the areas of the abdomen using the terminology of quadrants, as described previously.

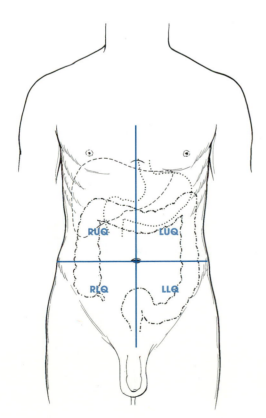

Fig. 3-3. Clinical divisions of the four quadrants of the abdomen.

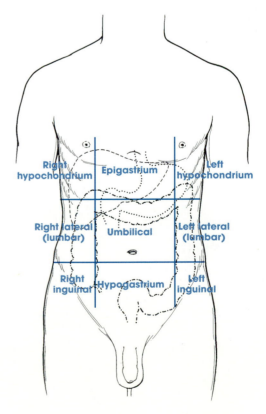

Fig. 3-4. Anatomic divisions of the nine regions of the abdomen.

Table 3-1. External landmarks related to body structures at the same level

Cervical area (see Fig. 3-5)

C1	Mastoid tip
C2, C3	Gonion (angle of mandible)
C3, C4	Hyoid bone
C5	Thyroid cartilage
C7	Vertebra prominens

Thoracic area (see Fig. 3-6)

T1	Approximately 5 cm (2 in) above level of jugular notch
T2, T3	Level of jugular notch and superior margins of scapulae
T4, T5	Level of sternal angle
T7	Level of inferior angles of scapulae
T10	Level of xiphoid process

Lumbar area

L3	Costal margin
L3, L4	Level of umbilicus on flat abdomen (lower on pendulent abdomen)
L4	Level of most superior aspect of crests of ilia

Sacrum and pelvic area

S1	Level of anterior superior iliac spines
Coccyx	Level of symphysis pubis and greater trochanters

SURFACE LANDMARKS

Most anatomic structures cannot be directly visualized. Thus the radiographer must use various protuberances, tuberosities, and other external indicators to accurately position the patient. These surface landmarks enable the radiographer to consistently obtain radiographs of optimal quality for a wide variety of body types. If surface landmarks are not used for radiographic positioning or if they are used incorrectly, the chance of having to repeat the radiograph greatly increases.

Many of the commonly used landmarks are listed in Table 3-1 and diagrammed in Figs. 3-5 and 3-6. It must be noted, however, that these landmarks are accepted *averages* for the majority of patients and should be used only as guidelines. Variations in anatomic build and/or pathologic conditions may warrant positioning compensation on an individual basis. The ability to do this comes with experience.

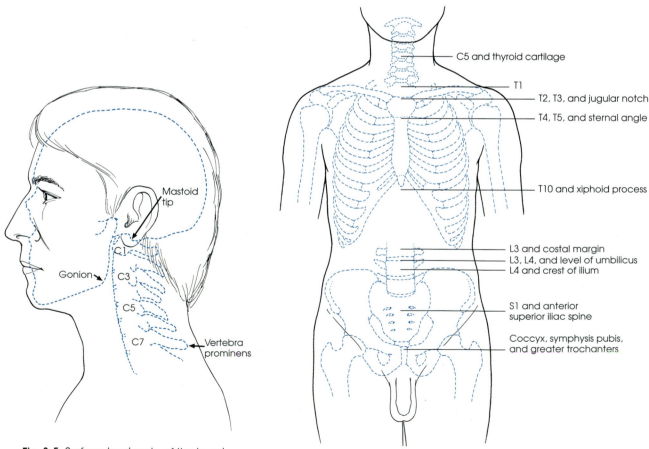

Fig. 3-5. Surface landmarks of the head and neck.

Fig. 3-6. Surface landmarks of the torso.

Body Habitus

The general form, or *habitus,* of the body determines the size, shape, position, tonus, and motility of the internal organs. After a study of a large number of subjects, Mills[1] classified numerous types of bodily habitus. The four major ones are the *hypersthenic, sthenic, hyposthenic,* and *asthenic.* Certain organs, such as the gall bladder, vary as much as 6 to 8 inches in position, both horizontally and vertically, between the two extreme types—hypersthenic and asthenic. For this reason, the radiographer must be familiar with the characteristics of the major types and be able to recognize their related intermediate types. An outline of the radiographically important characteristics of these four major types follows. The illustrations of the two extreme types should be studied and compared with the illustrations of the two dominant intermediate types.

The *hypersthenic* type of body is one of massive build (Fig. 3-7). This type represents the upper extreme, and only about 5% of persons fit into this classification. The thorax is broad and deep, the ribs assume an almost horizontal position, and the thoracic cavity is short. The lungs are short, narrowed above, and broad at their bases. The heart is short and wide, and its longitudinal axis is almost transverse. The diaphragm is high, resulting in a long abdomen. The upper part of the abdominal cavity is broad and capacious; the lower part is small. The stomach and gall bladder occupy high, almost horizontal positions, the latter being well away from the midline. The colon is also high and extends around the periphery of the abdominal cavity.

The *sthenic* habitus, a modification of the hypersthenic category, is the predominant type: it comprises approximately 50% of all persons (Fig. 3-8).

[1]Mills WR: The relation of bodily habitus to visceral form, position, tonus, and motility, AJR 4:155-169, 1917.

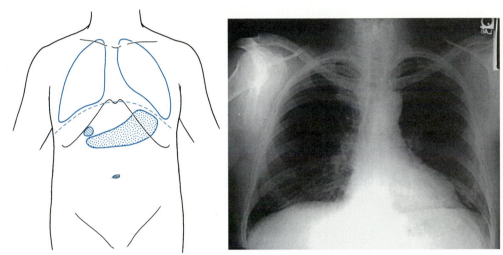

Fig. 3-7. Hypersthenic habitus. (Lungs, diaphragm, stomach, and gall bladder shown.)

(Courtesy Lois Baird, R.T.)

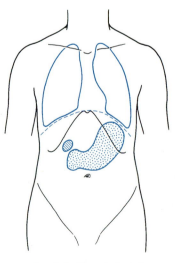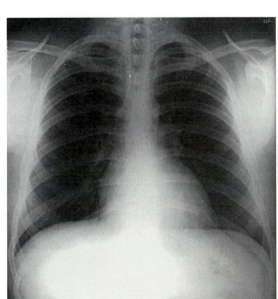

Fig. 3-8. Sthenic habitus.
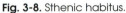

The *hyposthenic* habitus is a modification of the more extreme asthenic type; that is, it is more toward the sthenic type. Approximately 35% of individuals fit into this classification (Fig. 3-9).

The *asthenic* type of body is one of extremely slender build. This type represents the lower extreme and includes only about 10% of persons (Fig. 3-10). The asthenic thorax is narrow and shallow, the ribs slope sharply downward, and the cavity of the thorax is long. The lungs are long, extend well above the clavicles, and are broader above than at their bases. The heart is long and narrow, and its longitudinal axis is almost vertical. The diaphragm is low and the abdominal cavity short, its greatest capacity being in the lower portion. The stomach and gall bladder are low, vertical, and near the midline. The colon folds on itself and occupies a low, median position.

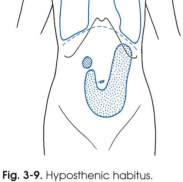

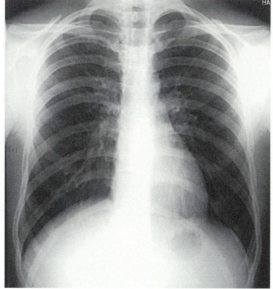

Fig. 3-9. Hyposthenic habitus.

(Courtesy Lois Baird, R.T.)

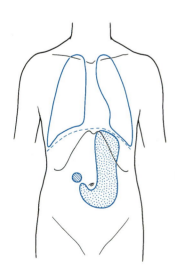

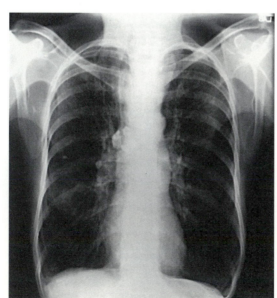

Fig. 3-10. Asthenic habitus.

SKELETAL ANATOMY

In the adult the skeleton is normally composed of 206 bones (which excludes small sesamoid and accessory or supernumerary bones in the skull) and, in certain places, pieces of cartilage. The bones and cartilage are united by ligaments in such a way that they form the supporting framework of the body, afford places of attachment for muscles, and protect the delicate visceral organs.

The bony framework of the body is divided into two main groups: the appendicular and the axial skeleton. The *appendicular skeleton* consists of the upper and lower limbs (extremities) and the respective shoulder and pelvic girdles. The *axial skeleton* includes the skull, vertebral column, sternum, and ribs. The anatomy of each of these divisions is discussed in the chapter dealing with the positioning of the particular region.

Bones are composed of an inner, trabeculated, portion called *spongy* (cancellous) *tissue* surrounded by an outer layer of compact bony tissue called the *cortex* (Fig. 3-11). The comparative amount of spongy (cancellous) tissue and cortex varies widely depending on each bone's location and function. Long bones have a central cylindrical cavity called the *medullary canal*. The medullary canal is filled with marrow, which contains blood vessels, immature blood cells, and fat. Except where covered by articular cartilage, the bones are covered by a tough fibrous membrane called the *periosteum*. The surfaces of the bones are smooth at points of articulation, have projections at points where muscles and ligaments attach, and present depressions for the passage of blood vessels and nerves.

Bones are classified by shape as either long, short, flat, or irregular.

Long bones consist of a body, or shaft, and two articular extremities. These bones are frequently curved for strength and narrowed to accommodate muscles. Until full maturity is attained, the articular ends are separated from the shaft by a layer of cartilage called the epiphyseal plate. The shaft is referred to as the *diaphysis,* and the articular ends as the *epiphyses.* Long bones are found only in the limbs (extremities).

Short bones consist mainly of spongy tissue and have only a thin outer layer of the compact cortex tissue. They are found where compactness, elasticity, and full range of motion are required. The carpals and tarsals of the wrists and ankles are examples of short bones.

Flat bones consist largely of compact cortex tissue in the form of two plates, or tables, that enclose a layer of spongy tissue, or *diploë* (which means "placed between two tables of cranial bone"), such as the bones of the cranium, or broad surfaces for muscle attachment, such as the scapulae.

Irregular bones, because of their peculiar shape, cannot be classified in any of the foregoing groups. The vertebrae, bones of the face, and sesamoids are typical bones of this group. *Sesamoid bones* are small bones embedded in tendons. Generally located near joints, the function of a sesamoid bone is to decrease the wear of tendons. Most of the sesamoid bones in the body are located in the hands and feet with the largest sesamoid in the body, the *patella* (kneecap), being the exception. These bones often can be demonstrated in radiographic examinations of the hands and feet. Sesamoid bones can be fractured; such fractures can cause the patient a great deal of pain.

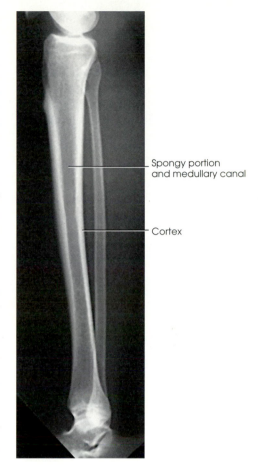

Spongy portion and medullary canal

Cortex

Fig. 3-11. Tibia and fibula showing bone composition.

(Courtesy Patti Chapman, R.T.)

ARTICULATIONS OR JOINTS

An *articulation,* or *joint,* expresses a relationship between two or more bones of the skeleton. The bones of the skeleton are joined together by ligaments, cartilages, or the dovetailing of bone (as in the sutures of the cranium). Articulations of the body are classified in two general ways, according to *function* and *structure.*

Functional classification

When articulations are classified according to their function, or mobility, the three classifications are: (1) *synarthroses,* or immovable joints; (2) *amphiarthroses,* or joints permitting limited, or slight, motion; and (3) *diarthroses,* or freely movable joints.

Structural classification

The more recent classification of joints is based on the structural details of the joint, where two or more bones are joined. The structural classifications are as follows:

Fibrous joints, or synarthrodial joints, exist when adjacent bones are held together by a thin layer of fibrous connective tissue or by a layer of cartilage. Fibrous joints include sutures, syndesmoses, and gomphoses. The immovable *sutures* of the skull are formed when the bones make contact with one another along interlocking edges (Fig. 3-12, *A*). *Syndesmoses* are very slightly movable joints such as the inferior tibiofibular joint where ligaments, or fibrous bands, connect adjacent bones (Fig. 3-12, *B*). A *gomphosis* is a specific joint between the root of a tooth and the alveolar process of the mandible (Fig. 3-12, *C*).

Cartilaginous joints, or amphiarthrodial joints, represent a transitional stage of holding bones together by cartilage. The two classifications of cartilaginous joints consist of both symphyses and synchondroses. A *symphysis* is defined as the joining together of two midline bones in the body by a plate of fibrocartilage. These cartilaginous joints are only slightly movable, such as those found between the vertebral bodies, and that of the symphysis pubis (Fig. 3-13, *A*). (Slight movement of the symphysis pubis during childbirth makes passage of the infant through the birth canal easier.) A *synchondrosis* is a joint in which two bones are joined by hyaline cartilage. The joints connecting the first ten ribs with the sternum are examples of synchondrosis-type joints (Fig. 3-13, *B*).

Synovial joints, or diarthrodial joints, provide free movement such as that seen in the knee. The articular surfaces of the bones are shaped for the movement required of the joint, covered by articular cartilage, and enclosed in a fibrous envelope called a *capsule.* The capsule consists of two layers of tissue: an outer fibrous layer and an inner layer lined by a *synovial membrane* which secretes *synovial fluid* (Fig. 3-14, *A*). The synovial fluid supplies lubricants and nutrients to the joint surfaces. Also found inside the fibrous capsule of certain joints are menisci and ligaments (Fig. 3-14, *B*). A *meniscus,* or an articular disk, consists of a crescent-shaped pad of fibrocartilage located between the ends of bones in selected joints. A *ligament* consists of a band of connective fibrous tissue that joins bones or cartilages.

Where the joint action is such that muscles or tendons slide over underlying parts, fluid-containing sacs called *bursae,* also lined with a synovial membrane, are interposed between the sliding surfaces to reduce friction. Important bursae are located at such joints as the shoulder, elbow, hip, and knee and under muscles such as the deltoid and trapezius.

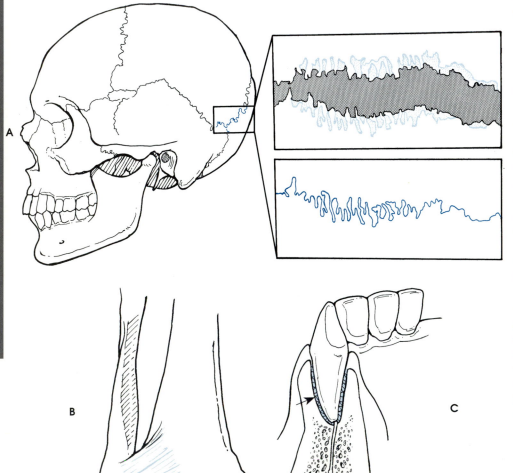

Fig. 3-12. Fibrous joints. **A,** Sutures (with disarticulated images). **B,** Syndesmosis *(arrow).* **C,** Gomphosis *(arrow).*

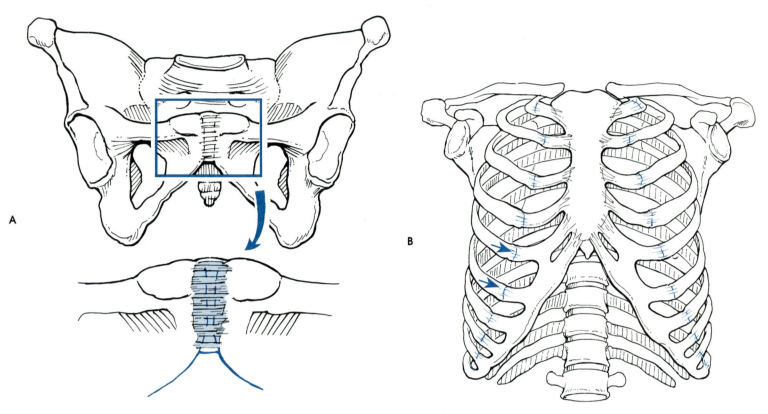

Fig. 3-13. Cartilaginous joints. **A,** Symphysis (with enlarged image). **B,** Synchondroses *(arrows).*

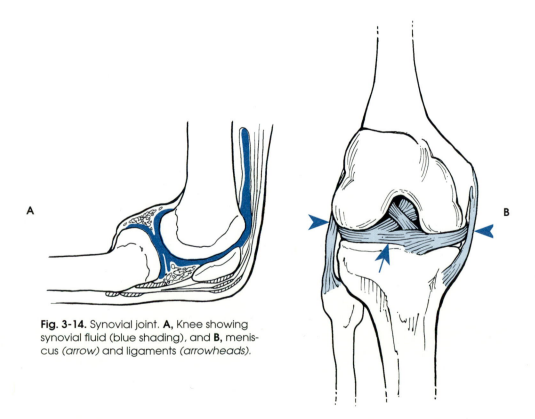

Fig. 3-14. Synovial joint. **A,** Knee showing synovial fluid (blue shading), and **B,** meniscus *(arrow)* and ligaments *(arrowheads).*

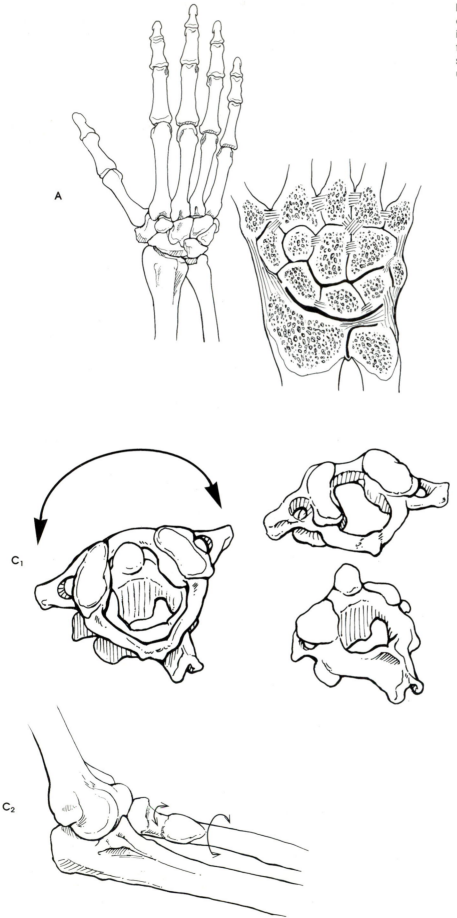

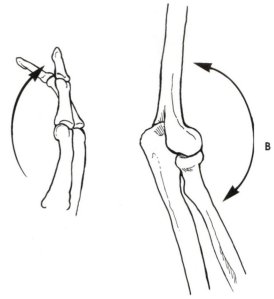

Fig. 3-15. Synovial, or diarthrodial, joints shown in order of increasing movement. **A,** Plane, or gliding, joint of wrist. **B,** Ginglymus, or hinge, joint of finger and elbow. **C,** Trochoidal, or pivot, joint showing dens (of axis) and the axis (with disarticulated drawing of dens and axis) and elbow.

Synovial joints: types of movement. All synovial joints provide for movement of a body part. As such, all synovial, or diarthrodial, joints permit one or more of the following six types of body movement. Here they are listed in order of increasing movement:

1. The *plane,* or *gliding, joint* provides for simple gliding or sliding motion without any angular movement. Examples of plane joints are the intercarpal and intertarsal joints found in the wrist and ankle (Fig. 3-15, *A*).

2. A *ginglymus,* or *hinge, joint* permits movement in only one plane such as flexion and extension. Examples of ginglymus joints are the elbow and finger (Fig. 3-15, *B*). To assist in flexion and extension of the joint, the articular capsule is thin on the bending surfaces and stronger on the lateral portion of the joint.

3. The *trochoidal,* or *pivot, joint* provides rotational movement around a single axis. Examples of trochoidal or pivot joints include the articulation of the dens (C_2) and the atlas (C_1) cervical vertebrae, permitting rotation of the head (Fig. 3-15, C_1), and the proximal radioulnar articulation near the elbow, permitting rotation of the hand (Fig. 3-15, C_2).

4. A *condyloid joint* permits movement in two directions at right angles to one another. The radiocarpal joint of the wrist is a condyloid joint, in which flexion and extension occur in one plane (Fig. 3-15, D_1) and abduction and adduction occur in the second plane (Fig. 3-15, D_2). Rotation does not occur in the condyloid joint. Circumduction movement does occur, however, which is the composite movement as a result of flexion, extension, abduction, and adduction. Examples of other condyloid joints are the metacarpophalangeal and the metatarsophalangeal joints of the fingers and toes, respectively.

5. The *sellar*, or *saddle*, *joint* also permits movement around two axes similar to the condyloid joint. In the sellar joint, the joining surfaces of the bones involved are complementing. Each has both a concave and a convex portion. An excellent example of a sellar joint is the carpometacarpal joint of the thumb, which permits opposing the thumb to the fingers (Fig. 3-15, E).

6. The *spheroidal*, or *ball and socket*, *joint* is the articulation permitting the greatest range of movement (i.e., flexion, extension, abduction, adduction, circumduction, and rotation; see definitions on p. 56). The center point of movement is near the center of the ball-shaped process that fits into a cup-shaped, concave socket. Examples of spheroidal joints include the shoulder and hip. The shoulder, having a shallow "socket" compared to that of the hip, is a weaker joint than the hip. However, the shallower the socket, the greater the amount of movement that is possible (Fig. 3-15, F).

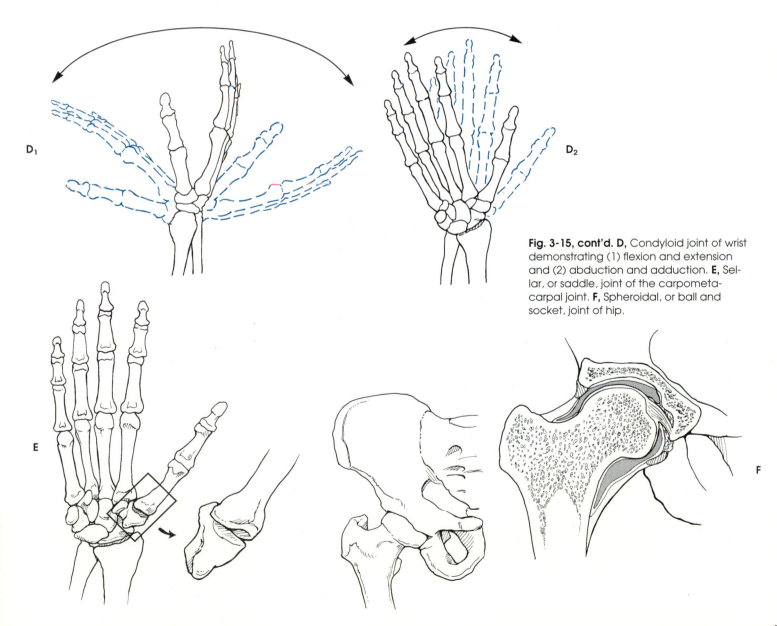

Fig. 3-15, cont'd. **D,** Condyloid joint of wrist demonstrating (1) flexion and extension and (2) abduction and adduction. **E,** Sellar, or saddle, joint of the carpometacarpal joint. **F,** Spheroidal, or ball and socket, joint of hip.

BONE MORPHOLOGY

In approximately the second month of embryonic life, the bones begin to develop in areas of fibrous membranes and cartilage. These areas of bone formation are termed *centers of ossification* and consist of bone-forming cells called *osteoblasts*. The time required for the bones to reach full development varies for the different regions of the skeleton.

In long bones, growth occurs in both the *diaphysis* and *epiphysis*. Remember: the *diaphysis* is the body (shaft) area of long bones, whereas the *epiphysis* is located at the end of long bones. Bone growth progresses from each diaphysis toward each epiphysis and vice versa. The diaphysis and epiphysis are separated by a layer of cartilage called the *epiphyseal plate,* which is often visible on pediatric radiographs (Fig. 3-16). Upon completion of bony maturation occurring between approximately 15 and 21 years, the epiphyseal plate is no longer radiographically visible. However, the time required for the bones to reach full development varies for different regions of the body and for different individuals. Full development occurs more rapidly in the female than in the male.

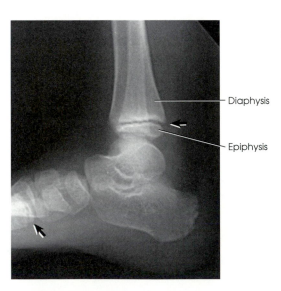

Fig. 3-16. Lateral ankle showing epiphyseal plates *(arrows).*

(Courtesy Lynn Rhatigan, R.T.)

ANATOMIC TERMS

The following anatomic terms are used to describe either processes or depressions.

Processes or **projections** that extend beyond or jut out from the main body of a structure are designated by the following terms:

condyle   A rounded process at an articular extremity.
coracoid or coronoid   A beaklike process.
cornu   A hornlike process on a bone.
crest   A ridgelike process.
epicondyle   A projection above a condyle.
facet   A small, smooth-surfaced process for articulation.
hamulus   A hook-shaped process.
head   Expanded end of a long bone.
malleolus   A club-shaped process.
protuberance or process   A bony projection.
spine   A sharp process.
styloid   A long, pointed process.
trochanter   Either of two large, rounded, and elevated processes (greater, or major, and lesser, or minor) located at junction of neck and shaft of femur.
tubercle   A small, rounded, elevated process.
tuberosity   A large, rounded, elevated process.

Depressions are hollow, or depressed, areas and are described by the following terms:

fissure   A cleft or groove.
foramen   A hole in a bone for transmission of blood vessels and nerves.
fossa   A pit, fovea, or hollow.
groove   A shallow, linear depression.
sinus   A recess, groove, cavity, or hollow space, such as:
   1. A recess or groove in bone, as used to designate a channel for venous blood on inner surface of cranium.
   2. An air cavity in bone or a hollow space in other tissue; used to designate a hollow space within a bone as in paranasal sinuses.
   3. A fistula or suppurating channel in soft tissues.
sulcus   A furrow, trench, or fissurelike depression.

BODY PART TERMINOLOGY

In addition to the general anatomic terms just described, other terms are used to describe the position of the patient. These terms are routinely used when radiographic examinations are performed, and the more common terms are defined and illustrated below (Figs. 3-17 and 3-18).

anterior and ventral Refer to forward or front part of body or to forward part of an organ; superior surface of foot is referred to as **dorsum** or **dorsal** surface.

caudal, caudad, and inferior Refer to parts *away* from the head of the body.

central Refers to the midarea or main part of an organ.

contralateral Refers to a part or parts on the opposite side of the body. Opposite of ipsilateral.

cranial, cephalic, and superior Refer to parts *toward* the head of the body.

deep Refers to a part far down or far from the surface.

distal Refers to parts farthest from the point of attachment, point of reference, origin, or beginning.

external Refers to a part outside of an organ or on the outside of the body. Opposite of internal.

internal Refers to a part within or on the inside of an organ. Opposite of external.

ipsilateral Refers to a part on the same side of the body. Opposite of contralateral.

lateral Refers to parts away from median plane of body or away from middle of a part to right or left.

medial and mesial Refer to parts toward median plane of body or toward middle of a part; opposite of lateral.

peripheral Refers to parts at or near the surface, edge, or outside of a body part.

plantar Refers to the sole of the foot.

posterior and dorsal Refer to the back of a part or organ.

proximal Refers to parts nearer the point of attachment, point of reference, origin, or beginning.

superficial Refers to a part near the skin or surface.

Radiographic Positioning Terminology

Radiography is the process of recording a body part on an image receptor (film). The terminology used in positioning the patient to obtain the radiograph appears to have developed through convention. Attempts to analyze the usage often lead to confusion, because the manner in which the terms are used does not follow one specific rule. In preparing this chapter, contact has been maintained with The American Registry of Radiologic Technologists (ARRT) and the Canadian Association of Medical Radiation Technologists (C.A.M.R.T.). The ARRT first distributed the "Standard Terminology for Positioning and Projection"[1] in 1978, and it has not been substantially revised since initially distributed.[2,3] Despite this title, the ARRT has not actually defined selected positioning terms.[4] When such terms are not defined by the ARRT, they are defined in this text.

---

[1]ARRT Educator's Handbook, ed 3, The American Registry of Radiologic Technologists, January 1990.
[2]ARRT personal correspondence, August 4, 1992.
[3]ARRT, Conventions specific to the radiographic examination, May 1993.
[4]ARRT personal correspondence, May 6, 1993.

Approval of Canadian positioning terminology is the responsibility of the C.A.M.R.T. Radiography Council on Education. This council provided information in developing this chapter and clearly identified the terminology differences between the United States and Canada.[5]

The four most commonly used positioning terms in radiology are *projection*, *position*, *view*, and *method*. Each is defined on the following pages.

---

[5]C.A.M.R.T. Council on Education, personal correspondence, July 20, 1993.

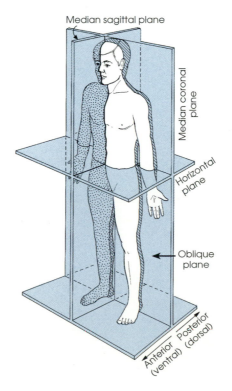

Fig. 3-17. Terms used to describe body part location.

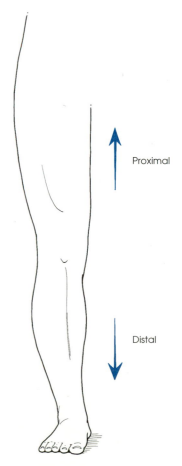

Fig. 3-18. Proximal and distal.

Table 3-2. Primary x-ray projections and body positions

Projections	Positions
AP	**Body positions**
PA	Upright
Lateral	Seated
AP oblique	Recumbent
PA oblique	Supine
Axial	Prone
AP axial	Trendelenberg
PA axial	
AP axial oblique	**Radiographic positions**
PA axial oblique	
Axiolateral	Right lateral
Axiolateral oblique	Left lateral
Transthoracic	Right posterior oblique (RPO)
Craniocaudal	Left posterior oblique (LPO)
Tangential	Right anterior oblique (RAO)
Inferosuperior	Left anterior oblique (LAO)
Superoinferior	Right lateral decubitus
Plantodorsal	Left lateral decubitus
Dorsoplantar	Ventral decubitus
Lateromedial	Dorsal decubitus
Mediolateral	Lordotic
Submentovertical	
Verticosubmental	
Parietoacanthial	
Orbitoparietal	
Parieto-orbital	

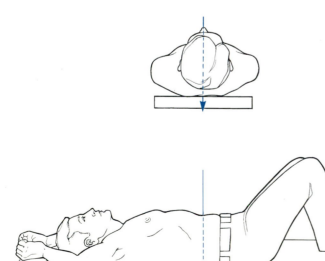

Fig. 3-19. AP (anteroposterior) projection.

PROJECTION

According to the ARRT,[1] the term *projection* is "restricted to the discussion of the path of the central ray" as it exits the x-ray tube and goes through the patient to the image receptor. The term projection continues to be standardized in this edition to describe the path of the central ray through the body part as though the body part were in the *anatomical position* (described on the first page of this chapter)— even when it is not (e.g., when the patient is *lying* supine on the radiographic table). Therefore if the patient is in the anatomical position and the central ray enters anywhere in the front (anterior) of the body surface and exits the back (posterior), an *AP (anteroposterior) projection* is obtained. Regardless of which body position the patient is in (e.g., supine, prone, upright, etc.), if the central ray enters the anterior body surface and exits the posterior body surface, the projection is termed *"AP projection."* This description is in agreement with both the ARRT[1] and C.A.M.R.T.[2]

All radiographic examinations described in this edition of the atlas have been standardized and titled by their *x-ray projection*. It is the x-ray projection that accurately and concisely defines each image produced. See Table 3-2 for a listing of the primary radiographic projections used in radiology.

AP Projection

In Fig. 3-19, the patient is placed in the supine (see the following section for definition), or dorsal recumbent, body position. The central ray is shown entering the anterior body surface and exiting the posterior body surface. This position correctly prepares the patient for an *AP projection*.

PA Projection

In Fig. 3-20, the patient is placed in the upright body position with the central ray entering the posterior and exiting the anterior body surface. This patient is properly positioned for a *PA (posteroanterior) projection*.

[1]ARRT Educator's Handbook, ed 3, The American Registry of Radiologic Technologists, January 1990.
[2]C.A.M.R.T. Council on Education, personal correspondence, July 20, 1993.

Axial projection

Previous editions of this atlas listed the term *axial* as a position. In response to the support offered by the professional community, axial has been changed and is now listed as a projection.

In an *axial projection* (Fig. 3-21) there is *longitudinal angulation* of the central ray with the long axis of the body. Some texts use the terms *semiaxial* (for a portion of an axial) and *half axial* (suggesting a 45-degree angle). To simplify the terminology, this atlas continues to use the term axial to refer to *all images obtained when the central ray is angled* 10 degrees or more along the long axis of the body or of the body part.

The ARRT[1] has no opinion or definition regarding the term axial. In *Canada,*[2] an axial image is properly referred to as a projection, because of the identification and angulation of the central ray.

Tangential projection

Previous editions of this text described the term *tangential* as a radiographic position. In response to the widespread support offered by colleagues, tangential is now listed as a projection.

A *tangential projection* (Fig. 3-22) is one in which the central ray is positioned so that it *skims* between body parts or *skims* the body surface, to profile a body part and project it free of superimposition. The ARRT[1] has not defined or offered an opinion regarding the term tangential. In *Canada,*[2] tangential is properly referred to as a view.

Lateral Projection

The term *lateral* is correctly used both as an x-ray projection and a body position (see next section for further description of lateral position). A *lateral projection* is one in which the central ray enters the side or lateral aspect of the body or body part, based on the anatomical position. A lateral projection needs further clarification as to which side of the body the central ray enters so the patient can be properly positioned. Lateral projections of the head, chest, and abdomen are further clarified with the specific positioning terms *left lateral position* or *right lateral position* as described in the next section. Lateral projections of the *limbs* are further

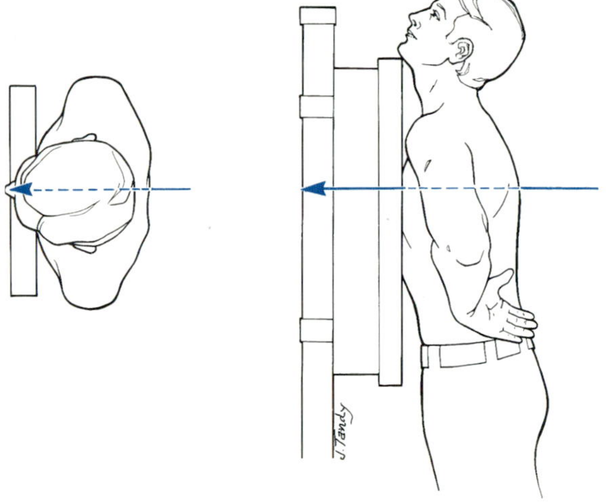

[1]ARRT personal correspondence, May 6, 1993.
[2]C.A.M.R.T. Council on Education, personal correspondence, July 20, 1993.

Fig. 3-20. PA (posteroanterior) projection.

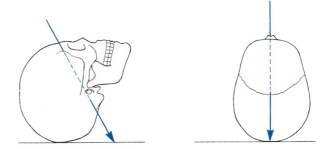

Fig. 3-21. Axial projection.

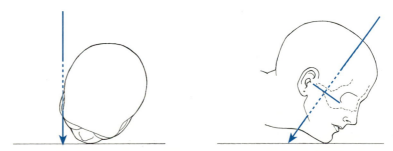

Fig. 3-22. Tangential projection.

clarified as to which aspect of the body the central ray enters (lateral or medial surface). The projection terms *lateromedial* or *mediolateral* are used to indicate the specific lateral projection in the limbs.

Oblique projection

The term *oblique*, like the term *lateral*, is also used both as an x-ray projection and a body position. An *oblique projection* is one in which the central ray enters the body or body part from a *side angle* into the anterior or posterior surface of the body. The central ray is most often perpendicular to the x-ray table, and the pa-

tient is rotated. However, for some examinations, the central ray is angled diagonally to enter the patient at a side angle, which also results in an oblique image.

In oblique projections, the central ray always enters the patient from either the anterior or posterior body surface. Therefore, the accurate terminology used is either *AP oblique projection* or *PA oblique projection*. Similar to the lateral projection, the oblique projection also needs an additional descriptive term to define the patient position. Oblique projections always need a position clarifier, as described in the next section.

POSITION

The term *position,* as used in radiology, has two relatively similar meanings. One meaning relates to a specific patient body position and the other meaning relates to the *act* of placing the patient in the appropriate position for a radiographic examination. See Table 3-2 for a listing of the primary positions used in radiology.

Body position

Body position refers to the manner in which the patient is placed in relation to the surrounding space. The following list describes the patient in several different body positions.

upright Erect or marked by a vertical position (Fig. 3-20).

recumbent Lying down in any position (Figs. 3-23, 3-24, 3-25).

supine (or dorsal recumbent) Lying on back (Fig. 3-23).

prone (or ventral recumbent) Lying face down (Fig. 3-24).

right lateral recumbent Lying on right side (Fig. 3-25).

Radiographic position

Radiographic position is the appropriate term used to describe a *specific position* of the body or body part in relation to the radiographic table or film: for example, *left lateral position* or *right anterior oblique position.*

In clinical practice, position and projection, unfortunately, are interchangeably used. Such use certainly leads to confusion for the student attempting to learn the correct terminology of the profession. Educators and clinicians are encouraged to use the term *projection* when referring to the path of the x-ray beam and also when generally describing any examination performed. The term *position* should be used

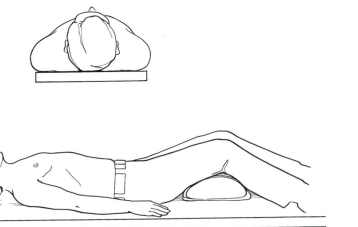

Fig. 3-23. Supine (dorsal recumbent) body position. (Knees flexed for patient comfort.)

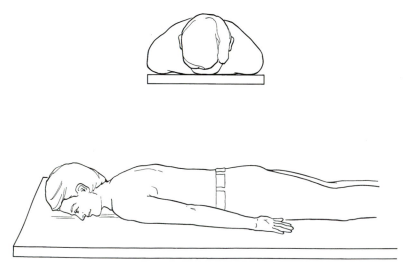

Fig. 3-24. Prone (ventral recumbent) body position.

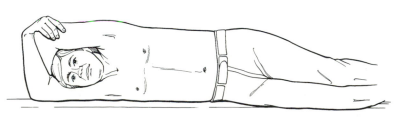

Fig. 3-25. Right lateral recumbent body position.

only when referring to the placement of the patient's body. These are two distinct and separate terms that should not be used interchangeably. For example, *"We are going to perform a PA projection of the chest with the patient in the upright position."*

Lateral position. *Lateral positions* are always named according to the side of the patient that is placed closest to the film, as demonstrated in the illustrations of the *left lateral position* (Fig. 3-26) and *right lateral position* (Fig. 3-27). The right or left lateral *positions* are indicated as subheadings in this atlas for all lateral x-ray projections where either the left or right side of the patient may be placed adjacent to

the image receptor. The specific side selected varies depending on the condition of the patient, the anatomic structure of clinical interest, and the purpose of the examination. Note in Figs. 3-26 and 3-27, the x-ray projection for the positions indicated is a *lateral projection*.

These lateral position illustrations are in agreement with the ARRT.[1] In Canada,[2] the laterally placed patient is named as above with the resulting image properly called a "view."

---

[1]ARRT personal correspondence, May 6, 1993.
[2]C.A.M.R.T. Council on Education, personal correspondence, July 20, 1993.

Oblique position. The term *oblique position* refers to a position in which the body or body part is *rotated* so it does not produce an AP, PA, or lateral image. Oblique positions, like lateral positions, are always named according to the side of the patient that is placed *closest to the film*. In Fig. 3-28, the patient is positioned to obtain a PA oblique projection. By rotating the patient to place the right anterior body surface in contact with the film, the patient is in the *right anterior oblique (RAO) position*. The RAO position is so named by the side (right) and the body surface (anterior) that is closest to the film. Similarly, Fig. 3-29 shows the patient positioned for a PA oblique projection. However, the patient is specifically placed in the *left anterior oblique (LAO) position*.

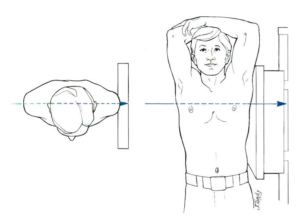

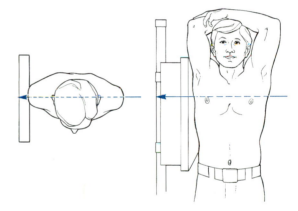

Fig. 3-26. Left lateral position resulting in a lateral projection.

Fig. 3-27. Right lateral position resulting in a lateral projection.

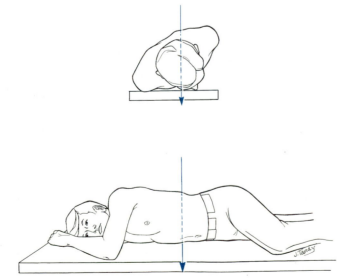

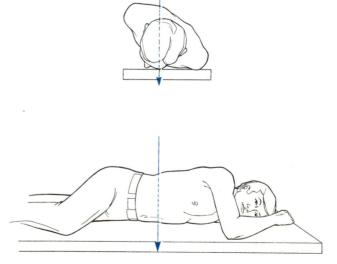

Fig. 3-28. RAO (right anterior oblique) position resulting in a PA oblique projection.

Fig. 3-29. LAO (left anterior oblique) position resulting in a PA oblique projection.

Following the same principle for all obliques, AP oblique projections require the patient to be placed in either the *LPO* (left posterior oblique) *position* or the *RPO* (right posterior oblique) *position* (Fig. 3-30 and 3-31) as illustrated.

The oblique positioning terminology used in this atlas has been standardized and is concisely listed using the RAO, LAO, LPO, or RPO position along with the appropriate AP or PA oblique projection. The degree of rotation changes depending upon the anatomic structures to be demonstrated. The number of degrees of body part rotation needed is specified for each individual radiographic position (e.g., rotated 45 degrees from the prone position).

For oblique projections of the limbs, the terms *medial rotation* or *lateral rotation* are standardized to designate which position the limbs have been turned from the anatomical position.

The ARRT is in confirmed agreement with the oblique position illustrations.[1] Canadian oblique positions are named as above; however, in *Canada*[2] the image of the oblique patient is properly called a view (e.g., an RAO view) indicating the right anterior body surface is closest to the film.

---

[1] ARRT personal correspondence, May 6, 1993.
[2] C.A.M.R.T. Council on Education, personal correspondence, July 20, 1993.

Decubitus positions. *Decubitus* (L. *decumbere,* to lie down) is defined as the act of or the position assumed in lying down. In radiographic positioning terminology, the term *decubitus* indicates that the patient is *lying down* and that the *central ray is horizontal,* or parallel to the floor. For most radiographic decubitus procedures, the patient is lying on the lateral body surface because the lateral position is most useful in the diagnosis of air-fluid levels in the chest and abdomen. It must be realized that the resulting image is most often an AP or PA projection achieved with the patient lying on his or her side.

Similar to lateral and oblique positions, decubitus positions are also named by the body surface on which the patient is lying.

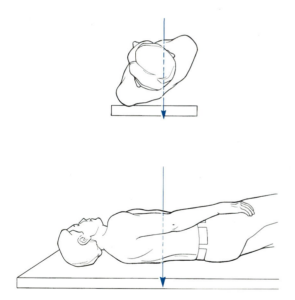

Fig. 3-30. LPO (left posterior oblique) position resulting in an AP oblique projection.

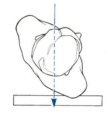

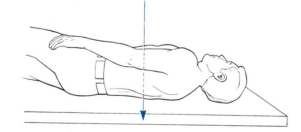

Fig. 3-31. RPO (right posterior oblique) position resulting in an AP oblique projection.

In Fig. 3-32, the patient is placed in the *left lateral decubitus position* (United States and Canada). Note that this body position, in relation to the horizontal central ray, results in an AP projection of the body part. Thus, Fig. 3-32 is accurately described as an AP projection with the body in the left lateral decubitus position. If the patient shown in Fig. 3-32 was to roll over and lie on the right side with the chest and abdomen against the x-ray cassette holder, the correct terminology would be described as a *PA projection with the patient in the right lateral decubitus position.*

In Fig. 3-33, the patient is placed in a *dorsal decubitus position,* and the resulting image is a *lateral projection.* Note that the x-ray tube is horizontal. In keeping with the previous example, the correct terminology would be described as a *lateral projection with the patient placed in the dorsal decubitus position.*

Positioning the patient *prone,* or the *ventral decubitus position,* produces a *lateral projection* of the body part, as demonstrated in Fig. 3-34. (The x-ray tube is not shown for purposes of the illustration.) Similar to the above examples, this positioning, used with a horizontal central ray, is accurately described as a *lateral projection with the patient in the ventral decubitus position.*

The ARRT[1] generally offers no opinion regarding decubitus positions. *In Canada,*[2] the decubitus image is properly called a position.

[1]ARRT personal correspondence, May 6, 1993.
[2]C.A.M.R.T. Council on Education, personal correspondence, July 20, 1993.

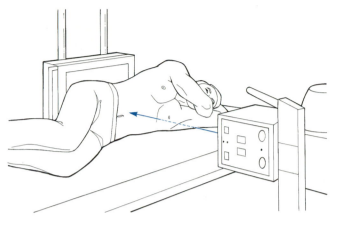

Fig. 3-32. Patient in the left lateral decubitus position resulting in an AP projection.

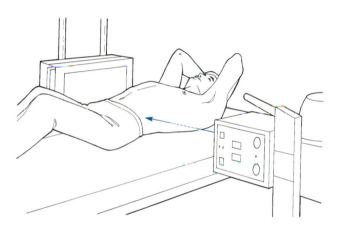

Fig. 3-33. Patient in the dorsal decubitus position resulting in a lateral projection.

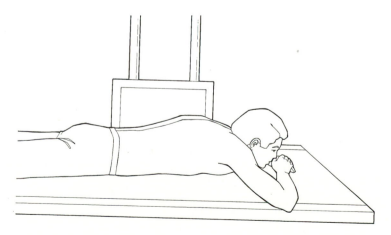

Fig. 3-34. Patient in the ventral decubitus position resulting in a lateral projection.

View

The ARRT defines radiographic *view* as "the body part as seen by an x-ray film or other recording media, such as a fluoroscopic screen. Restricted to the discussion of a *radiograph* or *image*."[1] In comparing the definitions of view and projection, it is noted that they are exact opposites. For many years view and projection were often used interchangeably, which led to confusion. For consistency, this text refers to all views as *images* or *radiographs*. In the United States, view is no longer a term used to describe a patient position. In Canada, however, view remains an acceptable positioning term.

---

[1]ARRT Educator's Handbook. The American Registry of Radiologic Technologists, S-1, January 1990.

Method

Some radiological procedures are named after individuals (e.g., Waters or Law) in recognition of their having developed a method to demonstrate a specific anatomic part. The *method* was first described in the fifth edition of this text, and it describes the body position of the patient in reference to established anatomic landmarks. The method additionally specifies placement of the film and central ray. In this atlas a method is first described using the standard anatomic positioning terminology. For example, the Waters method, useful to demonstrate the maxillary sinuses, is anatomically called a *parietoacanthial projection* (both in the United States and Canada) when the patient is positioned adjusting the orbitomeatal line to form an angle of 37 degrees from the plane of the film. Both the ARRT[2] and C.A.M.R.T.[3] use the standard anatomic projection terminology and list the originator in parentheses, e.g., parietoacanthial (Waters) projection.

---

[2]ARRT "Conventions specific to the radiography examination," revised May 1993.
[3]C.A.M.R.T. Council on Education, personal correspondence, July 20, 1993.

Body Movement Terminology

The following terms are used to describe movement related to the limbs (extremities). These terms are often used in positioning descriptions as well as in the patient history provided to the radiographer by the referring physician and must, therefore, be studied carefully.

Abduction and adduction (Fig. 3-35)

abduction Movement of a part away from central axis of body or body part.
adduction Movement of a part toward central axis of body or body part.

Flexion and extension (Fig. 3-36)

extension Straightening of a joint; stretching of a part; also, a backward bending movement; opposite of flexion (also see hyperextension).
flexion A bending movement of a joint whereby angle between contiguous bones is diminished; also, a forward bending movement; opposite of extension (also see hyperflexion).
hyperextension Forced or excessive extension of a limb or part.
hyperflexion Forced overflexion of a limb or part.

Inversion and eversion (Fig. 3-37)

evert or eversion Movement of the foot when turned outward at the ankle joint.
invert or inversion Movement of the foot when turned inward at the ankle joint.

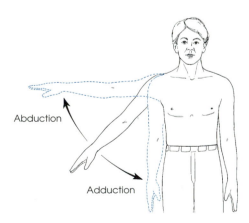

Fig. 3-35. Abduction and adduction.

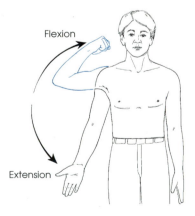

Fig. 3-36. Flexion and extension.

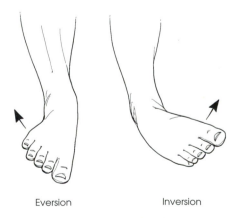

Fig. 3-37. Inversion and eversion.

Pronate, supinate, and rotate (Figs. 3-38 to 3-40).

pronate To turn forearm so that palm of hand faces backward.

supinate To turn forearm so that palm of hand faces forward.

rotate To turn around an axis. For example, the torso or the head is *rotated* from the frontal (AP or PA) body position to obtain an oblique radiographic image.

Medial—rotation of arm (or other body part) *toward* the midline of the body from the anatomical position.

Lateral—rotation of arm (or other body part) *away from* the midline of the body from the anatomical position.

Tilt (Fig. 3-41)

tilt The movement of the body part whereby the sagittal (longitudinal) plane is angled so it is *not* parallel with the long axis of the body. For example, the tangential projection to demonstrate the zygomatic arch (see Chapter 21) may be obtained by angling (i.e., tilting) the median sagittal plane of the head so it is not parallel with the long axis of the body. The term tilt is primarily used to describe angulation of the body part involving the skull.

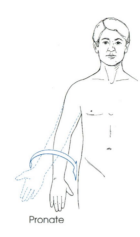

Pronate

Fig. 3-38. Pronation.

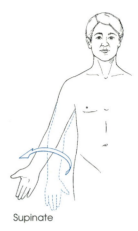

Supinate

Fig. 3-39. Supination.

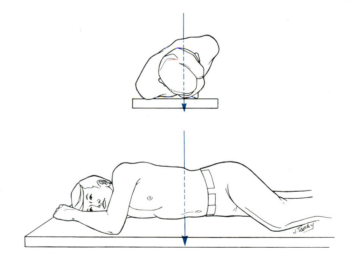

Fig. 3-40. Rotation of torso. (Arm and knee flexed for patient comfort.)

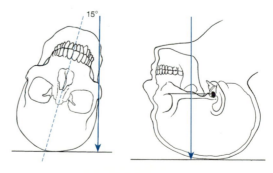

15°

Fig. 3-41. Tilt.

Medical Terminology

Plurals of some of the more common Greek and Latin nouns are formed as follows:

Singular	Plural	Example
a	ae	maxilla—maxillae
ex	ces	apex—apices
is	es	diagnosis—diagnoses
ix	ces	appendix—appendices
ma	mata	carcinoma—carcinomata
on	a	ganglion—ganglia
um	a	antrum—antra
us	i	ramus—rami

The selected examples of single and plural word forms shown below have been judged to be the most frequently misused.

Singular	Plural
acinus	acini
adnexus	adnexa
ala	alae
alveolus	alveoli
areola	areolae
bronchus	bronchi
calculus	calculi
coxa	coxae
diagnosis	diagnoses
diverticulum	diverticula
fenestra	fenestrae
fossa	fossae
gingiva	gingivae
haustrum	haustra
hilum	hila
ilium	ilia
labium	labia
lacuna	lacunae
lamina	laminae
loculus	loculi
lumen	lumina
mediastinum	mediastina
medulla	medullae
meninx	meninges
meniscus	menisci
metastasis	metastases
mucosa	mucosae
multipara	multiparae
naris	nares
natis	nates
nullipara	nulliparae
omentum	omenta
paralysis	paralyses
pleura	pleurae
plica	plicae
pneumothorax	pneumothoraces
ramus	rami
ruga	rugae
sulcus	sulci
theca	thecae
thrombus	thrombi
vertebra	vertebrae
viscus	viscera

Chapter 4

UPPER LIMB (EXTREMITY)

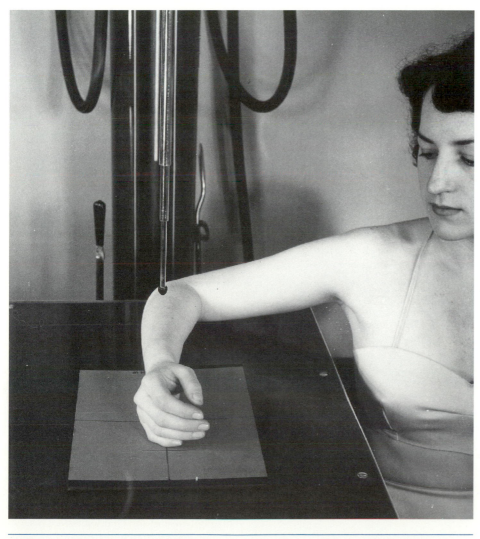

Patient positioned for a lateral hand radiograph; 1940s. Note that the patient was positioned with a cardboard film holder but no intensifying screen. The amount of exposure to radiation was significantly greater than it is in most modern procedures.

For purposes of study, anatomists divide the bones of the upper limbs, or extremities, into four main groups: the hand, forearm, arm, and shoulder girdle. The proximal arm and shoulder girdle are discussed in Chapter 5.

Hand

The hand consists of 27 bones, subdivided into three groups: the phalanges, or bones of the digits (fingers); metacarpals, or bones of the palm; and carpals, or bones of the wrist (Fig. 4-1).

DIGITS

The digits (fingers) are numbered and named; however, description by number is the more correct terminology. Beginning at the lateral (thumb) side, the numbers and names are: first digit, or thumb; second digit, or index finger; third digit, or middle finger; fourth digit, or ring finger; and fifth digit, or small (little) finger. There are 14 *phalanges* (*phalanx,* sing.) in the digits, three in each finger and two in the thumb. The phalanges of the first digit are described as first and second, or proximal (nearest the palm) and distal. Those of the other digits are described as first, second, and third, or proximal, middle, and distal. The phalanges are long bones consisting of a cylindrical body, or shaft, and two articular ends; they are slightly concave anteriorly. The distal phalanges are small and flattened and have a roughened rim around their distal anterior (ventral) end, which gives them a spatular appearance.

PALM

Five *metacarpals,* cylindrical in shape and slightly concave anteriorly, form the palm of the hand (Fig. 4-1). The metacarpals are numbered one to five, beginning at the lateral, or thumb, side of the hand. The metacarpals are long bones consisting of a body, or shaft, and two articular ends, the head distally and the base proximally. The metacarpal heads are seen on the dorsal hand and are commonly known as the knuckles.

WRIST

The wrist has *eight carpal bones.* They are fitted closely together and arranged in two horizontal rows (Fig. 4-1). With one exception, each of these bones has two or three names (see the box below on *Carpal Terminology Conversion*). The proximal row of carpals (those nearest the forearm) beginning at the lateral, or thumb, side are the *scaphoid* (navicular), the *lunate* (semilunar), the *triquetrum* (triquetral, cuneiform, or triangular), and the *pisiform.* In the distal row, beginning at the lateral side, are the *trapezium* (greater multangular), the *trapezoid* (lesser multangular), the *capitate* (os magnum), and the *hamate* (unciform). The carpals are classified as irregularly shaped short bones and are composed largely of cancellous tissue with an outer layer of compact bony tissue.

CARPAL TERMINOLOGY CONVERSION

Preferred	Synonyms
Proximal row:	
Scaphoid	Navicular
Lunate	Semilunar
Triquetrum	Triquetral, cuneiform, or triangular
Pisiform	(none)
Distal row:	
Trapezium	Greater multangular
Trapezoid	Lesser multangular
Capitate	Os magnum
Hamate	Unciform

Each carpal contains unique identifying characteristics. For instance, the *scaphoid,* the largest bone in the proximal carpal row, has a tubercle on the anterior and lateral aspect for muscle attachment. It is palpable near the base of the thumb. The secondary term used for the scaphoid is *navicular.* Anatomists specify that *scaphoid* is the preferred term for the carpal bone of the wrist, whereas *navicular* is the preferred term for the tarsal bone in the ankle. The *lunate* articulates with the radius proximally and is easy to recognize because of the characteristic crescent shape. The *triquetrum* is roughly pyramidal in shape and articulates anteriorly with the hamate. The *pisiform* is a pea-shaped bone situated anterior to the triquetrum; it is easily palpated.

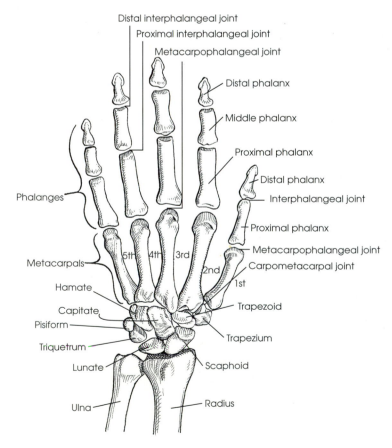

Fig. 4-1. Posterior aspect of hand and wrist.

Distal interphalangeal joint
Proximal interphalangeal joint
Metacarpophalangeal joint
Distal phalanx
Middle phalanx
Proximal phalanx
Distal phalanx
Interphalangeal joint
Proximal phalanx
Metacarpophalangeal joint
Carpometacarpal joint
Trapezoid
Trapezium
Scaphoid
Radius
Phalanges
Metacarpals
Hamate
Capitate
Pisiform
Triquetrum
Lunate
Ulna
5th 4th 3rd 2nd 1st

Beginning at the distal row of carpals on the thumb side is the *trapezium,* which exhibits a tubercle and groove on the anterior surface. The tubercle of the trapezium and the tubercle of the scaphoid comprise the lateral margin of the carpal groove. The *trapezoid* is irregularly shaped; the anterior surface is smaller than the posterior surface. The *capitate* is the largest of the carpals and articulates with the base of the third metacarpal, making it the most centrally located carpal. The *hamate* is known for its wedge-shaped design and exhibits a hook-like process, the *hamulus,* located on the anterior surface. The hamate and the pisiform are the two carpals that make up the medial margin of the carpal groove.

Located on the posterior surface of the wrist is a triangular depression that can be seen when the thumb is abducted and extended. This depression, known as the "anatomical snuff box," is formed by the tendons of the two major muscles of the thumb. The anatomical snuff box overlies the scaphoid bone and the radial artery, which carries blood to the dorsum of the hand. Tenderness in the snuff box area is a clinical sign suggesting fracture of the scaphoid—the most commonly fractured carpal bone.

Forearm

The forearm has two bones lying parallel to one another: the *radius* and *ulna.* Like other long bones, each consists of a body, or shaft, and two articular extremities. The radius is located on the lateral, or thumb, side of the forearm and the ulna on the medial side (Figs. 4-2 and 4-3).

ULNA

The *body* (shaft) of the ulna is long and slender and tapers inferiorly. The upper portion of the ulna is large and presents two beaklike processes and two concave depressions (Fig. 4-4). The proximal process, the *olecranon process,* is curved (concave) anteriorly and slightly inferiorly and forms the proximal portion of the *trochlear* (semilunar) *notch.* The slightly more distal *coronoid process* projects anteriorly from the anterior surface of the body (shaft) and curves slightly superiorly. It is triangular in shape and forms the lower portion of the trochlear (semilunar) notch. On the lateral aspect of the coronoid process is a depression called the *radial notch.*

The distal end of the ulna has a rounded process on its lateral side, the *head* of the ulna; and on the posteromedial side, a narrower conical projection called the *ulnar styloid process.* The head of the ulna is separated from the wrist joint by an articular disk.

RADIUS

The proximal end of the radius is small and presents a flat, disklike *head* above a constricted area called the *neck.* Just inferior to the neck, on the medial side of the body (shaft), is a roughened process called the *radial tuberosity.* The distal end of the radius is broad and flattened and has a conical projection on its lateral surface called the *radial styloid process.*

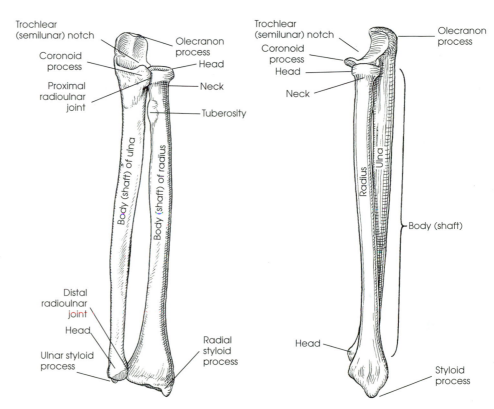

Fig. 4-2. Anterior aspect of radius and ulna.

Fig. 4-3. Lateral aspect of radius and ulna.

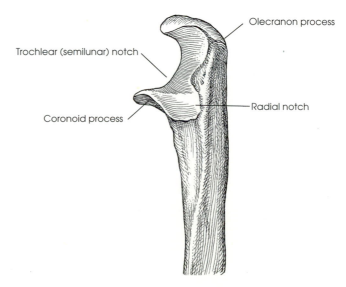

Fig. 4-4. Radial aspect of proximal ulna.

Arm

The arm has one bone, the *humerus,* which consists of a body, or shaft, and two articular ends (Figs. 4-5 and 4-6). The *body* is long and cylindrical. The proximal part of the humerus articulates with the shoulder girdle and is described in Chapter 5. The distal humerus is broad and flattened and presents numerous processes and depressions.

The distal end of the humerus is the *condyle.* There are two smooth elevations for articulation with the bones of the forearm, the *trochlea* on the medial side, and the *capitulum* (capitellum) on the lateral side. Superior to the condyle, and easily palpated, are the *medial* and *lateral epicondyles.* On the posterior and inferior surface of the medial epicondyle is a shallow groove for the ulnar nerve, which is called the *ulnar sulcus.* On the anterior surface, superior to the trochlea, is a shallow depression called the *coronoid fossa* for the reception of the coronoid process when the elbow is flexed. Lateral to the coronoid fossa and proximal to the capitulum (capitellum) is the relatively small *radial fossa,* which receives the radial head when the elbow is flexed. Immediately behind the coronoid fossa, on the posterior surface, is the *olecranon fossa,* a deep depression that accommodates the olecranon process when the elbow is extended.

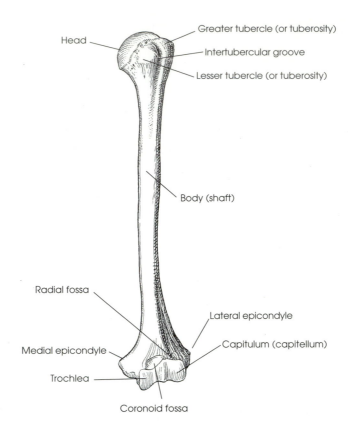

Fig. 4-5. Anterior aspect of humerus.

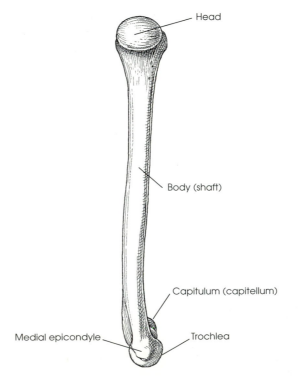

Fig. 4-6. Medial aspect of humerus.

Upper Limb Articulations

Beginning with the most distal portion of the upper limb, the articulations are as described in the following paragraphs.

The *interphalangeal* articulations between the *phalanges* are of the synovial (diarthrotic) ginglymus or hinge type, allowing only flexion and extension. The interphalangeal joints are named by location. The joints are differentiated as either proximal or distal; by the digit number; and as either right or left—for example, the proximal interphalangeal articulation of the fourth digit of the left hand (Fig. 4-7). The first digit, or thumb, has only two phalanges; therefore, the joint between these two phalanges is simply known as the interphalangeal joint.

The *metacarpals* articulate with the phalanges at their distal ends and the carpals at their proximal ends. The *metacarpophalangeal* articulations are synovial (diarthrotic) condyloid joints, having the movements of flexion, extension, abduction, adduction, and circumduction. Because of the less convex and wider surface of the metacarpophalangeal joint of the thumb, only limited abduction and adduction are possible. The *carpometacarpal* joint gives the thumb its freedom of motion.

The *carpals* articulate with each other, the metacarpals, and the radius of the forearm. All carpal articulations are synovial (diarthrotic) joints. In the *carpometacarpal* articulations, the first metacarpal and trapezium (greater multangular) form a sellar (saddle) joint, which permits the thumb to oppose the fingers (touch the fingertips). The articulations between the second, third, fourth, and fifth metacarpals and the trapezoid, capitate, and hamate form plane (gliding) joints of limited movement. The *intercarpal* articulations are also plane (gliding) joints. The *radiocarpal* articulation, the wrist joint proper, is of the condyloid type. This joint is formed by the articulation of the scaphoid (navicular), lunate (semilunar), and triquetrum (triquetral, cuneiform, or triangular) with the radius and the articular disk just distal to the ulna.

The dorsal surface of the articulated carpals is convex. The palmar surface is concave from side to side (Fig. 4-8), and the groove formed by the concavity is called the *carpal sulcus*. A strong fibrous band, the *flexor retinaculum,* attaches medially to the pisiform and the hamulus of the hamate, and laterally to the tubercles of the scaphoid and trapezium, and the groove of the trapezium. When closed by the flexor retinaculum, the *carpal sulcus* is referred to as the *carpal canal* or *carpal tunnel.* Passing through the carpal canal are the median nerve and the tendons of the flexor muscles of the digits.

Both the *distal* and *proximal radioulnar* articulations are synovial (diarthrotic) trochoidal (pivot) joints. The proximal head of the radius articulates with the radial notch of the ulna at the medial side. The distal ulna articulates with the ulnar notch of the distal radius. The movements of supination and pronation of the forearm and hand largely result from the combined rotary action of these two joints. In pronation the radius turns medially and crosses over the ulna at its upper third while the ulna makes a slight counterrotation, which obliques the humerus by rotating it medially.

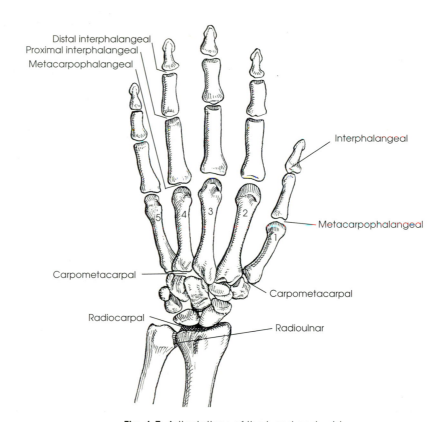

Fig. 4-7. Articulations of the hand and wrist.

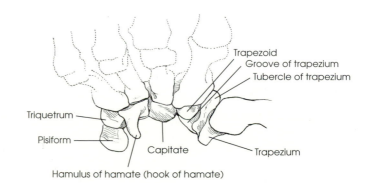

Fig. 4-8. Inferosuperior aspect of carpal sulcus.

The *elbow joint* proper includes the proximal radioulnar articulation as well as the articulations between the humerus and the radius and ulna. The three joints are enclosed in a common capsule. The *trochlea* of the humerus articulates with the ulna at the trochlear (semilunar) notch. The *capitulum* (capitellum) of the humerus articulates with the flattened head of the radius. The *humeroulnar* and *humeroradial* articulations form a synovial (diarthrotic) ginglymus (hinge joint), allowing flexion and extension movement only (Figs. 4-9 and 4-10).

Three small pockets of fat are associated with the distal humerus. The largest of these lies over the olecranon fossa, the smallest over the radial fossa, and the third, over the coronoid fossa. Normally these fat pads lie within their respective fossae. The fat pads become significant radiographically when an injury to the elbow causes joint effusion and displaces the fat superficially. Exposure factors designed to demonstrate soft tissue are extremely important on lateral radiographs of the elbow, because visualization of these fat pads may be the only evidence of injury.

The proximal humerus and its articulations are described with the shoulder girdle in Chapter 5.

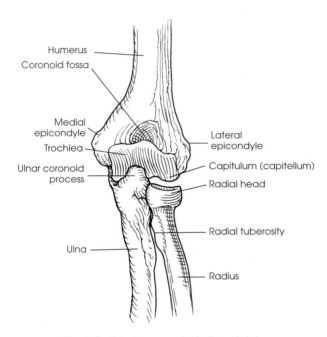

Fig. 4-9. Anterior aspect of elbow joint.

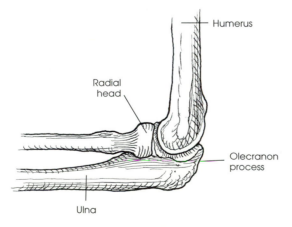

Fig. 4-10. Lateral aspect of elbow joint.

General Procedures

When the upper limb is radiographed, the following steps should be observed.

- Remove rings, watches and other radiopaque objects; place in secure storage during the procedure.
- Seat the patient at the side or the end of the table to avoid a strained or uncomfortable position.
- Place the cassette at a location and angle that will allow the patient to be positioned most comfortably. Because the degree of immobilization is limited, particularly of the hand and digits, it is important that the patient be comfortable so that he or she can relax and cooperate in maintaining the position.
- Unless otherwise specified, direct the central ray at right angles to the midpoint of the film. Because the joint spaces of the limbs are narrow, accurate centering is essential to avoid obscuring the joint spaces.
- When a bilateral examination of the hands and/or wrists is requested, radiograph *each side separately*. This prevents distortion, particularly of the joint spaces, as happens when both sides are placed on the cassette for simultaneous projections.
- Shield the gonad area from scattered radiation with a sheet of lead-impregnated rubber or lead apron placed over the patient's pelvis, as shown in Fig. 4-11. Close collimation should also be used. This technique is recommended for all upper limb radiographs.
- When radiographing the limbs, multiple exposures on one film are a common practice (see Fig. 1-15). Refer to Chapter 1 and review "Film Placement."
- The right or left markers should always be used, as appropriate, along with all other vital indentification markers.

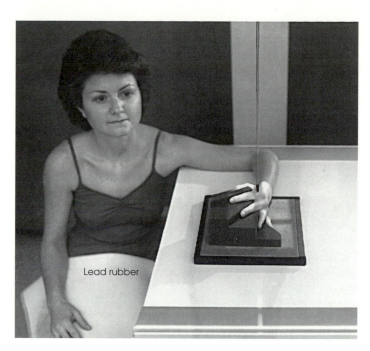

Lead rubber

Fig. 4-11. Properly shielded patient.

Digits (Second Through Fifth)

▲ PA PROJECTIONS

Film: 8 × 10 in (18 × 24 cm) crosswise for two or more images on one film.

Position of patient

- Seat the patient at the end of the radiographic table.

Position of part

When radiographing individual digits (except the first), take the following steps:
- Place the extended digit on the unmasked portion of the cassette with the palmar surface down.
- Separate the digits slightly and center the digit being examined to the midline portion of the film.
- Center the proximal interphalangeal joint to the film area (Figs. 4-12 to 4-15).
- *Shield gonads:* Place a lead shield over the patient's pelvis.

Central ray

- Direct the central ray perpendicular to the proximal interphalangeal joint (PIP) of the affected digit.
- Collimate to the digit being examined.

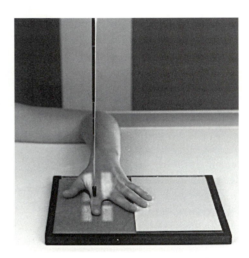

Fig. 4-12. PA second digit.

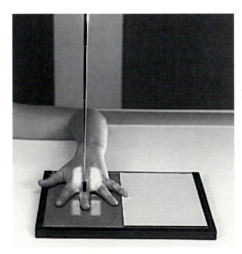

Fig. 4-13. PA third digit.

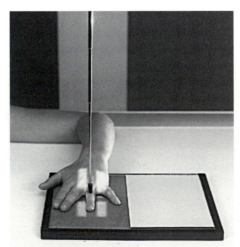

Fig. 4-14. PA fourth digit.

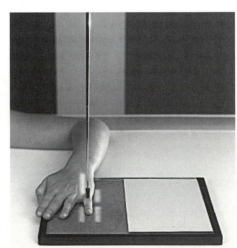

Fig. 4-15. PA fifth digit.

Structures shown

A PA projection of the appropriate digit is visualized (Figs. 4-16 to 4-19).

□ Evaluation criteria

The following should be clearly demonstrated:

- No rotation of the digit:
  - □ Concavity of the phalangeal shafts and equal amount of soft tissue on both sides of the phalanges.
  - □ The fingernail (if visualized and normal) centered over the distal phalanx.
- Entire digit from fingertip to distal portion of the adjoining metacarpal.
- No soft tissue overlap from adjacent digits.
- Open interphalangeal and metacarpophalangeal joint spaces without overlap of bones.
- Soft tissue and bony trabeculation.

NOTE: Digits that cannot be extended can be examined in small sections with dental films. If a joint is in question, an AP projection is recommended instead of a PA.

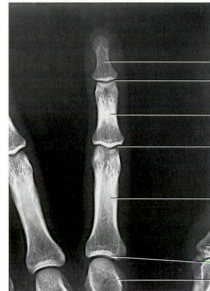

Distal phalanx
Distal interphalangeal joint
Middle phalanx
Proximal interphalangeal joint
Proximal phalanx
Thumb
Metacarpophalangeal joint
Head of metacarpal

Fig. 4-16. PA second digit.

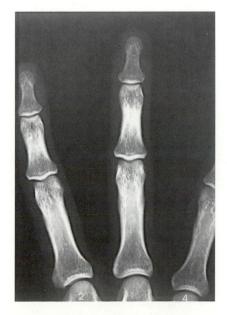

Fig. 4-17. PA third digit.

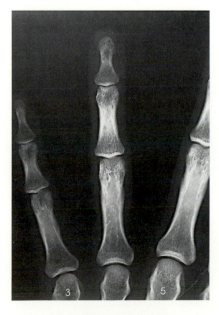

Fig. 4-18. PA fourth digit.

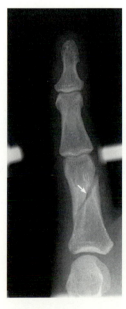

Fig. 4-19. Fractured fifth digit *(arrow)*.

(Courtesy Keith Shipman, R.T.)

Digits (Second Through Fifth)

LATERAL PROJECTION
Lateromedial or mediolateral

Film: 8 × 10 in (18 × 24 cm) crosswise for two or more images on one film.

Position of patient

- Seat the patient at the end of the radiographic table.

Position of part

- Because lateral digit positions are difficult to hold, tell the patient how the digit is to be adjusted on the cassette. Demonstrate with your own digit, and then let the patient assume the most comfortable arm position.
- Ask the patient to extend the digit to be examined, close the rest of the digits into a fist, and hold them in complete flexion with the thumb.
- When it is necessary to elevate the elbow to bring the digit into position, support it on sandbags or other suitable support as illustrated.
- With the digit to be examined extended and the other digits folded into a fist, the patient's hand should rest (1) on the lateral, or radial, surface for the second or third digit (Figs. 4-20 and 4-21) or (2) on the medial, or ulnar, surface for the fourth or fifth digit (Figs. 4-22 and 4-23).

- Before making the final adjustment of the digit position, place the cassette so that the midline of its unmasked portion is parallel with the long axis of the digit and center it to the proximal interphalangeal joint.
- The second and fifth digits rest directly on the cassette, but for an accurate image of the bones and joints, elevate the third and fourth digits to place their *long* axes parallel with the plane of the film. A radiolucent sponge may be used to support the digits.
- Immobilize the extended digit by placing a strip of adhesive tape, a tongue depressor, or other support against its palmar surface. The patient can hold the support with the opposite hand.
- Finally, adjust the anterior or posterior rotation of the hand to obtain a true lateral position of the digit.
- *Shield gonads:* Place a lead shield over the patient's pelvis.

Central ray

- Direct the central ray perpendicular to the proximal interphalangeal joint of the affected digit.
- Collimate to the digit being radiographed.

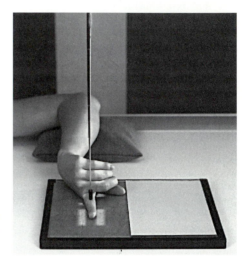

Fig. 4-20. Lateral second digit.

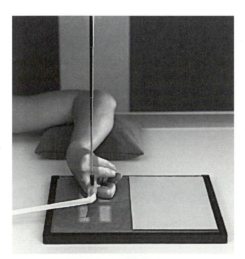

Fig. 4-21. Lateral third digit (adhesive tape).

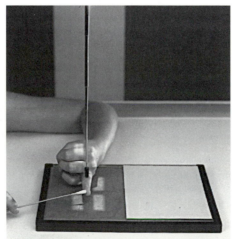

Fig. 4-22. Lateral fourth digit (cotton swab).

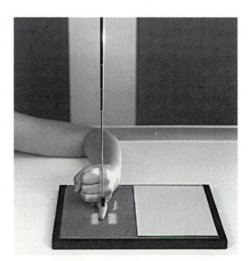

Fig. 4-23. Lateral fifth digit.

Structures shown

A lateral projection of the affected digit is seen (Figs. 4-24 to 4-27).

The following should be clearly demonstrated:

- ■ Entire digit in a true lateral position:
    - □ The fingernail, if visualized and normal, should be in profile.
    - □ Concave, anterior surface of the phalanges.
    - □ No rotation of the phalanges.
- ■ No obstruction of the proximal phalanx or metacarpophalangeal joint by adjacent digits.
- ■ Open interphalangeal and metacarpophalangeal joint spaces.
- ■ Soft tissue and bony trabeculation.

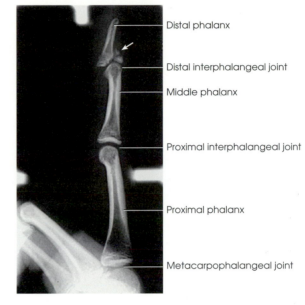

Distal phalanx

Distal interphalangeal joint

Middle phalanx

Proximal interphalangeal joint

Proximal phalanx

Metacarpophalangeal joint

Fig. 4-24. Lateral showing chip fracture *(arrow)* and dislocation involving the distal interphalangeal joint of second digit *(arrow).*

(Courtesy Ammar Saadeh, R.T.)

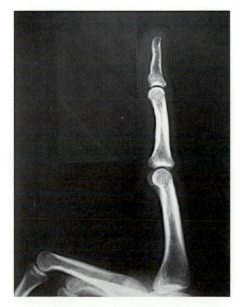

Fig. 4-25. Lateral third digit.

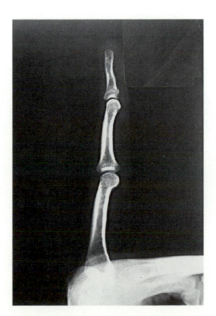

Fig. 4-26. Lateral fourth digit.

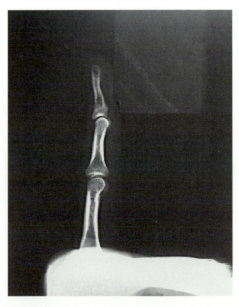

Fig. 4-27. Lateral fifth digit.

Digits (second through fifth)

Digits (Second Through Fifth)

PA OBLIQUE PROJECTION
Lateral rotation

Film: 8 × 10 in (18 × 24 cm) crosswise for two or more images on one film.

Position of patient

- Seat the patient at the end of the radiographic table.

Position of part

- Place the forearm on the table with the hand pronated and the palm resting on the cassette.
- Center the film at the level of the proximal interphalangeal joint.
- Rotate the hand laterally (externally) until the digits are separated and supported on a *45-degree* foam wedge. The wedge supports the digits in a position parallel with the film plane (Figs. 4-28 to 4-31) so the interphalangeal joint spaces will be open.
- *Shield gonads:* Place a lead shield over the patient's pelvis.

Central ray

- Direct the central ray perpendicular to the proximal interphalangeal joint of the affected digit.
- Collimate to the digit being examined.

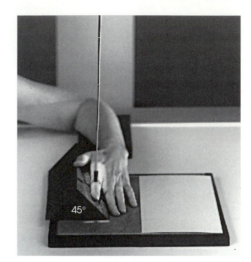

Fig. 4-28. PA oblique second digit.

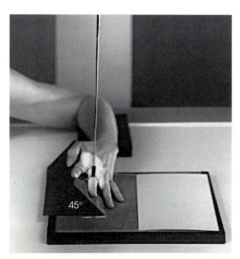

Fig. 4-29. PA oblique third digit.

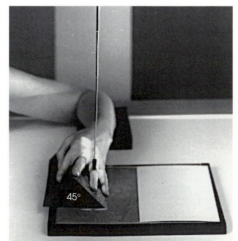

Fig. 4-30. PA oblique fourth digit.

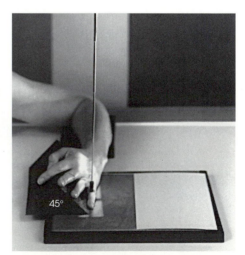

Fig. 4-31. PA oblique fifth digit.

Structures shown

The resultant images will show a PA oblique projection of the bones and soft tissue of the affected digit (Figs. 4-32 to 4-35).

□Evaluation criteria

The following should be clearly demonstrated:

- The entire digit rotated at a 45-degree angle, including the distal portion of the adjoining metacarpal.
- No superimposition of the adjacent digits over the proximal phalanx or metacarpophalangeal joint.
- Open interphalangeal and metacarpophalangeal joint spaces.
- Soft tissue and bony trabeculation.

OPTION: Some radiographers oblique the second digit medially from the prone position, as shown in Fig. 4-36. The advantage of medially rotating the digit is that the part is closer to the film for improved recorded detail. Care must be taken, however, to ensure the adjacent digits are not superimposed over the second digit. Similarly, medial rotation requires extending the digit, which can be painful to the patient with an injured digit.

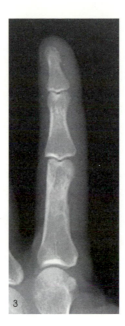

Fig. 4-32. PA oblique second digit.

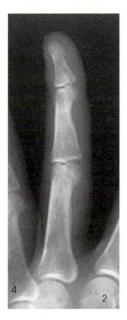

Fig. 4-33. PA oblique third digit.

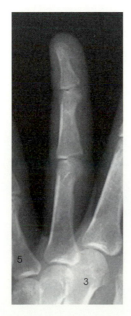

Fig. 4-34. PA oblique fourth digit.

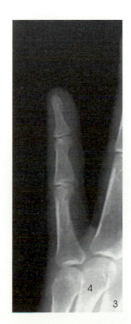

Fig. 4-35. PA oblique fifth digit.

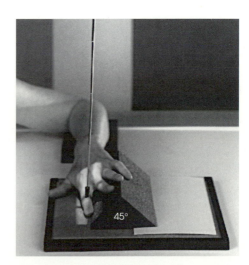

Fig. 4-36. PA oblique second digit (alternate method, medial rotation).

First Digit (Thumb)

AP, PA, LATERAL AND OBLIQUE PROJECTIONS

Film: 8 × 10 in (18 × 24 cm) crosswise for two or more images on one film.

 AP PROJECTION

Position of patient

- Seat the patient at the end of the radiographic table with the arm internally rotated.

Position of part

- To avoid motion or rotation demonstrate the desired position with your own hand. The patient can then, by adjusting the position of his or her body on the chair, place the hand in the correct position with the least amount of strain on the arm.
- With the patient's hand in position of extreme internal rotation, have the patient hold the extended digits back with tape or with the opposite hand. Rest the thumb on the cassette. If the elbow is elevated, place a support under it and have the patient rest the opposite forearm against the table for support (Fig. 4-37).
- With the long axis of the thumb parallel with the long axis of the cassette, center to the metacarpophalangeal joint. Adjust the position of the hand to secure a true AP projection of the thumb, being careful to have the fifth metacarpal back far enough to avoid superimposition.
- Lewis[1] suggested directing the central ray 10 to 15 degrees along the long axis of the thumb toward the wrist to demonstrate the first metacarpal free of the shadow of the sesamoids and of the soft tissue of the palm.
- *Shield gonads:* Place a lead shield over the patient's pelvis.

---

[1]Lewis S: New angles on the radiographic examination of the hand—II, Radiogr Today 54:29, 1988.

PA PROJECTION

Position of patient

- Seat the patient at the end of the radiographic table with the hand resting on its medial surface.

Position of part

- When it is necessary to take the PA projection of the first carpometacarpal joint and digit from the dorsal aspect, place the hand in the lateral position, rest the elevated and abducted thumb on a radiolucent support, and adjust the hand to place the dorsal surface of the digit parallel with the film.
- When the position requires that the wrist be elevated, support it on a small sandbag (Fig. 4-38).
- Center to the metacarpophalangeal joint.
- *Shield gonads:* Place a lead shield over the patient's pelvis.

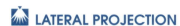 LATERAL PROJECTION

Position of patient

- Seat the patient at the end of the radiographic table with the relaxed hand placed on the cassette.

Position of part

- Place the hand in its natural arched position with the palmar surface down with the fingers flexed or resting on a sponge.
- Place the cassettes midline parallel with the long axis of the digit and center it to the metacarpophalangeal joint.
- Adjust the arching of the hand until a true lateral position of the thumb is obtained (Fig. 4-39).
- *Shield gonads:* Place a lead shield over the patient's pelvis.

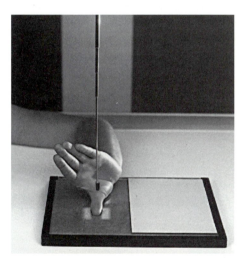

Fig. 4-37. AP first digit.

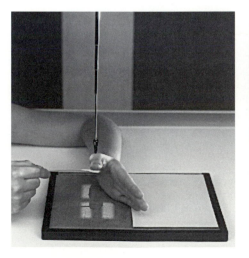

Fig. 4-38. PA first digit.

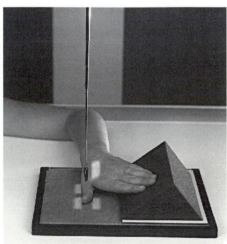

Fig. 4-39. Lateral first digit.

PA OBLIQUE PROJECTION

Position of patient

- Seat the patient at the end of the radiographic table with the palm of the hand resting on the cassette.

Position of part

- With the thumb abducted, place the palmar surface of the hand in contact with the cassette. This relatively normal placement positions the thumb in the oblique position.
- Align the longitudinal axis of the thumb with the long axis of the film and center to the metacarpophalangeal joint (Fig. 4-40).
- *Shield gonads:* Place a lead shield over the patient's pelvis.

Central ray

For the AP, PA, lateral, and oblique projections:
- Direct the central ray perpendicular to the metacarpophalangeal joint.
- Collimate to include entire first digit.

Structures shown

AP (Fig. 4-41), PA (Fig. 4-42), lateral (Fig. 4-43), and oblique (Fig. 4-44) projections of the thumb are demonstrated.

☐ Evaluation criteria

AP and PA thumb

The following should be clearly demonstrated:
- No rotation:
   ☐ Concavity of the phalangeal and metacarpal shafts and equal soft tissue on both sides.
   ☐ The thumbnail (if visualized) in the center of the distal thumb.
- Area from the distal tip of the thumb to the trapezium.
- Open interphalangeal and metacarpophalangeal joint spaces without overlap of bones.
- Overlap of soft tissue profile of the palm over the midshaft of the first metacarpal.
- Soft tissue and bony trabeculation.
- PA thumb projection somewhat magnified compared to the AP projection.

Lateral thumb

The following should be clearly demonstrated:
- First digit in a true lateral projection:
   ☐ The thumbnail (if visualized and normal) in profile.
   ☐ Concave anterior surface of the proximal phalanx.
   ☐ No rotation of the phalanges.
- Area from the distal tip of the thumb to the trapezium.
- Open interphalangeal and metacarpophalangeal joint spaces.
- Soft tissue and bony trabeculation.

Oblique thumb

The following should be clearly demonstrated:
- Proper rotation of phalanges, soft tissue, and first metacarpal.
- Area from the distal tip of the thumb to the trapezium.
- Open interphalangeal and metacarpophalangeal joint spaces.
- Soft tissue and bony trabeculation.

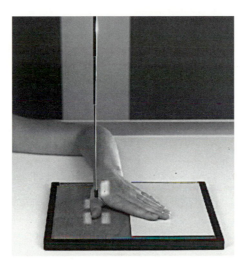

Fig. 4-40. PA oblique first digit.

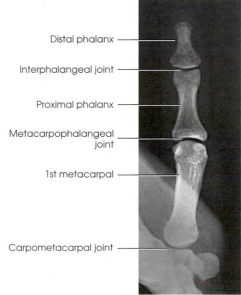

Distal phalanx

Interphalangeal joint

Proximal phalanx

Metacarpophalangeal joint

1st metacarpal

Carpometacarpal joint

Fig. 4-41. AP first digit.

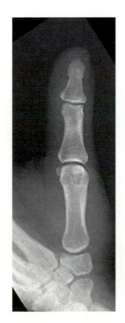 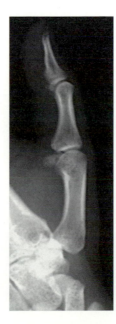 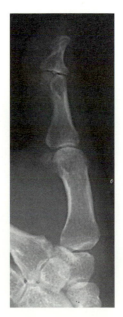

Fig. 4-42. PA first digit.   **Fig. 4-43.** Lateral first digit.   **Fig. 4-44.** PA oblique first digit.

(Courtesy Lois Baird, R.T.)

73

Hand

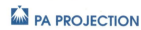

PA PROJECTION

Film: 8 × 10 in (18 × 24 cm) for hand of average size.

Position of patient

- Seat the patient at the end of the radiographic table.
- Adjust the patient's height so that the forearm is resting on the table (Fig. 4-45).

Position of part

- Rest the patient's forearm on the table and place the hand on the cassette with the palmar surface down.
- Center the film to the metacarpophalangeal joints and adjust the long axis of the film to be parallel with the long axis of the hand and forearm.
- Spread the fingers slightly (Figs. 4-45 and 4-46).

- Ask the patient to relax the hand to avoid motion. Prevent involuntary movement with the use of adhesive tape or positioning sponges. A sandbag may be placed over the distal forearm.
- *Shield gonads:* Shield the gonad area from scattered radiation with a sheet of lead-impregnated rubber over the patient's pelvis and close collimation, as shown in Fig. 4-45. This technique is recommended for all upper limb radiographs.

Central ray

- Direct the central ray perpendicular to the third metacarpophalangeal joint.

Structures shown

A PA projection (Fig. 4-47) of the carpals, metacarpals, and phalanges (except of the thumb); the interarticulations of the hand; and the distal radius and ulna is demonstrated. This image also demonstrates a PA oblique projection of the first digit (thumb).

□ Evaluation criteria

The following should be clearly demonstrated:

- No rotation of the hand.
  - □ Equal concavity of the metacarpal and phalangeal shafts on both sides.
  - □ Equal amount of soft tissue on both sides of the phalanges.
  - □ The fingernails (if visualized) in the center of each distal phalanx.
- Open metacarpophalangeal and interphalangeal joints, indicating that the hand was placed flat on the cassette.
- Slightly separated digits with no soft tissue overlap.
- All anatomy distal to the radius and ulna.
- Soft tissue and bony trabeculation.

NOTE: When the metacarpophalangeal joints are the point of interest and the patient cannot extend the hand enough to place its palmar surface in contact with the cassette, reverse the position of the hand for an AP projection. This position is also used for the metacarpals when, because of injury, a pathologic condition, or dressings, the hand cannot be extended.

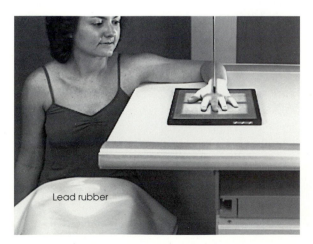

Fig. 4-45. Properly shielded patient.

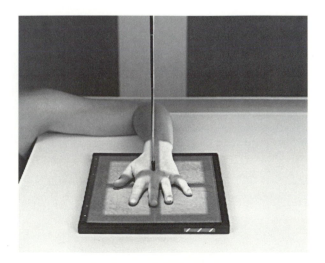

Fig. 4-46. PA hand.

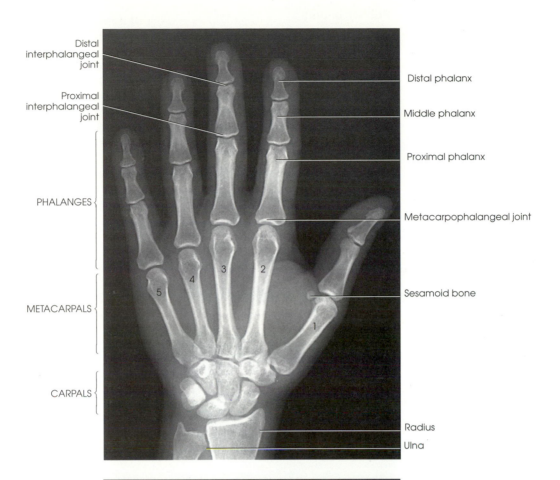

Distal interphalangeal joint

Proximal interphalangeal joint

PHALANGES

Distal phalanx

Middle phalanx

Proximal phalanx

Metacarpophalangeal joint

5   4   3   2

1

METACARPALS

Sesamoid bone

CARPALS

Radius

Ulna

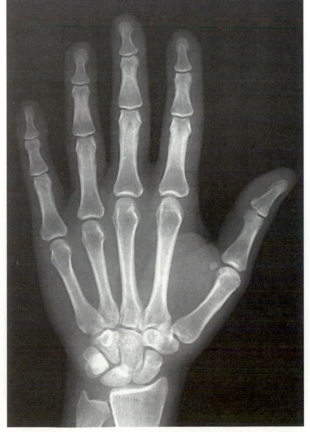

Fig. 4-47. PA hand.

Hand

PA OBLIQUE PROJECTION
Lateral rotation

Film: 8 × 10 in (18 × 24 cm) lengthwise.

Position of patient

- Seat the patient at the end of the radiographic table.
- Adjust the patient's height to rest the forearm on the table.

Position of part

- Rest the patient's forearm on the table with the hand pronated and the palm resting on the cassette.
- To demonstrate the interphalangeal joints, use a *45-degree* foam wedge to support the fingers in the extended position as in Figs. 4-48 and 4-49.
- When the metacarpals are the area of primary interest, obtain a PA oblique projection of the hand by rotating the patient's hand laterally (externally) from the pronated position until the fingertips touch the cassette as shown in Fig. 4-50.

- If it is not possible to obtain the correct position with all fingertips resting on the cassette, elevate the index finger and thumb on a suitable radiolucent material (Fig. 4-49). Elevation will open the joint spaces and reduce the degree of foreshortening of the phalanges.
- For either approach, center the film to the metacarpophalangeal joints and adjust the midline to be parallel with the long axis of the hand and forearm.
- Adjust the obliquity of the hand so the metacarpophalangeal joints form an angle of approximately *45 degrees* with the plane of the film.
- *Shield gonads:* Place a lead shield over the patient's pelvis.

Central ray

Direct the central ray perpendicular to the third metacarpophalangeal joint.

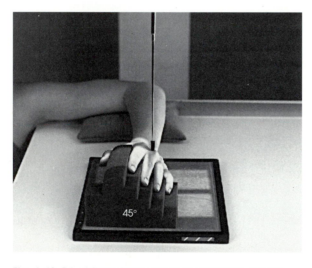

Fig. 4-48. PA oblique hand for demonstration of joint spaces.

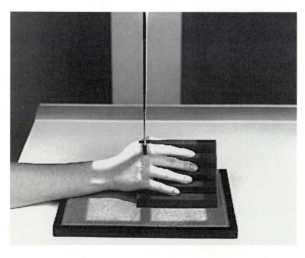

Fig. 4-49. PA oblique hand for demonstration of joint spaces.

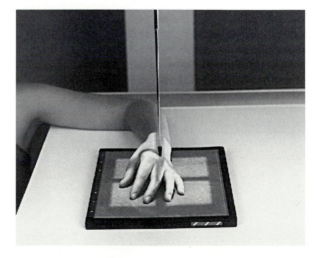

Fig. 4-50. PA oblique hand to demonstrate metacarpals.

Structures shown

The resulting image will show a PA oblique projection of the bones and soft tissues of the hand (Figs. 4-51 and 4-52). This supplemental position is used in the investigation of fractures and pathologic conditions.

☐ Evaluation criteria

The following should be clearly demonstrated:

- Minimal overlap of the third-fourth and fourth-fifth metacarpal shafts.
- Slight overlap of the metacarpal bases and heads.
- Separation of the second and third metacarpals.
- Open interphalangeal and metacarpophalangeal joints.
- Digits separated slightly; their soft tissues do not overlap.
- All anatomy distal to the distal radius and ulna.
- Soft tissue and bony trabeculation.

NOTE: Lane, et al[1] recommend the inclusion of a "reverse oblique" to better demonstrate severe metacarpal deformities or fractures. This projection is accomplished by having the patient rotate the hand 45 degrees medially (internally) from the palm down position.

[1]Lane CS, Kennedy JF, and Kuschner SH: The reverse oblique x-ray film: metacarpal fractures revealed, J Hand Surg 17A(3):504-506, 1992.

NOTE: Kallen[2] recommends using a tangential oblique projection to demonstrate metacarpal head fractures. From the PA hand position, the metacarpophalangeal joints are flexed 75 to 80 degrees with the dorsum of the digits resting on the cassette. Rotate the hand 40 to 45 degrees toward the ulnar surface then rotate the hand 40 to 45 degrees forward until the affected metacarpophalangeal joint is projected beyond its proximal phalanx. The perpendicular central ray is directed tangentially to enter the metacarpophalangeal joint of interest. Variations of rotation are described to demonstrate the second metacarpal head free of superimposition.

[2]Kallen MJ: Kallen projection reveals metacarpal head fractures, Radiol Technol 65(4):229-233, 1994.

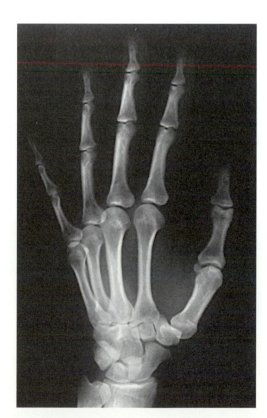

Fig. 4-51. PA oblique hand with digits on sponge to demonstrate open joints.

(Courtesy Lois Baird, R.T.)

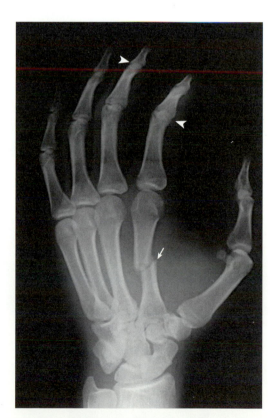

Fig. 4-52. PA oblique hand without support sponge showing fracture *(arrow)*. Note interphalangeal joints *(arrowheads)* not entirely open and foreshortening of phalanges.

(Courtesy Peter DeGraaf, R.T.)

Hand

 LATERAL PROJECTION
Mediolateral or lateromedial
In extension

Film: 8×10 in (18×24 cm) for hand of average size.

Position of patient

- Seat the patient at the end of the radiographic table with the forearm in contact with the table and the hand in the lateral position with the ulnar aspect down (Fig. 4-53).
- The hand may be optionally positioned with the radial side of the wrist against the film (Fig. 4-54), but this position is more difficult for the patient to assume.
- If the elbow is elevated, support it in position with sandbags as shown.

Position of part

- Extend the patient's digits and adjust the first digit (thumb) at a right angle to the palm.
- Place the palmar surface perpendicular to the cassette.
- Center the cassette to the metacarpophalangeal joints and adjust the midline to be parallel with the long axis of the hand and forearm. If the hand is resting on the ulnar surface, immobilization of the thumb may be necessary.
- The two positions described above result in superimposition of the phalanges. A modification of the above lateral hand is the "fan lateral," which eliminates superimposition of the phalanges for all except the proximal phalanges. For the fan lateral, place the digits on a sponge wedge as seen in Fig. 4-55. Abduct the thumb and place it on the radiolucent sponge for support.
- *Shield gonads:* Place a lead shield over the patient's pelvis.

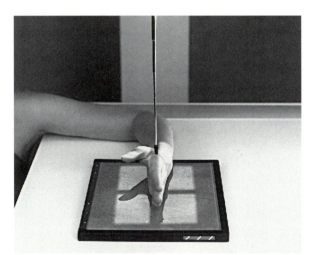

Fig. 4-53. Lateral hand with ulnar surface to film. Lateromedial.

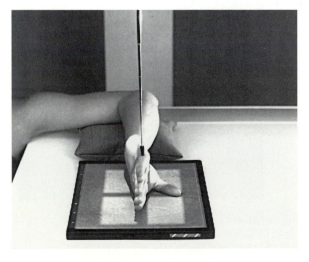

Fig. 4-54. Lateral hand with radial surface to film. Mediolateral.

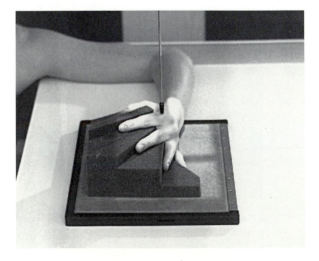

Fig. 4-55. Fan lateral hand.

Central ray

- Direct the central ray perpendicular to the second digit metacarpophalangeal joint.

Structures shown

- This image shows a lateral projection of the hand in extension (Fig. 4-56). This is the customary position for the localization of foreign bodies and metacarpal fracture displacement. The exposure technique will depend on the nature of the foreign body.
- While the fan lateral superimposes the metacarpals, the phalanges are individually demonstrated (Fig. 4-57), all except the most proximal portion of the proximal phalanges, which remain superimposed.

☐**Evaluation criteria**

The following should be clearly demonstrated:
- Hand should be in a true lateral position if the following are demonstrated:
  - ☐ Superimposed phalanges (individually demonstrated on fan lateral).
  - ☐ Superimposed metacarpals.
  - ☐ Superimposed distal radius and ulna.
- Extended digits.
- Thumb free of motion and superimposition.
- Each bone outlined through the superimposed shadows of the other metacarpals.

NOTE: To better demonstrate fractures of the fifth metacarpal, Lewis[1] recommends the hand be rotated 5 degrees posteriorly from the true lateral position. This positioning removes the shadows of the second through fourth metacarpals. The thumb is extended as much as possible, and the hand is allowed to become hollow, by relaxation. The central ray is angled so that it passes parallel to the extended thumb and enters the midshaft of the fifth metacarpal.

[1]Lewis S: New angles on the radiographic examination of the hand—III, Radiog Today 54(619):47-48, 1988.

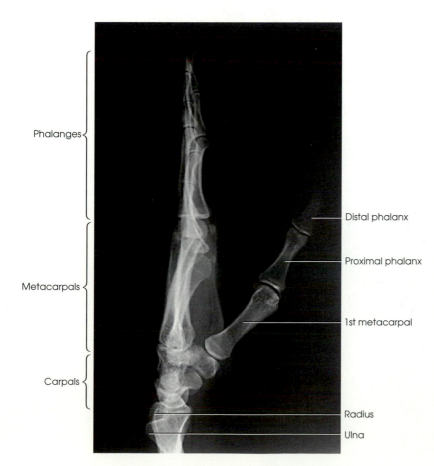

Phalanges

Distal phalanx

Proximal phalanx

Metacarpals

1st metacarpal

Carpals

Radius

Ulna

Fig. 4-56. Lateral hand.

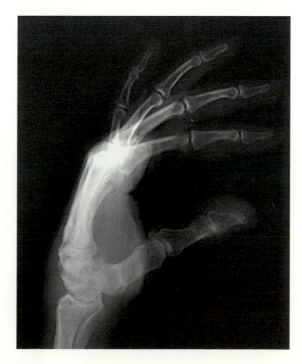

Fig. 4-57. Fan lateral hand.

(Courtesy John Syring, R.T.)

Hand

LATERAL PROJECTION
Lateromedial
In flexion

Film: 8 × 10 in (18 × 24 cm) lengthwise.

Position of patient

- Seat the patient at the end of the radiographic table.
- Ask the patient to rest the forearm on the table and place the hand on the film with the ulnar aspect down.

Position of part

- Center the cassette to the metacarpophalangeal joints and adjust it so that its midline is parallel with the long axis of the hand and forearm.
- With the patient relaxing the digits so as to maintain the natural arch of the hand, arrange them so that they are perfectly superimposed (Fig. 4-58).
- Have the patient hold the thumb parallel with the film. If he or she is unable to do so, immobilize the thumb with tape or a sponge.
- *Shield gonads:* Place a lead shield over the patient's pelvis.

Central ray

- Direct the central ray perpendicular to the metacarpophalangeal joints, entering the *second digit* metacarpophalangeal joint.

Structures shown

The resultant image will present a lateral image of the bony structures and soft tissues of the hand in their normally flexed position (Fig. 4-59).

This projection is used to demonstrate anterior or posterior displacement in fractures of the metacarpals.

□ Evaluation criteria

The following should be clearly demonstrated:
- Superimposed phalanges and metacarpals.
- Superimposed distal radius and ulna.
- Flexed digits.
- No motion or superimposition of the first digit.
- Radiographic density similar to frontal and oblique hand images. This requires increased exposure factors to compensate for greater part thickness.
- Clear outline of each bone through the superimposed shadows of the other metacarpals.

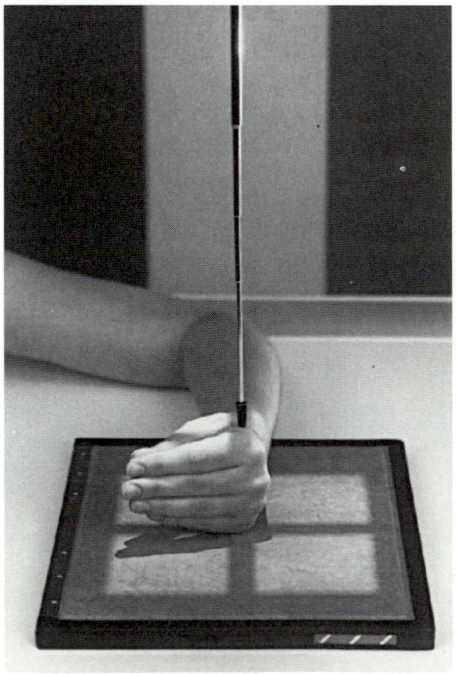

AP OBLIQUE PROJECTION
Medial rotation
NORGAARD METHOD[1,2]

This method, sometimes referred to as the "ball-catcher's" position, was described by Norgaard[1] and is useful in detecting early radiologic changes needed to diagnose rheumatoid arthritis. He reported that it is often possible to make an early diagnosis of rheumatoid arthritis by use of this position before laboratory tests are positive.[2] Norgaard also stated that extremely fine grain intensifying screens should be used to demonstrate high resolution. Low kVp is recommended (60 to 65) to obtain necessary contrast.

In a more recent article, Stapczynski[3] recommended this projection be used to demonstrate fractures of the base of the fifth metacarpal.

Film: 10 × 12 in (24 × 30 cm) crosswise.

Position of patient

- Seat the patient at the end of the radiographic table. Norgaard recommends that both hands be radiographed in the half-supinate position for comparison.

Position of part

- Have the patient place the palms of both hands together. Center the metacarpophalangeal joints on the medial aspect of both hands to the cassette; both hands will be in the lateral position.
- Place two 45-degree radiolucent sponge supports against the posterior aspect of each hand.
- Rotate the patient's hands to a half-supinate position until the dorsal surface of each hand rests against each 45-degree sponge support, as demonstrated in Fig. 4-60.
- The fingers should be extended and the thumbs slightly abducted to avoid superimposition over the fingers.

[1]Norgaard F: Earliest roentgenological changes in polyarthritis of the rheumatoid type: rheumatoid arthritis, Radiology 85:325-329, 1965.
[2]Norgaard F: Early roentgen changes in polyarthritis of the rheumatoid type, Radiology 92:299-303, 1969.
[3]Stapczynski JS: Fracture of the base of the little finger metacarpal: importance of the "Ball-Catcher" radiographic view. J Emerg Med, 9:145-149, 1991.

Fig. 4-58. Lateral hand in flexion.

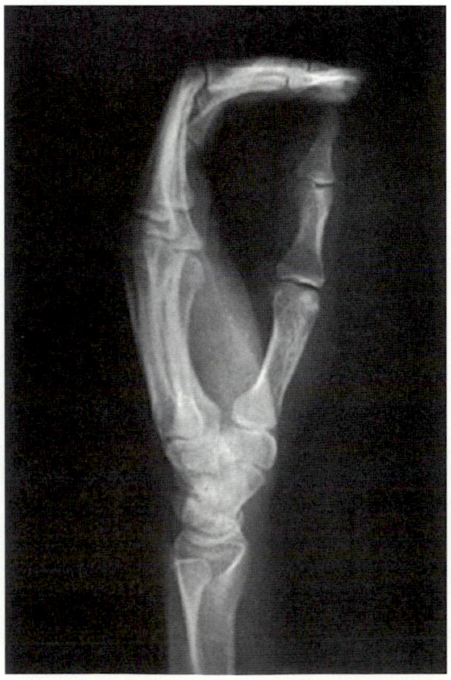

Fig. 4-59. Lateral hand in flexion.

- The original method of positioning the hands is often modified with the patient positioned similar to the method described except the fingers are not extended. Instead, the fingers are cupped as if the patient were going to catch a ball. This modification is demonstrated in Fig. 4-61. Comparable diagnostic information is demonstrated by either position.
- *Shield gonads:* Place a lead shield over the patient's pelvis.

Central ray

Direct the central ray perpendicular to the point midway between both hands at the level of the metacarpophalangeal joints for either of the two patient positions.

Structures shown

The resulting image shows an AP 45-degree oblique projection of both hands (Fig. 4-62). The early radiologic change significant in making the diagnosis of rheumatoid arthritis is a symmetrical, very slight indistinctness of the outline of the bone corresponding to the insertion of the joint capsule dorsoradial on the proximal end of the first phalanx of the four fingers. Additionally, there is always associated demineralization of the bone structure in an area directly below the contour defect.

□ Evaluation criteria

The following should be clearly demonstrated:
- Both hands included from the carpal area to the tips of the digits.
- Metacarpal heads, free of superimposition.
- A useful level of density over the heads of the metacarpals.

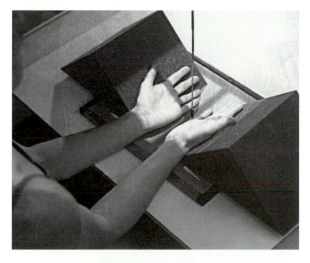

Fig. 4-60. AP oblique hands, half-supinate position.

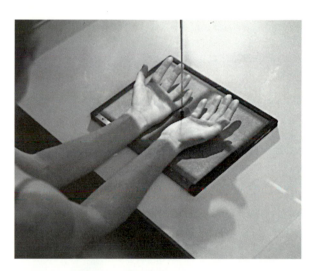

Fig. 4-61. "Ball-catcher" position.

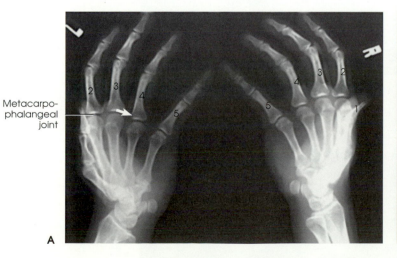

Metacarpo-
phalangeal
joint

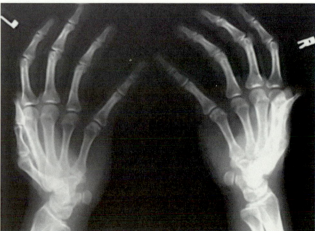

Fig. 4-62. A, AP oblique hands, "ball catcher" position showing where area of indistinctness occurs *(arrow)*. **B,** "Ball catcher" position.

(Courtesy Cheryl Stillberger, R.T.)

Wrist

First Carpometacarpal Joint

AP AXIAL PROJECTION
Radial shift position

When dorsiflexion of the wrist is not contraindicated, Burman[1] states that this projection gives a clearer image of the first carpometacarpal joint than does the standard AP projection.

Film: 8 × 10 in (18 × 24 cm) crosswise or lengthwise.

Position of patient

• Seat the patient at the end of the table in such a way that the forearm can be adjusted to lie approximately parallel with the long axis of the film.

Position of part

• Hyperextend the hand and have the patient hold it in this position with the opposite hand or with a bandage looped around the digits.
• Rotate the hand to place the first digit (thumb) in the horizontal position.
• Place the cassette under the wrist and digit and center 1 inch proximal to the first carpometacarpal joint; the joint will be projected to the center of the film (Fig. 4-63).
• *Shield gonads:* Place a lead shield over the patient's pelvis.

---

[1]Burman M: Anteroposterior projection of the carpometacarpal joint of the thumb by radial shift of the carpal tunnel view, J Bone Joint Surg 40A:1156-1157, 1958.

Central ray

• Direct the central ray to a point about 1 inch distal to the first carpometacarpal joint at an angle of 45 degrees toward the elbow.

Structures shown

This image shows the concavoconvex outline of the first carpometacarpal joint (Fig. 4-64).

☐ **Evaluation criteria**

The following should be clearly demonstrated:

■ The trapezium.
■ First metacarpal.
■ The first carpometacarpal joint, unobscured by adjacent carpals.

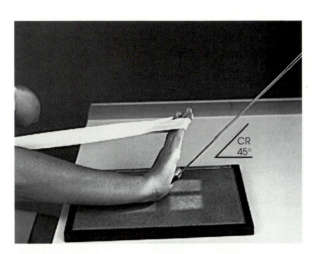

Fig. 4-63. AP axial wrist, radial shift.

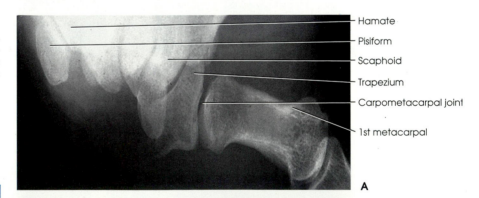

Hamate
Pisiform
Scaphoid
Trapezium
Carpometacarpal joint
1st metacarpal

A

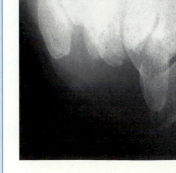

B

Fig. 4-64. A and **B,** AP axial wrist, radial shift.

(Courtesy Dr. Michael Burman.)

CARPAL TERMINOLOGY CONVERSION	
Preferred	**Synonyms**
Proximal row:	
Scaphoid	Navicular
Lunate	Semilunar
Triquetrum	Triquetral, cuneiform, or triangular
Pisiform	(none)
Distal row:	
Trapezium	Greater multangular
Trapezoid	Lesser multangular
Capitate	Os magnum
Hamate	Unciform

Wrist

PA PROJECTION

Film: 8 × 10 in (18 × 24 cm) crosswise for two or more images on one film.

Position of patient

- Seat the patient low enough to place the axilla in contact with the table, or elevate the limb to shoulder level on a suitable support. This places the shoulder, elbow, and wrist joints in the same plane to permit right-angle rotation of the ulna and the radius for the lateral position.

Position of part

- Have the patient rest the forearm on the table and center the wrist to the film area.
- When it is difficult to determine the exact location of the carpals because of a swollen wrist, ask the patient to flex the wrist slightly, and then center to the point of flexion. When the wrist is in a cast or a splint, the exact point of centering can be determined by comparison with the opposite side.
- Adjust the hand and forearm to lie parallel with the long axis of the film.
- Slightly arch the hand at the metacarpophalangeal joints by flexing the digits to place the wrist in close contact with the film (Fig. 4-65).
- When necessary, place a support under the digits to immobilize them.
- *Shield gonads:* Place a lead shield over the patient's pelvis.

Central ray

- Direct the central ray perpendicular to the midcarpal area.

Structures shown

A PA projection of the carpals, the distal radius and ulna, and the proximal metacarpals is shown (Fig. 4-66).

The PA projection gives a slightly oblique rotation to the ulna. When the ulna is the point of interest, the AP projection should be taken.

☐ Evaluation criteria

The following should be clearly demonstrated:

- Distal radius and ulna and the proximal half of the metacarpals, along with the carpals.
- No rotation in carpals, metacarpals, and radius.
- Soft tissue and bony trabeculation.
- No excessive flexion to overlap and obscure metacarpals with digits.

NOTE: To better demonstrate the scaphoid and capitate, Daffner, et al[1] recommend angling the central ray when the patient is positioned for a PA radiograph. A central ray angle of 30 degrees toward the elbow reportedly elongates the scaphoid and capitate, while an angle of 30 degrees toward the fingertips also elongates the capitate.

---

[1]Daffner RH, Emmerling EW, and Buterbaugh GA: Proximal and distal oblique radiography of the wrist: value in occult injuries, J Hand Surg Am 17:499-503, 1992.

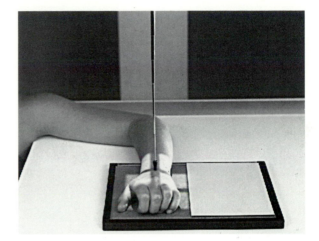

Fig. 4-65. PA wrist.

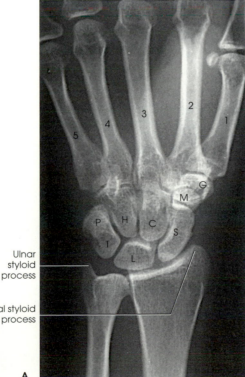
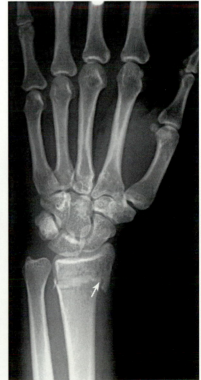

Ulnar styloid process

Radial styloid process

A

B

Fig. 4-66. A, PA wrist. *S,* scaphoid; *L,* lunate; *T,* triquetrum; *P,* pisiform; *G,* trapezium; *M,* trapezoid; *C,* capitate; and *H,* hamate. **B,** PA wrist showing fracture *(arrow).*

(Courtesy Keith Shipman, R.T.)

Wrist

AP PROJECTION

Film: 8 × 10 in (18 × 24 cm) crosswise for two or more images on one film.

Position of patient

- Seat the patient at the end of the table.

Position of part

- Have the patient rest the forearm on the table with the arm and hand supinated.
- Place the cassette under the wrist and center to the carpals.
- Elevate the digits on a suitable support to place the wrist in close contact with the cassette.
- Have the patient lean laterally to prevent rotation of the wrist (Fig. 4-67).
- *Shield gonads:* Place a lead shield over the patient's pelvis.

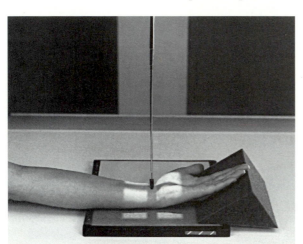

Fig. 4-67. AP wrist.

Central ray

- Direct the central ray perpendicular to the midcarpal area.

Structures shown

The *carpal interspaces* are better demonstrated in the AP than the PA image. Because of the interspaces' oblique direction, they are more nearly parallel with the divergence of the x-ray beam (Fig. 4-68).

☐ Evaluation criteria

The following should be clearly demonstrated:

- Distal radius and ulna and the proximal half of the metacarpals, along with the carpals.
- No rotation of the carpals, metacarpals, radius, and ulna.
- Well demonstrated soft tissue and bony trabeculation.
- No overlapping or obscuring of the metacarpals as a result of excessive flexion.

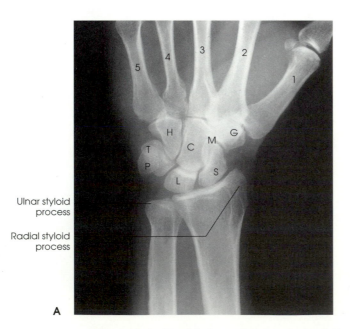

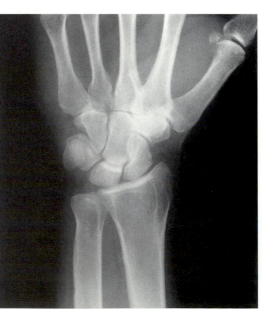

Fig. 4-68. A, AP wrist. *S,* scaphoid; *L,* lunate; *T,* triquetrum; *P,* pisiform; *G,* trapezium; *M,* trapezoid; *C,* capitate; and *H,* hamate. **B,** AP wrist.

Wrist

✦ LATERAL PROJECTION
Lateromedial

Film: 8 × 10 in (18 × 24 cm) for two images.

Position of patient

- Seat the patient at the end of the radiographic table.
- Have the patient rest the arm and forearm on the table to ensure a lateral wrist.

Position of part

- Have the patient flex the elbow 90 degrees to rotate the ulna to the lateral position.
- Center the film to the carpals and adjust the forearm and hand so the wrist is in a true lateral position (Fig. 4-69).
- *Shield gonads:* Place a lead shield over the patient's pelvis.

Central ray

- Direct the central ray perpendicular to the wrist joint.

Structures shown

This image shows a lateral projection of the proximal metacarpals, the carpals, and the distal radius and ulna (Fig. 4-70). An image obtained with the radial surface against the film (Fig. 4-71) is shown for comparison. This position can also be used to demonstrate anterior or posterior displacement in fractures.

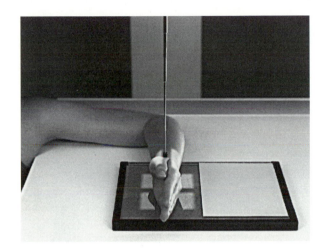

Fig. 4-69. Lateral wrist with ulnar surface to film.

CARPAL TERMINOLOGY CONVERSION	
Preferred	**Synonyms**
Proximal row:	
Scaphoid	Navicular
Lunate	Semilunar
Triquetrum	Triquetral, cuneiform, or triangular
Pisiform	(none)
Distal row:	
Trapezium	Greater multangular
Trapezoid	Lesser multangular
Capitate	Os magnum
Hamate	Unciform

A

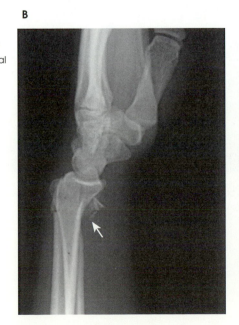

- 1st metacarpal
- Trapezium
- Scaphoid
- Capitate
- Lunate
- Radius
- Ulna

B

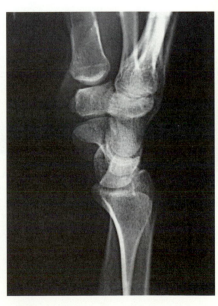

Fig. 4-70. A, Lateral wrist (ulnar surface to film). **B,** Lateral with fracture *(arrow).* Same patient as in Fig. 6-66, *B.*

(Courtesy Keith Shipman, R.T.)

Fig. 4-71. Lateral wrist (radial surface to film).

□ **Evaluation criteria**

The following should be clearly demonstrated:

- Distal radius and ulna, carpals, and the proximal half of the metacarpals.
- Superimposed distal radius and ulna.
- Superimposed metacarpals.
- Radiographic density similar to PA or AP and oblique radiographs. This requires increased exposure factors to compensate for greater part thickness.

NOTE: Burman et al.[1] suggest that the lateral position of the scaphoid be made with the wrist in palmar flexion, because this action rotates the bone anteriorly into a dorsovolar position (Fig. 4-72, *A*). This position, however, is of value only when sufficient flexion is permitted.

NOTE: Fiolle[2,3] was the first to describe a small bony growth occurring on the dorsal surface of the third carpometacarpal joint. He termed the condition "carpe bossu," or carpal boss, and found that it could be demonstrated to best advantage in a lateral position with the wrist in palmar flexion (Fig. 4-72, *B*).

[1]Burman MS, et al: Fractures of the radial and ulnar axes, AJR 51:455-480, 1944.
[2]Fiolle J: Le "carpe bossu," Bull. Soc. Chir. Paris 57:1687, 1931.
[3]Fiolle J, and Ailland: Nouvelle observation de "carpe bossu," Bull. Soc. Chir. Paris 58:187-188, 1932.

CARPAL TERMINOLOGY CONVERSION

Preferred	Synonyms
Proximal row:	
Scaphoid	Navicular
Lunate	Semilunar
Triquetrum	Triquetral, cuneiform, or triangular
Pisiform	(none)
Distal row:	
Trapezium	Greater multangular
Trapezoid	Lesser multangular
Capitate	Os magnum
Hamate	Unciform

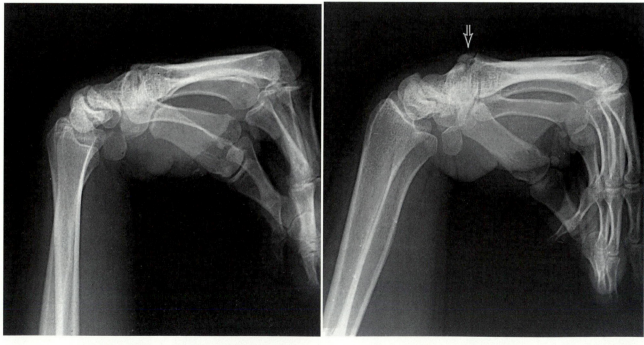

A   B

Fig. 4-72. A, Lateral wrist with palmar flexion of normal wrist. **B,** Lateral wrist with palmar flexion of wrist showing carpal boss *(arrow).*

Wrist

 PA OBLIQUE PROJECTION
Lateral rotation

Film: 8 × 10 in (18 × 24 cm) crosswise for two images on one film.

Position of patient

- Seat the patient at the end of the radiographic table with the axilla in contact with the table.

Position of part

- Rest the palmar surface of the wrist on the cassette.
- Adjust the cassette so its center point will be under the scaphoid when the wrist is rotated from the pronated position.
- From the pronated position, rotate the wrist laterally (externally) until it forms an angle of approximately 45 degrees with the plane of the film. For exact positioning and to ensure duplication in follow-up examinations, place a 45-degree foam wedge under the elevated side of the wrist.
- Extend the wrist just slightly, and, if the digits do not touch the table, support them in place (Fig. 4-73).
- When the scaphoid is the point of interest, adjust the wrist in ulnar flexion. Place a sandbag across the forearm.
- *Shield gonads:* Place a shield over the patient's pelvis.

Central ray

- Direct the central ray perpendicular to the midcarpal area. It enters just distal to the radius.

Structures shown

This projection demonstrates the carpals on the lateral side of the wrist, particularly the trapezium and the scaphoid. The scaphoid is superimposed on itself in the direct PA projection (Figs. 4-74 and 4-75).

Evaluation criteria

The following should be clearly demonstrated:

- A well-demonstrated scaphoid.
- Distal radius and ulna and the proximal half of the metacarpals, along with the carpals.
- Usually adequate amount of obliquity exists when there is:
  - Slight interosseus space between the third-fourth and fourth-fifth metacarpal shafts.
  - Slight overlap of the distal radius and ulna.
- Soft tissue and bony trabeculation.

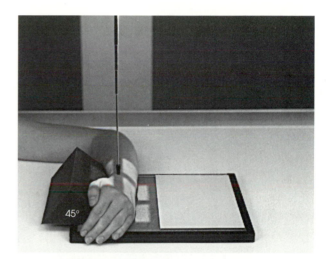

Fig. 4-73. PA oblique wrist. Lateral rotation.

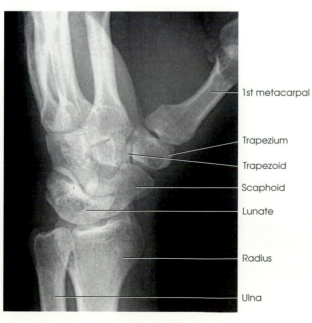

1st metacarpal

Trapezium

Trapezoid

Scaphoid

Lunate

Radius

Ulna

Fig. 4-74. PA oblique wrist.

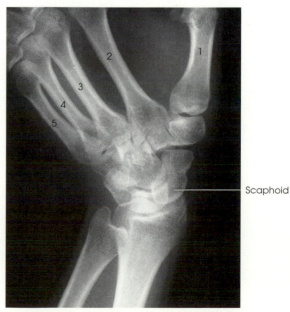

Scaphoid

Fig. 4-75. PA oblique wrist with ulnar flexion.

Wrist

AP OBLIQUE PROJECTION[1]
Medial rotation

Film: 8 × 10 in (18 × 24 cm) crosswise for two images on one film.

Position of patient

• Seat the patient at the end of the radiographic table.
• Have the patient rest the forearm on the table in the lateral position.

Position of part

• Place the cassette under the wrist and center it at the dorsal surface of the wrist.

[1]McBride E: Wrist joint injuries, a plea for greater accuracy in treatment, J Okla Med Assoc 19:67-70, 1926.

• Next rotate the wrist medially (internally) until it forms a semi-supinated position of approximately 45 degrees to the film (Fig. 4-76).
• *Shield gonads:* Place a lead shield over the patient's pelvis.

Central ray

• Direct the central ray perpendicular to the midcarpal area. It enters the anterior surface of the wrist midway between its medial and lateral borders.

Structures shown

This position separates the pisiform from the adjacent carpal bones. It also gives a more distinct radiograph of the triquetrum and hamate (unciform) (compare Figs. 4-77 and 4-78).

□ Evaluation criteria

The following should be clearly demonstrated:

■ Carpals on medial side of wrist; the triquetrum, hamate, and pisiform free of superimposition and in profile.
■ Distal radius and ulna and proximal half of metacarpals included along with the carpals.
■ Radiographic quality soft tissue and bony trabeculation.

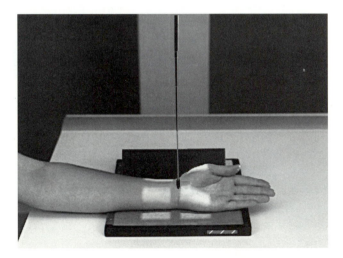

Fig. 4-76. AP oblique wrist. Medial rotation.

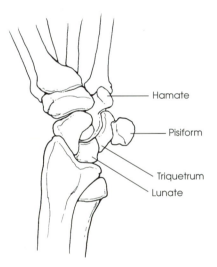

Fig. 4-77. AP oblique wrist.

CARPAL TERMINOLOGY CONVERSION	
Preferred	**Synonyms**
Proximal row:	
Scaphoid	Navicular
Lunate	Semilunar
Triquetrum	Triquetral, cuneiform, or triangular
Pisiform	(none)
Distal row:	
Trapezium	Greater multangular
Trapezoid	Lesser multangular
Capitate	Os magnum
Hamate	Unciform

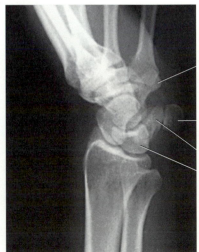
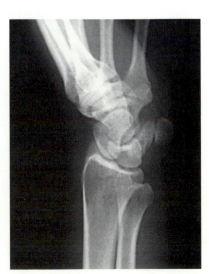

Fig. 4-78. AP oblique wrist.

Wrist

⛰ PA PROJECTION
Ulnar flexion

Film: 8 × 10 in (18 × 24 cm) for two images.

Position of patient

- Seat the patient at the end of the radiographic table with the arm and forearm resting on the table.

Position of part

- Position the wrist on the cassette for a PA projection.
- With one hand cupped over the joint to hold it in position, move the elbow away from the patient's body, and then turn the hand outward until the wrist is in extreme ulnar flexion, sometimes nebulously called "radial deviation" (Fig. 4-79).
- *Shield gonads:* Place a lead shield over the patient's pelvis.

Central ray

- Direct the central ray perpendicular to the scaphoid; according to the direction of the fracture line (clear delineation sometimes requires central ray angulation of 10 to 15 degrees proximally or distally).

Structures shown

This position corrects the foreshortening of the scaphoid, which is obtained with a perpendicular central ray and opens the spaces between the adjacent carpals (Fig. 4-80).

□ Evaluation criteria

The following should be clearly demonstrated:
- Scaphoid with adjacent articulations open.
- No rotation of wrist.
- Extreme ulnar flexion, as revealed by angle formed between longitudinal axes of forearm compared to metacarpals.
- Soft tissue and bony trabeculation.

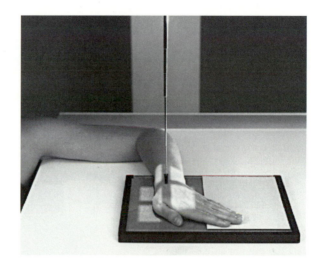

Fig. 4-79. PA wrist in ulnar flexion.

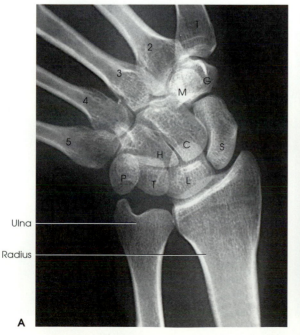

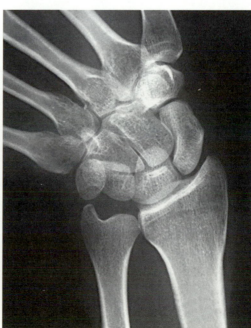

Ulna

Radius

A

B

Fig. 4-80. A, PA wrist in ulnar flexion. *S,* scaphoid; *L,* lunate; *T,* triquetrum; *P,* pisiform; *G,* trapezium; *M,* trapezoid; *C,* capitate; and *H,* hamate. **B,** Wrist in ulnar flexion.

Wrist

PA PROJECTION
Radial flexion

Film: 8 × 10 in (18 × 24 cm) for two images.

Position of patient

- Seat the patient at the end of the radiographic table.

Position of part

- Position the wrist on the cassette for a PA projection.
- Cup one hand over the wrist joint to hold it in position and then move the elbow toward the patient's body and the hand medially until the wrist is in extreme radial flexion, sometimes nebulously called "ulnar deviation" (Fig. 4-81).
- *Shield gonads:* Place a lead shield over the patient's pelvis.

Central ray

- Direct the central ray perpendicular to the midcarpal area.

Structures shown

Radial flexion opens the interspaces between the carpals on the medial side of the wrist (Fig. 4-82).

□ **Evaluation criteria**

The following should be clearly demonstrated:
- Carpals and their articulations on the medial side of the wrist.
- No rotation of wrist.
- Extreme radial flexion, as revealed by the angle formed between longitudinal axes of forearm compared to metacarpals.
- Soft tissue and bony trabeculation.

CARPAL TERMINOLOGY CONVERSION	
Preferred	**Synonyms**
Proximal row:	
Scaphoid	Navicular
Lunate	Semilunar
Triquetrum	Triquetral, cuneiform, or triangular
Pisiform	(none)
Distal row:	
Trapezium	Greater multangular
Trapezoid	Lesser multangular
Capitate	Os magnum
Hamate	Unciform

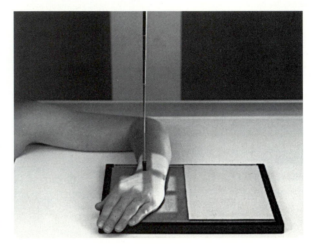

Fig. 4-81. PA wrist in radial flexion.

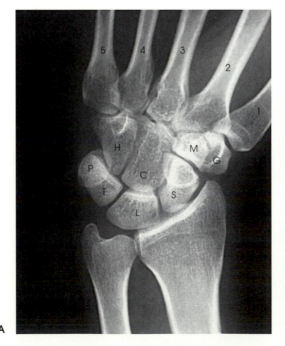

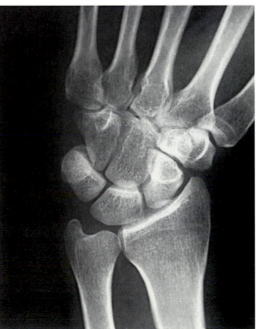

Fig. 4-82. A, PA wrist in radial flexion. *S,* scaphoid; *L,* lunate; *T,* triquetrum; *P,* pisiform; *G,* trapezium; *M,* trapezoid; *C,* capitate; and *H,* hamate. **B,** Wrist in radial flexion.

Wrist

Scaphoid

 ### PA AXIAL PROJECTION
STECHER METHOD

Film: 8 × 10 in (18 × 24 cm)

Position of patient

- Seat the patient at the end of the radiographic table with the arm and axilla in contact with table.
- Rest forearm on the table.

Position of part

- Place one end of the cassette on a support and adjust it so the finger end of the cassette is elevated 20 degrees (Fig. 4-83).
- Adjust the wrist on the cassette for a PA projection and center the wrist approximately ½ inch above the midpoint of the cassette. Bridgman[1] suggests that the wrist be positioned in ulnar flexion for this radiograph.
- *Shield gonads:* Place a lead shield over the patient's pelvis.

---

[1]Bridgman CF: Radiography of the carpal navicular bone, Med Radiogr Photogr 25:104-105, 1949.

Central ray

- With the central ray perpendicular to the table, direct it to enter the scaphoid.

Structures shown

The 20-degree angulation of the wrist places the scaphoid at right angles to the central ray so that it is projected without self-superimposition (Figs. 4-84 and 4-85).

□ Evaluation criteria

The following should be clearly demonstrated:

- Scaphoid.
- No rotation of carpals, metacarpals, radius, and ulna.
- Distal radius and ulna and the proximal half of the metacarpals, along with the carpals.
- Soft tissue and bony trabeculation.

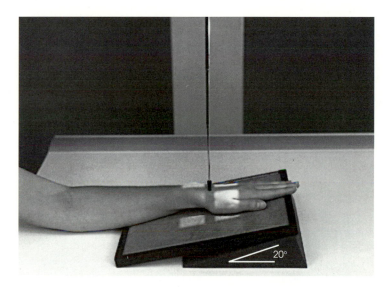

Fig. 4-83. PA axial wrist for scaphoid (Stecher method).

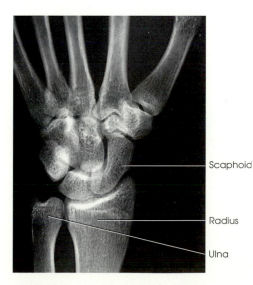

Scaphoid

Radius

Ulna

Fig. 4-84. PA axial wrist for scaphoid (Stecher method).

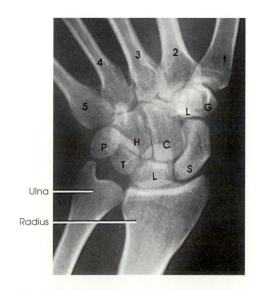

Ulna

Radius

Fig. 4-85. PA axial wrist for scaphoid (Bridgeman method), ulnar flexion. *S,* scaphoid; *L,* lunate; *T,* triquetrum; *P,* pisiform; *G,* trapezium; *M,* trapezoid; *C,* capitate; and *H,* hamate.

Variations

1. Stecher[1] recommends the previous method as being the preferable one; however, he says that a similar position can be obtained by placing the film and wrist horizontally and directing the central ray 20 degrees toward the elbow (Fig. 4-86).

   To demonstrate a fracture line that angles superoinferiorly, these positions may be reversed; that is, the wrist may be angled inferiorly, or from the horizontal position the central ray may be angled toward the digits.

[1]Stecher WR: Roentgenography of the carpal navicular bone, AJR 37:704-705, 1937.

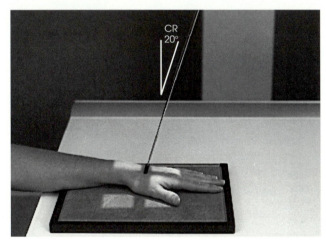

Fig. 4-86. PA axial wrist for scaphoid, Stecher method: angulation of central ray.

2. A third method recommended by Stecher is to have the patient clench the fist. This tends to elevate the distal end of the scaphoid so that it will lie parallel with the film; it also tends to widen the fracture line. The wrist is positioned as for the PA, and no central ray angulation is used.

Wrist

Trapezium

PA AXIAL OBLIQUE PROJECTION
CLEMENTS-NAKAYAMA METHOD[2]

Although fractures of the trapezium are rare, an undiagnosed fracture can lead to functional difficulties. In certain cases it is also important that the articular surfaces of the trapezium be evaluated to treat the osteoarthritic patient.

Film: 8 × 10 in (18 × 24 cm)

Position of patient

- With the patient seated at the end of the radiographic table, place the hand on the cassette in the lateral position.

Position of part

- Place the wrist in the lateral position, resting on the ulnar surface, over the center of the cassette.
- Place a 45-degree sponge wedge against the anterior surface, and rotate the hand to come in contact with the sponge.
- If the patient is able to achieve ulnar flexion, adjust the cassette so the long axis of the cassette and the forearm are aligned with the central ray (Fig. 4-87).
- If the patient is unable to comfortably achieve ulnar flexion, align the straight wrist to the cassette and rotate the elbow end of the cassette and arm 20 degrees away from the central ray (Fig. 4-88).
- *Shield gonads:* Place a lead shield over the patient's pelvis.

Central ray

- Direct the central ray 45 degrees distally to enter the anatomic snuff-box of the wrist and pass through the trapezium.

[2]Clements R and Nakayama H: Radiography of the polyarthritic hands and wrists, Radiol Technol 53:203-217, 1981.

Structures shown

The image clearly demonstrates the trapezium and the articulations with the adjacent carpal bones (Fig. 4-89). The articulation of the trapezium and scaphoid is not demonstrated on this image.

☐ Evaluation criteria

The following should be clearly demonstrated:

■ The trapezium will be projected free of the other carpal bones with the exception of the articulation with the scaphoid.

CARPAL TERMINOLOGY CONVERSION

Preferred	Synonyms
Proximal row:	
Scaphoid	Navicular
Lunate	Semilunar
Triquetrum	Triquetral, cuneiform, or triangular
Pisiform	(none)
Distal row:	
Trapezium	Greater multangular
Trapezoid	Lesser multangular
Capitate	Os magnum
Hamate	Unciform

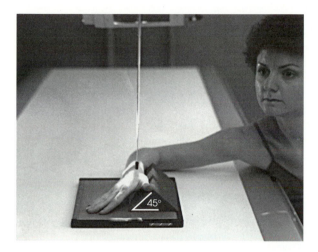

Fig. 4-87. PA axial oblique wrist for trapezium. Alignment with ulnar flexion.

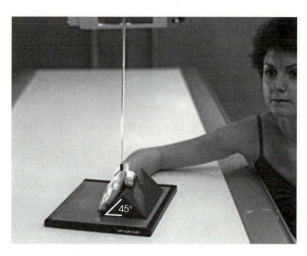

Fig. 4-88. PA axial oblique wrist for trapezium. Alignment without ulnar flexion.

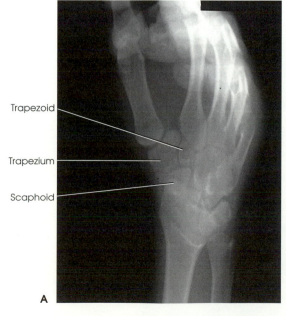

Trapezoid

Trapezium

Scaphoid

A

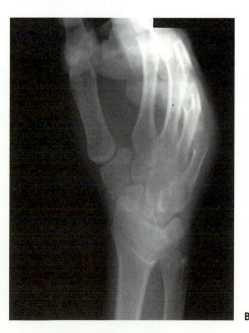

B

Fig. 4-89. A and **B,** PA axial oblique wrist for trapezium.

(Courtesy Roland Clements, R.T., F.A.S.R.T.)

Carpal Canal
TANGENTIAL PROJECTIONS
GAYNOR-HART METHOD

The carpal canal contains the tendons of the flexors of the fingers and the median nerve. Compression of this nerve results in pain. Radiography is performed to identify any abnormality of the bones or soft tissue of the canal.

Fractures of the hamulus of the hamate, pisiform, and trapezium are increasingly seen in athletes. The tangential projection is helpful in identifying fractures of these carpal bones.

Film: 8 × 10 in (18 × 24 cm).

Tangential projection (inferosuperior)

Position of patient

- Seat the patient at the end of the table in such a way that the forearm can be adjusted to lie parallel with the long axis of the table.

Position of part

- Hyperextend the wrist and center the cassette to the joint at the level of the radial styloid process.
- Place a radiolucent pad approximately ¾ inch thick under the lower forearm for support.
- Adjust the position of the hand to make its long axis as vertical as possible.
- To prevent superimposition of the shadows of the hamate and pisiform bones, rotate the hand slightly toward the radial side.
- Have the patient grasp the digits with the opposite hand, or use a suitable device to hold the wrist in the extended position (Fig. 4-90).
- *Shield gonads:* Place a lead shield over the patient's pelvis.

Central ray

- Direct the central ray to the palm of the hand, to a point approximately 1 inch distal to the base of the third metacarpal, at an angle of 25 to 30 degrees to the long axis of the hand.

Structures shown

This image of the carpal canal (carpal tunnel) shows the palmar aspect of the trapezium, the tubercle of the trapezium, the scaphoid, the capitate, the hamulus of hamate (hook of the hamate), the triquetrum, and the entire pisiform (Fig. 4-91).

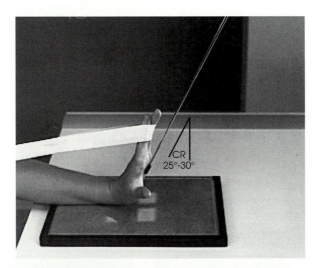

Fig. 4-90. Tangential (inferosuperior) carpal canal.

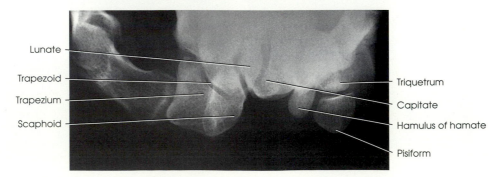

Lunate

Trapezoid

Trapezium

Scaphoid

Triquetrum

Capitate

Hamulus of hamate

Pisiform

Fig. 4-91. Tangential (inferosuperior) carpal canal.

Tangential Projection (Superoinferior)

When the patient cannot assume or maintain the previously described wrist position, a similar but not identical image may be obtained by adjusting the wrist as shown in Fig. 4-92. Have the patient dorsiflex the wrist as much as is tolerable and lean forward to place the carpal canal tangent to the film. The canal is easily palpable on the palmar aspect of the wrist as the concavity between the trapezium laterally and the hamulus of the hamate and pisiform medially.

When dorsiflexion of the wrist is limited, Marshall[1] suggests placing a 45-degree angle sponge under the palmar surface of the hand, slightly elevating the wrist, in order to place the carpal canal tangent to the central ray. A slight degree of magnification exists because of the increased OID (Fig. 4-93).

Central ray

- Direct the central ray tangent to the carpal canal at the level of the midpoint of the wrist.
- Angle the central ray toward the hand approximately 20 to 35 degrees from being parallel with the long axis of the forearm.

[1]Marshall J: Imaging the carpal tunnel, Radiog Today 56:11-13, 1990.

□ **Evaluation criteria**

With either approach, the following should be clearly demonstrated:

- Carpals in an arch arrangement.
- Pisiform in profile and free from superimposition.
- Hamulus of the hamate (unciform).
- Visualization of all carpals.

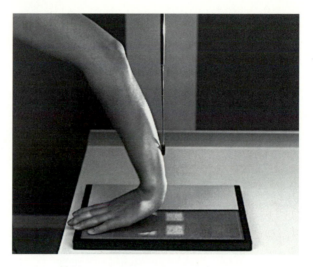

Fig. 4-92. Tangential (superoinferior) carpal canal.

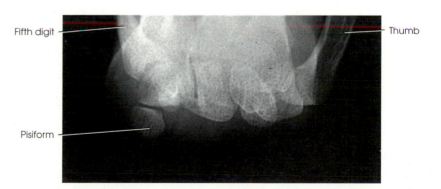

Fifth digit   Thumb

Pisiform

Fig. 4-93. Tangential (superoinferior) carpal canal.

Carpal Bridge
TANGENTIAL PROJECTION

Film: 8 × 10 in (18 × 24 cm) lengthwise.

Position of patient

- Seat or stand the patient at the side of the table to permit the required manipulation of the arm or x-ray tube.

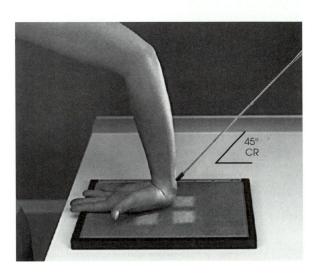

Fig. 4-94. Tangential carpal bridge, original method.

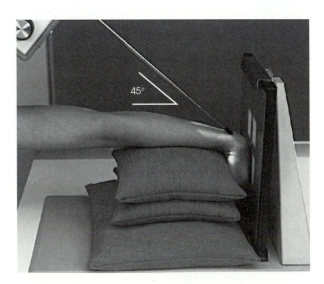

Fig. 4-95. Tangential carpal bridge, modified method.

Position of part

- The originators[1] of this projection recommend that the hand lie palm upward on the cassette, with the hand forming a right angle to the forearm, as shown in Fig. 4-94.
- When the wrist is too painful to be adjusted in the above position, a similar but not identical image can be obtained by elevating the forearm on sandbags or other suitable support. Then, with the wrist flexed to a right-angle position, place the film in the vertical position, as shown in Fig. 4-95.
- *Shield gonads:* Place a lead shield over the patient's pelvis.

Central ray

- Direct the central ray to a point about 1½ inches proximal to the wrist joint at a caudal angle of 45 degrees.

[1]Lentino W et al: The carpal bridge view, J Bone Joint Surg 39A:88-90, 1957.

CARPAL TERMINOLOGY CONVERSION	
Preferred	**Synonyms**
Proximal row:	
Scaphoid	Navicular
Lunate	Semilunar
Triquetrum	Triquetral, cuneiform, or triangular
Pisiform	(none)
Distal row:	
Trapezium	Greater multangular
Trapezoid	Lesser multangular
Capitate	Os magnum
Hamate	Unciform

Structures shown

The carpal bridge is demonstrated on the image (Figs. 4-96 and 4-97). The originators recommend this procedure for the demonstration of (1) fractures of the scaphoid, (2) lunate dislocations, (3) calcifications and foreign bodies in the dorsum of the wrist, and (4) chip fractures of the dorsal aspect of the carpal bones.

□**Evaluation criteria**

The following should be clearly demonstrated:

- Dorsal aspect of the wrist.
- The carpals.
- The dorsal surface of the carpals, free of superimposition by the metacarpal bases.

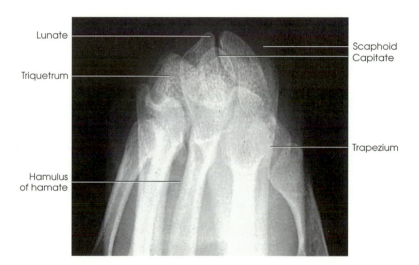

Lunate

Triquetrum

Scaphoid
Capitate

Trapezium

Hamulus
of hamate

Fig. 4-96. Tangential carpal bridge, original method.

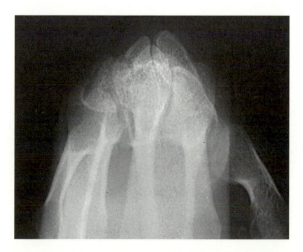

Fig. 4-97. Tangential carpal bridge, modified method.

Forearm

AP PROJECTION

Select a film long enough to include the entire forearm from the olecranon process of the ulna to the styloid process of the radius. Both images of the forearm may be taken on one film by alternately covering one half with a lead mask. Allow space for patient identification marker so as not to cut off any radiographic image.

Film: 10 × 12 in (24 × 30 cm) or 11 × 14 in (30 × 35 cm).

Position of patient

• Seat the patient close to the table and low enough to place the entire limb in the same plane.

Position of part

• Supinate the hand, extend the elbow, and center the unmasked half of the cassette to the forearm. Ensure that the joint of interest is included.
• Adjust the cassette so that the long axis is parallel with that of the forearm.
• Have the patient lean laterally until the forearm is in a true supinated position (Fig. 4-98).

• Because it is common for the proximal forearm to be rotated in this position it is important to palpate and adjust the humeral epicondyles to be equidistant from the film.
• Ensure that the hand is supinated (Fig. 4-99). Pronation of the hand crosses the radius over the ulna at its proximal third and rotates the humerus medially, resulting in an oblique projection of the forearm (Fig. 4-100).
• *Shield gonads:* Place a lead shield over the patient's pelvis.

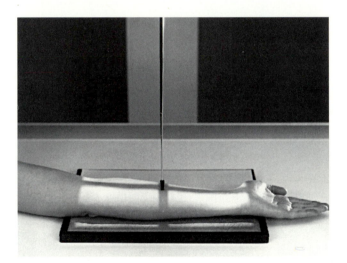

Fig. 4-98. AP forearm.

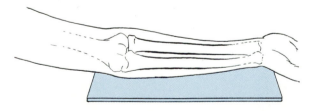

Fig. 4-99. AP forearm with hand supinated.

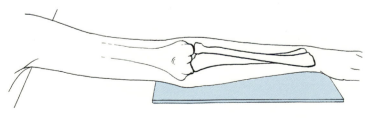

Fig. 4-100. AP forearm with hand pronated, incorrect.

Central ray

- Direct the central ray perpendicular to the midpoint of the forearm.

Structures shown

An AP projection of the forearm demonstrates the elbow joint, the radius and ulna, and the proximal row of slightly distorted carpal bones (Fig. 4-101).

□ Evaluation criteria

The following should be clearly demonstrated:

- Wrist and distal humerus.
- Slight superimposition of the radial head, neck, and tuberosity over the proximal ulna.
- No elongation or foreshortening of the humeral epicondyles.
- Partially open elbow joint (if the shoulder was placed in the same plane as the forearm).
- Similar radiographic densities of the proximal and distal forearm.

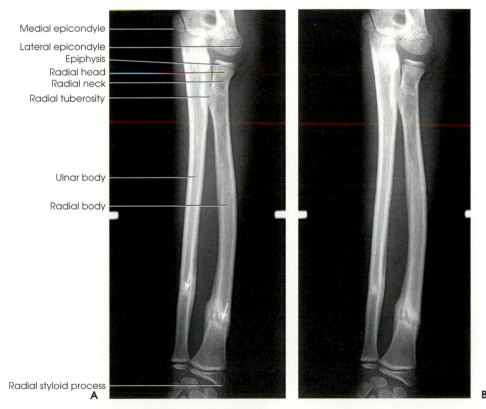

Medial epicondyle
Lateral epicondyle
Epiphysis
Radial head
Radial neck
Radial tuberosity

Ulnar body

Radial body

Radial styloid process

A   B

Fig. 4-101. A, AP forearm with fractured radius and ulna *(arrows)*. **B,** AP forearm. (Elbow not able to be exactly perpendicular as a result of patient condition.)

(Courtesy Ammar Saadeh, R.T.)

Forearm

LATERAL PROJECTION
Lateromedial

Film: 10 × 12 in (24 × 30 cm) or 11 × 14 in (30 × 35 cm) for two exposures on one film or a 7 × 17 in (18 × 43 cm) for the tall patient.

Position of patient

• Seat the patient close to the table and low enough so the humerus, shoulder joint, and elbow lie in the same plane; this permits the ulna to rotate to the lateral position.

Position of part

• Flex the elbow 90 degrees, and center the forearm over the unmasked half of the cassette, parallel with its long axis.
• Make sure the entire joint of interest is included.
• Adjust the limb in a true lateral position. The thumb side of the hand must be up (Fig. 4-102).
• *Shield gonads:* Place a lead shield over the patient's pelvis.

Central ray

• Direct the central ray perpendicular to the midpoint of the forearm.

Structures shown

The lateral projection demonstrates the bones of the forearm, the elbow joint, and the proximal row of carpal bones (Fig. 4-103).

☐ **Evaluation criteria**

The following should be clearly demonstrated:

■ Wrist and distal humerus.
■ Superimposition of the radius and ulna at their distal end.
■ Superimposition by the radial head over the coronoid process.
■ Radial tuberosity facing anteriorly.
■ Superimposed humeral epicondyles.
■ Elbow flexed 90 degrees.
■ Soft tissue and bony trabeculation along the entire length of the radial and ulnar shafts.

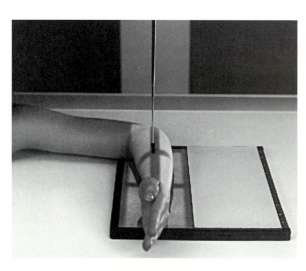

Fig. 4-102. Lateral forearm.

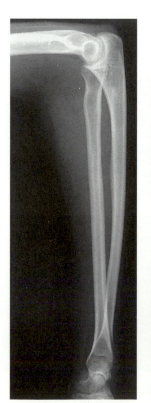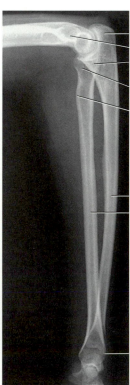

Olecranon process
Humeral epicondyle
Coronoid process

Radial head

Radial tuberosity

Ulnar body
Radial body

Ulnar styloid process

Fig. 4-103. Lateral forearm.

Elbow

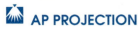
AP PROJECTION

Film: 8 × 10 in (18 × 24 cm) or 10 × 12 in (24 × 30 cm) crosswise.

Position of patient

- Seat the patient near the table and low enough to place the shoulder joint, humerous, and elbow joint in the same plane.

Position of part

- Extend the elbow, supinate the hand, and center the cassette to the elbow joint.
- Adjust the cassette to make it parallel with the long axis of the part (Fig. 4-104).
- Have the patient lean laterally until the humeral epicondyles and the anterior surface of the elbow are parallel with the plane of the film.
- The hand must be supinated to prevent rotation of the bones of the forearm.
- *Shield gonads:* Place a lead shield over the patient's pelvis.

Central ray

- Direct the central ray perpendicular to the elbow joint.

Structures shown

An AP projection of the elbow joint, the distal arm, and the proximal forearm is presented (Fig. 4-105).

□ Evaluation criteria

The following should be clearly demonstrated:

- Radial head, neck, and tuberosity slightly superimposed over the proximal ulna.
- Elbow joint open and centered to the central ray.
- Humeral epicondyles, not rotated.
- Soft tissue and bony trabeculation.

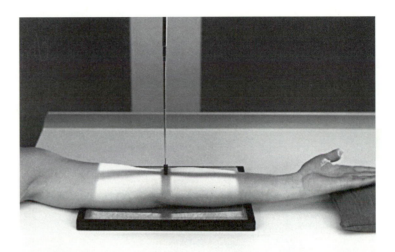

Fig. 4-104. AP elbow.

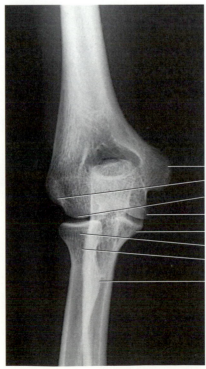
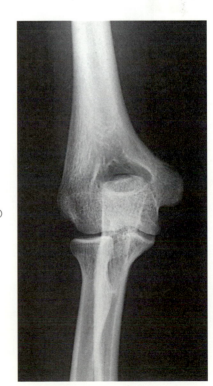

Medial epicondyle
Lateral epicondyle
Capitulum (capitellum)
Trochlea
Proximal ulna
Radial head
Radial neck
Radial tuberosity

Fig. 4-105. AP elbow.

Elbow

 ## LATERAL PROJECTION
Lateromedial

Griswold[1] gives two reasons for the importance of flexing the elbow 90 degrees: (1) the olecranon process can be seen in profile, and (2) the elbow fat pads are the least compressed. It must be realized that in partial or complete extension the posterior elbow fat pad is elevated by the olecranon process and can simulate joint pathology.

Film: 8 × 10 in (18 × 24 cm) or 10 × 12 in (24 × 30 cm) crosswise.

Position of patient

- Seat the patient at the end of the radiographic table low enough to place the humerous and elbow joint in the same plane.

[1]Griswold R: Elbow fat pads: a radiography perspective, Radiol Technol 53:303-307, 1982.

Position of part

- From the supine position, flex the elbow 90 degrees and place the humerus and forearm in contact with the table.
- Center the cassette to the elbow joint and adjust it so that its long axis is parallel with the long axis of the forearm, as shown in Figs. 4-106 and 4-107. On patients with muscular forearms, it may be necessary to elevate the wrist to place the forearm parallel with the film.
- To include more of the arm and forearm, adjust the cassette diagonally, as shown in Fig. 4-108.
- To obtain a lateral projection of the elbow (1) adjust the hand in the lateral position and (2) ensure that the humeral epicondyles are perpendicular to the plane of the film.
- *Shield gonads:* Place a lead shield over the patient's pelvis.

Central ray

- Direct the central ray perpendicular to the elbow joint, regardless of its location on the film.

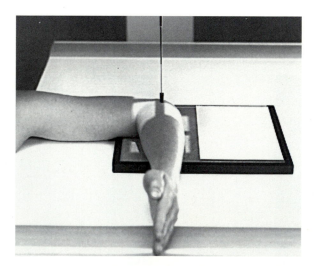

Fig. 4-106. Lateral elbow.

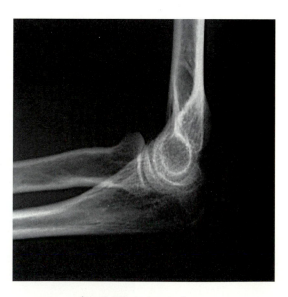

Fig. 4-107. Lateral elbow.

(Courtesy Leon Montgomery, C.R.T.)

Structures shown

The lateral projection demonstrates the elbow joint, the distal arm, and the proximal forearm (Figs. 4-107 and 4-108).

□Evaluation criteria

The following should be clearly demonstrated:

- Open elbow joint centered to the central ray.
- Elbow flexed 90 degrees.
- Superimposed humeral epicondyles.
- Anterior-facing radial tuberosity.
- Radial head partially superimposing the coronoid process.
- Olecranon process, seen in profile.
- Bony trabeculation seen, as well as any elevated fat pads in the soft tissue at the anterior and posterior distal humerus and the anterior proximal forearm.

NOTE: When the soft tissue about the elbow is in question, the joint should be flexed only 30 or 35 degrees as shown in Fig. 4-109. This partial flexion does not compress or stretch the soft structures as in the full 90-degree lateral.

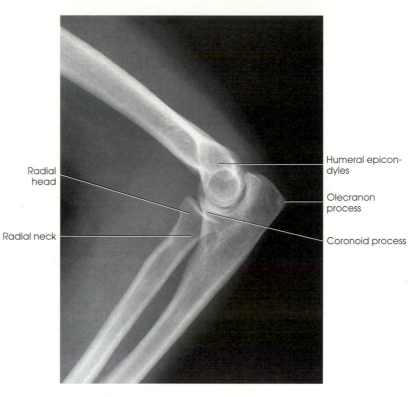

Radial head
Radial neck

Humeral epicondyles
Olecranon process
Coronoid process

Fig. 4-108. Lateral elbow.

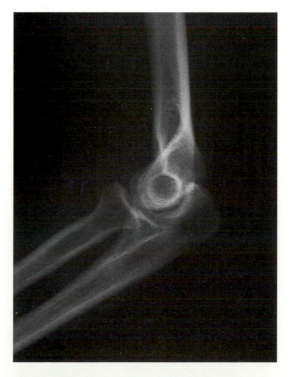

Fig. 4-109. Lateral elbow in partial flexion position for soft tissue.

Elbow

AP OBLIQUE PROJECTION
Medial rotation

Film: 8 × 10 in (18 × 24 cm) or 10 × 12 in (24 × 30 cm) crosswise.

Position of patient

• Seat the patient at the end of the radiographic table with the arm extended and in contact with the table.

Position of part

• Extend the limb in position for an AP projection and center the midpoint of the cassette to the elbow joint (Fig. 4-110).

• Medially (internal) rotate or pronate the hand and adjust the elbow to place its anterior surface at an angle of 40 to 45 degrees. This degree of obliquity will usually clear the coronoid process of the radial head.

• *Shield gonads:* Place a lead shield over the patient's pelvis.

Central ray

• Direct the central ray perpendicular to the elbow joint.

Structures shown

The image shows an oblique projection of the elbow with the coronoid process projected free of superimposition (Fig. 4-111).

□ **Evaluation criteria**

The following should be clearly demonstrated:

- Coronoid process in profile.
- Elongated medial humeral epicondyle.
- Ulna superimposed by the radial head and neck.
- Olecranon process within olecranon fossa.
- Soft tissue and bony trabeculation.

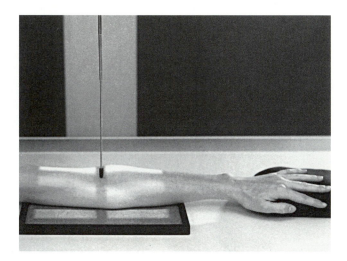

Fig. 4-110. AP oblique elbow. Medial rotation.

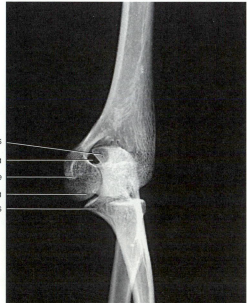

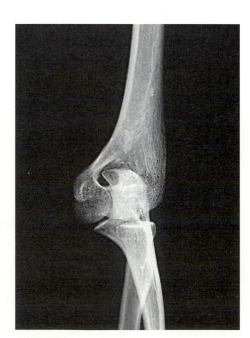

Olecranon process
Olecranon fossa
Medial epicondyle
Trochlea
Coronoid process

Fig. 4-111. AP oblique elbow.

Elbow

AP OBLIQUE PROJECTION
Lateral rotation

Film: 8 × 10 in (18 × 24 cm) or 10 × 12 in (24 × 30 cm) crosswise.

Position of patient

- Seat the patient at the end of the radiographic table with the arm extended and in contact with the table.

Position of part

- Extend the limb in position for an AP projection and center the midpoint of the cassette to the elbow joint.
- Rotate the hand laterally (external) to place the posterior surface of the elbow at an angle of 40 degrees (Fig. 4-112). When proper lateral rotation is achieved, the patient's thumb and second digit should touch the table.
- *Shield gonads:* Place a lead shield over the patient's pelvis.

Central ray

- Direct the central ray perpendicular to the elbow joint.

Structures shown

The image shows an oblique projection of the elbow with the radial head and neck projected free of superimposition of the ulna (Fig. 4-113).

□ Evaluation criteria

The following should be clearly demonstrated:

- Radial head, neck, and tuberosity, projected free of the ulna.
- Open elbow joint.
- Soft tissue and bony trabeculation.

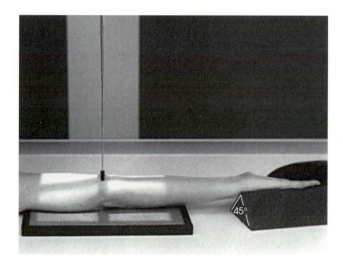

Fig. 4-112. AP oblique elbow. Lateral rotation.

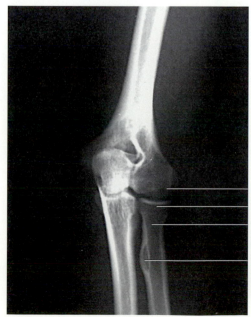
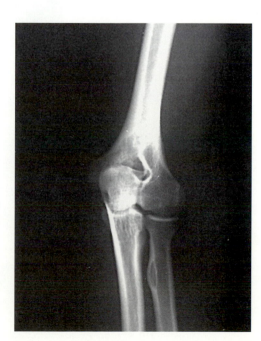

Capitulum (capitellum)

Radial head

Radial neck

Radial tuberosity

Fig. 4-113. AP oblique elbow.

(Courtesy Lois Baird, R.T.)

Elbow

 ## AP PROJECTION
Partial flexion

When the patient is unable to completely extend the elbow, the lateral position is easily performed, but it is necessary to obtain two AP radiographs to avoid distortion.

Film: Both exposures can be made on one 8 × 10 in (18 × 24 cm) film, or on one film placed crosswise by alternately covering one half of the film with a lead mask.

Distal humerus

Position of patient

- Seat the patient low enough to place the entire humerus in the same plane. Support the elevated forearm.

Position of part

- If possible, the hand should be supinated. Place the cassette under the elbow and center to the condyloid area of the humerus (Fig. 4-114).
- *Shield gonads.*

Central ray

- Direct the central ray perpendicular to the humerus, traversing the elbow joint.
- Depending on the degree of flexion, it may be necessary to angle the central ray distally into the joint.

Structures shown

This projection shows the distal humerus when the elbow cannot be fully extended (Figs. 4-115 and 4-116).

□ Evaluation criteria

The following should be clearly demonstrated:

- Distal humerus without rotation or distortion.
- Proximal radius superimposed over the ulna.
- Closed elbow joint.
- Greatly foreshortened proximal forearm.
- Trabecular detail on the distal humerus.

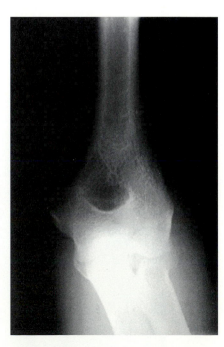

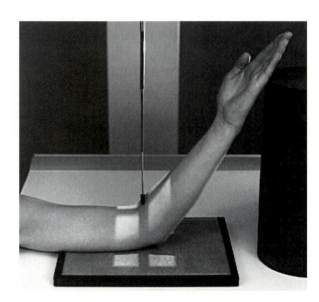

Fig. 4-114. AP elbow, partially flexed.

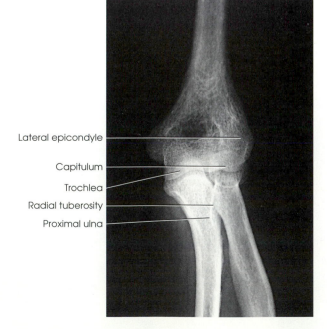

Lateral epicondyle
Capitulum
Trochlea
Radial tuberosity
Proximal ulna

Fig. 4-115. AP elbow, partially flexed, demonstrating distal humerus.

Fig. 4-116. AP elbow, partially flexed, demonstrating distal humerus.

(Courtesy Fayette Capik, R.T.)

Proximal forearm

Position of patient

- Seat the patient at the end of the radiographic table with the hand supinated.

Position of part

- Seat the patient high enough to permit the dorsal surface of the forearm to rest on the table (Fig. 4-117). If this is not possible, elevate the limb on a support, adjust it in the lateral position, place the cassette in the vertical position behind the upper end of the forearm, and direct the central ray horizontal.
- *Shield gonads.*

Central ray

- Direct the central ray perpendicular to the elbow joint and the long axis of the forearm.
- Adjust the cassette so that the central ray will pass to its midpoint.

Structures shown

This projection demonstrates the proximal forearm (Fig. 4-118) when the elbow cannot be fully extended (Fig. 4-119).

☐ Evaluation criteria

The following should be clearly demonstrated:

- Proximal radius and ulna, without rotation or distortion.
- Radial head, neck, and tuberosity slightly superimposed over the proximal ulna.
- Partially open elbow joint.
- Foreshortened distal humerus.
- Trabecular detail on the proximal forearm.

NOTE: Holly[1] has described a method for obtaining the AP projection of the radial head. The patient is positioned as described for the distal humerus. Extend the elbow as much as possible and support the forearm. Holly states that the forearm should be supinated enough to place the horizontal plane of the wrist at an angle of 30 degrees with the horizontal.

---

[1]Holly EW: Radiography of the radial head, Med Radiogr Photogr 32:13-14, 1956.

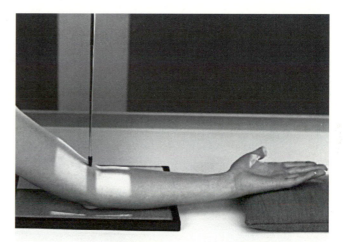

Fig. 4-117. AP elbow, partially flexed.

(Courtesy Fayette Capik, R.T.)

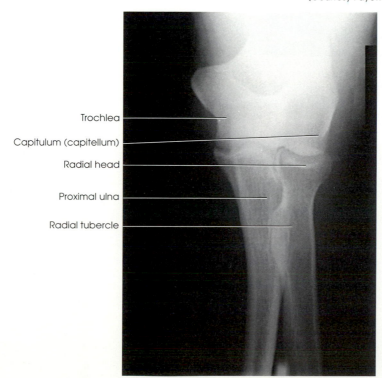

Trochlea

Capitulum (capitellum)

Radial head

Proximal ulna

Radial tubercle

Fig. 4-118. AP elbow, partially flexed, demonstrating proximal forearm. Dislocated elbow on same patient as shown in Fig. 4-119.

(Courtesy Fayette Capik, R.T.)

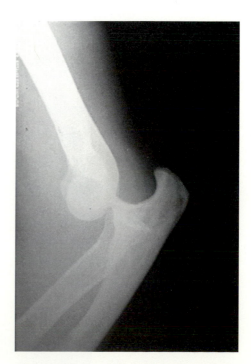

Fig. 4-119. Lateral elbow showing dislocation on same patient as shown in Figs. 4-116 and 4-118.

(Courtesy Fayette Capik, R.T.)

Elbow

Acute Flexion Sequence

When fractures around the elbow are being treated using the Jones method (complete flexion), the lateral position offers little difficulty, but the frontal projection must be made through the superimposed bones of the AP arm and PA forearm.

Distal humerus
AP PROJECTION

Film: 8 × 10 in (18 × 24 cm). Film may be divided for two images on one film.

Position of patient

- Seat the patient at the end of the radiographic table with the elbow fully flexed, unless contraindicated.

Position of part

- Center the cassette proximal to the epicondylar area of the humerus. The long axis of the arm and forearm should be parallel with the long axis of the film (Figs. 4-120 and 4-121).
- Adjust the arm or the radiographic tube and film to prevent rotation.
- *Shield gonads:* Place a lead shield over the patient's pelvis.

Central ray

- Direct the central ray perpendicular to the humerus approximately 2 inches superior to the olecranon process.

Structures shown

This position superimposes the bones of the forearm and arm. The olecranon process should be clearly demonstrated (Fig. 4-122).

☐ Evaluation criteria

The following should be clearly demonstrated:

- Forearm and humerus superimposed.
- No rotation.
- Olecranon process and distal humerus.
- Soft tissue outside the olecranon process.

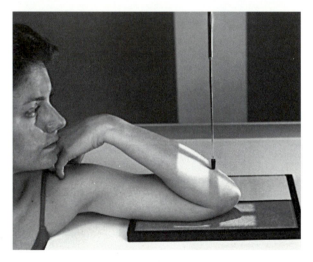

Fig. 4-120. AP distal humerus (acute flexion of elbow).

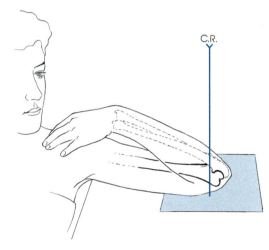

Fig. 4-121. AP distal humerus (acute flexion of elbow).

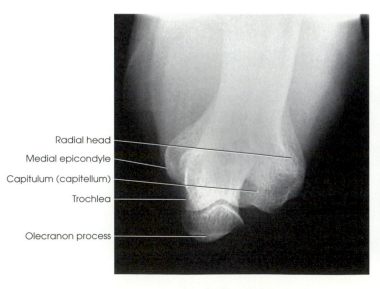
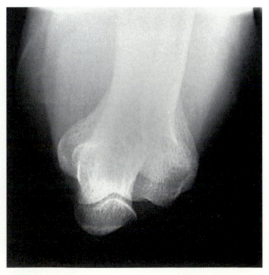

Radial head
Medial epicondyle
Capitulum (capitellum)
Trochlea
Olecranon process

Fig. 4-122. AP distal humerus (acute flexion of elbow).

(Courtesy Leon Montgomery, C.R.T.)

Proximal forearm
PA PROJECTION

Film: 8 × 10 in (18 × 24 cm).

Position of patient

• Seat the patient at the end of the radiographic table with the elbow fully flexed.

Position of part

• Center the flexed elbow joint to the center of the film. The long axis of the superimposed forearm and arm should be parallel with the long axis of the film (Figs. 4-123 and 4-124).

• Move the cassette toward the shoulder so the central ray will pass to the midpoint.

• *Shield gonads:* Place a lead shield over the patient's pelvis.

Central ray

• Direct the central ray perpendicular to the flexed forearm entering approximately 2 inches distal to the olecranon process.

Structures shown

The superimposed bones of the arm and forearm are outlined (Fig. 4-125). The elbow joint should be more open than for the distal humerus.

☐ Evaluation criteria

The following should be clearly demonstrated:

■ Forearm and humerus superimposed.
■ No rotation.
■ Proximal radius and ulna.

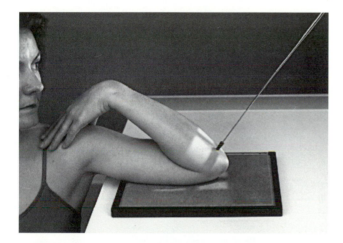

Fig. 4-123. PA proximal forearm (full flexion of elbow).

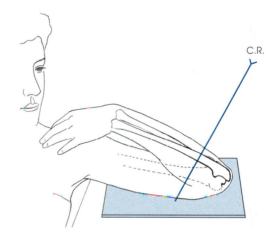

Fig. 4-124. PA proximal forearm (full flexion of elbow).

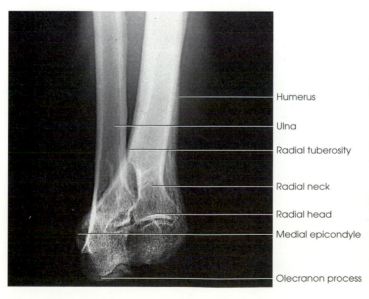

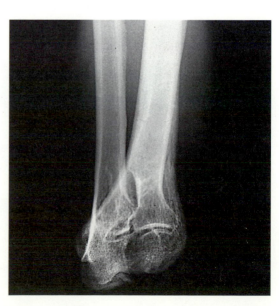

Humerus

Ulna

Radial tuberosity

Radial neck

Radial head

Medial epicondyle

Olecranon process

Fig. 4-125. PA proximal forearm (full flexion of elbow).

Elbow

Radial Head
LATERAL PROJECTION
Lateromedial

Four Position Series

Place the cassette in position and cover the unused part of the film area with sheet lead. To demonstrate the entire circumference of the radial head free of superimposures, perform four projections, varying the position of the hand.

Film: 8 × 10 in (18 × 24 cm) or 10 × 12 in (24 × 30 cm) for two or four exposures on one film.

Position of patient

- Seat the patient low enough to place the entire limb in the same horizontal plane.

Position of part

- Flex the elbow 90 degrees, center the joint to the unmasked cassette, and place it in the lateral position.
- Make the first exposure with the hand supinated as much as is possible in this position (Fig. 4-126).
- Shift the film and make the second exposure with the hand in the lateral position, that is, with the thumb surface up (Fig. 4-127).

- Shift the film and make the third exposure with the hand pronated (Fig. 4-128).
- Shift the film and make the fourth exposure with the hand in extreme internal rotation, that is, resting on the thumb surface (Fig. 4-129).
- *Shield gonads:* Place a lead shield over the patient's pelvis.

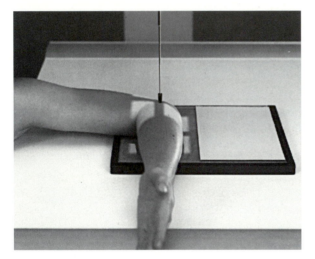

Fig. 4-126. Lateral elbow, radius with hand supinated (as much as possible).

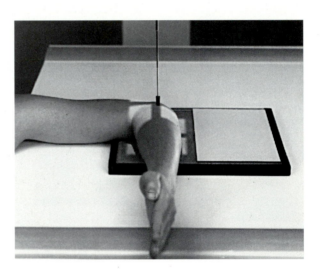

Fig. 4-127. Lateral elbow, radius with hand lateral.

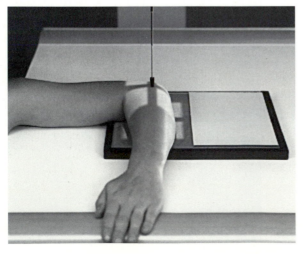

Fig. 4-128. Lateral elbow, radius with hand pronated.

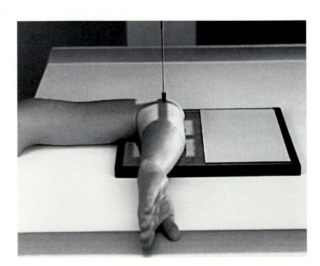

Fig. 4-129. Lateral elbow, radius with hand internally rotated.

Central ray

- Direct the central ray perpendicular to the elbow joint.

Structures shown

The radial head is projected in varying degrees of rotation (Figs. 4-130 to 4-133). The portion of the radial head demonstrated corresponds to the respective illustrations.

□ Evaluation criteria

The following should be clearly demonstrated:

- Radial tuberosity should face anteriorly for first and second images and posteriorly for the third and fourth images (Figs. 4-130 to 4-133).
- Elbow flexed 90 degrees.
- Radial head partially superimposing the coronoid process, but seen in all images.

NOTE: Greenspan and Norman[1] reported the radial head can be projected more clearly with reduced superimposition by directing the central ray 45 degrees medially (toward the shoulder) when positioned as in Figs. 4-126 to 4-129. The resulting radiograph is seen in Fig. 4-134.

[1]Greenspan A and Norman A: The radial head, capitellum view: useful technique in elbow trauma. AJR 138:1186-1188, 1982.

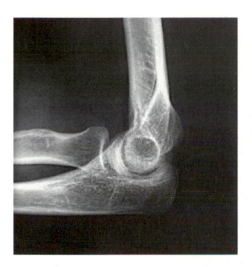

Fig. 4-130. Lateral elbow, radius with hand supinated.

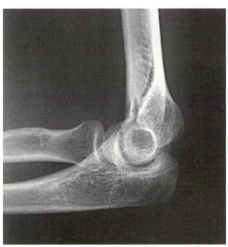

Fig. 4-131. Lateral elbow, radius with hand lateral.

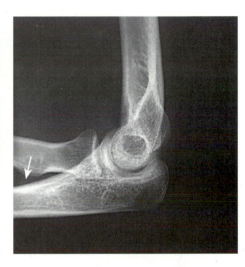

Fig. 4-132. Lateral elbow, radius with hand pronated (radial tuberosity, *arrow*).

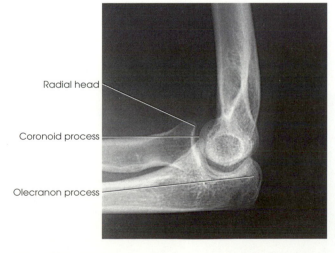

Radial head

Coronoid process

Olecranon process

Fig. 4-133. Lateral elbow, radius with hand internally rotated.

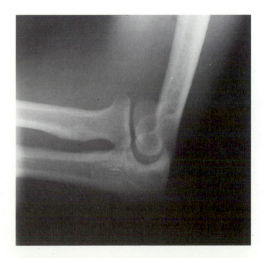

Fig. 4-134. Lateral elbow, radial head with central ray angled 45 degrees medially as described by Greenspan and Norman.

(Courtesy Thomas White, R.T.)

Distal Humerus

PA AXIAL PROJECTION

Film: 8 × 10 in (18 × 24 cm) for one or two images on one film.

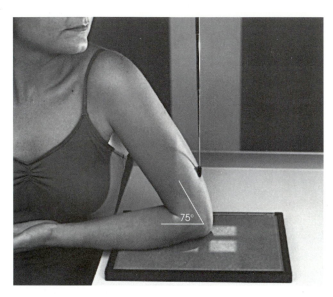

Fig. 4-135. PA axial distal humerus.

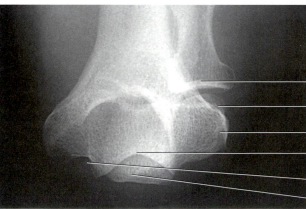

Radial head

Capitulum

Lateral epicondyle

Trochlea

Ulnar sulcus

Olecranon process

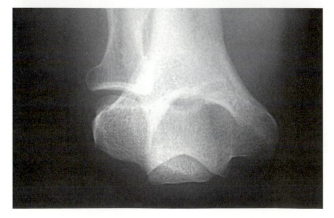

Fig. 4-136. PA axial distal humerus.

Position of patient

- Seat the patient high enough to enable the forearm to rest on the table with the arm in the vertical position.
- The patient must be seated so that the forearm can be adjusted parallel to the long axis of the table.

Position of part

- Ask the patient to rest the forearm on the table, and then adjust it so that its long axis is parallel with the table.
- Center a point midway between the epicondyles to the center of the film.
- Flex the patient's elbow to place the arm in a near vertical position so the humerus forms an angle of approximately 75 degrees from the forearm (approximately 15 degrees between the central ray and the long axis of the humerus).
- Confirm that the patient is not leaning anteriorly or posteriorly.
- Supinate the hand to prevent rotation of the humerus and ulna, and have the patient immobilize it with the opposite hand (Fig. 4-135).
- *Shield gonads:* Place a lead shield over the patient's pelvis.

Central ray

- Direct the central ray perpendicular to the ulnar sulcus, a point just medial to the olecranon process.

Structures shown

This projection demonstrates the epicondyles, trochlea, ulnar sulcus (the groove between the medial epicondyle and the trochlea), and the olecranon fossa (Fig. 4-136). It is used in radiohumeral bursitis (tennis elbow) to detect otherwise obscured calcifications located in the ulnar sulcus.

☐ Evaluation criteria

The following should be clearly demonstrated:

- ▪ Outline of the ulnar sulcus (groove).
- ▪ Soft tissue outside the distal humerus.
- ▪ Forearm and humerus superimposed.
- ▪ No rotation.

Olecranon Process

PA AXIAL PROJECTION

Film: 8 × 10 in (18 × 24 cm)

Position of patient

- Seat the patient at the end of the radiographic table, high enough so the forearm can rest flat on the cassette.

Position of part

- Adjust the arm at an angle of 45 to 50 degrees from the vertical position and ensure there is no anterior or posterior leaning.
- Supinate the hand and have the patient immobilize it with the opposite hand.
- Center midway between the epicondyles to the center of the film.
- *Shield gonads:* Place a lead shield over the patient's pelvis.

Central ray

- Direct the central ray to the olecranon process (1) perpendicular to demonstrate the dorsum of the olecranon process and (2) at an angle of 20 degrees toward the wrist to demonstrate the curved extremity and articular margin of the olecranon process (Fig. 4-137).

Structures shown

The projection demonstrates the olecranon process and the articular margin of the olecranon and the humerus (Figs. 4-138 to 4-140).

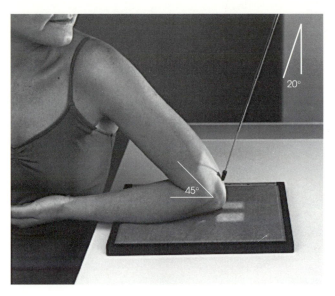

Fig. 4-137. PA axial olecranon process with central ray angled 20 degrees.

□Evaluation criteria

The following should be clearly demonstrated:

- Olecranon process in profile.
- Soft tissue outside the olecranon process.
- Forearm and humerus superimposed.
- No rotation.

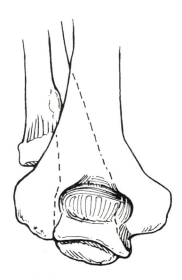

Fig. 4-138. PA axial olecranon process.

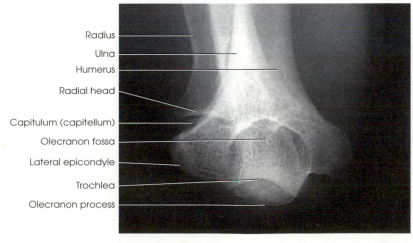

Radius
Ulna
Humerus
Radial head
Capitulum (capitellum)
Olecranon fossa
Lateral epicondyle
Trochlea
Olecranon process

Fig. 4-139. PA axial olecranon process with central ray angulation of 0 degrees.

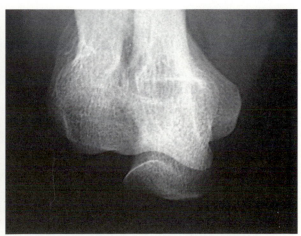

Fig. 4-140. PA axial olecranon process with central ray angulation of 20 degrees.

Humerus

AP PROJECTION
Upright

Shoulder and arm abnormalities, whether traumatic or pathologic in origin, are extremely painful. For this reason an upright position, either standing or seated, should be used whenever possible. By rotation of the patient's body as required, the arm can be positioned quickly and accurately with minimum discomfort to the patient and, in the presence of fracture, with no danger of fragment displacement.

The film selected should be long enough to include the humerus from its head to its condyle. An 11 × 14 in (30 × 35 cm) film is adequate for most adults when the arm can be abducted enough for diagonal placement on the film. If a longer film is needed, a 7 × 17 in (18 × 43 cm) cassette is adequate.

Film: 11 × 14 in (30 × 35 cm) or 7 × 17 in (18 × 43 cm).

Position of patient

- Place the patient in a seated or standing position facing the x-ray tube.

Fig. 4-141 illustrates the body position used for an AP projection of the freely movable arm. The body position, whether oblique or facing toward or away from the film, is unimportant as long as a true frontal radiograph of the arm is obtained.

Position of part

- Adjust the height of the cassette to place the upper margin of the film about 1½ inches above the head of the humerus.
- Locate the epicondyles and, while holding them between the thumb and index fingers of one hand, adjust the position of the arm or have the patient turn slowly until the desired position is reached. A coronal plane passing through the epicondyles will be parallel with the plane of the film for the AP (or PA) projection (Fig. 4-141).
- *Shield gonads:* Place a lead shield over the patient's pelvis.
- Ask patient to suspend respiration for the exposure.

Central ray

- Direct the central ray perpendicular to the center of the long axis of the humerus positioned midway between the elbow and shoulder joints.

Structures shown

The AP projection demonstrates the entire length of the humerus. The accuracy of the position is shown by the epicondyles (Fig. 4-142).

□ **Evaluation criteria**

The following should be clearly demonstrated:

- Elbow and shoulder joints.
- Maximal visibility of epicondyles without rotation.
- Humeral head and greater tubercle seen in profile.
- Outline of the lesser tubercle, located between the humeral head and the greater tubercle.
- Beam divergence possibly partially closing the elbow joint.
- No great variation in radiographic densities of the proximal and distal humerus.

NOTE: Radiographs of the humerus and shoulder may be taken with or without a grid. The patient's size and the radiographer's and physician's preference are factors often considered in reaching a decision. Most medical facilities establish a policy for the initial procedures, and, whether the policy is to use a grid or not, the positioning of the body part remains the same.

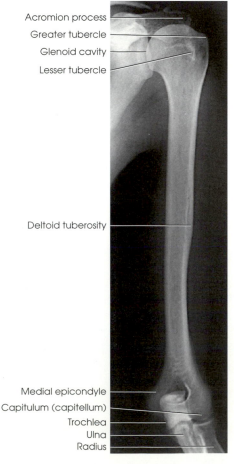

Fig. 4-142. Upright AP humerus.

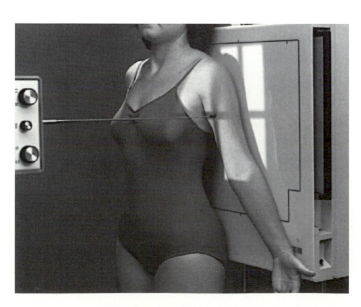

Fig. 4-141. Upright AP humerus.

Humerus

LATERAL PROJECTION
Lateromedial: upright

Film: 11 × 14 in (30 × 35 cm) or 7 × 17 in (18 × 43 cm). The film selected for the lateral must be long enough to include the humerus from the head to the condyle.

Position of patient

- Place the patient in a seated or standing position facing the x-ray tube. The body position, whether oblique or facing toward or away from the film, is not critical, as long as a true projection of the lateral arm is obtained.

Position of part

- Place the top margin of the film approximately 1½ inches above the level of the head of the humerus.
- Unless contraindicated by possible fracture, internally rotate the limb, flex the elbow approximately 90 degrees, and place the hand on the patient's hip. When so positioned, the coronal plane passing through the epicondyles will be perpendicular with the plane of the film (Fig. 4-143).
- *Shield gonads:* Place a lead shield over the patient's pelvis.
- Ask patient to suspend respiration for the exposure.

Central ray

- Direct the central ray perpendicular to the center of the long axis of the humerus.

Structures shown

The lateral projection demonstrates the entire length of the humerus. A true lateral image is confirmed by superimposed epicondyles (Fig. 4-144).

□ Evaluation criteria

The following should be clearly demonstrated:
- Elbow and shoulder joints.
- Superimposed epicondyles.
- Lesser tubercle in profile.
- Greater tubercle superimposed over the humeral head.
- Beam divergence possibly partially closing the elbow joint.
- No great variation in radiographic densities of the proximal and distal humerus.

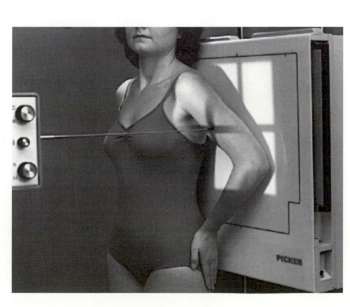

Fig. 4-143. Upright lateral humerus.

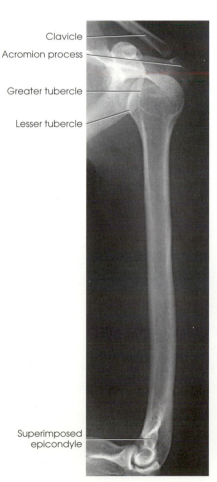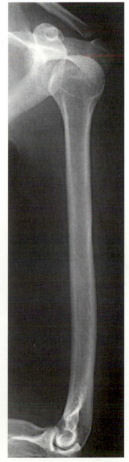

Clavicle
Acromion process
Greater tubercle
Lesser tubercle

Superimposed epicondyle

Fig. 4-144. Upright lateral humerus.

Humerus

AP PROJECTION
Recumbent

The cassette size selected should be long enough to include the bone from its head to its condyle inclusively.

Film: 11 × 14 in (30 × 35 cm), 7 × 17 in (18 × 43 cm), or 14 × 17 in (35 × 43 cm)

Position of patient

- With the patient in the supine position, adjust the cassette to include the entire length of the humerus.

Position of part

- Place the upper margin of the film approximately 1½ inches above the humeral head.
- Elevate the opposite shoulder on a sandbag to place the affected arm in contact with the cassette, or elevate the arm and cassette on sandbags.
- Unless contraindicated, supinate the hand and adjust the extremity to place the epicondyles parallel with the plane of the film (Fig. 4-145).
- *Shield gonads:* Place a lead shield over the patient's pelvis.
- Ask patient to suspend respiration for the exposure.

Central ray

- Direct the central ray perpendicular to the midpoint of the humerus.

Structures shown

An AP projection of the entire humerus is presented (Fig. 4-146).

☐ Evaluation criteria

The following should be clearly demonstrated:
- Elbow and shoulder joints.
- Maximum visibility and no rotation of the epicondyles.
- Humeral head and greater tubercle in profile.
- Outline of the lesser tubercle located between the humeral head and the greater tubercle.
- No great variation in radiographic densities of the proximal and distal humerus.
- Possible partial closure of the elbow joint (by beam divergence).

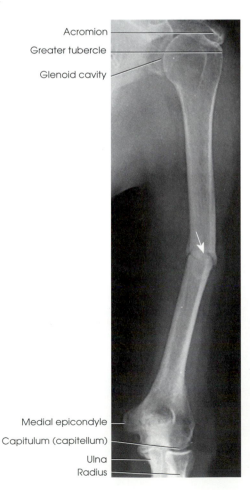

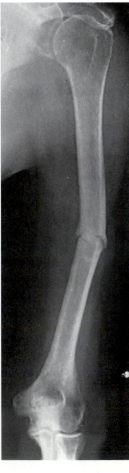

Acromion
Greater tubercle
Glenoid cavity

Medial epicondyle
Capitulum (capitellum)
Ulna
Radius

Fig. 4-146. Recumbent AP humerus showing healing fracture mid-shaft *(arrow)*.

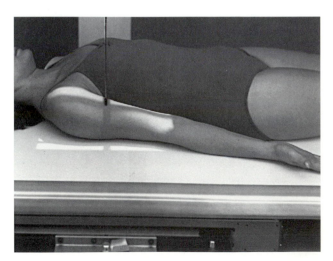

Fig. 4-145. Recumbent AP humerus.

LATERAL PROJECTION
Lateromedial: recumbent

Film: 11 × 14 in (30 × 35 cm) or 7 × 17 in (18 × 43 cm). The film selected for the lateral must be long enough to include the humerus from the head to the condyle.

Position of patient

- Place the patient in the supine position with the humerus centered to the film or bucky.

Position of part

- Adjust the top of the film to be approximately 1½ inches above the level of the head of the humerus. Unless contraindicated by possible fracture, abduct the arm somewhat and center the cassette under it.
- Rotate the forearm medially to place the epicondyles perpendicular to the plane of the film, and rest the hand against the patient's side. The elbow may be flexed for comfort.

- Adjust the position of the cassette to include the entire length of the humerus (Fig. 4-147).

 Lateral recumbent position

- When known or suspected fracture exists, position the patient in the lateral recumbent position, place the cassette close to the axilla and center the humerus to its midline.
- Unless contraindicated, flex the elbow, turn the thumb surface of the hand up, and rest it on a suitable support (Fig. 4-148).
- Adjust the position of the body to place the lateral surface of the humerus perpendicular to the central ray.

- *Shield gonads:* Place a lead shield over the patient's pelvis.
- Ask patient to suspend respiration for the exposure.

Central ray

- Direct the central ray perpendicular to the midpoint of the humerus.

Structures shown

The lateral projection demonstrates the entire humerus (Fig. 4-149).

□ **Evaluation criteria**

The following should be clearly demonstrated:
- Elbow and shoulder joints.
- Superimposed epicondyles.
- Lesser tubercle in profile.
- Greater tubercle superimposed over the humeral head.
- No great variations in radiographic densities of the proximal and distal humerus.

Humerus

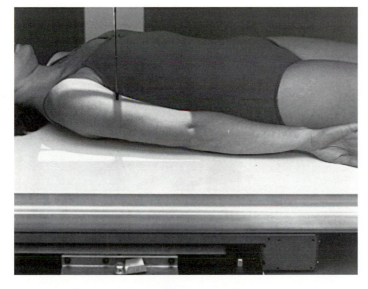

Fig. 4-147. Recumbent lateral humerus.

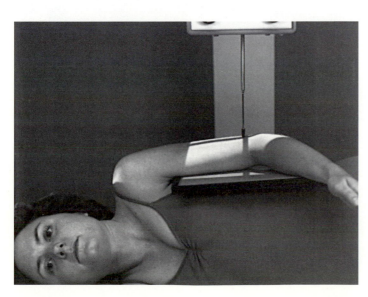

Fig. 4-148. Lateral recumbent body position, for lateral humerus.

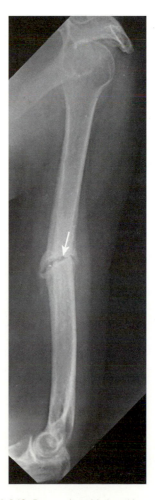

Fig. 4-149. Recumbent lateral humerus showing healing fracture *(arrow).*

Upper limb (extremity)

Proximal Humerus

 TRANSTHORACIC LATERAL PROJECTION
R or L position
LAWRENCE METHOD[1]

The Lawrence method is used when the arm cannot be abducted for the AP or lateral projections described on the preceeding pages.

Film: 8 × 10 in (18 × 24 cm) or 10 × 12 in (24 × 30 cm) lengthwise.

Position of patient

- Although this position can be carried out with the patient in the supine or upright position, the upright position facilitates accurate adjustment of the shoulder.
- Seat or stand the patient in the lateral position before a vertical grid device.

Position of part

- Have the patient raise the uninjured arm, rest the forearm on his or her head, and elevate the shoulder as much as possible. Elevation of the uninjured shoulder will give the desired depression of the injured side, thus separating the shoulders to prevent superimposition.
- Center the cassette to the region of the surgical neck of the affected humerus (Fig. 4-150).
- While holding the humeral epicondyles between the thumb and forefinger of one hand, adjust the rotation of the patient's body to project the humerus between the vertebral column and sternum. The epicondyles should be perpendicular to the plane of the film. This step may, however, be contraindicated by humeral fracture or dislocation.
- When the patient is able to hold his or her breath for 5 or 6 seconds, lung detail may be blurred considerably by the action of the heart. When this is possible, maintain the usual mAs factor but convert to a low mA–long exposure time combination.

- *Shield gonads:* Place a lead shield over the patient's pelvis.
- Respiration: Instruct the patient to hold his or her breath at full inspiration when you are ready to make the exposure. Having the lungs full of air improves the contrast and decreases the exposure necessary to penetrate the body.
- If the patient can be sufficiently immobilized to prevent voluntary motion, breathing motion can be used. In this case, instruct the patient and have him or her practice slow, deep breathing. An exposure time of 7 to 10 seconds will give excellent results while using a low mA.

Central ray

- Direct the central ray perpendicular to the film at the level of the surgical neck.
- If the patient cannot elevate the unaffected shoulder as described above, the central ray may be angled 10 to 15 degrees cephalad to achieve a comparable radiograph.

Structures shown

The resultant image will show a lateral projection of the proximal half or two thirds of the humerus, projected through the thorax. Although recorded detail may be poor, the outline of the humerus is clearly shown (Fig. 4-151).

☐ Evaluation criteria

The following should be clearly demonstrated:

- Proximal portion of the humerus.
- Lesser tubercle in profile on the anterior surface of the humeral head.
- Outline of the greater tubercle superimposed on the humeral head.
- Outline of the humerus clearly demonstrated through the ribs and lung fields.
- No overlap of the area of interest by the unaffected humerus and shoulder. (It may be necessary to direct the central ray 10 to 20 degrees cephalic for some patients.)
- No superimposition of the upper thoracic vertebrae by the humerus.

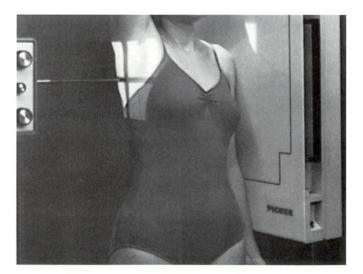

Fig. 4-150. Transthoracic lateral for proximal humerus.

---

[1]Lawrence, WS: A method of obtaining an accurate lateral roentgenogram of the shoulder joint, AJR 5:193-194, 1918.

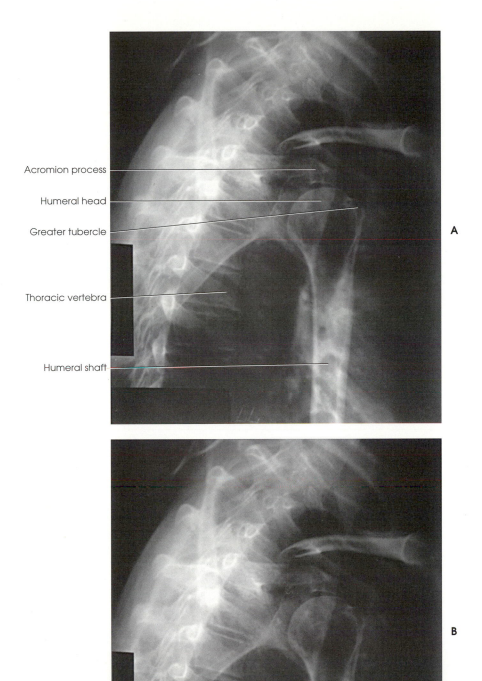

Acromion process

Humeral head

Greater tubercle

Thoracic vertebra

Humeral shaft

A

B

Fig. 4-151. Transthoracic lateral for proximal humerus.

(Courtesy Laurie Funk, R.T.)

Chapter 5

SHOULDER GIRDLE

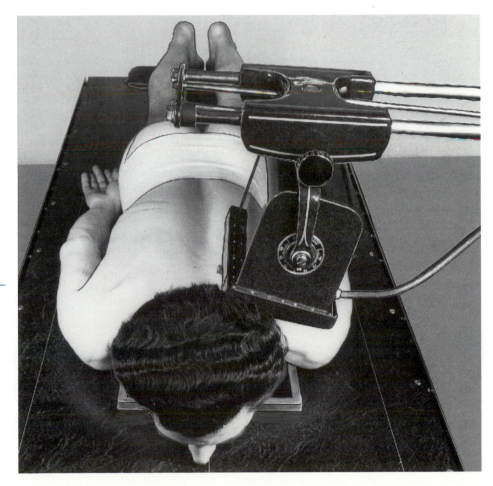

Patient positioned for sternoclavicular articulation. The cone on the radiographic tube has been removed, and the tube placed in contact with the posterior body surface. This procedure selectively magnifies (blurs) the posterior ribs and allows a view of the sternoclavicular joint. This technique is illegal under current radiation safety regulations.

The shoulder girdle, formed by the clavicle and scapula, connects the upper limb to the trunk. Although the alignment of these two bones is considered a girdle, it is incomplete both in front and behind. The girdle is completed in front by the sternum, which articulates with the medial end of the clavicle. The two scapulae are widely separated in the back. The proximal humerus is part of the upper limb and not the shoulder girdle proper; however, since the proximal portion of the humerus is included in the shoulder joint, its anatomy is considered with that of the shoulder girdle.

Clavicle

The *clavicle* (Fig. 5-1), classified as a long bone, has a *body* (shaft), and two articular extremities. The clavicle lies in a horizontal oblique plane just above the first rib and forms the anterior part of the shoulder girdle. The lateral, or *acromial extremity* articulates with the acromion process of the scapula, and the medial, or *sternal extremity* articulates with the manubrium of the sternum. The clavicle, which serves as a fulcrum for the movements of the arm, is doubly curved for strength. The curvature is more acute in males than in females.

Scapula

The *scapula* (Fig. 5-2), classified as a flat bone, forms the posterior part of the shoulder girdle. Triangular in shape, the scapula has two surfaces, three borders, and three angles. Lying on the superoposterior thorax between the second and seventh ribs, the scapula's *medial* (vertebral) *border* runs parallel with the vertebral column. The *body* (ala or wing) of the bone is arched from top to bottom for greater strength, and its surfaces serve for the attachment of numerous muscles.

The *costal* (anterior) *surface* of the scapula is slightly concave and contains the *subscapular fossa*. It is almost entirely filled by the attachment of the subscapularis muscle. The serratus anterior muscle attaches to the medial (vertebral) border of the costal surface from the *superior* (medial) to the *inferior angle*.

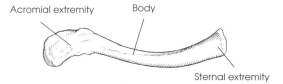

Fig. 5-1. Superior aspect of right clavicle.

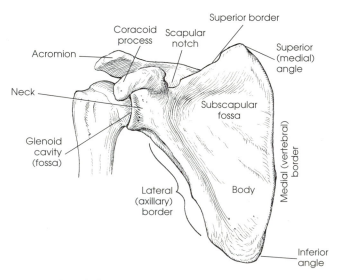

Fig. 5-2. Costal surface (anterior aspect) of scapula.

The *dorsal* (posterior) *surface* (Fig. 5-3) is divided into two portions by a prominent spinous process. The *crest of the spine* arises at the superior third of the medial border from a smooth, triangular area and runs obliquely superior to end in a flattened, ovoid projection called the *acromion*. The area above the spine is called the *supraspinous* (supraspinatus) *fossa* and gives origin to the supraspinatus muscle. The infraspinous muscle arises from the portion below the spine, which is called the *infraspinatus fossa*. The teres minor muscle arises from the superior two thirds of the lateral border of the dorsal surface and the teres major from the distal third and the inferior angle. The dorsal surface of the medial border affords attachment of the levator scapulae, rhomboideus major, and rhomboideus minor muscles.

The *superior border* extends from the superior angle to the *coracoid process* and, at its lateral end, has a deep depression, the *scapular notch*. The *medial* (vertebral) *border* extends from the superior (medial) to the inferior angles. The *lateral* (axillary) *border* extends from the *glenoid cavity* (fossa) to the inferior angle.

The *superior* (medial) *angle* is formed by the junction of the superior and medial (vertebral) borders. The *inferior angle* is formed by the junction of the medial (vertebral) and lateral (axillary) borders and lies over the seventh rib. The *lateral angle,* the thickest part of the body of the scapula, ends in a shallow, oval depression called the *glenoid cavity* (fossa). The constricted region around the glenoid cavity (fossa) (Fig. 5-4) is called the *neck* of the scapula. The coracoid process arises from a thick base that extends from the scapular notch to the superior portion of the neck of the scapula. This process projects first anteriorly and medially and then curves on itself to project laterally. The coracoid process can be palpated just distal and slightly medial to the acromioclavicular articulation.

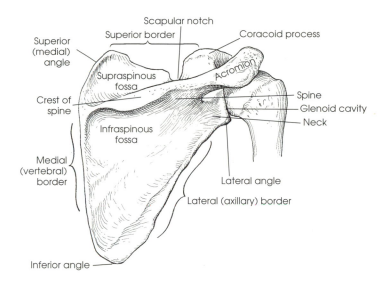

Fig. 5-3. Dorsal surface (posterior aspect) of scapula.

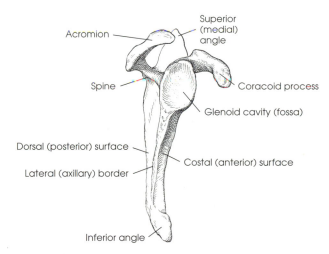

Fig. 5-4. Lateral aspect of scapula.

Humerus

The proximal end of the *humerus* (Fig. 5-5) consists of a head, an anatomic neck, two prominent processes called the greater and lesser tubercles (tuberosities), and the surgical neck. The *head* is large, smooth, and rounded, and lies in an oblique plane on the superomedial side of the humerus. Just below the head, lying in the same oblique plane, is the narrow, constricted *anatomic neck*. The constriction of the body (shaft) just below the tubercles (tuberosities) is called the *surgical neck,* the site of many fractures.

The *lesser tubercle* (tuberosity) (Figs. 5-5 and 5-6) is situated on the anterior surface of the bone, immediately below the anatomic neck. The tendon of the subscapularis muscle inserts at the lesser tubercle (tuberosity). The *greater tubercle* (tuberosity) is located on the lateral surface of the bone, just below the anatomic neck, and is separated from the lesser tubercle (tuberosity) by a deep depression called the *intertubercular* (bicipital) *groove.* The superior surface of the greater tubercle (tuberosity) slopes posteriorly at an angle of approximately 25 degrees and has three flattened impressions for muscle insertions. The anterior impression is the highest of the three and affords attachment to the tendon of the supraspinatus muscle. The middle impression is the point of insertion of the infraspinatus muscle. The tendon of the upper fibers of the teres minor muscle inserts at the posterior impression (the lower fibers insert into the body (shaft) of the bone immediately below this point).

Bursae are small synovial fluid-filled sacs that relieve pressure and reduce friction in tissue. They are often found between the bones and the skin and allow the skin to move easily when the joint is moved. Bursae also are found between bones and ligaments, muscles, or tendons. One of the largest bursae of the shoulder is the *subacromial* (deltoid) *bursa* (Fig. 5-7). It is located under the acromion process and lies between the deltoid muscle and the shoulder joint capsule. It does not normally communicate with the joint. Other bursae of the shoulder are found superior to the acromion, between the coracoid process and the joint capsule, and between the capsule and the tendon of the subscapularis muscle. Bursae become important radiographically when injury or age causes the deposition of calcium.

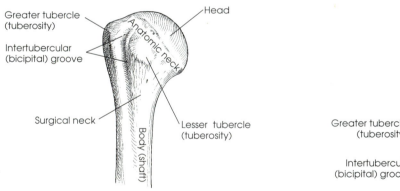

Fig. 5-5. Anterior aspect of proximal humerus.

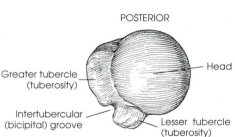

Fig. 5-6. Superior aspect of humerus.

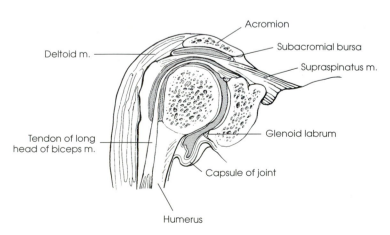

Fig. 5-7. Shoulder bursae.

Shoulder Girdle Articulations

SHOULDER ARTICULATION

The *scapulohumeral* articulation between the *glenoid cavity* (fossa) and the *head of the humerus* forms a synovial (diarthrotic) joint of the spheroidal (ball and socket) type, allowing movement in all directions (Fig. 5-8). Although many muscles connect with, support, and enter into the function of the shoulder joint, radiographers are chiefly concerned with the insertion points of the short rotator cuff muscles (Figs. 5-9 and 5-10). The insertion points of these muscles—the subscapularis, supraspinatus, infraspinatus, and teres minor—have already been described.

An *articular capsule* completely encloses the shoulder joint. The tendon of the long head of the biceps brachii muscle, which arises from the superior margin of the glenoid cavity (fossa), passes through the capsule of the shoulder joint, between its fibrous and synovial layers, arches over the head of the humerus, and descends through the intertubercular (bicipital) groove. The short head of the biceps arises from the coracoid process and, with the long head of the muscle, inserts in the radial tuberosity. Because it crosses with both the shoulder and elbow joints, the biceps help synchronize their action.

The interaction of movement between the wrist, elbow and shoulder joints makes the *position of the hand* important in radiography of the upper limb. Any rotation of the hand also rotates the joints. The best approach to the study of the mechanics of joint and muscle action is to perform all movements ascribed to each joint and carefully note the reaction in remote parts.

ACROMIOCLAVICULAR ARTICULATION

The articulation between the *acromion* process of the scapula and the acromial extremity of the *clavicle* is a synovial (diarthrotic) plane (gliding) joint. It permits both gliding and rotary (elevation, depression, protraction and retraction) movement. Because the end of the clavicle rides higher than the adjacent surface of the acromion, the slope of the surfaces tends to favor displacement of the acromion downward and under the clavicle.

STERNOCLAVICULAR ARTICULATION

The union of the medial end of the *clavicle* with the *manubrium* of the sternum is the only bony union between the upper limb and trunk. This articulation is synovial (diarthrotic) with the form of a plane (gliding) joint. However the joint is adapted by a fibrocartilaginous disc to provide movements similar to a ball and socket joint: circumduction, elevation, depression, and forward and backward movements. The clavicle carries the scapula with it through any movement.

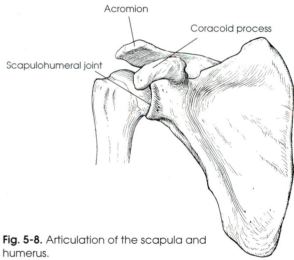

Fig. 5-8. Articulation of the scapula and humerus.

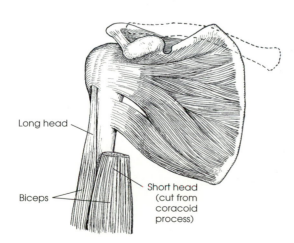

Fig. 5-9. Muscles on costal (anterior) surface of scapula and proximal humerus.

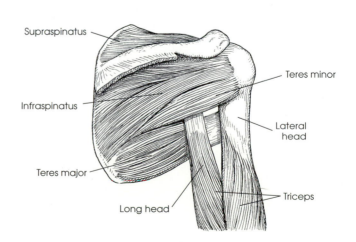

Fig. 5-10. Muscles on dorsal (posterior) surface of scapula and proximal humerus.

Radiation Protection

Protection of the patient from unnecessary radiation is a professional responsibility of the radiographer (see Chapter 1 for specific guidelines). In this chapter, the *"Shield gonads"* statement at the end of the "Position of part" section indicates that the patient is to be protected from unnecessary radiation by using proper collimation *and* the placing of lead shielding between the gonads and the radiation source to restrict the radiation beam.

Shoulder

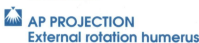

AP PROJECTION
External rotation humerus

NOTE: *Do not have the patient rotate the arm in cases of suspected fracture and/or dislocation.*

Film: 10×12 in (24×30 cm) crosswise or lengthwise, according to the area to be included.

Position of patient

• Examine the patient in the upright or the supine position. It must be recalled, however, that shoulder and arm lesions, whether traumatic or pathologic in origin, are extremely sensitive to movement and pressure. For this reason the upright position should be used whenever possible so that the patient's body position can be adjusted to require little or no manipulation of the arm.

Position of part

• Adjust the position of the cassette and the patient's body to center the film to a point 1 in (2.5 cm) inferior and 1 in (2.5 cm) medial to the coracoid process.
• To overcome the curve of the back and the resultant obliquity of the shoulder structures, it may be necessary to rotate the patient enough to place the body of the scapula parallel with the plane of the film.
• When the patient is in the supine position, support the elevated shoulder and hip on sandbags.
• When the patient is in this basic body position, locate the epicondyles, and, while holding them between the thumb and index fingers of one hand, adjust the arm as follows:
• Unless contraindicated, ask the patient to supinate the hand.
• Abduct the arm slightly and rotate it so that the coronal plane of the epicondyles is parallel with the plane of the film.

• When the patient is upright, immobilize the arm by resting the hand against an IV standard or the back of a chair. Externally rotating the entire arm from the neutral position places the shoulder and entire humerus in the true anatomical position (Fig. 5-11).
• *Shield gonads.*
• Ask the patient to suspend respiration for each exposure.

Central ray

• Direct the central ray perpendicular to a point 1 in (2.5 cm) inferior and 1 in (2.5 cm) medial to the coracoid process.

Structures shown

External rotation of the humerus allows demonstration of the bony and soft structures of the shoulder and proximal humerus in the anatomic position (Fig. 5-12). The scapulohumeral joint relationship and the region of the subacromial bursa are seen. The greater tubercle of the humerus and the site of insertion of the supraspinatus tendon are visualized.

□ Evaluation criteria

The following should be clearly demonstrated:

■ Superior scapula, lateral half of the clavicle, and proximal humerus.
■ Soft tissue around the shoulder, along with bony trabecular detail.
■ Humeral head in profile.
■ Greater tubercle in profile on the lateral aspect of the humerus.
■ Scapulohumeral joint visualized with slight overlap of humeral head on glenoid cavity.
■ Outline of lesser tubercle between humeral head and greater tubercle.

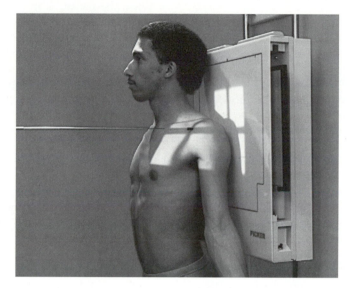

Fig. 5-11. AP shoulder. External rotation humerous.

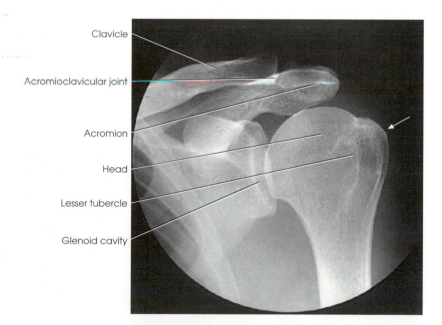

Clavicle

Acromioclavicular joint

Acromion

Head

Lesser tubercle

Glenoid cavity

Fig. 5-12. AP shoulder. External rotation humerus; greater tubercle (arrow).

127

Shoulder

AP PROJECTION
Neutral rotation humerus

Film: 10 × 12 in (24 × 30 cm) crosswise or lengthwise, according to the area to be included.

Position of patient

- Examine the patient in the upright or the supine position. It must be recalled, however, that shoulder and arm lesions, whether traumatic or pathologic in origin, are extremely sensitive to movement and pressure. For this reason the upright position should be used whenever possible so that the patient's body position can be adjusted to require little or no manipulation of the arm.

Position of part

- Adjust the position of the cassette and the patient's body to center the film to a point 1 in (2.5 cm) inferior and 1 in (2.5 cm) medial to the coracoid process.
- To overcome the curve of the back and the resultant obliquity of the shoulder structures, it may be necessary to rotate the patient enough to place the body of the scapula parallel with the plane of the film.

- When the patient is in the supine position, support the elevated shoulder and hip on sandbags.
- When the patient is in this basic body position, locate the epicondyles, and, while holding them between the thumb and index fingers of one hand, adjust the arm as follows:
- Ask the patient to rest the palm of his or her hand against the thigh. This position of the arm rolls the humerus slightly internal into a neutral position, placing the coronal plane of the epicondyles at an angle of about 45 degrees with the plane of the film (Fig. 5-13).
- *Shield gonads.*
- Ask the patient to suspend respiration for each exposure.

Central ray

- Direct the central ray perpendicular to a point 1 in (2.5 cm) inferior and 1 in (2.5 cm) medial to the coracoid process.

Structures shown

Fig. 5-14 demonstrates the posterior part of the supraspinatus insertion, sometimes profiling small calcific deposits not otherwise visualized.

□ Evaluation criteria

The following should be clearly demonstrated:

- Superior scapula, lateral half of the clavicle, and proximal humerus.
- Soft tissue around the shoulder, along with bony trabecular detail.
- Greater tubercle partially superimposing the humeral head.
- Humeral head in partial profile.
- Slight overlap of the humeral head on the glenoid cavity.

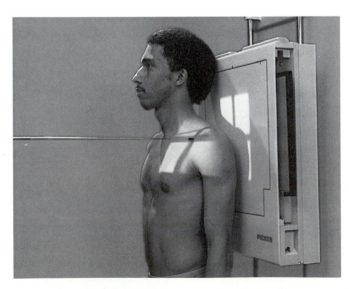

Fig. 5-13. AP shoulder. Neutral rotation humerus.

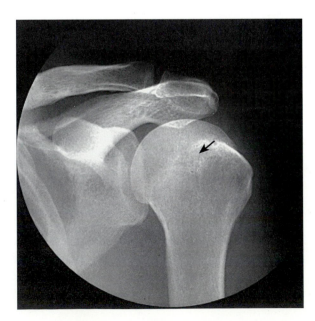

Fig. 5-14. AP shoulder. Neutral rotation humerus; greater tubercle (*arrow*).

Shoulder

 ## AP PROJECTION
Internally rotated humerus

Film: 10 × 12 in (24 × 30 cm) crosswise or lengthwise, according to the area to be included.

Position of patient

- Examine the patient in the upright or the supine position. It must be recalled, however, that shoulder and arm lesions, whether traumatic or pathologic in origin, are extremely sensitive to movement and pressure. For this reason the upright position should be used whenever possible so that the patient's body position can be adjusted to require little or no manipulation of the arm.

Position of part

- Adjust the position of the cassette and the patient's body to center the film to a point 1 in (2.5 cm) inferior and 1 in (2.5 cm) medial to the coracoid process.
- To overcome the curve of the back and the resultant obliquity of the shoulder structures, it may be necessary to rotate the patient enough to place the body of the scapula parallel with the plane of the film.

- When the patient is in the supine position, support the elevated shoulder and hip on sandbags.
- When the patient is in this basic body position, locate the epicondyles, and, while holding them between the thumb and index fingers of one hand, adjust the arm as follows:
- Ask the patient to flex the elbow somewhat, rotate the arm internally, and rest the back of the hand on the hip.
- Adjust the arm to place the coronal plane of the epicondyles perpendicular to the plane of the film. (When the shoulder is too painful for adequate internal rotation of the arm, the patient may turn somewhat away from the film. However, if the object-to-image receptor distance becomes too great, the patient should be turned for adjustment from a PA projection.) This adjustment of the arm in the internal rotation position rolls the humerus into the true lateral position (Fig. 5-15).
- *Shield gonads.*
- Ask the patient to suspend respiration for each exposure.

Central ray

- Direct the central ray perpendicular to a point 1 in (2.5 cm) inferior and 1 in (2.5 cm) medial to the coracoid process.

Structures shown

With the arm in internal rotation, the region of the subacromial bursa is demonstrated. When the arm can be abducted enough to clear the lesser tubercle of the head of the scapula, a profile image of the site of the insertion of the subscapularis tendon is seen (Fig 5-16).

□Evaluation criteria

The following should be clearly demonstrated:
- Superior scapula, lateral half of the clavicle, and proximal humerus.
- Soft tissue around the shoulder, along with bony trabecular detail.
- Lesser tubercle in profile and pointing medially.
- Outline of the greater tubercle superimposing the humeral head.
- Greater amount of humeral overlap of the glenoid cavity than in the external and neutral positions.

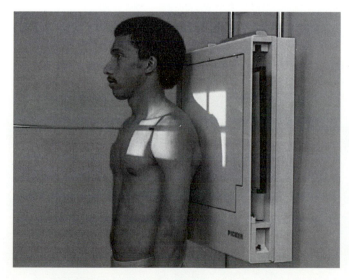
Fig. 5-15. AP shoulder. Internal rotation humerus.

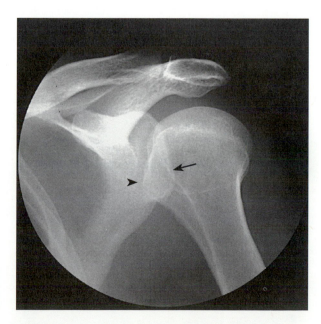
Fig. 5-16. AP shoulder. Internal rotation humerus. Greater tubercle (*arrow*); *lesser* tubercle shown in profile (*arrowhead*).

Shoulder

 TRANSTHORACIC LATERAL PROJECTION
R or L position
LAWRENCE METHOD[1]

The Lawrence method is used when the arm cannot be rotated or abducted due to injury or the inability of the patient to move the arm.

Film: 10 × 12 in (24 × 30 cm) lengthwise.

Position of patient

Although this position can be carried out with the patient in the upright or the supine position, the upright position facilitates accurate adjustment of the shoulder. For upright positioning:
- Seat or stand the patient in the lateral position before a vertical grid device (Fig 5-17).
- If an upright position is not possible, place the patient in a recumbent position on the table with radiolucent pads elevating the head and shoulders (Fig. 5-18).

---

[1]Lawrence WS: A method of obtaining an accurate lateral roentgenogram of the shoulder joint. AJR 5:193-194, 1918.

Position of part

- Have the patient raise the uninjured arm, rest the forearm on the head, and elevate the shoulder as much as possible (Fig. 5-17). Elevation of the uninjured shoulder will give the desired depression of the injured side, separating the shoulders to prevent superimposition. Ensure that median coronal plane is perpendicular to the film.
- No attempt should be made to rotate or otherwise move the injured arm.
- Center the cassette to the surgical neck of the affected humerus.
- *Shield gonads.*
- *Respiration options:*
  - For control of *respiration,* instruct the patient to hold his or her breath at *full inspiration* when ready to make the exposure. Having the lungs full of air improves the contrast and decreases the exposure necessary to penetrate the body.
  - When the patient is able to hold his or her breath for 5 or 6 seconds, lung detail may be blurred considerably by the action of the heart. When this is possible, maintain the usual mAs factor but convert to a low mA–long exposure time combination.
  - If the patient can be sufficiently immobilized to prevent voluntary motion, breathing motion can be utilized. In this case, instruct the patient in, and have him or her practice, slow, deep breathing. An exposure time of 4 to 5 seconds will give excellent results.

Central ray

- Direct the central ray perpendicular to the median coronal plane, exiting the surgical neck of the affected humerus.
- If the patient cannot elevate the unaffected shoulder, angle the central ray 10 to 15 degrees cephalad to obtain a comparable radiograph.

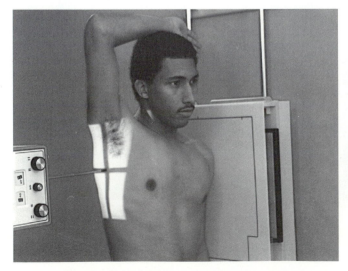

Fig. 5-17. Upright transthoracic lateral shoulder.

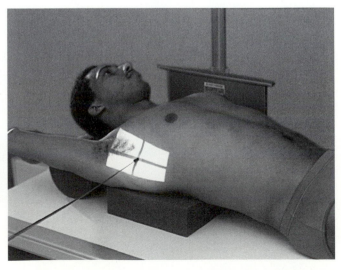

Fig. 5-18. Recumbent transthoracic lateral shoulder.

Structures shown

A lateral image of the shoulder and proximal humerus is seen, projected through the thorax (Figs. 5-19 and 5-20).

□ Evaluation criteria

The following should be clearly demonstrated:

- Proximal humerus.
- Scapula, clavicle, and humerus seen through the lung field.
- Scapula superimposed over the thoracic spine.
- Unaffected clavicle and humerus projected above the shoulder closest to the film.

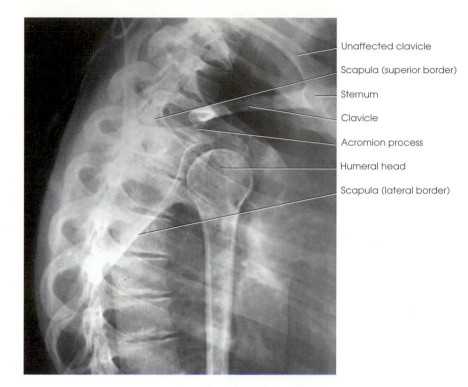

Unaffected clavicle
Scapula (superior border)
Sternum
Clavicle
Acromion process
Humeral head
Scapula (lateral border)

Fig. 5-19. Transthoracic lateral shoulder.

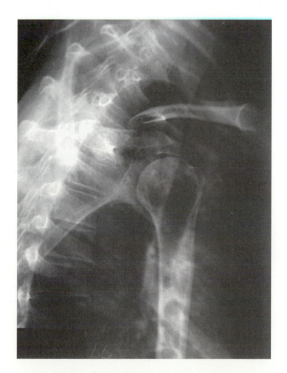

Fig. 5-20. Transthoracic lateral shoulder (patient breathing).

(Courtesy Laurie Funk, R.T.)

Shoulder Joint

INFEROSUPERIOR AXIAL PROJECTION
LAWRENCE METHOD

When abduction is limited, inferosuperior radiographs of the shoulder may be more easily obtained with the patient in the seated position. If necessary, a mobile x-ray unit may be helpful. The upright body position is contraindicated for trauma patients unless the injured arm is moved by the physician.

Film: 8 × 10 in (18 × 24 cm) placed in the vertical position in contact with the superior surface of the shoulder.

Position of patient

- With the patient in the supine position, elevate the head, shoulders and elbow about 3 or 4 inches.

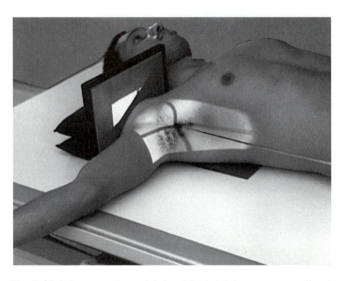

Fig. 5-21. Inferosuperior axial shoulder joint: Lawrence method.

Position of part

- As nearly as possible, abduct the arm of the affected side at right angles to the long axis of the body.
- Keep the humerus in external rotation, and adjust the forearm and hand in a comfortable position, grasping a vertical support or extended on sandbags or a firm pillow. Support may be needed under the forearm and hand. Provide patient with an extension board.
- Have the patient turn the head away from the side being examined, if necessary, to permit the cassette to be against the neck.
- Place the cassette on edge over the shoulder and as close as possible to the neck.
- Support the cassette in position with sandbags or vertical cassette holder (Figs. 5-21 and 5-22).
- *Shield gonads.*
- Ask the patient to suspend respiration for the exposure.

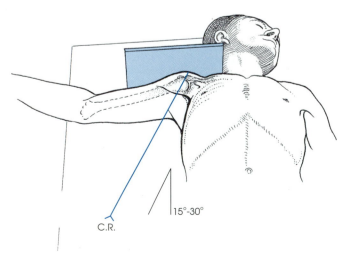

15°-30°

C.R.

Fig. 5-22. Lawrence method with medial CR angulation.

Central ray

- Direct the central ray horizontally through the axilla to the region of the acromioclavicular articulation.
- The degree of medial angulation of the central ray depends on the degree of abduction of the arm. The degree of medial angulation is often between 15 and 30 degrees. The greater the abduction, the greater the angle.

Structures shown

An inferosuperior axial image shows the proximal humerus, scapulohumeral joint, the lateral portion of the coracoid process, and the acromioclavicular articulation. The insertion site of the subscapularis tendon on the lesser tubercle of the humerus and the point of insertion of the teres minor tendon on the greater tubercle of the humerus are also shown (Figs. 5-23 and 5-24).

□Evaluation criteria

The following should be clearly demonstrated:

- Scapulohumeral joint with slight overlap.
- Coracoid process, pointing anteriorly.
- Lesser tubercle in profile and directed anteriorly.
- Acromioclavicular joint, acromion, and acromial end of clavicle projected through the humeral head.
- Soft tissue in the axilla with bony trabecular detail.
- Axillary structures.

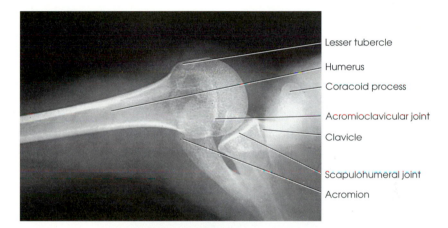

Lesser tubercle
Humerus
Coracoid process
Acromioclavicular joint
Clavicle
Scapulohumeral joint
Acromion

Fig. 5-23. Inferosuperior axial shoulder joint: Lawrence method.

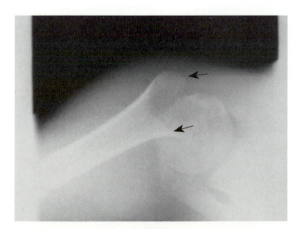

Fig. 5-24. Inferosuperior axial shoulder joint: Lawrence method with little arm abduction due to fracture of surgical neck *(arrows)*.

(Courtesy Roland W. Clements, R.T., F.A.S.R.T.)

Shoulder Joint

INFEROSUPERIOR AXIAL PROJECTION
WEST POINT METHOD[1]

Film: 8 × 10 in (18 × 24 cm) placed in the vertical position in contact with the superior surface of the shoulder.

Position of patient

- Adjust the patient in the prone position with approximately a 3-inch pad under the shoulder being examined.
- Turn the patient's head away from the side being examined.

[1]Rokous JR, Feagin JA, and Abbott HG: Modified axillary roentgenogram, Clin Orthop 82:84-86, 1972.

Position of part

- Abduct the arm of the affected side *90 degrees* and rotate so the forearm rests over the edge of the table, or a Bucky tray, which may be used for support.
- Turn the patient's palm down (Figs. 5-25 and 5-26).
- Place a vertically supported cassette against the superior aspect of the shoulder with the edge of the cassette in contact with the neck.
- Support the cassette with sandbags or a vertical cassette holder.
- *Shield gonads.*
- Ask the patient to suspend respiration for the exposure.

Central ray

- Direct the central ray at a dual angle of 25 degrees *anteriorly* from the horizontal and 25 degrees *medially*. The central ray enters approximately 5 in (12 to 14 cm) inferior, and 1½ in (3 to 4 cm) medial, to the acromial edge and exits the glenoid cavity.

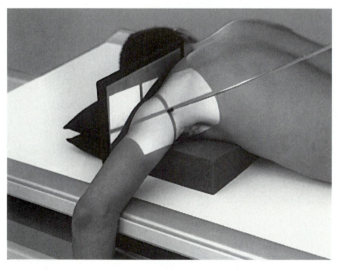

Fig. 5-25. Inferosuperior axial shoulder joint: West Point method.

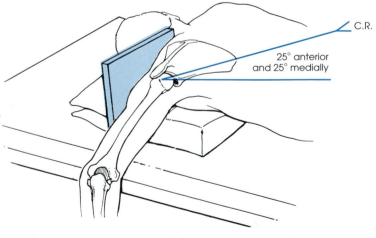

Fig. 5-26. West Point method with anterior and medial CR angulation.

Structures shown

The resulting image will show bony abnormalities of the glenoid rim in patients with instability of the shoulder (Fig. 5-27).

The following should be clearly demonstrated:

- The humeral head, projected free of the coracoid process.
- Articulation between the head of the humerus and the glenoid cavity.
- Acromion superimposed over the posterior portion of humeral head.

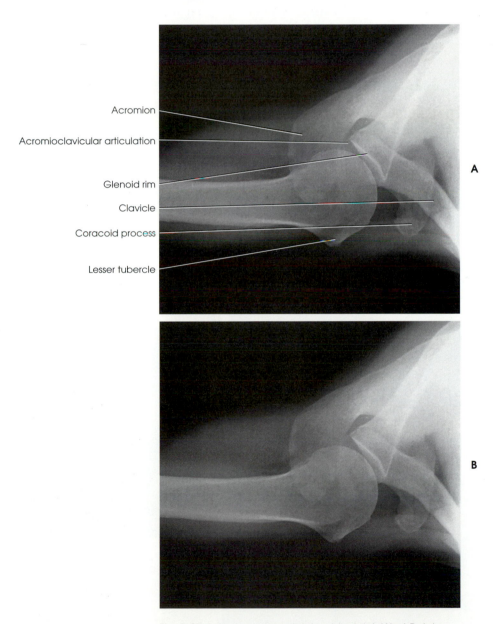

Acromion

Acromioclavicular articulation

Glenoid rim

Clavicle

Coracoid process

Lesser tubercle

A

B

Fig. 5-27. Inferosuperior axial shoulder joint: West Point method.

(Courtesy Julianne M. Curtin, R.T.)

Shoulder Joint
INFEROSUPERIOR AXIAL PROJECTION
CLEMENTS MODIFICATION[1]

Film: 8 × 10 in (18 × 24 cm) placed in the vertical position in contact with the superior surface of the shoulder.

Position of patient

- When the prone or supine position is not possible, Clements[1] suggests the patient be radiographed in the lateral recumbent position lying on the unaffected side.
- Flex the patient's hips and knees.

---

[1]Clements RW: Adaptation of the technique for radiography of the glenohumeral joint in the lateral position. Radiol Technol 51:305-312, 1979.

Position of part

- Abduct the affected arm 90 degrees and point it toward the ceiling.
- Place the cassette against the superior aspect of the patient's shoulder, holding it in place by the unaffected arm or by securing it appropriately (Fig. 5-28, *A*).
- *Shield gonads.*
- Ask the patient to suspend respiration for the exposure.

Central ray

- Direct the central ray horizontal to the median coronal plane, passing through the midaxillary region of the shoulder.
- Angle the central ray 5 to 15 degrees medially when the patient cannot abduct the arm a full 90 degrees (Fig. 5-28, *B*). The resulting radiograph is seen in Fig. 5-29.

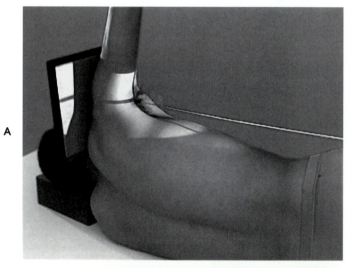
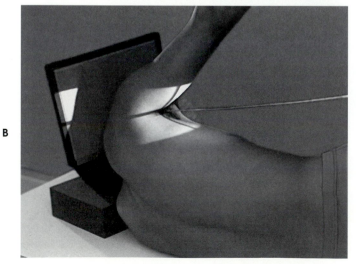

Fig. 5-28. Inferosuperior axial shoulder joint: Clements modification. **A,** Arm abducted 90 degrees. **B,** Arm partially abducted.

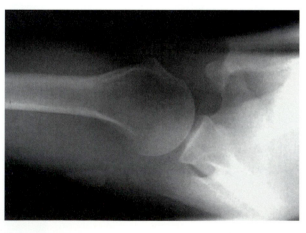

Fig. 5-29. Inferosuperior axial shoulder joint: Clements modification.

(Courtesy Roland W. Clements, R.T., F.A.S.R.T.)

Shoulder Joint

SUPEROINFERIOR AXIAL PROJECTION

Before undertaking this position verify the patient's ability to abduct the arm to a near right angle to the long axis of the body and the advisability of doing so.

Film: 8 × 10 in (18 × 24 cm) film placed lengthwise for accurate centering to the shoulder joint. A curved cassette may be used for this position to reduce the object-to-image receptor distance.

Position of patient

- Seat the patient at the end of the table on a stool or chair high enough to enable him or her to extend the shoulder being examined well over the cassette.
- Center the shoulder to the midline of the cassette.

Position of part

- Place the cassette near the end of the table and parallel with its long axis.
- Ask the patient to hold the hand of the affected side and raise the arm to a position as near as possible at right angles to the long axis of the body. Then have the patient lean laterally over the cassette until the shoulder joint is over the midpoint of the film.
- Bring the elbow to rest on the table.
- Flex the patient's elbow 90 degrees and place the hand in the prone position (Figs. 5-30 and 5-31).
- Have the patient tilt the head toward the unaffected shoulder.
- To obtain a direct lateral of the head of the humerus, adjust any anterior or posterior leaning of the body to place the humeral epicondyles in the vertical position.
- *Shield gonads.*
- Ask the patient to suspend respiration for the exposure.

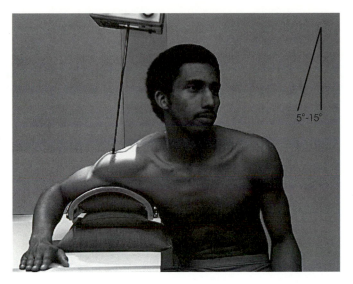

Fig. 5-30. Superoinferior axial shoulder joint: curved cassette.

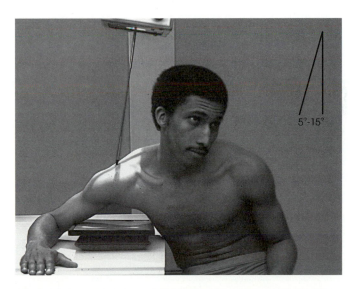

Fig. 5-31. Superoinferior axial shoulder joint: standard cassette.

SUPEROINFERIOR AXIAL PROJECTION, cont'd

Central ray

• Direct the central ray to the shoulder joint at an angle of 5 to 15 degrees toward the elbow.

Structures shown

A superoinferior axial image shows the joint relationship of the proximal end of the humerus and the glenoid cavity (Figs. 5-32 and 5-33). The acromioclavicular articulation, the outer portion of the coracoid process, and the points of insertion of the subscapularis and (body of scapula) teres minor (inferior axillary border) are demonstrated. Depending on the flexibility of the patient, a greater or lesser portion of the medial structures is shown.

☐ Evaluation criteria

The following should be clearly demonstrated:

■ Open scapulohumeral joint; not open on patients with limited flexibility.
■ Coracoid process projected above the clavicle.
■ Lesser tubercle in profile.
■ Acromioclavicular joint through the humeral head.
■ Soft tissue in the axilla with bony trabecular detail.

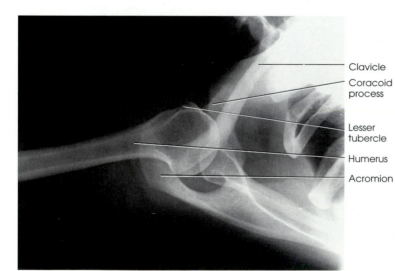

Clavicle
Coracoid process
Lesser tubercle
Humerus
Acromion

Fig. 5-32. Superoinferior axial shoulder joint.

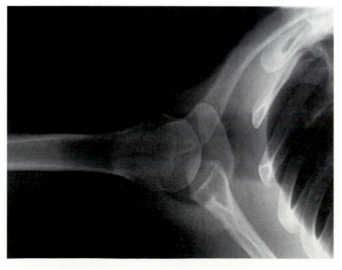

Fig. 5-33. Superoinferior axial shoulder joint.

Shoulder Joint

ROLLED-FILM AXIAL PROJECTION
CLEAVES METHOD

Cleaves[1] devised a method of obtaining an axial projection of the shoulder joint for use with patients who cannot or should not abduct the arm enough for one of the preliminary axial radiographs.

Film: 8 × 10 in (18 × 24 cm).

This position requires that an 8 × 10 in film be enclosed in a lightproof envelope and gently curved around a small tube approximately 2 inches in diameter. A tube smaller than 2 inches will cause too much distortion on the radiograph, and a tube that is too large will be difficult to place high in the axilla.

To reduce radiation exposure to the patient, the envelope used to enclose the film may include flexible intensifying screens. The loaded envelope is curved around the tube and secured at each end. If screens are used, extreme care must be taken to avoid damaging them when loading and unloading.

---

[1]Cleaves EN: A new film holder for roentgen examination of the shoulder, AJR 45:288-290, 1941.

Position of patient

- Seat the patient laterally at the end of the table. When necessary, adapt this position for the supine patient.

Position of part

- Place the film roll as high in the axilla as possible and adjust it so that it is horizontal (Fig. 5-34). Ensure that the forearm is resting on the tabletop if the sitting position is used.
- *Shield gonads.*
- Ask the patient to suspend respiration for the exposure.

Central ray

- Direct the central ray perpendicular to the shoulder, entering 1 cm posterior to the acromioclavicular joint (Fig. 5-35).

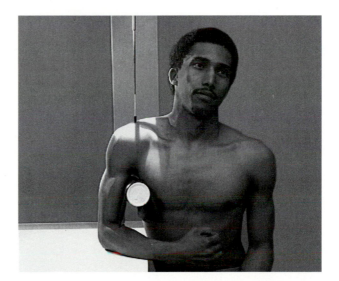

Fig. 5-34. Axial shoulder joint: Cleaves method. Rolled film.

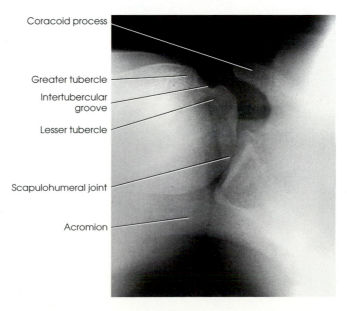

Fig. 5-35. Axial shoulder joint: Cleaves method. Angulation of 0 degrees.

Variations

- Direct the central ray to the acromio-clavicular articulation (1) at a 5-degree medial angulation to demonstrate the lesser tubercle and intertubercular (bicipital) groove (Fig. 5-36), and (2) at a 5-degree lateral angulation to demonstrate the coracoid process (Fig. 5-37).

Structures shown

An axial image demonstrates the scapulohumeral joint, greater and lesser tubercles, intertubercular (bicipital) groove, and coracoid process (Figs. 5-35 to 5-37).

□ Evaluation criteria

The following should be clearly demonstrated:

- Scapulohumeral joint open and visualized.
- Coracoid, intertubercular (bicipital) groove, and humeral tubercles.

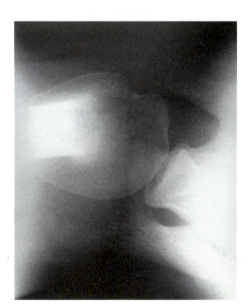

Fig. 5-36. Axial shoulder joint: Cleaves method. Medial angulation of 5 degrees.

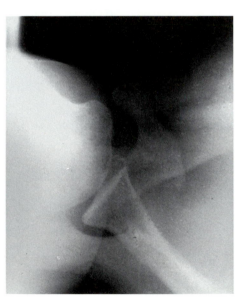

Fig. 5-37. Axial shoulder joint: Cleaves method. Lateral angulation of 5 degrees.

Shoulder Joint

AP AXIAL PROJECTION

Film: 8 × 10 in (18 × 24 cm) crosswise.

Position of patient

- Position the patient in the upright or supine body position.

Position of part

- Center the scapulohumeral joint of the shoulder being examined to the midline of the grid (Fig. 5-38).
- *Shield gonads.*
- Ask the patient to suspend respiration for the exposure.

Central ray

- Direct the central ray through the scapulohumeral joint at a cephalic angle of 35 degrees.

Structures shown

The axial image shows the relationship of the head of the humerus to the glenoid cavity. This is useful in diagnosing cases of posterior dislocation (Fig. 5-39).

□ Evaluation criteria

The following should be clearly demonstrated:

- ■ Scapulohumeral joint.
- ■ Proximal humerus.
- ■ Clavicle projected above superior angle of scapula.

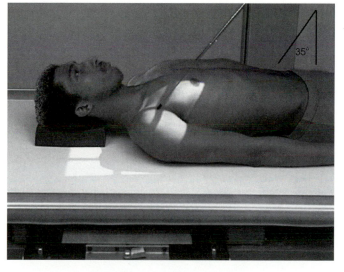

Fig. 5-38. AP axial shoulder joint.

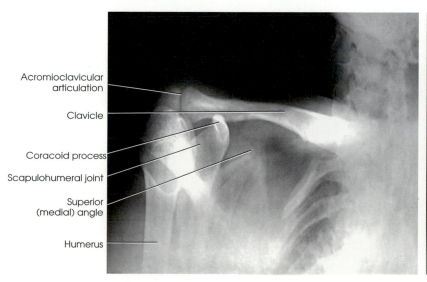
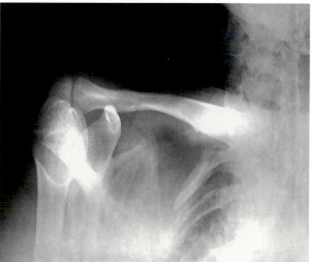

Acromioclavicular articulation

Clavicle

Coracoid process

Scapulohumeral joint

Superior (medial) angle

Humerus

Fig. 5-39. AP axial shoulder joint.

Shoulder Joint

 **PA OBLIQUE PROJECTION
RAO or LAO position
SCAPULAR Y**

This projection, described by Rubin, Gray, and Green,[1] obtained its name as a result of the appearance of the scapula. The body of the scapula forms the vertical component of the Y and the acromion and coracoid processes form the upper limbs. The projection is useful in the evaluation of suspected shoulder dislocations.

Film: 10 × 12 in (24 × 30 cm)

Position of patient

- The patient may be radiographed in the upright or recumbent body position; the upright position is preferred if the shoulder is tender.
- When the patient is severely injured, the anterior oblique position can be modified by placing the patient in the posterior oblique position.

[1]Rubin SA, Gray RL, and Green WR: The scapular Y: a diagnostic aid in shoulder trauma, Radiol. 110:725-726, 1974.

Position of part

- With the anterior surface of the shoulder being examined centered to the cassette, rotate the patient so the median coronal plane forms an angle of 60 degrees from the film. The position of the arm is not critical since it does not alter the relationship of the humeral head to the glenoid cavity (Fig. 5-40).
- *Shield gonads.*
- Ask the patient to suspend respiration for the exposure.

Central ray

- Direct the central ray perpendicular to the shoulder joint at the level of the scapulohumeral joint.

Structures shown

The scapular Y is demonstrated on an oblique image of the shoulder. In the normal shoulder, the humeral head is directly superimposed over the junction of the Y (Fig. 5-41). In anterior (subcoracoid) dislocations, the humeral head is beneath the coracoid process (Fig. 5-42); in posterior (subacromial) dislocations, it is projected beneath the acromion process. An AP shoulder projection is shown for comparison (Fig. 5-43).

□Evaluation criteria

The following should be clearly demonstrated:
- No superimposition of the scapular body over the bony thorax.
- Acromion projected laterally and free of superimposition.
- Coracoid possibly superimposed or projected below the clavicle.
- Scapula in lateral profile.

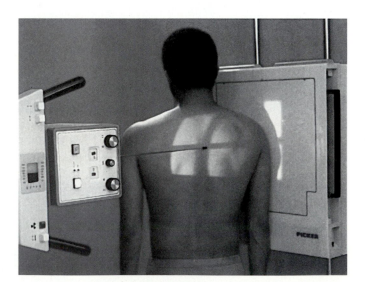

Fig. 5-40. PA oblique shoulder joint.

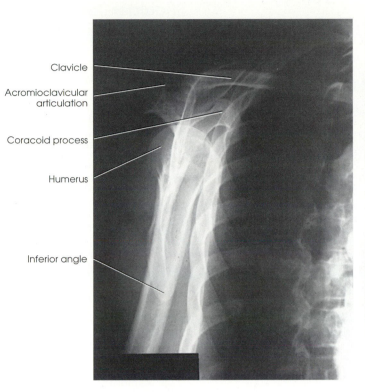

Clavicle

Acromioclavicular articulation

Coracoid process

Humerus

Inferior angle

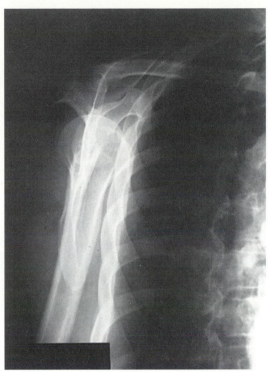

Fig. 5-41. PA oblique shoulder joint. Note the scapular Y components—body, acromian, and coracoid.

(Courtesy Roland W. Clements, R.T., F.A.S.R.T.)

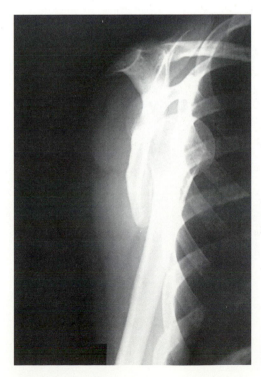

Fig. 5-42. PA oblique shoulder joint showing anterior dislocation (humeral head projected beneath coracoid process).

(Courtesy Roland W. Clements, R.T., F.A.S.R.T.)

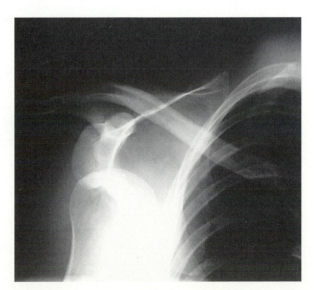

Fig. 5-43. AP shoulder (same patient as shown in Fig. 5-42).

(Courtesy Roland W. Clements, R.T., F.A.S.R.T.)

143

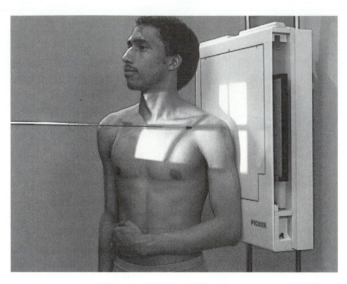

Fig. 5-44. Upright AP oblique glenoid cavity: Grashey method.

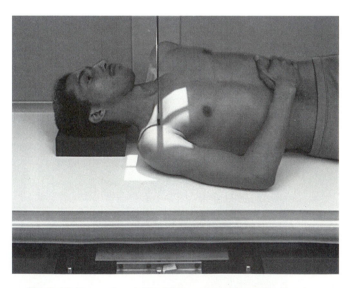

Fig. 5-45. Recumbent AP oblique glenoid cavity: Grashey method.

Shoulder Joint

AP OBLIQUE PROJECTION:
Glenoid Cavity
RPO or LPO position
GRASHEY METHOD

Film: 8 × 10 in (18 × 24 cm) or 10 × 12 in (24 × 30 cm) crosswise.

Position of patient

- Although to demonstrate the glenoid cavity, this position can be achieved with the patient in the supine or upright position, the upright position is more comfortable for the patient and facilitates accurate adjustment of the part.

Position of part

- Center the cassette to the scapulohumeral joint.
- Rotate the body approximately 35 to 45 degrees toward the affected side (Fig. 5-44).
- Adjust the degree of rotation to place the scapula parallel with the plane of the film and the head of the humerus in contact with it.
- If the patient is in the supine position, the body may need to be rotated more than 45 degrees to place the scapula parallel to the film.
- In addition, support the elevated shoulder and hip on sandbags (Fig. 5-45).
- Abduct the arm slightly in internal rotation. Place palm of the hand on the abdomen.
- *Shield gonads.*
- Ask the patient to suspend respiration.

Central ray

- Direct the central ray perpendicular to the glenoid cavity at a point 2 inches medial and 2 inches distal to the superolateral border of the shoulder.

Structures shown

The joint space between the humeral head and the glenoid cavity (scapulohumeral joint) is shown (Fig. 5-46).

□ **Evaluation criteria**

The following should be clearly demonstrated:

- Open joint space between the humeral head and glenoid cavity.
- Glenoid cavity in profile.
- Soft tissue at the scapulohumeral joint along with trabecular detail on the glenoid and humeral head.

NOTE: Kornguth and Salazar[1] reported a projection similar to the 45-degree AP oblique shoulder just described. For their apical oblique projection, the central ray enters the coracoid process with a caudal angulation of 45 degrees. The patient remains in a 45-degree oblique position with the affected shoulder against the film.

[1]Kornguth PJ and Salazar AM: The apical oblique view of the shoulder: its usefulness in acute trauma, AJR 149:113-116, July 1987.

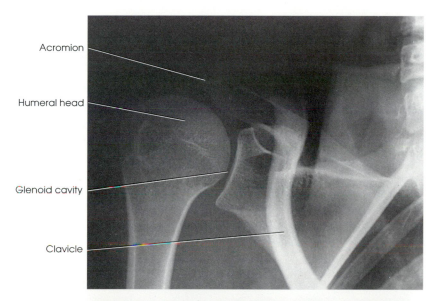

Acromion

Humeral head

Glenoid cavity

Clavicle

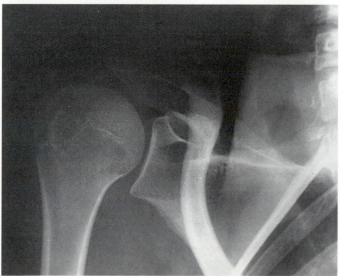

Fig. 5-46. AP oblique glenoid cavity: Grashey method.

Shoulder Joint
TANGENTIAL PROJECTION:
Supraspinatus "Outlet"[1,2]:
RAO or LAO position

This radiographic projection is useful to tangentially demonstrate the coracoacromial arch for diagnostic information needed to diagnose shoulder impingement. The tangential image is obtained by projecting the x-ray beam under the acromion and acromioclavicular joint, which defines the superior border of the coracoacromial outlet.

Film: 10×12 in (24×30 cm).

Position of patient

- Place the patient in a seated or standing position facing the radiographic film.

---

[1]Neer CS II: Acromioplasty for the chronic impingement syndrome in the shoulder: a preliminary report, J Bone Joint Surg 54-A, 41-50, 1972.
[2]Neer CS II: Shoulder reconstruction, WB Saunders, Philadelphia, pp. 14-24, 1990.

Position of part

- With the patient's affected shoulder centered and in contact with the film, rotate the patient's unaffected side away from the film until the palpated affected scapula is perpendicular to the film.
- The degree of patient obliquity varies from patient to patient. The average degree of patient rotation varies from 50 to 60 degrees from the plane of the film (Fig. 5-47).
- *Shield gonads.*
- Ask the patient to suspend respiration for the exposure.

Central ray

- Direct the central ray 10 to 15 degrees caudad, entering the medial aspect of the humeral head and exiting the posterosuperior surface of the clavicle.

Structures shown

The tangential outlet image demonstrates the posterior surface of the acromion and the acromioclavicular joint identified as the superior border of the coracoacromial outlet (Figs. 5-48 and 5-49).

☐Evaluation criteria

The following should be clearly demonstrated:
- Humeral head projected below the acromioclavicular joint.
- Humeral head and acromioclavicular joint with bony detail.
- The humerus and scapular body, generally parallel.

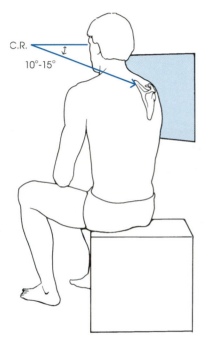

Fig. 5-47. Tangential supraspinatus "outlet" projection.

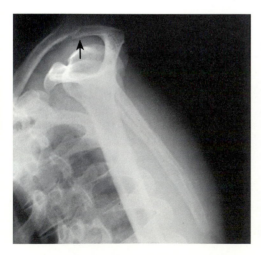

Fig. 5-48. Tangential supraspinatus "outlet" on patient showing impingement of the shoulder outlet *(arrow)*.

(Courtesy Karen J. Bauer, R.T.)

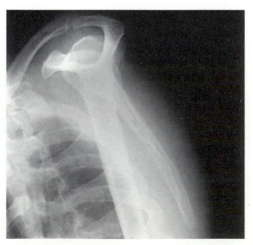

Fig. 5-49. Radiograph on same patient as Fig. 5-48 after surgical removal of posterolateral surface of clavicle.

(Courtesy Karen Bauer, R.T.)

Proximal Humerus

AP AXIAL PROJECTION
Humeral Notch[1]

Dislocations of the shoulder are frequently caused by posterior defects involving the head of the humerus. Such defects are often not demonstrated using conventional radiographic positions. Hall, Isaac, and Booth[2] described the notch projection, from ideas expressed by Stryker,[1] as being useful in identifying the cause of shoulder dislocation.

Film: 10 × 12 in (24 × 30 cm).

Position of patient

- Place the patient on the radiographic table in the supine position.

---

[1]This position was credited to its originator, Commander William S. Stryker, United States Naval Hospital, Corona, CA, in 1953. All individuals requested to avoid eponymous designation.
[2]Hall RH, Isaac F, and Booth CR: Dislocations of the shoulder with special reference to accompanying small fractures, J Bone Joint Surg 41-A(3): 489-494, 1959.

Position of part

- With the coracoid process of the affected shoulder centered to the table, ask the patient to flex the arm slightly beyond 90 degrees and place the palm of the hand on top of the head with the fingertips resting on the top of the head. (This hand position places the humerus in a slight internal rotation position.) The body (shaft) of the humerus is adjusted to be vertical so that it is parallel with the median sagittal plane of the body (Fig. 5-50).
- *Shield gonads.*
- Ask the patient to suspend respiration for the exposure.

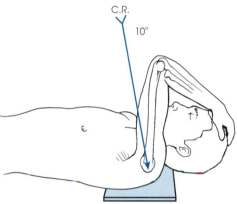

C.R.

10°

Fig. 5-50. AP axial humeral notch.

Central ray

- Direct the central ray 10 degrees cephalad, entering the coracoid process.

Structures shown

The resulting image will show the posterosuperior and anteroinferior areas of the humeral head (Fig. 5-51).

☐ Evaluation criteria

The following should be clearly demonstrated:

- Overlapping of coracoid process and clavicle.
- The long axis of the humerus aligned with the long axis of the patient's body.
- Bony trabeculation of the head of the humerus.

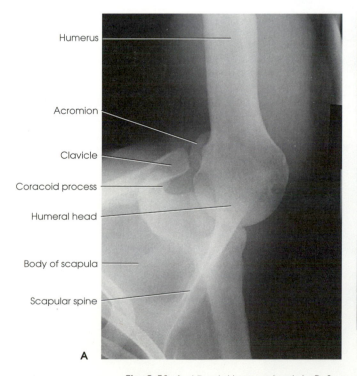

Humerus

Acromion

Clavicle

Coracoid process

Humeral head

Body of scapula

Scapular spine

A

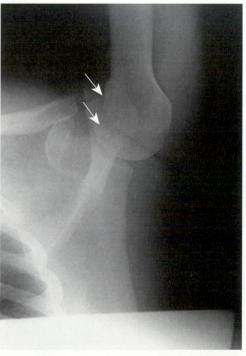

B

Fig. 5-51. A, AP axial humeral notch. **B,** Same projection on patient with small Hill-Sachs defect *(arrows)*.

(Courtesy April S. Apple, R.T.)

Proximal Humerus

TANGENTIAL PROJECTION
Intertubercular Groove

In recent years, various modifications of the intertubercular groove image have been devised. In all cases, the central ray is aligned to be tangent to the intertubercular groove, which lies on the anterior surface of the humerus.

A regular or a flexible cassette (the type used for panoramic examinations containing intensifying screens) may be used. The flexible cassette allows the film to be placed closer to the shoulder than with a rigid cassette.

A limitation in performing this examination can be the x-ray tube head assembly. Some radiographic units have large collimators and/or handles that limit flexibility in positioning. A mobile radiographic unit may be used to reduce this difficulty.

Film: 8×10 in (24×30 cm).

Position of patient

- Place the patient in the supine, seated, or standing position.
- Extending the chin or rotating the head away from the affected side permits improved centering.

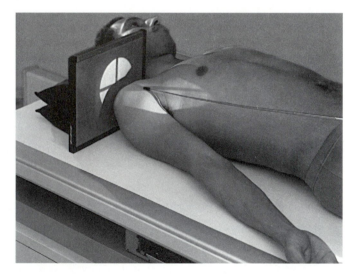

Fig. 5-52. Supine tangential intertubercular groove.

Position of part

- With the patient supine, palpate the anterior surface of the shoulder to locate the intertubercular groove.
- With the patient's hand in the supinated position, place the film against the superior surface of the shoulder and immobilize the film as seen in Fig. 5-52.
- *Shield gonads.*
- Ask the patient to suspend respiration for the exposure.

Fisk[1] first described this position with the patient standing at the end of the radiographic table; this employs a greater object-to-image receptor distance. The following steps are then taken with Fisk's technique:

- Instruct the patient to flex the elbow and lean forward far enough to place the posterior surface of the forearm on the table.
- The patient supports and grasps the cassette as depicted in Fig. 5-53.
- For radiation protection and to reduce the backscatter to the film from the forearm, place a lead shielding between the cassette back and the forearm.
- Place a sandbag under the hand to place the film horizontal.
- Have the patient lean forward or backward as required to place the humerus at an angle of 10 to 15 degrees, open anteriorly from the vertical.

---

[1]Fisk C: Adaptation of the technique for radiography of the bicipital groove, Radiol Technol 34:47-50, 1965.

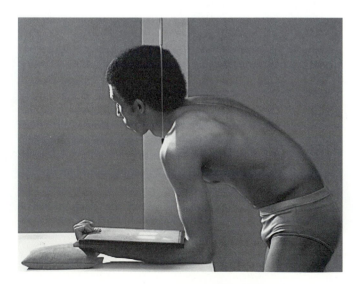

Fig. 5-53. Standing tangential intertubercular groove.

Central ray

- Direct the central ray 10 to 15 degrees posterior (down from horizontal) to the long axis of the humerus for the supine position (Fig. 5-52).
- Direct the central ray perpendicular to the film when the patient is leaning forward and the humerus 10 to 15 degrees (Fig. 5-53).

Structures shown

The tangential image profiles the intertubercular groove free of superimposition of the surrounding shoulder structures (Figs. 5-54 and 5-55).

□ Evaluation criteria

The following should be clearly demonstrated:

- Intertubercular groove in profile.
- Soft tissue; enhanced visibility of the intertubercular groove.

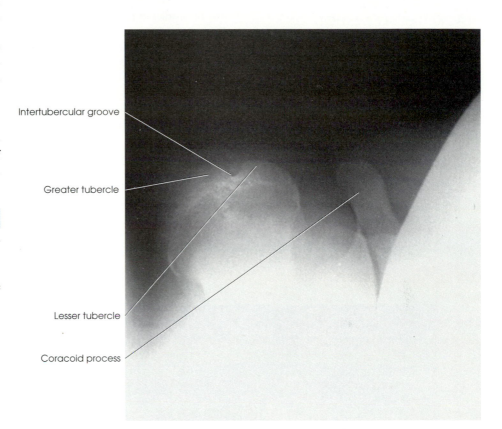

Intertubercular groove

Greater tubercle

Lesser tubercle

Coracoid process

Fig. 5-54. Supine tangential intertubercular groove.

(Courtesy Heide Galli, R.T.)

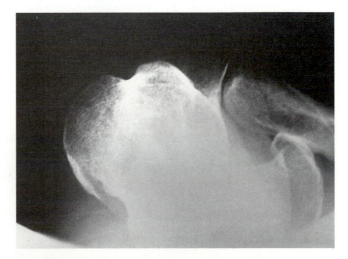

Fig. 5-55. Standing tangential intertubercular groove.

Proximal Humerus

PA PROJECTION:
Teres Minor Insertion
BLACKETT-HEALY METHOD

Film: 8 × 10 in (18 × 24 cm) crosswise.

Position of patient

- Adjust the patient in the prone position, the arms along the sides of the body and the head resting on the cheek of the affected side.
- Place support under the ankles for the patient's comfort.

Position of part

- Place the cassette under the shoulder and center it to a point about 1 inch below the coracoid process.
- Turn the arm to a position of extreme internal rotation and, if possible, flex the elbow and place the hand on the patient's back (Figs. 5-56 and 5-57).
- *Shield gonads.*
- Ask the patient to suspend respiration at the end of exhalation for a more uniform density.

Central ray

- Direct the central ray perpendicular to the head of the humerus.

Structures shown

This position rotates the head of the humerus so the greater tubercle is brought anteriorly, giving a tangential image of the insertion of the teres minor at the outer edge of the bone just below the articular surface of the head (Fig. 5-58).

□ Evaluation criteria

The following should be clearly demonstrated:

- Outline of the greater tubercle superimposing the humeral head.
- Lesser tubercle in profile and pointing medially.
- Soft tissue around the humerus along with trabecular detail on the humeral head.

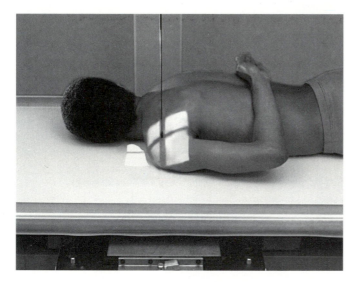

Fig. 5-56. PA teres minor insertion.

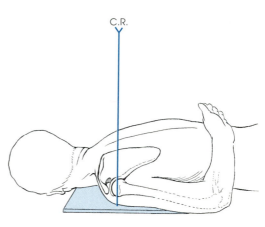

Fig. 5-57. PA teres minor insertion.

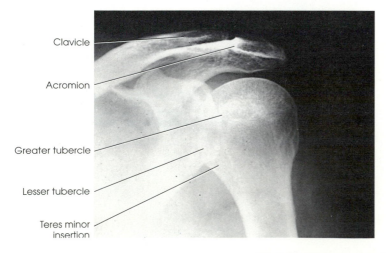

Clavicle

Acromion

Greater tubercle

Lesser tubercle

Teres minor insertion

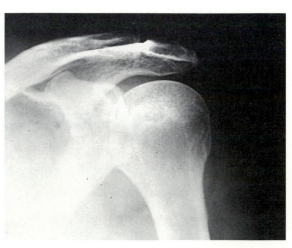

Fig. 5-58. PA teres minor insertion.

Proximal Humerus

AP PROJECTION:
Subscapularis Insertion
BLACKETT-HEALY METHOD

Film: 8 × 10 in (18 × 24 cm) or 10 × 12 in (24 × 30 cm) crosswise.

Position of patient

- Place the patient in the supine position, arms resting along the sides of the body.

Position of part

- Align the body so the affected shoulder joint is centered to the midline of the table.
- The opposite shoulder may be elevated approximately 15 degrees and supported with a sandbag.

- Abduct the affected arm to the long axis of the body, flex the elbow, and rotate the arm internally by pronating the hand (Figs. 5-59 and 5-60).
- Place one sandbag under the hand and another on top, if necessary, for immobilization.
- *Shield gonads.*
- Ask the patient to suspend respiration at the end of exhalation.

Central ray

- Direct the central ray perpendicular to the shoulder joint, entering the coracoid process.

Structures shown

This method provides an image of the insertion of the subscapularis at the lesser tubercle (Fig. 5-61).

☐ Evaluation criteria

The following should be clearly demonstrated:

- Lesser tubercle in profile and pointing inferiorly.
- Outline of the greater tubercle superimposing the humeral head.
- Soft tissue around the humerus along with trabecular detail on the humeral head.

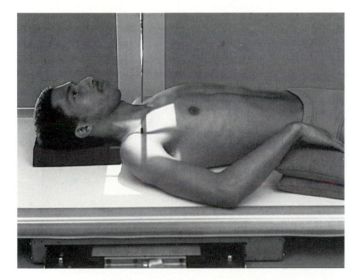

Fig. 5-59. AP subscapularis insertion.

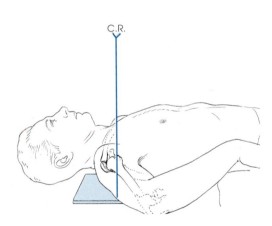

Fig. 5-60. AP subscapularis insertion.

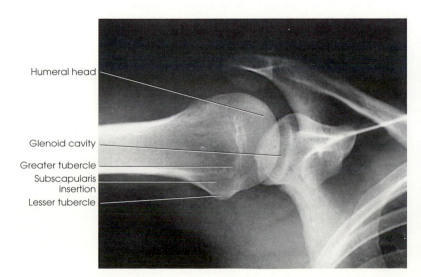

Humeral head

Glenoid cavity

Greater tubercle

Subscapularis insertion

Lesser tubercle

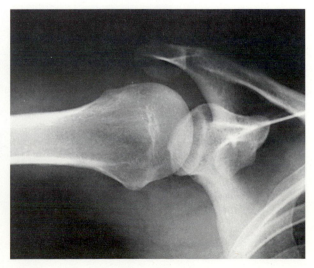

Fig. 5-61. AP subscapularis insertion.

Proximal Humerus
AP AXIAL PROJECTION:
Infraspinatus Insertion

Place the patient in the supine position with the affected arm by the patient's side and turn in external rotation to open the subacromial space (Fig. 5-62, *A*). Rotate the arm to the neutral position (Fig. 62, *B*), and in complete internal rotation (Fig. 5-62, *C*) to allow full evaluation of the humeral head. Direct the central ray to enter the coracoid process at an angle of 25 degrees caudad. The image profiles the greater tubercle, the site of insertion of the infraspinatus tendon, and opens the subacromial space.

Acromioclavicular Articulations

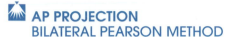
AP PROJECTION
BILATERAL PEARSON METHOD

Film: 7 × 17 in (18 × 43 cm) or two 8 × 10 in (18 × 24 cm) films, as needed to fit the patient.

Position of patient

Because a dislocation, partial or complete, of the acromioclavicular (A-C) joint tends to reduce itself in the recumbent position, demonstration of this condition requires an AP projection in the upright body position. This projection must therefore be made seated or standing, if the patient's condition permits. The positioning is easily modified to obtain a PA projection.

Position of part

- Place the patient in the upright position before a vertical grid device, and adjust the height of the cassette so that the midpoint of the cassette lies at the level of the acromioclavicular joints. (Fig. 5-63)
- Center the midline of the body to the midline of the grid.
- Ensure that the weight of the body is equally distributed on the feet to avoid rotation.
- With the patient's arms hanging by the sides, adjust the shoulders to lie in the same horizontal plane. It is important that the arms hang unsupported.
- It is common for two exposures to be made: one with the patient standing upright without holding weights, and a second exposure made with equal weights (5-8 lb) affixed[1,2] to each wrist.
- Slowly affix the weights to the patient's wrist using a band or strap.
- Instruct the patient not to favor (tense up) the injured shoulder.
- *Avoid having the patient hold weights in each hand;* this tends to make the shoulder muscles contract, thus reducing the possibility of demonstrating a small acromioclavicular separation.
- If separated, the joint will be wider on the separated side.
- *Shield gonads.*
- Ask the patient to suspend respiration.

[1]Allman FL: Fractures and ligamentous injuries of the clavicle and its articulations, J Bone Joint Surg 49-A:774-784, 1967.
[2]Rockwood CA and Green DP: Fractures in adults, 3rd ed, Philadelphia, JB Lippincott, 1991.

A
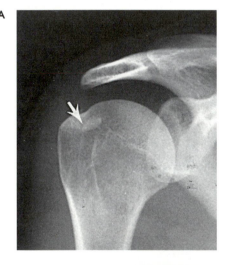

B
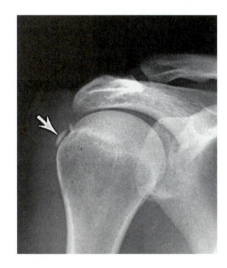

C
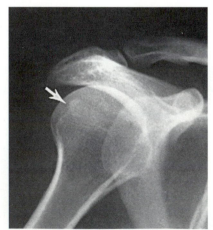

Fig. 5-62. AP axial 25-degree caudal angulation demonstrating calcareous peritendinitis *(arrows).* **A,** External rotation. **B,** Neutral position. **C,** Internal rotation.

(Courtesy Dr. Hudson J. Wilson, Jr.)

Central ray

- Direct the central ray perpendicular to the midline of the body, at the level of the acromioclavicular joints, for a single projection.
- When two separate exposures are needed for broad-shouldered patients, the central ray enters each respective acromioclavicular joint. Ensure that weights are attached to both arms for single exposure.
- Use a 72-inch SID to compensate for the increased object-to-image receptor distance when positioned for an AP projection.

Structures shown

Bilateral images of the acromioclavicular joints are presented (Figs. 5-64 and 5-65). This projection is used to demonstrate dislocation, separation, and function of the joints.

□ Evaluation criteria

The following should be clearly demonstrated:
- Acromioclavicular joints visualized with some soft tissue and without excessive density.
- Both acromioclavicular joints entirely included on one or two single radiographs.
- If the patient has broad shoulders, two small cassettes exposed individually.
- No rotation or leaning by the patient.
- Right or left and weight or non-weight markers.

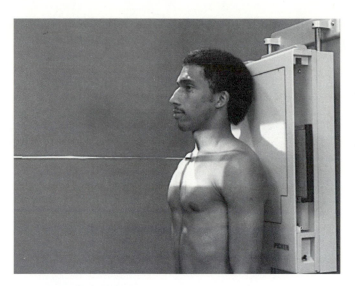

Fig. 5-63. Bilateral AP acromioclavicular articulations.

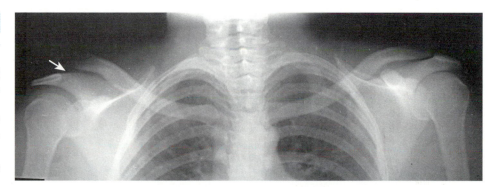

Fig. 5-64. Bilateral AP acromioclavicular joints demonstrating normal left joint, separation of joint on right (arrow).

(Courtesy Cindy Wedel, R.T.)

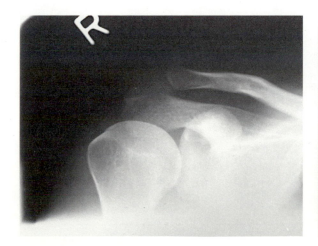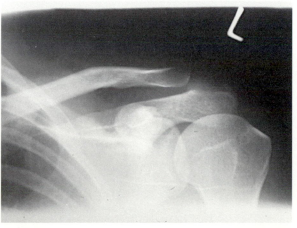

Fig. 5-65. Normal acromioclavicular joints requiring two separate radiographs.

(Courtesy Cheryl Stillberger, R.T.)

Acromioclavicular Articulations

AP AXIAL PROJECTION
ALEXANDER METHOD

Alexander[1] suggested that both AP and lateral projections be used in cases of suspected acromioclavicular subluxation or dislocation. Each side is examined separately.

Film: 8 × 10 in (18 × 24 cm) lengthwise.

Position of patient

- Place the patient in the upright position, either standing or seated.

[1]Alexander OM: Radiography of the acromioclavicular articulation, Med Radiogr Photogr 30:34-39, 1954.

Position of part

- Have the patient place his or her back against the vertical grid device and to sit or stand upright.
- Center the shoulder being examined to the grid.
- Adjust the height of the cassette so that the midpoint of the film is at the level of the acromioclavicular joint.
- Adjust the patient's position to center the coracoid process to the film (Fig. 5-66).
- *Shield gonads.*
- Ask the patient to suspend respiration at the end of exhalation.

Central ray

- Direct the central ray to the coracoid process at a cephalic angle of 15 degrees (Fig. 5-67). This angulation projects the shadow of the acromioclavicular joint above that of the acromion.

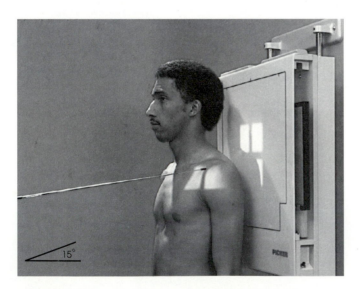

Fig. 5-66. Unilateral AP axial acromioclavicular articulation: Alexander method.

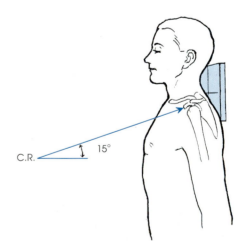

Fig. 5-67. AP axial acromioclavicular articulation.

Structures shown

The resulting image will show the acromioclavicular joint projected slightly superiorly when compared to an AP projection (Fig. 5-68).

□ Evaluation criteria

The following should be clearly demonstrated:
- Acromioclavicular joint and clavicle projected above the acromion.
- Acromioclavicular joint visualized with some soft tissue and without excessive density.

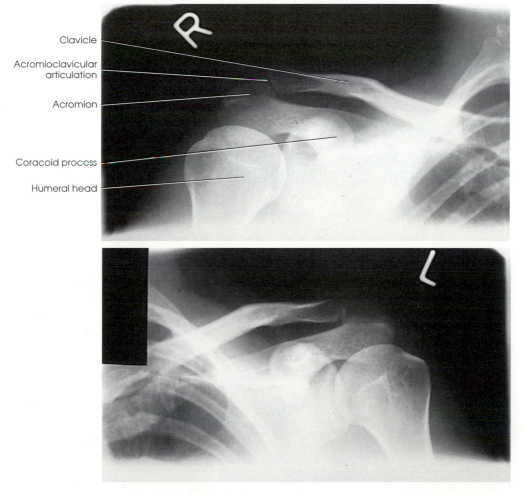

Clavicle
Acromioclavicular articulation
Acromion
Coracoid process
Humeral head

Fig. 5-68. AP axial acromioclavicular articulation: Alexander method.

Acromioclavicular Articulations

PA AXIAL OBLIQUE PROJECTION
RAO or LAO position

Film: 8 × 10 in (18 × 24 cm) lengthwise.

Position of part

- Stand or sit the patient facing the film and place the hand of the affected side well up under the opposite axilla.

- Rotate the unaffected side 30 to 35 degrees away from the film. (RAO or LAO.)
- Adjust the patient's position to center the acromioclavicular joint to the midline of the grid (Fig. 5-69).
- Just before making the exposure, have the patient lean the shoulder being examined against the cassette stand with the arm pulled firmly across the chest. Placing the arm across the chest draws the scapula laterally and forward. The slight obliquity of the chest and the pressure against the scapulohumeral joint further rotates the scapula laterally and anteriorly. The scapula and acromioclavicular joint are thus placed in the lateral position.
- *Shield gonads.*
- Ask the patient to suspend respiration.

Central ray

- Direct the central ray through the coracoid process at an angle of 15 degrees caudad.

Structures shown

The PA axial oblique image demonstrates the acromioclavicular joint and the relationship of the bones of the shoulder (Fig. 5-70).

☐ Evaluation criteria

The following should be clearly demonstrated:

- Acromioclavicular articulation in profile.
- Acromioclavicular joint visualized with some soft tissue without excessive density.

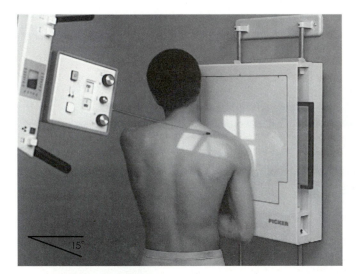

Fig. 5-69. PA axial oblique acromioclavicular articulation.

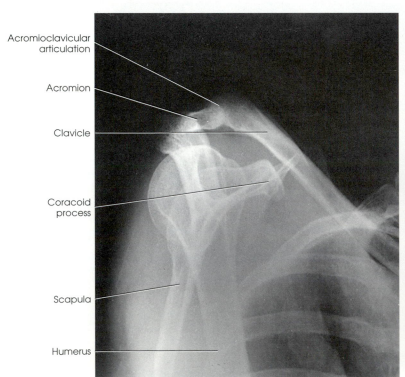
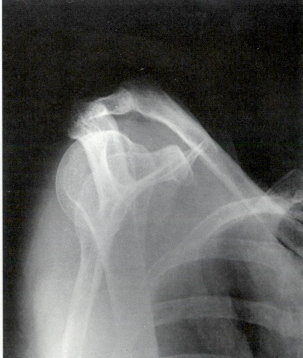

Acromioclavicular articulation

Acromion

Clavicle

Coracoid process

Scapula

Humerus

Fig. 5-70. PA axial oblique acromioclavicular articulation.

Clavicle

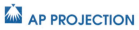 **AP PROJECTION**

Film: 10×12 in (24×30 cm) crosswise.

Position of patient

- Place the patient in the supine or upright position.
- If the clavicle is being examined for a fracture or a destructive disease and if the patient cannot be placed in the upright position, use the supine position to obviate the possibility of fragment displacement or additional injury.

Position of part

- Adjust the body to center the clavicle to the midline of the table or vertical grid device.
- Place the arms along the sides of the body, and adjust the shoulders to lie in the same horizontal plane.
- Center the cassette to a point midway between the midline of the body and the lateral border of the shoulder at the level of the coracoid process (Fig. 5-71).
- *Shield gonads.*
- Ask the patient to suspend respiration at the end of exhalation for a more uniform density.

Central ray

- Direct the central ray perpendicular to the midshaft of the clavicle.

Structures shown

This projection demonstrates a frontal image of the clavicle (Fig. 5-72).

□Evaluation criteria

The following should be clearly demonstrated:
- Entire clavicle.
- A density that is not excessive at the lateral third of the clavicle but that is sufficient to demonstrate the medial third through the thorax.
- The lateral half of the clavicle above the scapula, with the medial half superimposing the thorax when the central ray is perpendicular to film.
- A radiograph centered at the level of the coracoid process.

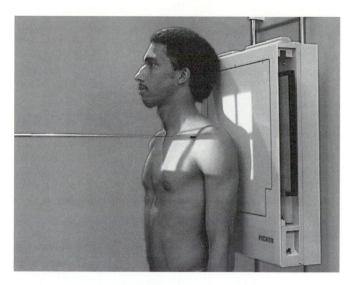

Fig. 5-71. AP clavicle.

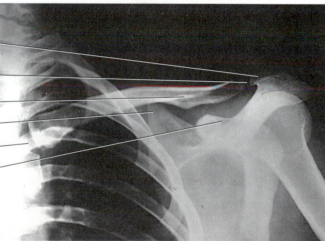

Acromion
Acromioclavicular articulation
Clavicle
Superior angle of scapula
Sternoclavicular articulation
Coracoid process

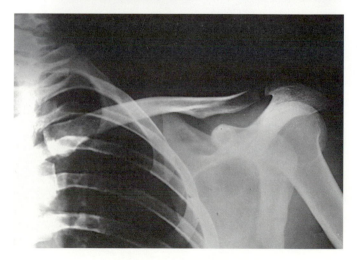

Fig. 5-72. AP clavicle.

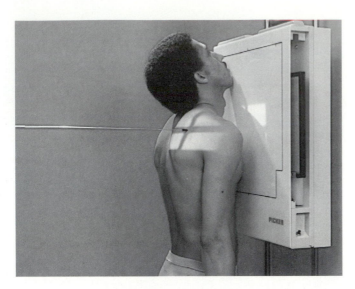

Fig. 5-73. PA clavicle.

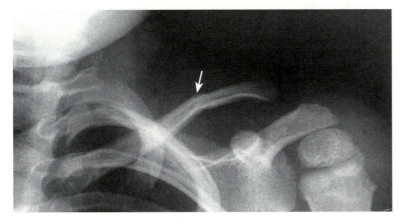

Fig. 5-74. PA clavicle on 3-year-old child showing fracture *(arrow)*. See Fig. 5-77 for AP axial of same patient.

Clavicle

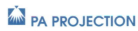 **PA PROJECTION**

The PA projection is generally well accepted by the patient who is able to stand, and it is most useful when improved recorded detail is desired. The advantage of the PA is that the clavicle is closer to the film, thus reducing the object-to-image receptor distance. The PA clavicle is positioned similarly to the AP clavicle just described. The differences are:

- The patient is standing upright (back toward the x-ray tube) or prone (Fig. 5-73).
- The clavicle is centered to the film.
- The perpendicular central ray exits mid-shaft of the clavicle (Fig. 5-74).
- Structures shown and evaluation criteria are the same as for the AP described above.

Clavicle

⛭ AP AXIAL PROJECTION

NOTE: If the patient is injured or unable to assume the lordotic position, a slightly distorted image results when radiographing the patient in the supine or upright position. An optional approach for improved recorded detail is the PA axial clavicle.

Film: 10 × 12 in (24 × 30 cm) crosswise.

Position of patient

- Place the patient who is unable to stand and assume the lordotic position supine on the table.

or

- Place the patient facing the x-ray tube, standing or seated, approximately 1 foot in front of the vertical film device.

Position of part

For the standing lordotic approach:
- While temporarily supporting the patient to simulate the lordotic position, estimate the required central ray angulation, and have the patient reassume the upright position while the equipment is adjusted.
- With the patient's arms in a comfortable position, place one hand against the patient's lumbar region to provide patient support.
- Have the patient lean backwards in a position of extreme lordosis, and rest the neck and shoulder against the vertical grid device. The neck will be in extreme flexion (Figs. 5-75 and 5-76).
- Center the clavicle approximately to the center of the cassette (Fig. 5-76).

For the supine approach:
- Center the casssette to the clavicle.
- *Shield gonads.*
- Ask the patient to suspend respiration at the end of full inhalation to further elevate and angle the clavicle.

Central ray

- Direct the central ray to enter the midshaft of the clavicle.
- Cephalic central ray angulation can vary from 15 to 45 degrees from the long axis of the torso; thinner patients require more angulation to project the clavicle off the scapula and ribs.
  - For the standing lordotic patient, 15 to 25 degrees is recommended (Fig. 5-75).
  - For the supine patient, 25 to 30 degrees is recommended (Fig. 5-76).

Structures shown

An axial image of the clavicle projected above the ribs (Fig. 5-77).

□ Evaluation criteria

The following should be clearly demonstrated:
- Most of the clavicle projected above the ribs and scapula with the medial end overlapping the first or second ribs.
- Clavicle in a horizontal placement.
- Entire clavicle along with the acromioclavicular and sternoclavicular joints.

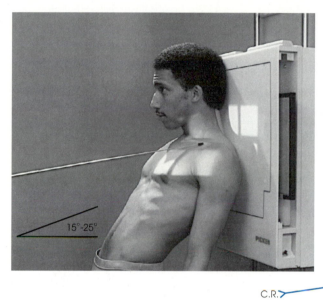

15°-25°

A

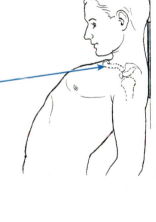

C.R.

B

Fig. 5-75. **A** and **B**, AP axial clavicle.

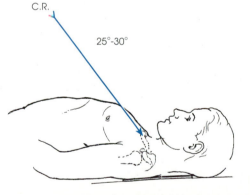

C.R.

25°-30°

Fig. 5-76. AP axial clavicle.

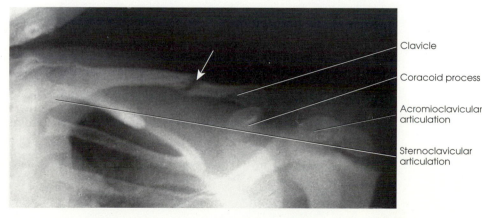

Clavicle

Coracoid process

Acromioclavicular articulation

Sternoclavicular articulation

Fig. 5-77. AP clavicle axial of 3-year-old child showing fracture *(arrow)*. Same patient as Fig. 5-74.

Clavical
PA AXIAL PROJECTION

The PA axial clavicle is positioned similarly to the AP axial just described. The differences are:

- The patient is prone or standing, facing the vertical grid device.
- The clavicle is centered to the grid device.
- The central ray is angled the same number of degrees as for the AP axial clavicle, but angled caudad (Fig. 5-78).

Structures shown and evaluation criteria are the same as for the AP axial described previously.

Clavicle
TANGENTIAL PROJECTION

The tangential projection is similar to the AP axial described on the previous page. However, the increased angulation of the central ray required for this tangential approach places the central ray nearly parallel with the rib cage. The clavicle is thus projected free of the chest wall.

Film: 8 × 10 in (18 × 24 cm) crosswise.

Position of patient

- With the patient in the supine position, place the arms along the sides of the body.

Position of part

- Depress the shoulder, if possible, to place the clavicle in a horizontal plane.
- Have the patient turn the head away from the side being examined.
- Place the cassette on edge at the top of the shoulder and support it in position. The cassette should be as close to the neck as possible (Figs. 5-79 and 5-80).
- *Shield gonads.*
- Ask the patient to suspend respiration for the exposure.

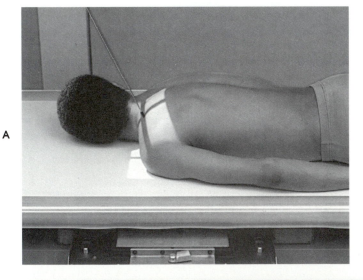

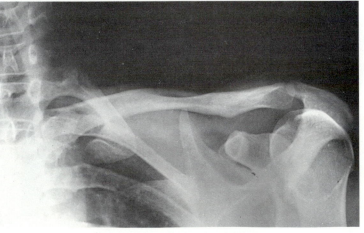

Fig. 5-78. A and **B,** PA axial clavicle.

Central ray

- Angle the tube so the central ray will pass between the clavicle and the chest wall, perpendicular to the plane of the film. The angulation will be about 25 to 40 degrees from the horizontal.
- If the medial third of the clavicle is in question, it is also necessary to angle the central ray laterally; 15 to 25 degrees is usually sufficient.

Structures shown

An inferosuperior image of the clavicle is demonstrated, projected free of superimposition (Fig. 5-81).

□ Evaluation criteria

The following should be clearly demonstrated:

- Midclavicle without superimposition.
- The acromial and sternal ends superimposed.
- Entire clavicle along with the acromioclavicular and sternoclavicular joints.

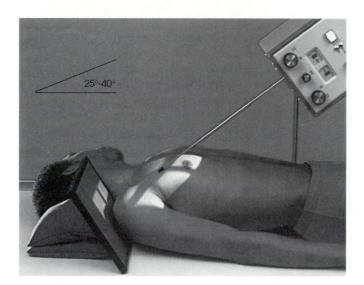

Fig. 5-79. Tangential clavicle.

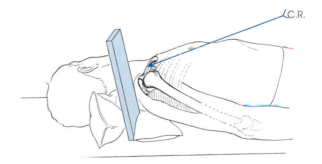

Fig. 5-80. Tangential alignment for clavicle.

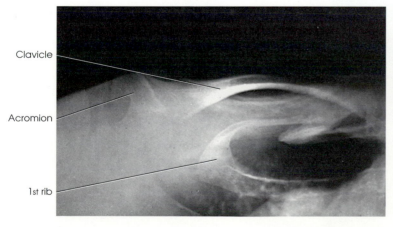
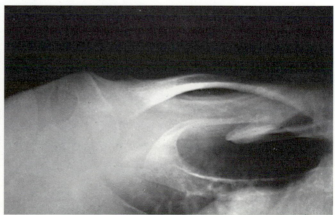

Clavicle

Acromion

1st rib

Fig. 5-81. Tangential clavicle.

Clavicle

TANGENTIAL PROJECTION
TARRANT METHOD

The Tarrant method[1] is particularly useful with patients who have multiple injuries or who cannot assume the lordotic or recumbent position.

Film: 10 × 12 in (24 × 30 cm) crosswise.

Position of patient

- Place the patient in a seated position.

[1]Tarrant RM: The axial view of the clavicle, Xray Techn 21:358-359, 1950.

Position of part

- Adjust a sheet of leaded rubber over the gonad area as illustrated. A folded pillow or blankets may be placed on the patient's lap to support the horizontally placed cassette if needed.
- Center the cassette to the projected clavicle area, using the collimator light as the indicator, and have the patient hold the cassette in position.
- Ask the patient to lean slightly forward (Fig. 5-82).
- *Shield gonads.*
- Ask the patient to suspend respiration for the exposure.

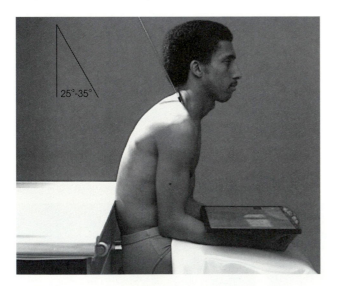

Fig. 5-82. Tangential clavicle: Tarrant method.

Central ray

- Direct the central ray anterior and inferior to the midshaft of the clavicle at a 25- to 35-degree angle. It should pass perpendicular to the longitudinal axis of the clavicle.
- Because of the considerable object-to-image receptor distance, an increased SID is recommended to reduce magnification.

Structures shown

The clavicle above the thoracic cage is demonstrated (Fig. 5-83).

□ **Evaluation criteria**

The following should be clearly demonstrated:

- Most of the clavicle above the ribs and scapula with the medial end overlapping the first or second ribs.
- Clavicle in a horizontal orientation.
- Entire clavicle, along with the acromioclavicular and sternoclavicular joints.

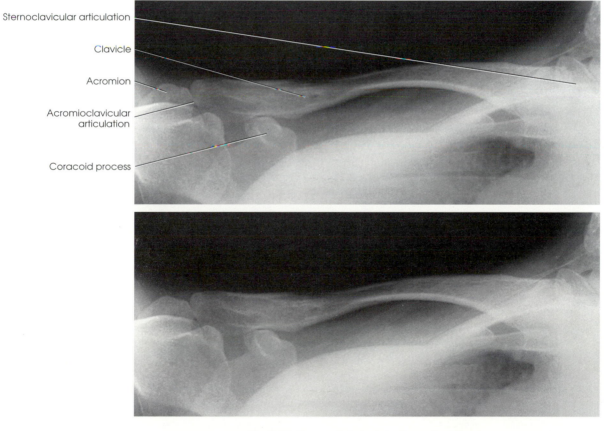

Sternoclavicular articulation

Clavicle

Acromion

Acromioclavicular articulation

Coracoid process

Fig. 5-83. Tangential clavicle: Tarrant method.

Scapula

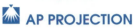 **AP PROJECTION**

Film: 10 × 12 in (24 × 30 cm) lengthwise.

Position of patient

- Place the patient in the upright or supine position. The upright position is preferred if the shoulder is tender.

Position of part

- Adjust the patient's body and center the affected scapula to the midline of the grid.
- Abduct the arm to a right angle with the body to draw the scapula laterally; then flex the elbow and support the hand in a comfortable position.
- Do not rotate the body toward the affected side for this projection, because the resultant obliquity would offset the effect of drawing the scapula laterally (Fig. 5-84).
- *Shield gonads.*
- *Respiration:* Make this exposure during shallow breathing to obliterate lung detail.

Central ray

- Direct the central ray to the midscapular area, perpendicular to a point approximately 2 inches inferior to the coracoid process.

Structures shown

An AP projection of the scapula is demonstrated (Fig. 5-85).

Evaluation criteria

The following should be clearly demonstrated:
- Lateral portion of the scapula free of superimposition from the ribs.
- Scapula horizontal and not obliqued.
- Scapular detail visualized through the superimposed lung and ribs. Shallow breathing should help obliterate lung detail.
- Acromion process and inferior angle.

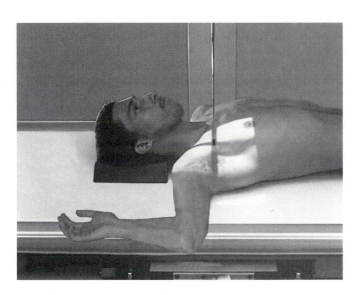

Fig. 5-84. AP scapula.

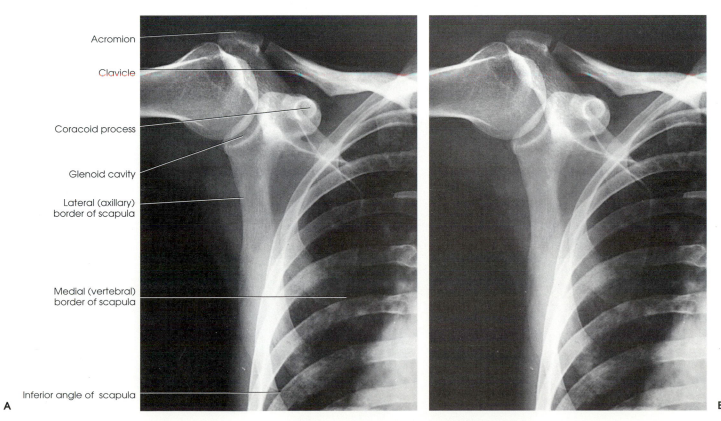

Acromion

Clavicle

Coracoid process

Glenoid cavity

Lateral (axillary)
border of scapula

Medial (vertebral)
border of scapula

Inferior angle of scapula

A

B

Fig. 5-85. A and **B,** AP scapula.

165

Scapula

 ## LATERAL PROJECTION
RAO or LAO body position

Film: 10 × 12 in (24 × 30 cm) length-wise.

Position of patient

- Place the patient in the upright position, standing or seated, facing a vertical grid device.
- When a patient cannot be placed in the upright position, a lateral position of the scapula can be obtained by adjusting the degree of body rotation and the placement of the arm from the prone or supine position.

Position of part

- Adjust the patient in an RAO or LAO position, with the affected scapula centered to the grid.
- Place the arm according to the area of the scapula to be demonstrated.
- For the delineation of the body of the scapula, the elbow is flexed and the hand placed on the anterior or posterior thorax at a level that will prevent the shadow of the humerus from overlapping that of the scapula (Figs. 5-86 and 5-87). Mazujian[1] suggests that the arm may be adjusted across the upper chest by grasping the opposite shoulder as seen in Fig. 5-88.

[1]Mazujian M: Lateral profile view of the scapula, Xray Techn 25:24-25, 1953.

- For the demonstration of the acromion and coracoid processes, ask the patient to extend the arm upward and rest the forearm on the head (Fig. 5-89).
- For the demonstration of the scapulo-humeral joint, to prove or disprove posterior, or anterior, dislocation, McLaughlin[2] recommends that the arm hang beside the body and be adjusted to have it superimposed by the wing of the scapula. (See Scapular Y method, pp. 142-143 and Figs. 5-40 to 5-42.)
- After placing the arm for any of the above positions, grasp the lateral and medial borders of the scapula between the thumb and index fingers of one hand.
- Adjust the body rotation to place the body of the scapula perpendicular to the plane of the film.
- *Shield gonads.*
- Ask the patient to suspend respiration for the exposure.

[2]McLaughlin HL: Posterior dislocation of the shoulder, J Bone Joint Surg 34A:584-590, 1952.

Central ray

- Direct the central ray perpendicular to the medial border of the protruding scapula.

Structures shown

A true lateral image of the scapula is demonstrated by this projection. The placement of the arm determines what portion of the superior scapula is superimposed over the humerus.

□Evaluation criteria

The following should be clearly demonstrated:
- Lateral and medial borders superimposed.
- No superimposition of the scapular body on the ribs.
- No superimposition of the humerus on the area of interest.
- Inclusion of the acromion process and inferior angle.
- Lateral thickness of scapula with proper density.

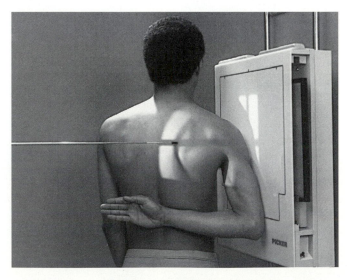

Fig. 5-86. Lateral scapula with patient in RAO body position.

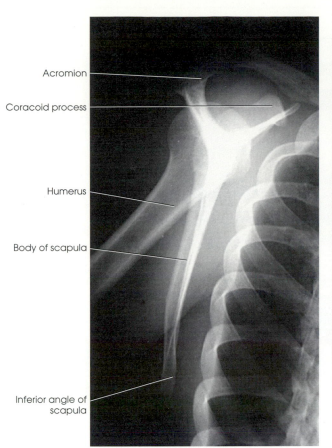
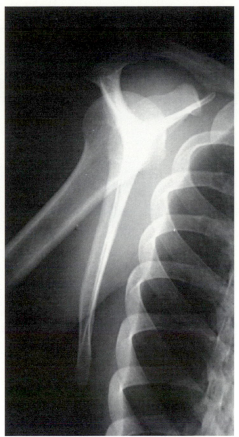

Acromion

Coracoid process

Humerus

Body of scapula

Inferior angle of scapula

Fig. 5-87. Lateral scapula with arm on posterior chest.

(Courtesy Thomas White, R.T.)

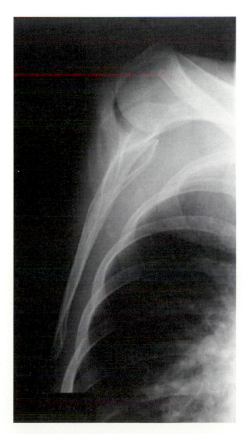
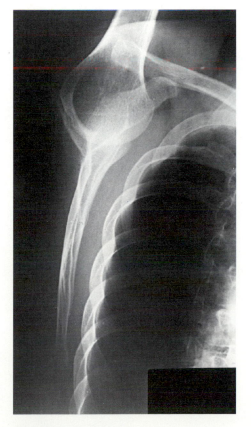

Fig. 5-88. Lateral scapula with arm across upper anterior thorax.

(Courtesy Linda Willman, R.T.)

Fig. 5-89. Lateral scapula with arm extended above head.

(Courtesy M.G. Rauckis, R.T.)

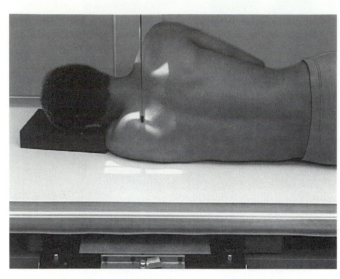

Fig. 5-90. PA oblique scapula: Lorenz method.

Scapula
PA OBLIQUE PROJECTION
RAO or LAO position
LORENZ AND LILIENFELD METHODS

Film: 10 × 12 in (24 × 30 cm) length-wise.

Position of patient

- Place the patient in the upright or lateral recumbent position.
- When the shoulder is painful, use the upright position if possible.

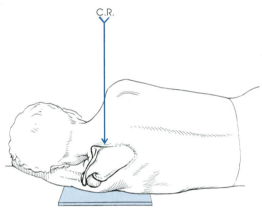

Fig. 5-91. PA oblique scapula: Lilienfeld method.

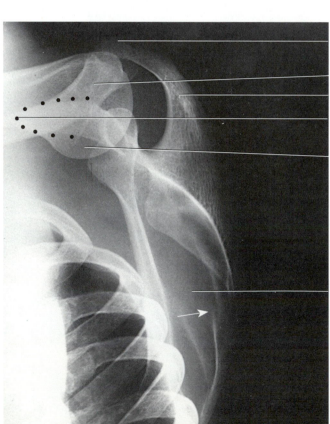

Acromioclavicular articulation

Clavicle

Acromion

Coracoid process

Humeral head

Fig. 5-92. Lorenz method scapula showing fracture *(arrow)*.

Body of scapula

Inferior angle of scapula

Position of part

- With the patient in the lateral position, upright or recumbent, align the body and center the scapula to the midline of the grid device.
- Adjust the arm according to the projection desired.
- For the Lorenz method, adjust the arm of the affected side at a right angle to the long axis of the body, flex the elbow, and rest the hand against the patient's head.
  - Rotate the body slightly forward, and have the patient grasp the side of the table or the stand for support (Fig. 5-90).

- For the Lilienfeld method, extend the arm of the affected side obliquely upward, and have the patient rest the hand on his or her head.
  - Rotate the body slightly forward, and have the patient grasp the side of the table or the stand for support (Fig. 5-91).
- For either method, grasp the lateral and medial borders of the scapula between the thumb and index fingers of one hand, and adjust the rotation of the body so that the scapula will be projected free of the rib cage.
- *Shield gonads.*
- Ask the patient to suspend respiration for the exposure.

Central ray

- Direct the central ray perpendicular to the film, between the chest wall and the midarea of the protruding scapula.

Structures shown

An oblique image of the scapula is shown. The degree of obliquity depends on the position of the arm. Compare the delineation of the different parts of the bone in the two obliques shown in Figs. 5-92 and 5-93.

☐ Evaluation criteria

The following should be clearly demonstrated:

- ■ Oblique scapula.
- ■ Medial border adjacent to the ribs.
- ■ Acromion process and inferior angle.

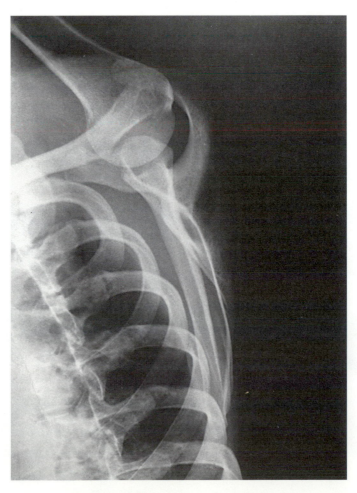

Fig. 5-93. PA oblique scapula: Lilienfeld method.

Scapula

AP OBLIQUE PROJECTION
RPO or LPO position

Film: 10 × 12 in (24 × 30 cm) lengthwise.

Position of patient

- Place the patient in the supine or upright position. The upright position should be used when the shoulder is painful.

Position of part

- Align the body and center the affected scapula to the midline of the grid.
- For moderate AP oblique projection, ask the patient to extend the arm superiorly, flex the elbow, and place the supinated hand under the head or have the patient extend the affected arm across the anterior chest.
- Have the patient turn away from the affected side enough to oblique the shoulder 15 to 25 degrees (Fig. 5-94).
- For a steeper oblique projection, ask the patient to extend the arm and rest the flexed elbow on the forehead.
- Rotate the body *away* from the affected side 25 to 35 degrees (Fig. 5-95).
- Grasp the lateral and medial borders of the scapula between the thumb and index fingers of one hand, and adjust the rotation of the body to project the scapula free of the rib cage.

- For a direct lateral position, draw the arm across the chest, and adjust the body rotation to place the scapula perpendicular to the plane of the film as previously described and shown in Figs. 5-86 to 5-89.
- *Shield gonads.*
- Ask the patient to suspend respiration for the exposure.

Central ray

- Direct the central ray perpendicular to the lateral border of the rib cage at the midscapular area.

Structures shown

Oblique images of the scapula are presented, projected free or nearly free of rib superimposition (Figs. 5-96 to 5-97).

☐Evaluation criteria

The following should be clearly demonstrated:

- Oblique scapula.
- Lateral border adjacent to the ribs.
- Acromion process and inferior angle.

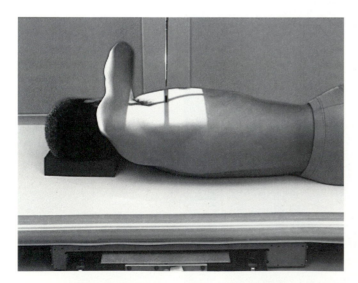

Fig. 5-94. AP oblique scapula, 20 degrees.

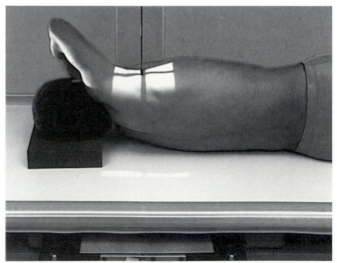

Fig. 5-95. AP oblique scapula, 35 degrees.

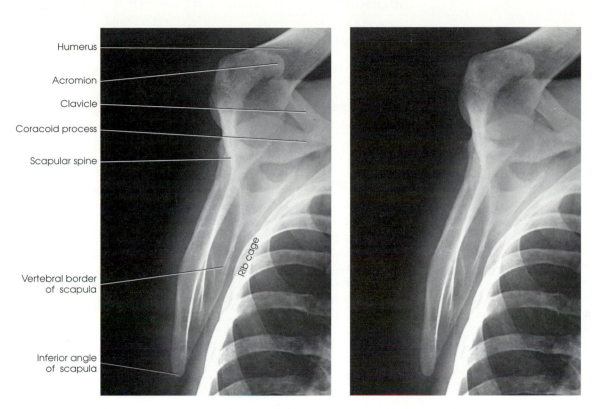

Humerus

Acromion

Clavicle

Coracoid process

Scapular spine

Rib cage

Vertebral border
of scapula

Inferior angle
of scapula

Fig. 5-96. AP oblique scapula, 15- to 25-degree rotation.

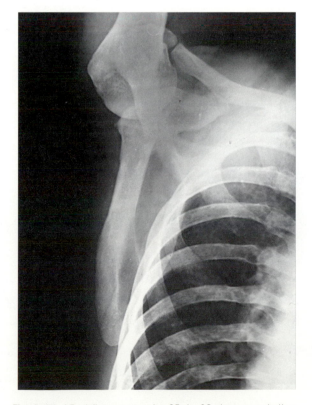

Fig. 5-97. AP oblique scapula, 25- to 30-degree rotation.

Scapula

AP AXIAL PROJECTION:
Coracoid Process

Film: 8 × 10 in (18 × 24 cm) or 10 × 12 in (24 × 30 cm) crosswise.

Position of patient

- Place the patient in the supine position with his or her arms along the sides of the body.

Position of part

- Adjust the position of the body, and center the affected coracoid process to the midline of the grid.
- Position the cassette so that the midpoint of the film will coincide with the central ray.
- Adjust the shoulders to lie in the same horizontal plane.
- Abduct the arm of the affected side slightly, and supinate the hand, immobilizing it with a sandbag across the palm (Fig. 5-98).
- *Shield gonads.*
- Ask the patient to suspend respiration at the end of exhalation for a more uniform density.

Central ray

- Direct the central ray to enter the coracoid process at an angle of 15 to 45 degrees cephalad. Kwak et al.[1] recommend 30 degrees. The degree of angulation depends on the shape of the patient's back; round-shouldered patients will require a greater angulation than those who have a straight back (Fig. 5-99).

Structures shown

A slightly elongated inferosuperior image of the coracoid process is shown (Fig. 5-100). Because the coracoid is curved on itself, it casts a small, oval shadow in the direct AP projection of the shoulder.

□ Evaluation criteria

The following should be clearly demonstrated:
- Coracoid process with minimal self-superimposition.
- Clavicle slightly superimposing the coracoid process.

[1]Kwak DL, Espiniella JL, and Kattan KR: Angled anteroposterior views of the shoulder, Radiol Technol 53:590-593, 1982.

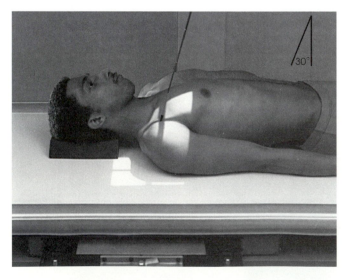

Fig. 5-98. AP axial coracoid process.

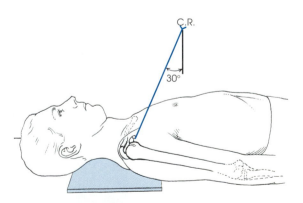

Fig. 5-99. AP axial coracoid process.

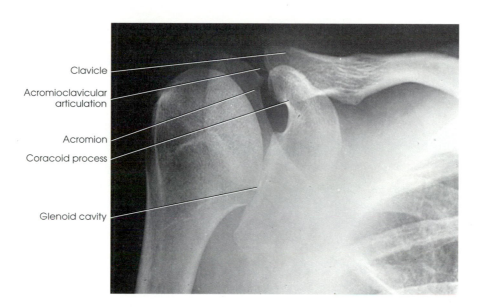

Clavicle

Acromioclavicular
articulation

Acromion
Coracoid process

Glenoid cavity

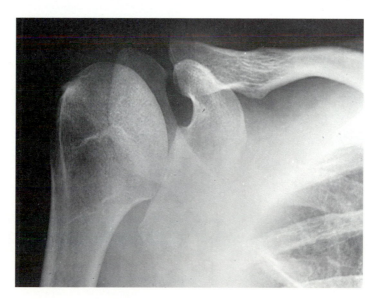

Fig. 5-100. AP axial coracoid process.

Scapular Spine
TANGENTIAL PROJECTION
LAQUERRIÈRE-PIERQUIN METHOD

Film: 8 × 10 in (18 × 24 cm) crosswise.

Position of patient

- As described by the originators,[1] place the patient in the supine position.

Position of part

- Center the shoulder to the midline of the grid.
- Adjust the patient's rotation to place the body of the scapula in a horizontal position. When this requires elevation of the opposite shoulder, support it on sandbags or radiolucent sponges.

---

[1]Laquerrière and Pierquin: De la nécessité d'employer une technique radiographique spéciale pour obtenir certains détails squelettiques, J Radiol Electr 3:145-148, 1918.

- Turn the head away from the shoulder being examined enough to prevent superimposition (Fig. 5-101).
- Funke[1] found that in the examination of patients with small breasts, clavicular superimposition can be prevented by using a 15-degree radiolucent wedge to angle the shoulder caudally.
- *Shield gonads.*
- Ask the patient to suspend respiration for the exposure.

---

[1]Funke T: Tangential view of the scapular spine, Med Radiogr Photogr 34:41-43, 1958.

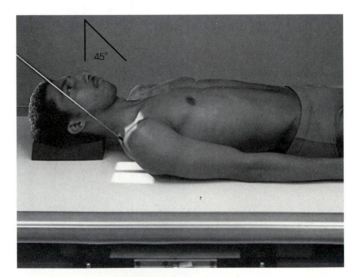

Fig. 5-101. Tangential scapular spine.

Central ray

- Direct the central ray through the posterosuperior region of the shoulder at an angle of 45 degrees caudad. A 35-degree angulation suffices for obese and round-shouldered subjects.
- After the adjustment of the x-ray tube, position the cassette so that it is centered to the central ray.

Structures shown

The spine of the scapula is shown in profile and free of bony superimposition except for the lateral end of the clavicle (Figs. 5-102 and 5-103).

□Evaluation criteria

The following should be clearly demonstrated:
- Scapular spine superior to the scapular body.
- Scapular spine with some soft tissue around it and without excessive density.

NOTE: When the shoulder is too painful to tolerate the supine position, this projection can be obtained with the patient in the prone or upright position, as described on the following page.

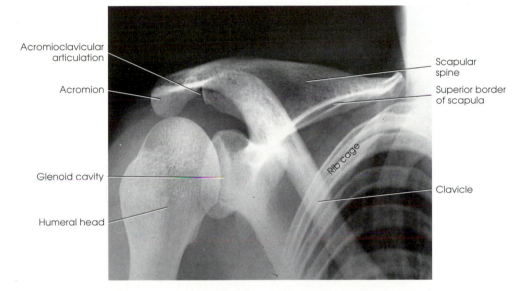

Fig. 5-102. Tangential scapular spine with 45-degree cental ray angulation.

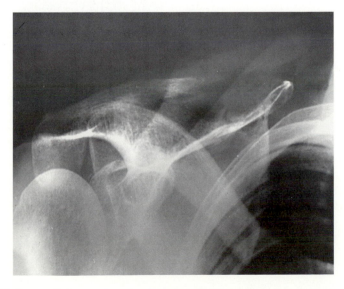

Fig. 5-103. Tangential scapular spine image with 35-degree central ray angulation.

(Courtesy Dr. Hudson J. Wilson, Jr.)

Scapular Spine

TANGENTIAL PROJECTION

Film: 8 × 10 in (18 × 24 cm) crosswise.

Prone position

Position of part

- Place the patient in the prone position, and center the shoulder to the midline of the grid.
- Place the arms along the sides of the body, and adjust the shoulders to lie in the same horizontal plane.
- Take care to prevent lateral rotation of the scapula.
- Have the patient rest his or her head on the chin or the cheek of the affected side.

- Supinate the hand of the affected side (Fig. 5-104).
- Adjust a radiolucent wedge under the side of the shoulder and upper arm to place the scapula in the horizontal position.
- *Shield gonads*.
- Ask the patient to suspend respiration for the exposure.

Central ray

- Direct the central ray through the scapular spine at an angle of 45 degrees cephalad. It exits at the anterosuperior aspect of the shoulder.

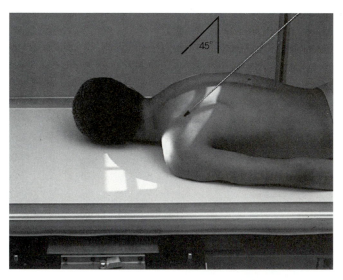

Fig. 5-104. Prone tangential scapular spine.

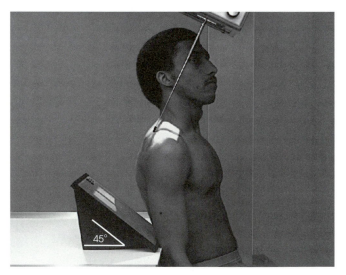

Fig. 5-105. Upright tangential scapular spine.

Upright position

An increased SID is recommended because of the greater object-to-image receptor distance.

Position of part

- Seat the patient with his or her back toward and resting against the end of the table.
- Place the cassette on the table, center it in line with the shoulder, and adjust the cassette on a support to place it at an angle of 45 degrees (Fig. 5-105).
- *Shield gonads.*
- Ask the patient to suspend respiration for the exposure.

Central ray

- Direct the central ray through the anterosuperior aspect of the shoulder at a posteroinferior angle of 45 degrees. The central ray should be perpendicular to the plane of the film.

Structures shown

The tangential image shows the scapular spine in profile and free of superimposition of the scapular body (Figs. 5-106 and 5-107).

□Evaluation criteria

The following should be clearly demonstrated:
- Scapular spine above the scapular wing.
- Scapular spine with some soft tissue around it and without excessive density.

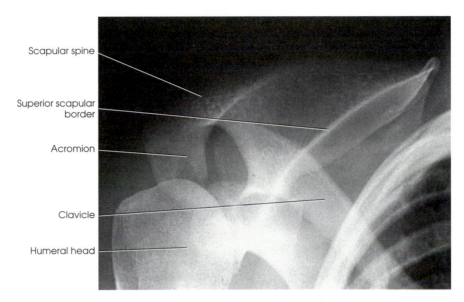

Scapular spine

Superior scapular border

Acromion

Clavicle

Humeral head

Fig. 5-106. Prone tangential scapular spine.

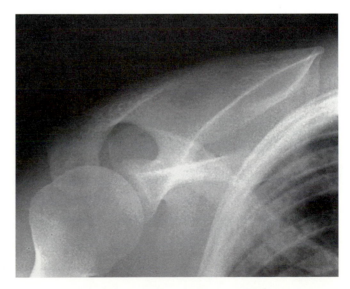

Fig. 5-107. Upright tangential scapular spine.

Chapter 6

LOWER LIMB (EXTREMITY)

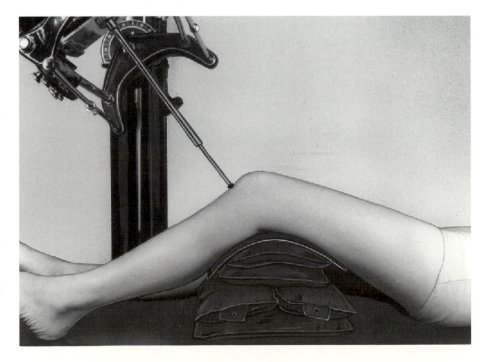

Patient positioned to show the intercondyloid fossa using the Béclerè method. Notice how the cardboard film holder is used without intensifying screens in order to place the film closer to the anatomy.

The lower limb (extremity) and its girdle (considered in Chapter 7) is studied in four parts: (1) the foot, (2) the leg, (3) the thigh, and (4) the hip. The bones are composed, shaped, and placed so that they can carry the body in the upright position and transmit its weight to the ground with a minimum amount of stress to the individual parts.

Foot

The *foot* consists of 26 bones (Figs. 6-1 and 6-2), subdivided into three parts: (1) the phalanges, or bones of the toes; (2) the metatarsals, or bones of the instep; and (3) the tarsals, or bones of the ankle. For descriptive purposes, the foot is sometimes divided into (1) the forefoot, which includes the metatarsals and toes; (2) the midfoot, which includes the cuneiforms, navicular, and cuboid; and (3) the hindfoot, which includes the talus (astragalus) and calcaneus (os calcis). The bones of the foot are shaped and joined together to form a series of longitudinal and transverse arches. This results in a considerable variation in the thickness of the component parts of the foot. To overcome the resulting difference in radiopacity, it is necessary to balance the exposure factors to obtain the greatest possible range of tissue density. The superior (anterior) surface of the foot is termed the *dorsum* or *dorsal surface*, and the inferior (posterior) aspect of the foot is termed the *plantar surface*.

PHALANGES

There are 14 *phalanges* in the toes, two in the great toe and three in each of the other toes. The phalanges of the great toe are termed the distal and proximal phalanges. Those of the other toes are termed the proximal, middle, and distal phalanges. Each phalanx is composed of a *body* or *shaft* and two expanded articular ends— the proximal base and the distal head. The distal phalanges are small and flattened and have a roughened rim of cancellous tissue at their distal end for the support of the nail.

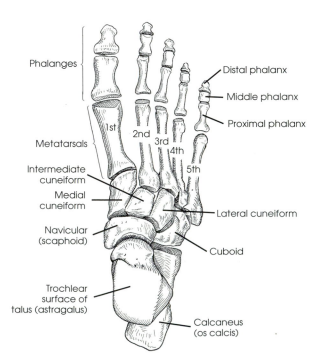

Fig. 6-1. Dorsal (superior) aspect of foot in normal anatomic position.

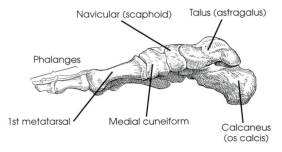

Fig. 6-2. Medial aspect of foot.

METATARSALS

The five *metatarsals* are numbered one to five beginning at the medial, or great toe, side of the foot. The metatarsals consist of a *body,* or shaft, and two articular extremities. The proximal extremities, the *bases,* articulate with the cuboid and cuneiforms. The distal extremities of the metatarsals, the *heads,* form the ball of the foot. The first metatarsal is the shortest and thickest, and there are commonly sesamoid bones located near the plantar surface of the head of the first metatarsal. The second metatarsal is the longest, and the fifth presents a prominent *tuberosity* at the lateral side on its base.

TARSALS

There are seven *tarsals* in the ankle (Fig. 6-1): the calcaneus (os calcis), talus (astragalus), navicular (scaphoid), cuboid, and three cuneiforms. Beginning at the medial side of the foot, the cuneiforms are described as: the medial, intermediate, and lateral; the first, second, and third; or the internal, middle, and external.

The *calcaneus* (os calcis, or heel) (Fig. 6-3), the largest and strongest tarsal bone, is more or less cuboidal in shape. It projects posteriorly and medially at the distal part of the foot. Directed inferiorly, the long axis of the calcaneus forms an angle of approximately 30 degrees, open forward, with the sole of the foot. The posterior and inferior portion of the calcaneus contains the posterior *tuberosity.* Superiorly, three *articular surfaces* exist and join with the talus. Between the middle and posterior talar articular surfaces is a groove, the *calcaneal sulcus,* which corresponds to a similar groove on the inferior surface of the talus. Collectively these sulci comprise the *sinus tarsi.* The medial aspect of the calcaneus extends outward as a shelf-like overhang termed the *sustentaculum tali.* The lateral surface of the calcaneus contains the *trochlea.*

The *talus,* irregular in form and occupying the highest position, is the second largest of the tarsal bones. The superior surface, the *trochlear surface,* articulates with the tibia. The head of the talus is directed anteriorly and has articular surfaces to join the navicular and calcaneus. On the inferior surface is a groove, the *sulcus tali,* which forms the roof of the sinus tarsi. Posterior to the sinus tali is the posterior articular surface for articulation with the calcaneus.

The *cuboid* lies on the lateral side of the foot between the calcaneus and the fourth and fifth metatarsals. The *navicular* (scaphoid) lies on the medial side of the foot between the talus and the three cuneiforms. The *cuneiforms* lie at the central and medial aspect of the foot between the navicular and the first, second, and third metatarsals. The *medial* cuneiform is the largest, and the *intermediate* is the smallest of the three cuneiforms.

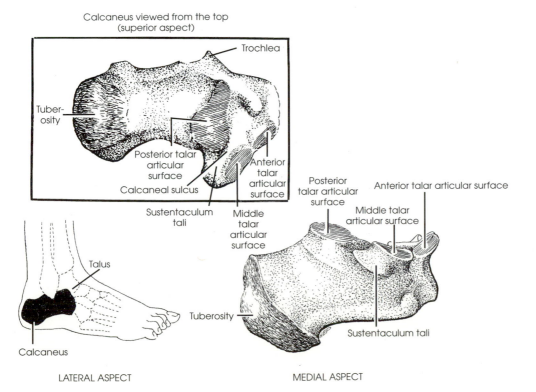

Calcaneus viewed from the top (superior aspect)

Trochlea

Tuberosity

Posterior talar articular surface

Calcaneal sulcus

Sustentaculum tali

Middle talar articular surface

Anterior talar articular surface

Posterior talar articular surface

Anterior talar articular surface

Middle talar articular surface

Talus

Calcaneus

Tuberosity

Sustentaculum tali

LATERAL ASPECT

MEDIAL ASPECT

Fig. 6-3. Articular surfaces of calcaneus.

Foot

Leg

The leg has two bones: the tibia and fibula. The tibia, the second largest bone in the body, is situated on the medial side of the leg. Slightly posterior in position to the tibia, and on the lateral side of the leg, is the fibula.

TIBIA

The *tibia* (Figs. 6-4 to 6-6) is the larger of the two bones of the leg and consists of a *body* (shaft) and two expanded extremities. The proximal end of the tibia presents two prominent processes, the *medial* and *lateral condyles*. The superior surfaces of the condyles form smooth facets for articulation with the condyles of the femur. Between the two articular surfaces is a sharp projection, the *intercondylar eminence* (tibial spine), which terminates in two peaklike processes called the medial and lateral intercondylar tubercles. The lateral condyle has a facet at its distal posterior surface for articulation with the *head* of the fibula. On the anterior surface of the tibia, just below the condyles, is a prominent process called the *tibial tuberosity,* to which the ligamentum patellae attaches. Extending along the anterior surface of the body (shaft) beginning at the tuberosity is a

sharp ridge called the *anterior border* (crest). The distal end of the tibia is broad, and its medial surface is prolonged into a large process called the *medial malleolus*. The lateral surface is flattened and presents a triangular depression for the inferior tibiofibular articulation. The undersurface of the distal tibia is smooth and shaped for articulation with the talus.

FIBULA

The *fibula* is slender in comparison to its length and consists of a *body* (shaft) and two articular extremities. The proximal end of the fibula is expanded into a *head,* which articulates with the lateral condyle of the tibia. At the lateroposterior aspect of the head is a conical projection called the *apex* (styloid process). The enlarged distal end of the fibula is the *lateral malleolus*. The lateral malleolus is pyramidal in shape and marked by several depressions at its inferior and posterior surfaces.

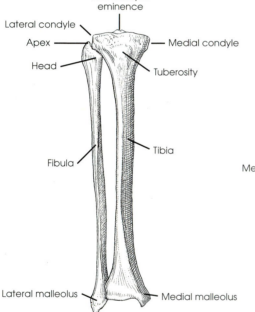

Fig. 6-4. Anterior aspect of tibia and fibula.

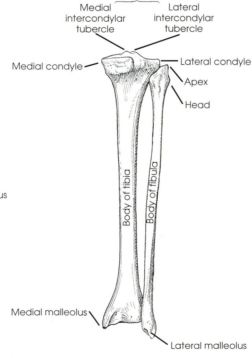

Fig. 6-5. Posterior aspect of tibia and fibula.

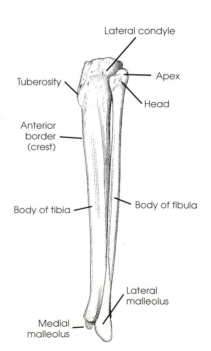

Fig. 6-6. Lateral aspect of tibia and fibula.

Thigh

The *femur* (thigh bone) is the largest, strongest, and heaviest bone in the body (Figs. 6-7 to 6-9). This bone consists of a body shaft and two articular extremities. The *body* (shaft) is cylindrical in form, slightly convex anteriorly, and slants obliquely, inferiorly, and medially. The degree of medial inclination depends on the breadth of the pelvic girdle. The superior portion of the femur articulates with the acetabulum of the hip joint and is considered with the pelvic girdle in Chapter 7.

The distal end of the femur is broadened and presents two large eminences: the larger *medial condyle* and the smaller *lateral condyle*. Anteriorly the condyles are separated by the *patellar surface* (intercondylar sulcus), a shallow, triangular depression. Posteriorly the condyles are separated by a deep depression called the *intercondylar fossa* (notch). A slight prominence above and within the curve of each condyle forms the *medial* and *lateral epicondyles*. The triangular area superior to the intercondylar fossa on the posterior femur is the *popliteal surface,* over which pass the popliteal blood vessels and nerves.

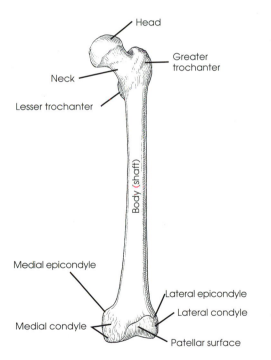

Fig. 6-7. Anterior aspect of femur.

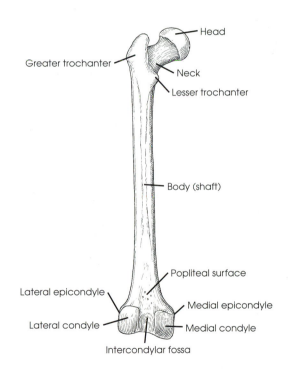

Fig. 6-8. Posterior aspect of femur.

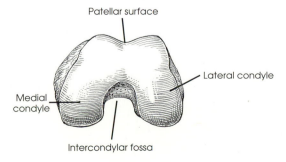

Fig. 6-9. Inferior aspect of femur.

Patella

The *patella* (kneecap) (Fig. 6-10) is the largest and most constant sesamoid bone in the body (see Chapter 3). The patella is a flat, triangular bone situated at the distal anterior surface of the femur. The patella develops in the tendon of the quadriceps femoris muscle between the ages of 3 and 5 years. The *apex,* or tip, is directed inferiorly, lies slightly above the joint space of the knee, and is attached to the tuberosity of the tibia by the patellar ligament.

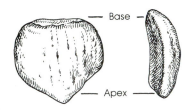

Fig. 6-10. Anterior and lateral aspects of patella.

Lower Limb Articulations

Beginning with the most distal portion of the lower limb, the articulations are as follows.

The interphalangeal articulations between the *phalanges* are of the synovial, ginglymus, or hinge type (diarthrotic), allowing only flexion and extension. The joints between the distal and middle phalanges are the distal interphalangeal joints (DIP). Articulations between the middle and proximal phalanges are proximal interphalangeal joints (PIP). With only two phalanges in the great toe, the joint is known simply as the interphalangeal joint.

The distal heads of each *metatarsal* articulate with the proximal ends of the phalanges at the metatarsophalangeal articulations to form synovial condyloid joints (diarthrotic) that have movements of flexion, extension, and slight adduction and abduction. The proximal bases of the metatarsals articulate with one another (intermetatarsal articulations) and with the distal tarsals (tarsometatarsal articulations) to form synovial condyloid joints (diarthrotic) that permit flexion, extension, adduction, and abduction movements.

Two *sesamoid bones* are usually present on the plantar surface of the first metatarsophalangeal joint, and occasionally there are more. Frequently sesamoids are found on the plantar surface at one or more of the other metatarsophalangeal joints and at the interphalangeal joints of the first and second toes. These sesamoids begin to appear between the ages of 8 and 12 years.

The *calcaneus* supports the talus, articulating with it by an irregularly shaped, three-faceted joint surface forming the *subtalar* (talocalcaneal) *joint.* Anteriorly, the calcaneus articulates with the cuboid. The *talus* rests on top of the calcaneus. It articulates with the navicular anteriorly, supports the tibia above, and articulates with the malleoli of the tibia and fibula at its sides (see Fig. 6-3).

The *intertarsal* articulations allow only slight gliding movements between the bones and are classified as synovial plane or gliding (diarthrotic) joints. The joint spaces are narrow and obliquely situated. Those lying in the horizontal plane slant inferiorly and posteriorly at an angle of approximately 15 degrees to the vertical. When the joint surfaces of these bones are in question, it is necessary to angle the tube or adjust the foot to place the joint spaces parallel with the central ray. Several positions with varying central ray angulations are required to demonstrate the subtalar (talocalcaneal) joint (Fig. 6-11). Each of the three parts of the subtalar joint is formed by reciprocally shaped facets on the inferior surface of the talus and the superior surface of the calcaneus. Study of the superior and medial aspects of the calcaneus (Fig. 6-3) will help the radiographer to better understand the problems involved in radiography of this joint.

The *ankle,* or *mortise joint,* (talocrural articulation) is formed by the articulations between the lateral malleolus of the fibula, and the inferior surface and medial malleolus of the tibia. These form a socket type of structure that articulates with the superior portion (trochlea) of the talus. The articulation is a synovial, ginglymus, or hinge-type joint (diarthrodial). The primary action of the ankle joint is dorsiflexion (flexion) and plantar flexion (extension); however, in full plantar flexion (full extension), a small amount of rotation and abduction-adduction is permitted. Other movements at the ankle largely depend on the gliding movements of the intertarsal joints, particularly the one between the talus and calcaneus (Fig. 6-12).

The *fibula* articulates with the *tibia* at both its distal and proximal ends. The distal tibiofibular joint is a syndesmosis, a fibrous joint allowing slight movement. The head of the fibula articulates with the posteroinferior surface of the lateral condyle of the tibia that forms the proximal tibiofibular joint, which is a synovial plane or gliding joint (diarthrotic).

The *patella* articulates with the patellar surface of the femur and functions to protect the front of the knee joint. When the knee is extended and relaxed, the patella is freely movable over the patellar surface of the femur. When the knee is flexed the patella is locked in position in front of the patellar surface.

The *knee* joint, which is of the synovial ginglymus or hinge type (diarthrotic), is the largest joint in the body. Two menisci, one medial and one lateral, are interposed between the articular surfaces of the tibia and the condyles of the femur. The joint is enclosed in an articular capsule and held together by numerous ligaments. There are many bursae around the anterior, posterolateral, and medial surfaces of the joint (Fig. 6-13).

The articulations of the hip joint are considered with the pelvic girdle in Chapter 7.

Radiation Protection

Protection of the patient from unnecessary radiation is a professional responsibility of the radiographer (see Chapter 1 for specific guidelines). In this chapter, the *"Shield gonads"* statement at the end of the "Position of part" section indicates the patient is to be protected from unnecessary radiation by restricting the radiation beam, using proper collimation *and* placing lead shielding between the gonads and the radiation source.

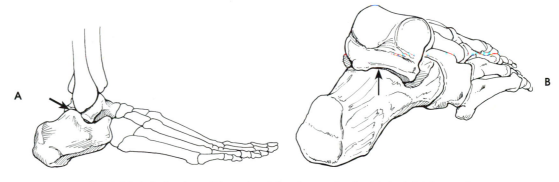

Fig. 6-11. A, Lateral, and **B,** posterolateral aspects of subtalar joint *(arrows).*

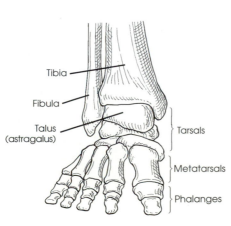

Tibia
Fibula
Talus (astragalus)
Tarsals
Metatarsals
Phalanges

Fig. 6-12. Anterior aspect of ankle joint.

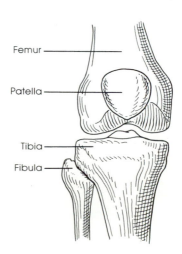

Femur
Patella
Tibia
Fibula

Fig. 6-13. Anterior aspect of knee joint.

Toes

 ### AP OR AP AXIAL PROJECTIONS

Because of the natural curve of the toes, the interphalangeal joint spaces are not best demonstrated on the AP projection. When demonstration of these joint spaces is not critical, an AP projection may be performed (Figs. 6-14 and 6-15). An AP axial projection is recommended to open the joint spaces and reduce foreshortening (Figs. 6-16 and 6-17).

Film: 8 × 10 in (18 × 24 cm) crosswise for two images on one film.

Position of patient

- Have the patient seated or placed supine on the table.

Position of part

- With the patient in the supine or seated position, flex the knees, separate the feet about 6 inches, and touch the knees together for immobilization.
- Center the toes directly over one half of the cassette (Figs. 6-14 and 6-16), or place a 15-degree foam wedge well under the foot to rest the toes near the elevated base of the wedge (Fig. 6-18).
- Adjust the cassette half with its midline parallel with the long axis of the foot, and center it to the second metatarsophalangeal joint.
- *Shield gonads.*

NOTE: Some institutions may demonstrate the entire foot while others radiograph only the toe(s) of interest.

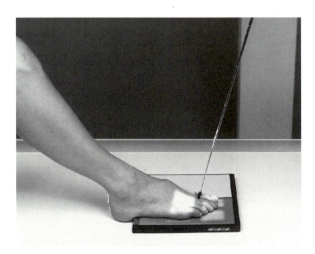

Fig. 6-14. AP toes with perpendicular central ray.

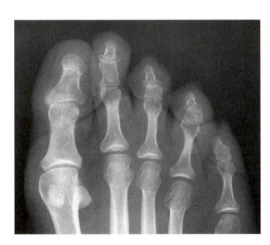

Fig. 6-15. AP toes with perpendicular central ray.

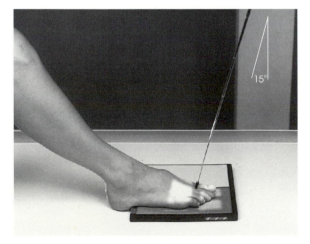

Fig. 6-16. AP axial toes with central ray angulation of 15 degrees.

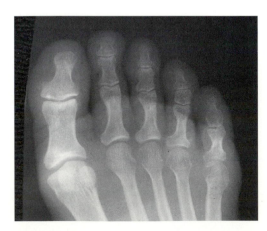

Fig. 6-17. AP axial toes with central ray angulation of 15 degrees.

(Courtesy Paul T. Ichino, R.T.)

Central ray

- When demonstration of the joint spaces is not critical, direct the central ray perpendicular through the second metatarsophalangeal joint (Fig. 6-15). To open the joint spaces, either direct the central ray 15 degrees cephalad through the second metatarsophalangeal joint (Fig. 6-17), or if the 15-degree foam wedge is used, direct the central ray perpendicular (Fig. 6-19).

Structures shown

The images will demonstrate the 14 phalanges of the toes, the distal portions of the metatarsals, and, on the axial projections, the interphalangeal joints.

□ Evaluation criteria

The following should be clearly demonstrated:
- No rotation of phalanges.
- Open interphalangeal and metatarsophalangeal joint spaces on the axial projections.
- Toes separated from each other.
- Distal ends of the metatarsals.
- Soft tissues and bony trabecular detail.

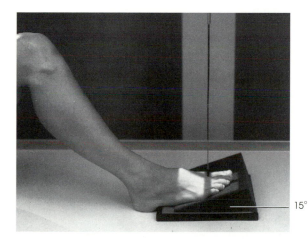

Fig. 6-18. AP axial with 15-degree foam wedge.

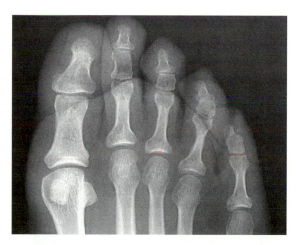

Fig. 6-19. AP axial with toes on 15-degree wedge.

Toes

187

Toes

PA PROJECTION

Film: 8 × 10 in (18 × 24 cm) crosswise for two images on one film.

Position of patient

- Have patient lie prone on the table. This position will naturally turn the foot over so the dorsal aspect is in contact with the cassette.

Position of part

- Place the toes in the appropriate position by elevating the toes on one or two small sandbags and adjusting the support to place the toes horizontal.
- Place the cassette half under the toes with the midline parallel with the long axis of the foot, and center it to the second metatarsophalangeal joint (Fig. 6-20).
- *Shield gonads.*

NOTE: Some institutions may demonstrate the entire foot while others radiograph only the toe(s) of interest.

Central ray

- Direct the central ray perpendicular to the midpoint of the film, entering the second metatarsophalangeal joint (Fig. 6-20). The interphalangeal joint spaces are shown well because the natural divergence of the x-ray beam coincides closely with the position of the toes (Fig. 6-21).

Structures shown

This projection will demonstrate the 14 phalanges of the toes, the interphalangeal joints, and the distal portions of the metatarsals.

□ Evaluation criteria

The following should be clearly demonstrated:

- No rotation of phalanges.
- Open interphalangeal and metatarsophalangeal joint spaces.
- Toes separated from each other.
- Distal ends of the metatarsals.
- Soft tissues and bony trabecular detail.

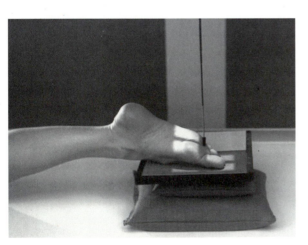

Fig. 6-20. PA toes.

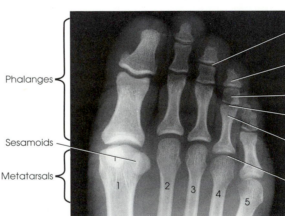

Fig. 6-21. PA toes.

Toes

AP OBLIQUE PROJECTION
Medial rotation

Film: 8 × 10 in (18 × 24 cm) crosswise for two images on one film.

Position of patient

- Place the patient in either the supine or seated position on the radiographic table.
- Flex the knee of the affected side enough to have the sole of the foot resting firmly on the table.

Position of part

- Position the cassette half under the toes.
- Medially rotate the lower leg and foot, and adjust the plantar surface of the foot to form a 30- to 45-degree angle from the plane of the film (Fig. 6-22).
- Center the proximal phalanx of the third toe to the cassette.
- *Shield gonads.*

Central ray

- Direct the central ray perpendicular to enter the third metatarsophalangeal joint.

NOTE: Oblique positions of individual toes may be obtained by centering the affected toe to the portion of the cassette being used and collimating closely. The foot may be placed in a medial oblique position for the first and second toes and in a lateral oblique position for the fourth and fifth toes. Either oblique position is adequate for the third (middle) toe.

Structures shown

An AP oblique projection of the phalanges shows the toes and the distal portion of the metatarsals rotated medially (Fig. 6-23).

□ Evaluation criteria

The following should be clearly demonstrated:

- All phalanges.
- Oblique toes.
- Open interphalangeal and second through fifth metatarsophalangeal joint spaces.
- First metatarsophalangeal joint (not always opened).
- Toes separated from each other.
- Distal ends of the metatarsals.
- Soft tissue and bony trabecular detail.

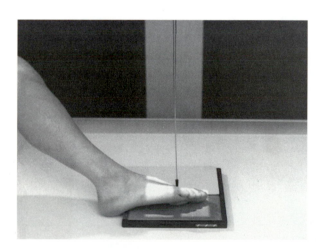

Fig. 6-22. AP oblique toes. Medial rotation.

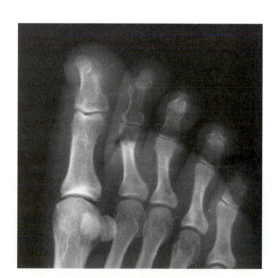

Fig. 6-23. AP oblique toes.

(Courtesy Lynn Rhatigan, R.T.)

Toes

PA OBLIQUE PROJECTION
Lateral rotation

Film: 8 × 10 in (18 × 24 cm) crosswise for two exposures on one film.

Position of patient

- Have the patient lie in the lateral recumbent position on the affected side.

Position of part

- Adjust the affected limb in a partially extended position.
- Have the patient turn toward the prone position until the ball of the foot forms an angle of approximately 30 degrees with the horizontal, or have the patient rest the foot against a foam wedge or sandbag (Fig. 6-24).
- Center the cassette half to the second metatarsophalangeal joint and adjust it so that its central line is parallel with the long axis of the foot.
- *Shield gonads.*

Central ray

- Direct the central ray perpendicular to the second metatarsophalangeal joint.

Structures shown

A PA oblique projection of the phalanges shows the toes and the distal portion of the metatarsals rotated laterally (Fig. 6-25).

□**Evaluation criteria**

The following should be clearly demonstrated:

- All phalanges.
- Oblique toes.
- Open interphalangeal and second through fifth metatarsophalangeal joint spaces.
- First metatarsophalangeal joint (not always opened).
- Toes separated from each other.
- Distal ends of the metatarsals.
- Soft tissue and bony trabecular detail.

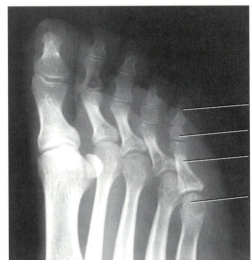

Distal phalanx
Middle phalanx
Proximal phalanx
Metatarsal head

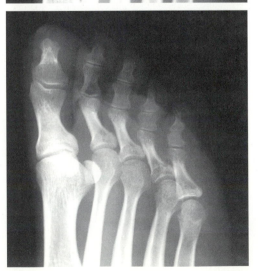

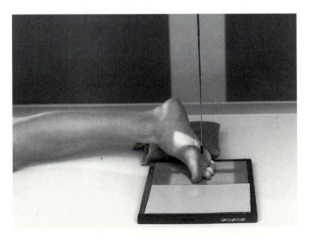

Fig. 6-24. PA oblique toes. Lateral rotation.

Fig. 6-25. PA oblique toes.

Toes

 LATERAL PROJECTIONS
Mediolateral or lateromedial

Film: 8 × 10 in (18 × 24 cm) crosswise for multiple exposures on one film.

Position of patient

- Have the patient lie in the lateral recumbent position on the *unaffected* side.
- Support the affected limb on sandbags and adjust it in a comfortable position.
- To prevent superimposition, tape the toe or toes above the one being examined into a flexed position. A 4 × 4 inch gauze pad may also be used to separate the toes.

Position of part

Great toe, second toe

- Place an 8 × 10 in (18 × 24 cm) cassette under the toe and center to the proximal phalanx.
- Grasp the limb by the heel and knee, and adjust its position to place the toe in a true lateral position.
- Adjust the cassette so that it is parallel with the long axis of the toe (Figs. 6-26 to 6-28).

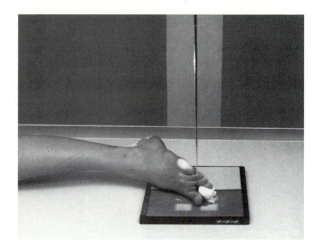

Fig. 6-26. Lateral great toe.

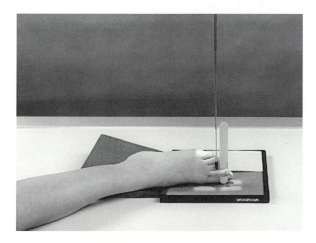

Fig. 6-27. Lateral second toe.

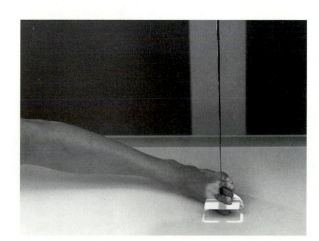

Fig. 6-28. Lateral, second toe using occlusal film.

Toes

Third, fourth, fifth toes

- Place the patient on the *affected* side for these three toes.
- Select an 8 × 10 in (18 × 24 cm) cassette or an occlusal film.
- If the occlusal film is used, place it with the pebbled surface up between the toe being examined and the subadjacent toe.
- Adjust the position of the limb to place the toe of interest and the film in a parallel position, placing the toe as close to the film as possible.
- Support the elevated heel on a sandbag or sponge for immobilization (Figs. 6-29 to 6-31).
- *Shield gonads.*

Central ray

- Direct the central ray perpendicular to the plane of the film, entering the metatarsophalangeal joint of the great toe or the proximal interphalangeal joint of the lesser toes.

Structures shown

The resulting images will show a lateral projection of the phalanges of the toe and the interphalangeal articulations, projected free of the other toes (Figs. 6-32 to 6-36).

□ **Evaluation criteria**

The following should be clearly demonstrated:
- Phalanges in profile; toenail should appear lateral.
- Phalanx, without superimposition of adjacent toes. When superimposition cannot be avoided, the proximal phalanx must be demonstrated.
- Open interphalangeal and metatarsophalangeal joint spaces.
- Soft tissue and bony trabecular detail.

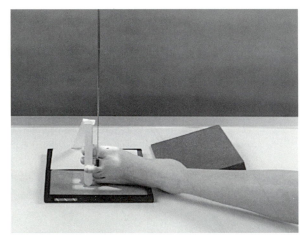

Fig. 6-29. Lateral third toe.

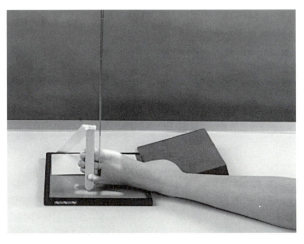

Fig. 6-30. Lateral fourth toe.

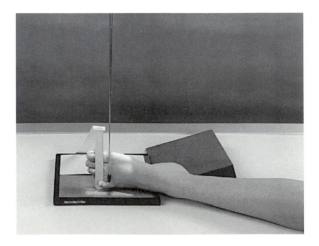

Fig. 6-31. Lateral fifth toe.

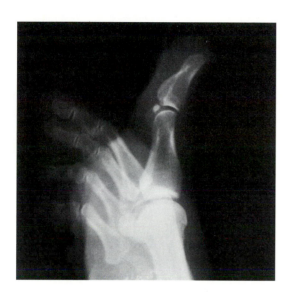

Fig. 6-32. Lateral great toe.

(Courtesy Lois Baird, R.T.)

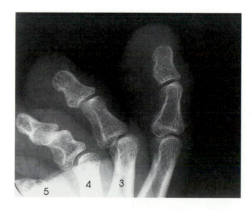

Fig. 6-33. Lateral second toe.

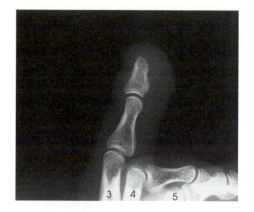

Fig. 6-34. Lateral third toe.

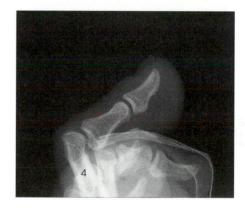

Fig. 6-35. Lateral fourth toe.

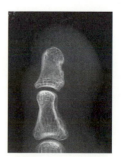

Fig. 6-36. Lateral fifth toe.

Sesamoids

TANGENTIAL PROJECTION
LEWIS[1] AND HOLLY[2] METHODS

Film: 8 × 10 in (18 × 24 cm) crosswise for multiple exposures on one film.

[1]Lewis RW: Non-routine views in roentgen examination of the extremities, Surg Gynecol Obstet 69:38-45, 1938.
[2]Holly EW: Radiography of the tarsal sesamoid bones. Med Radiogr Photogr 31:73, 1955.

Position of patient

- Place the patient in the prone position.
- Elevate the ankle of the affected side on sandbags for stability if needed. A folded towel may be placed under the knee for comfort.

Position of part

- Rest the great toe on the table in a position of dorsiflexion and adjust it to place the ball of the foot perpendicular to the horizontal plane. Place an 8 × 10 in (18 × 24 cm) cassette crosswise.
- Center the cassette to the second metatarsal (Fig. 6-37).
- *Shield gonads.*

Central ray

- Direct the central ray perpendicular and tangential to the first metatarsophalangeal joint.

Structures shown

The resulting image will show a tangential projection of the metatarsal head in profile and the sesamoids (Fig. 6-38).

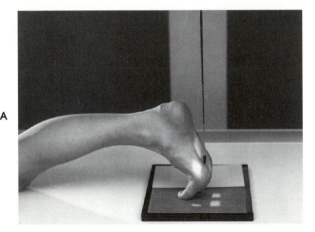

A

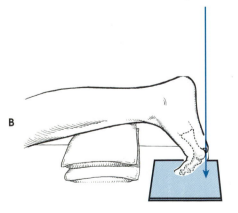

B

Fig. 6-37. A and **B,** Tangential sesamoids: Lewis-method.

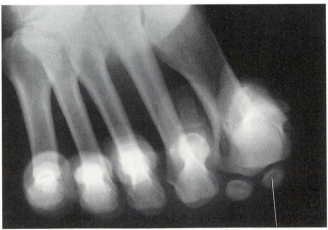

Sesamoid

Fig. 6-38. Tangential sesamoids (Lewis method) with toes against cassette.

(Courtesy Annette Wendt, R.T.)

Lower limb (extremity)

□ Evaluation criteria

The following should be clearly demonstrated:

- Sesamoids free of any portion of the first metatarsal.
- Metatarsal heads.

NOTE: Holly[2] described a position that he believes is more comfortable for the patient. With the patient seated on the table, adjust the foot so that the medial border is vertical and the plantar surface is at an angle of 75 degrees with the plane of the film. The patient holds the toes in a flexed position with a strip of gauze bandage. The central ray is directed perpendicularly to the head of the first metatarsal bone (Figs. 6-39 and 6-40).

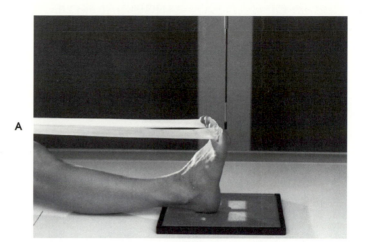

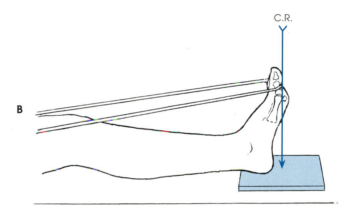

Fig. 6-39. A and **B,** Tangential sesamoids: Holly method.

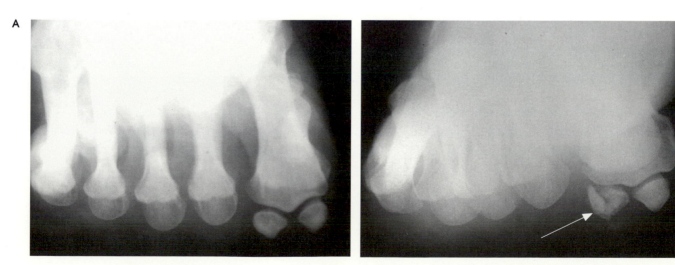

Fig. 6-40. A, Tangential sesamoids (Holly method) with heel against cassette. **B,** Sesamoid with fracture *(arrow).*

Sesamoids

TANGENTIAL PROJECTION
CAUSTON METHOD[1]

Film: 8 × 10 in (18 × 24 cm).

[1]Causton J: Projection of sesamoid bones in the region of the first metatarsophalangeal joint. Radiology 9:39, 1943.

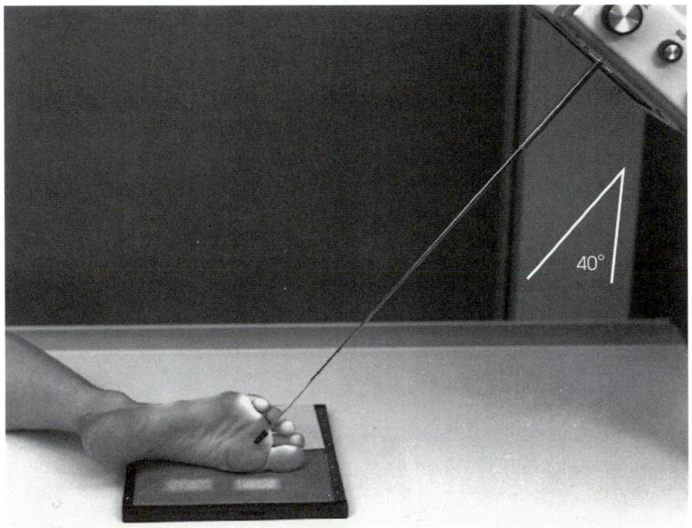

Position of patient

- Place the patient in the lateral recumbent position on the unaffected side and flex the knees.

Position of part

- Partially extend the limb being examined and put sandbags under the knee and foot.
- Adjust the height of a sandbag under the knee to place the foot in the *lateral position* with the first metatarsophalangeal joint perpendicular to the horizontal.
- Place the cassette under the distal metatarsal region and adjust it so that the midpoint will coincide with the central ray (Figs. 6-41 and 6-42).
- *Shield gonads.*

Fig. 6-41. Tangential sesamoids.

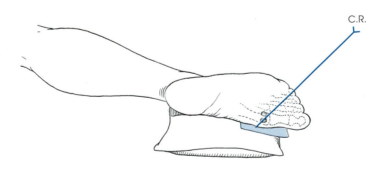

Fig. 6-42. Tangential sesamoids using occlusal film.

Central ray

• Direct the central ray to the prominence of the first metatarsophalangeal joint at an angle of 40 degrees toward the heel.

Structures shown

The tangential image will show the sesamoid bones projected axiolaterally with a slight overlap (Fig 6-43).

□Evaluation criteria

The following should be clearly demonstrated:

■ First metatarsophalangeal sesamoids with little overlap.

Occlusal film technique

For improved detail a similar projection may be taken using an occlusal film. The film is placed on a sandbag as illustrated (Fig. 6-42) and appropriately processed.

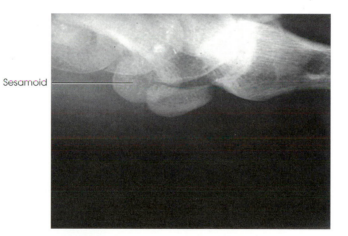

Sesamoid

Fig. 6-43. Tangential sesamoids.

Lower limb (extremity)

Foot

AP OR AP AXIAL PROJECTION

Similar radiographs may be obtained by directing the central ray perpendicular to the plane of the film or by angling the central ray 10 degrees posteriorly. The tarsometatarsal joint spaces of the midfoot are usually demonstrated better when a posterior angulation is used (Figs. 6-44 and 6-45).

Film: 8 × 10 in (18 × 24 cm) or 10 × 12 in (24 × 30 cm), depending on the length of the foot.

Position of patient

- Place the patient in the supine position.
- Flex the knee of the affected side enough to rest the sole of the foot firmly on the table.

Position of part

- Position the cassette under the foot, center it to the base of the third metatarsal, and adjust it so that its midline is parallel with the long axis of the foot.
- Hold the leg in the vertical position by having the patient flex the opposite knee and lean it against the knee of the affected side.
- In this foot position the entire plantar surface rests on the cassette; thus it is necessary to take precautions against the cassette slipping.
- *Shield gonads.*

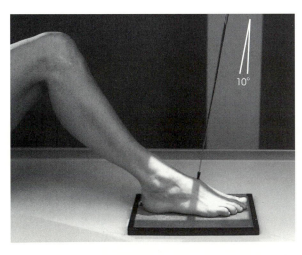

Fig. 6-44. AP axial foot with posterior angulation of 10 degrees.

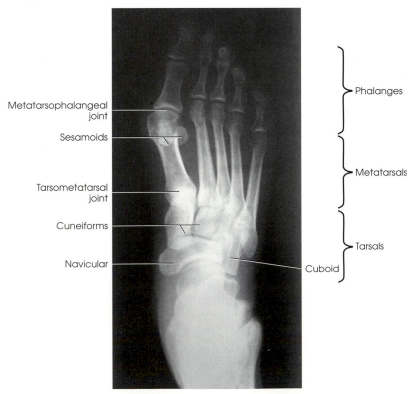

Fig. 6-45. AP axial foot with posterior angulation of 10 degrees.

(Courtesy John Syring, R.T.)

Metatarsophalangeal joint

Sesamoids

Tarsometatarsal joint

Cuneiforms

Navicular

Phalanges

Metatarsals

Tarsals

Cuboid

Central ray

- Direct the central ray one of two ways: (1) 10 degrees toward the heel to the base of the third metatarsal (Fig. 6-44) or (2) perpendicular to the cassette directed to the base of the third metatarsal (Fig. 6-46).

Structures shown

The resulting image will show an AP (dorsoplantar) projection of the tarsals anterior to the talus, the metatarsals, and the phalanges (Figs. 6-45, 6-47, and 6-48). This projection is used for foreign body localization, for determining the location of fragments in fractures of the metatarsals and anterior tarsals, and as a general survey of the bones of the foot.

☐ Evaluation criteria

The following should be clearly demonstrated:

- No rotation of the foot.
- Equal amount of space between the adjacent mid-shafts of the second through fourth metatarsals.
- Overlap of the second through fifth metatarsal bases.
- Visualization of the phalanges and tarsals distal to the talus as well as the metatarsals.

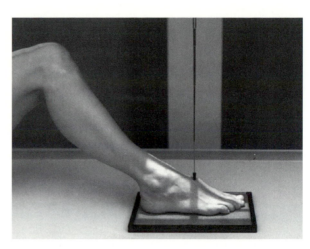

Fig. 6-46. AP foot with perpendicular central ray.

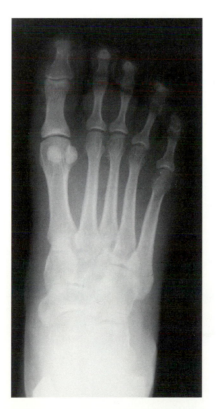

Fig. 6-47. AP foot with perpendicular central ray.

(Courtesy Lynn Rhatigan, R.T.)

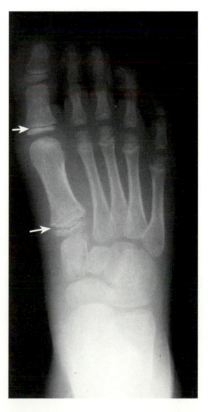

Fig. 6-48. AP foot of 6-year-old. Note epiphyseal centers of ossification *(arrows)*.

(Courtesy Javier Pagan, R.T.)

Foot

Lower limb (extremity)

Foot

AP OBLIQUE PROJECTION
Medial rotation

Film: 8 × 10 in (18 × 24 cm) or 10 × 12 in (24 × 30 cm), depending on the length of the foot.

Position of patient

- Place the patient in the supine position.
- Flex the knee of the affected side enough to have the plantar surface of the foot rest firmly on the table.

Position of part

- Place the cassette under the foot, parallel with its long axis, and center it to the midline of the foot at the level of the base of the third metatarsal.
- Rotate the leg medially until the plantar surface of the foot forms an angle of 30 degrees to the plane of the film (Fig. 6-49).
- *Shield gonads.*

Central ray

- Direct the central ray perpendicular to the base of the third metatarsal.

Structures shown

The resulting image will show the interspaces between the cuboid and calcaneus, between the cuboid and the fourth and fifth metatarsals, between the cuboid and the lateral cuneiform, and between the talus and the navicular. The sinus tarsi is also well shown (Fig. 6-50).

□Evaluation criteria

The following should be clearly demonstrated:

- Third through fifth metatarsal bases free of superimposition.
- The lateral tarsals with less superimposition than in the AP projection.
- Lateral tarsometatarsal and intertarsal joints.
- Sinus tarsi.
- Tuberosity of the fifth metatarsal.
- Bases of the first and second metatarsals.
- An equal amount of space between the shafts of the second through fifth metatarsals.
- Sufficient density to demonstrate the phalanges, metatarsals, and tarsals.

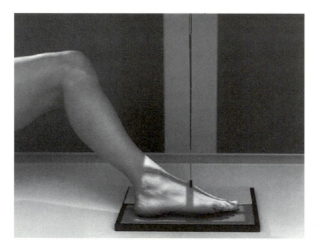

Fig. 6-49. AP oblique foot. Medial rotation.

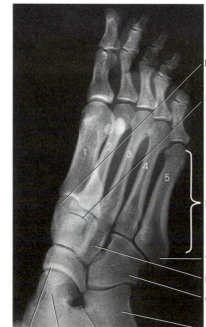

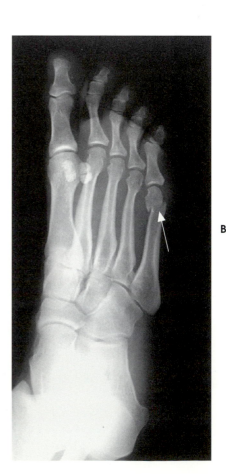

Fig. 6-50. A and **B,** AP oblique projection foot, medial rotation. **B,** Fracture of the distal aspect of the fifth metatarsal (*arrow*).

(**B,** Courtesy Ammar Saadeh, R.T.)

Medial cuneiform · Intermediate cuneiform · Metatarsals · Tuberosity · Lateral cuneiform · Cuboid · Calcaneus · Navicular · Talus · Sinus tarsi

200

Foot

AP OBLIQUE PROJECTION
Lateral rotation

Film: 8 × 10 in (18 × 24 cm) or 10 × 12 in (24 × 30 cm), depending on the length of the foot.

Position of patient

- Place the patient in the supine position.
- Flex the knee of the affected side enough for the plantar surface of the foot to rest firmly on the table.

Position of part

- Place the cassette under the foot, parallel with its long axis, and center it to the midline of the foot at the level of the base of the third metatarsal.
- Rotate the leg laterally until the plantar surface of the foot forms an angle of 30 degrees to the film.
- Support the elevated side of the foot on a 30-degree foam edge to ensure consistent results (Fig. 6-51).
- *Shield gonads.*

Central ray

- Direct the central ray perpendicular to the base of the third metatarsal.

Structures shown

The resulting image will show the interspaces between the first and second metatarsals and between the medial and intermediate cuneiforms (Fig. 6-52).

☐ Evaluation criteria

The following should be clearly demonstrated:

- Separate first and second metatarsal bases.
- No superimposition of the medial and intermediate cuneiforms.
- Navicular more clearly demonstrated than in the medial rotation.
- Sufficient density to demonstrate the phalanges, metatarsals, and tarsals.

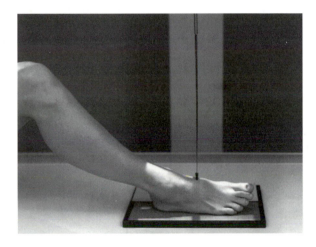

Fig. 6-51. AP oblique foot. Lateral rotation.

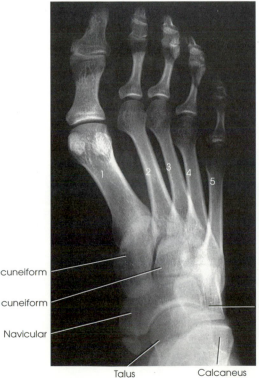

Medial cuneiform

Intermediate cuneiform

Navicular

Cuboid

Talus   Calcaneus

Fig. 6-52. AP oblique foot.

Foot

PA OBLIQUE PROJECTIONS
Medial or lateral rotation
GRASHEY METHODS

Film: 8 × 10 in (18 × 24 cm) or 10 × 12 in (24 × 30 cm), depending on the length of the foot.

Position of patient

• Place the patient in the prone position.
• Elevate the affected foot on sandbags. If desired, place a folded towel under the knee.

Position of part

• Adjust the elevation of the foot to place its dorsal surface in contact with the cassette.
• Position the cassette under the foot, parallel with its long axis, and center it to the base of the third metatarsal.
• To demonstrate the interspace between the first and second metatarsals, rotate the *heel* medially approximately 30 degrees (Figs. 6-53 and 6-54).
• To demonstrate the interspaces between the second and third, the third and fourth, and the fourth and fifth metatarsals, adjust the foot so that the heel is rotated laterally approximately 20 degrees (Fig. 6-54).
• *Shield gonads.*

Central ray

• Direct the central ray perpendicular to the base of the third metatarsal.

Structures shown

The resulting image will show a PA oblique projection of the bones of the foot and of the interspaces of the proximal ends of the metatarsals.

□ Evaluation criteria

The following should be clearly demonstrated:

Thirty-degree medial rotation.
■ First and second metatarsal bases free of superimposition.
■ Medial cuneiform projected without superimposition.
■ Navicular seen in profile.
Twenty-degree lateral rotation.
■ Third through fifth metatarsal bases free of superimposition.
■ Tuberosity of the fifth metatarsal and cuboid.

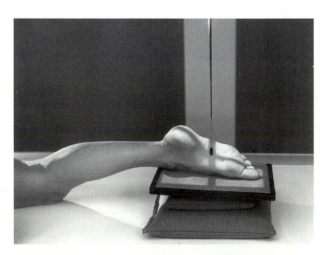

Fig. 6-53. PA oblique foot with heel medially rotated 30 degrees.

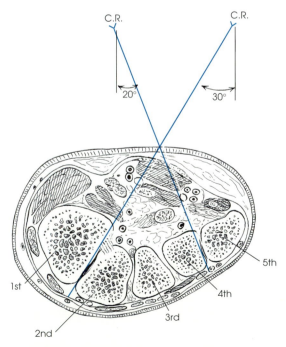

Fig. 6-54. Coronal section near base of metatarsals of right foot.

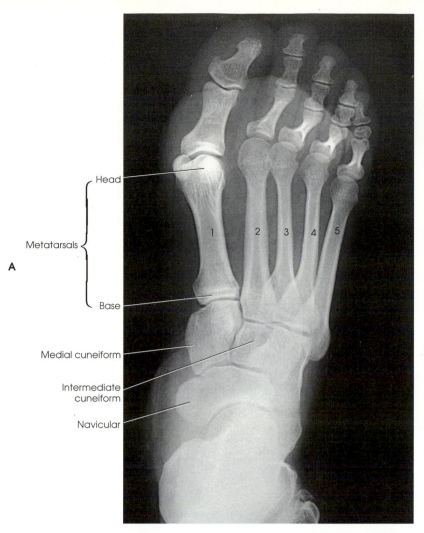

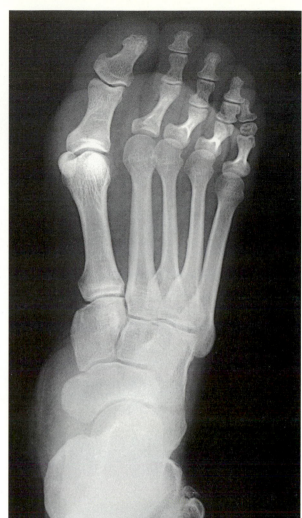

Head

Metatarsals {

A

Base

Medial cuneiform

Intermediate
cuneiform

Navicular

B

Foot

Fig. 6-55. PA oblique foot with heel medially rotated 30 degrees.

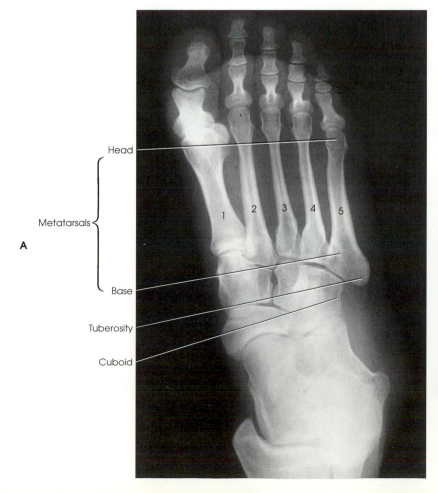

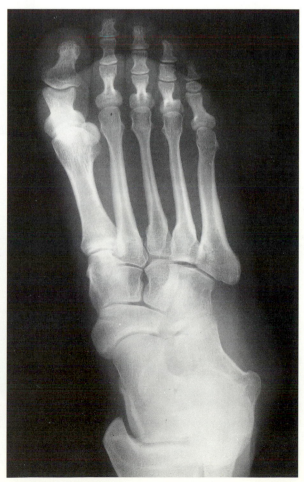

Head

Metatarsals {

A

Base

Tuberosity

Cuboid

B

Fig. 6-56. PA oblique foot with heel laterally rotated 20 degrees.

Foot

PA OBLIQUE PROJECTION
Medial rotation

Film: 8 × 10 in (18 × 24 cm) or 10 × 12 in (24 × 30 cm), depending on the length of the foot.

Position of patient

- Place the patient in the lateral recumbent position on the affected side and flex the knees.

Position of part

- Fully extend the leg of the side being examined.
- Have the patient turn toward the prone position until the plantar surface of the foot forms an angle of 45 degrees to the plane of the film.
- Center the cassette opposite the base of the fifth metatarsal and adjust it so that its midline is parallel with the long axis of the foot.
- Rest the dorsum of the foot against a foam wedge. The general survey study is usually made with the foot at an angle of 45 degrees to obtain uniform results (Fig. 6-57).
- *Shield gonads.*

Central ray

- Direct the central ray perpendicular to the midline of the foot at the level of the base of the fifth metatarsal.

Structures shown

The resulting image will show a PA oblique projection of the bones of the foot. The articulations between the cuboid and the adjacent bones—the calcaneus, lateral cuneiform, and fourth and fifth metatarsals—are clearly shown (Fig. 6-58). The articulations between the talus and navicular, between the navicular and cuneiforms, and between the sustentaculum tali and talus are usually shown.

☐Evaluation criteria

The following should be clearly demonstrated:

- A greater oblique projection than compared to the Grashey method.
- Third through fifth metatarsal bases and the tarsals.
- Tarsometatarsal and intertarsal joints.
- Tuberosity of the fifth metatarsal.
- Some superimposition of the first and second metatarsals.
- Sufficient density to demonstrate the phalanges, metatarsals, and tarsals.

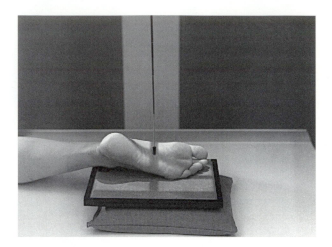

Fig. 6-57. PA oblique foot. Medial rotation.

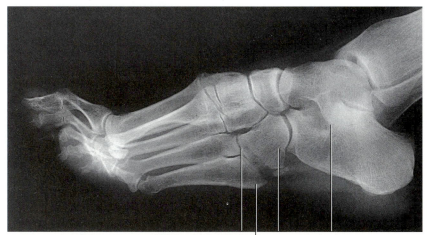

Tarsometatarsal joint   Cuboid   Calcaneus
Fifth metatarsal tuberosity

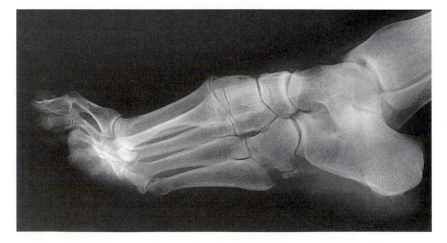

Fig. 6-58. PA oblique foot.

Foot

 LATERAL PROJECTION
Mediolateral

The lateral (mediolateral) projection is routinely used in most radiology departments because it is a comfortable position for the patient to assume. The *latero-medial* projection, however, is the recommended alternative when the patient's condition permits.

> **Film** 8 × 10 in (18 × 24 cm) or 10 × 12 in (24 × 30 cm), depending on the size of the foot.

Position of patient

- Place the patient on the table and have him or her turn toward the affected side until the leg and foot are lateral.

Position of part

- Elevate the knee enough to place the patella perpendicular to the horizontal plane, and adjust a sandbag support under the knee (Fig. 6-59).
- Center the cassette to the mid-area of the foot and adjust it so that the midline is parallel with the long axis of the foot.
- Dorsiflex the foot enough to rest it on its lateral surface, and adjust it so that the plantar surface is perpendicular to the film.
- *Shield gonads.*

Central ray

- Direct the central ray perpendicular to the base of the third metatarsal.

Structures shown

The resulting image will show the entire foot in profile, the ankle joint, and the distal ends of the tibia and fibula (Figs. 6-60).

□Evaluation criteria

The following should be clearly demonstrated:
- Metatarsals nearly superimposed.
- Distal leg.
- Fibula overlapping the posterior portion of the tibia.
- Tibiotalar joint.
- Sufficient density to demonstrate the superimposed tarsals and metatarsals.

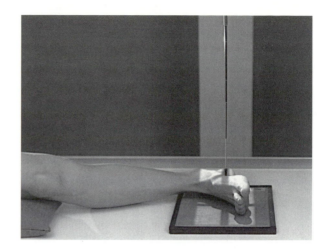

Fig. 6-59. Lateral foot.

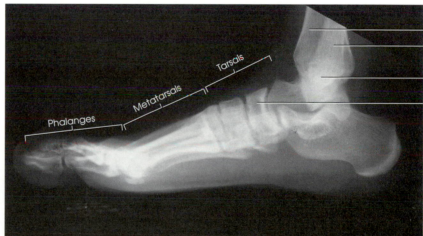

Fig. 6-60. Lateral foot.

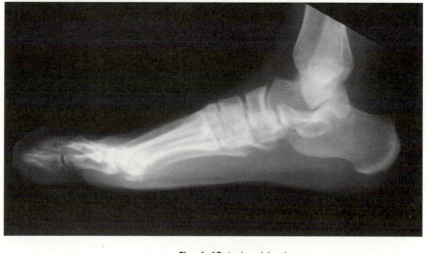

(Courtesy Colleen Gillespie, R.T.)

Foot

LATERAL PROJECTION
Lateromedial

Whenever possible, lateral projections of the foot are recommended to be made with the medial side in contact with the cassette. In the absence of an unusually prominent medial malleolus, hallux valgus, or other deformity, the foot assumes an exact or nearly exact lateral position when resting on its medial side. Although the medial position may be more difficult for some patients to achieve, true lateral projections are more easily and consistently obtained with the foot in this position.

Film: 8 × 10 in (18 × 24 cm) or 10 × 12 in (24 × 30 cm), depending on the length of the foot.

Position of patient

- Place the patient in the supine position.
- Turn the patient onto the *unaffected* side until the affected leg and foot are laterally placed. The patient's body will be in an LPO or RPO position.

Position of part

- Elevate the knee enough to place the patella perpendicular to the horizontal plane, and support the knee on a sandbag or sponge (Fig. 6-61).
- Center the cassette to the mid-area of the foot, and adjust it so that its midline is parallel with the long axis of the foot.
- Adjust the foot so that the plantar surface is perpendicular to the film.
- *Shield gonads.*

Central ray

- Direct the central ray perpendicular to the base of the third metatarsal.

Structures shown

The resulting image will show a true lateromedial projection of the foot, ankle joint, and distal ends of the tibia and fibula (Fig. 6-62).

☐ Evaluation criteria

The following should be clearly demonstrated:
- Metatarsals usually more superimposed than in the mediolateral image, depending on the transverse arch of the foot.
- Distal leg.
- Fibula overlapping the posterior portion of the tibia.
- Tibiotalar joint.
- Sufficient density to demonstrate the superimposed tarsals and metatarsals.

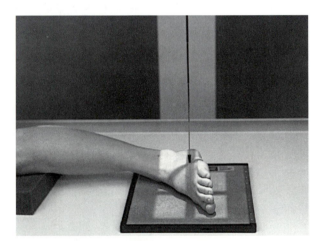

Fig. 6-61. Lateral foot.

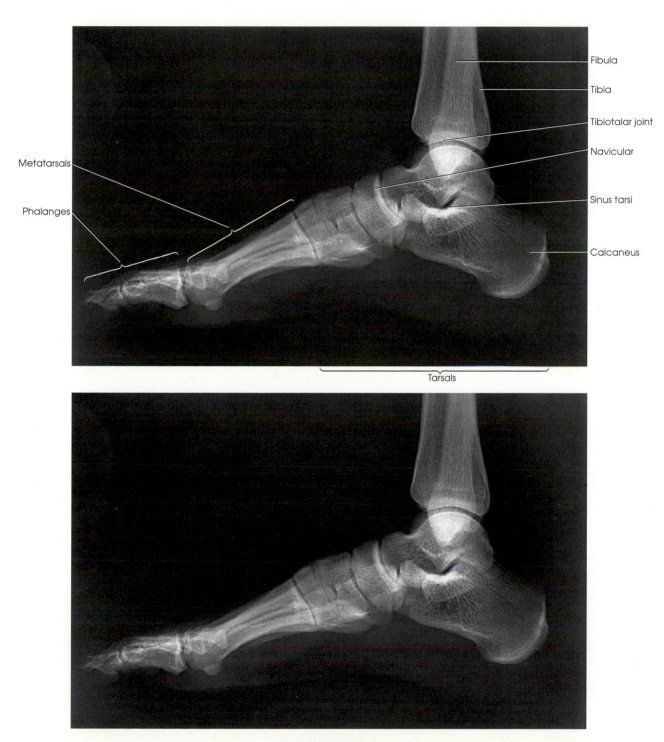

Fibula

Tibia

Tibiotalar joint

Navicular

Sinus tarsi

Calcaneus

Metatarsals

Phalanges

Tarsals

Fig. 6-62. Lateral foot.

Foot

LATERAL PROJECTION:
Longitudinal Arch
Lateromedial
WEIGHT-BEARING

Film: 8 × 10 in (18 × 24 cm) or 10 × 12 in (24 × 30 cm) film, depending on the length of the foot and whether a unilateral or a bilateral examination is being performed.

Position of patient

- Place the patient in the upright position, preferably on a low stool that has a film well. If such a stool is not available, use blocks to elevate the feet to tube level (Figs. 6-63 and 6-64).
- If needed, use a mobile unit to allow the patient to stand comfortably.

Position of part

- Place the cassette in the cassette groove of the stool or between blocks with a sheet of leaded rubber to protect its lower half.
- Have the patient stand in a natural position, one foot on each side of the cassette, with the weight of the body equally distributed on the feet.
- Adjust the cassette so that it is centered to the base of the fifth metatarsal.
- After the first exposure has been made, remove the cassette, turn it over to face the opposite foot, and place it back into the cassette groove, being careful to center to the same point.
- Rotate the tube 180 degrees to the opposite side, and make the second exposure.
- *Shield gonads.*

Central ray

- Direct the central ray perpendicular to a point just above the base of the fifth metatarsal.

Structures shown

The resulting image will show a lateromedial projection of the bones of the foot with weight bearing. The projection is used to demonstrate the structural status of the longitudinal arch. The right and left sides are examined for comparison (Fig. 6-65).

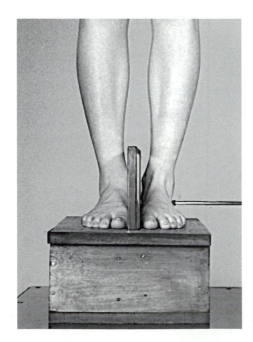

Fig. 6-63. Weight-bearing lateral foot.

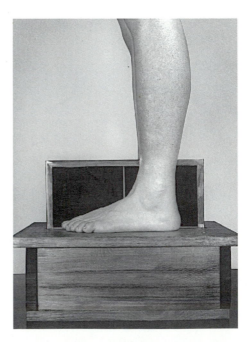

Fig. 6-64. Weight-bearing lateral foot.

□ Evaluation criteria

The following should be clearly demonstrated:

- Superimposed plantar surfaces of the metatarsal heads.
- Entire foot and distal leg.
- Fibula overlapping the posterior portion of the tibia.
- Sufficient density to visualize the superimposed tarsals and metatarsals.

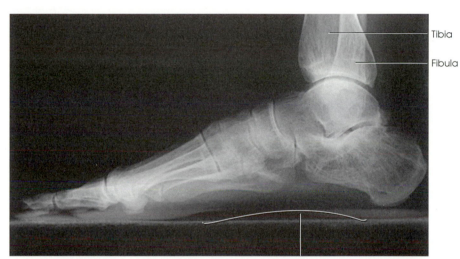

Tibia

Fibula

Longitudinal arch

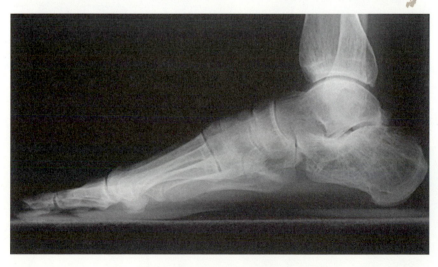

Fig. 6-65. Weight-bearing lateral foot.

(Courtesy John Syring, R.T.)

Foot

AP AXIAL PROJECTION
WEIGHT-BEARING COMPOSITE

Film: 8 × 10 in (18 × 24 cm) or 10 × 22 in (24 × 30 cm), depending on the length of the foot.

Position of patient

- Place the patient in the standing-upright position. A mobile unit allows the patient to stand at a comfortable height on a low stool or on the floor.

Position of part

- With the patient standing upright, adjust the cassette under the foot and center its midline to the long axis of the foot.
- To prevent superimposition of the leg shadow on that of the ankle joint, have the patient place the opposite foot one step backward for the exposure of the forefoot, and one step forward for the exposure of the hindfoot or calcaneus.
- *Shield gonads.*

Central ray

- To use the masking effect of the leg, direct the central ray along the plane of alignment of the foot in both exposures.

- With the tube in front of the patient and adjusted for a posterior angulation of 15 degrees, center to the base of the third metatarsal for the first exposure (Figs. 6-66 and 6-67).
- Caution the patient to carefully maintain the position of the affected foot, and then have him or her place the opposite foot one step forward in preparation for the second exposure.
- Move the tube behind the patient, adjust it for an anterior angulation of 25 degrees, and direct the central ray to the posterior surface of the ankle. The central ray emerges on the plantar surface at the level of the lateral malleolus (Figs. 6-68 and 6-69). An increase in technical factors is recommended for this exposure.

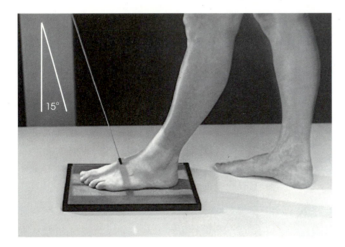

Fig. 6-66. Composite AP axial foot with posterior angulation of 15 degrees.

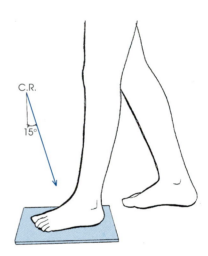

Fig. 6-67. Composite AP axial foot with posterior angulation of 15 degrees.

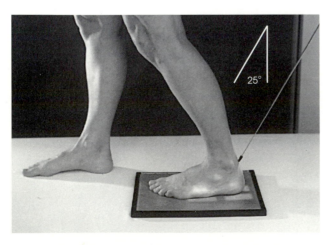

Fig. 6-68. Composite AP axial foot with anterior angulation of 25 degrees.

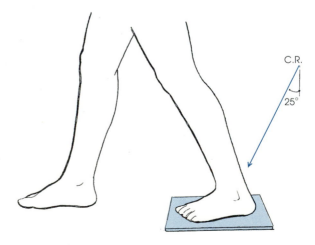

Fig. 6-69. Composite AP axial foot with anterior angulation of 25 degrees.

Structures shown

The resulting image will show a weight-bearing, AP axial projection of all of the bones of the foot. The full outline of the foot is projected free of the leg (Fig. 6-70).

□Evaluation criteria

The following should be clearly demonstrated:
- All tarsals.
- Shadow of leg not overlapping the tarsals.
- Foot not rotated.
- Tarsals, metatarsals, and toes with similar densities.

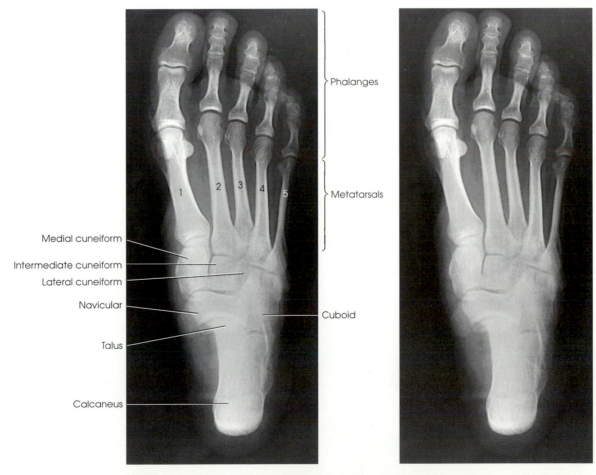

Fig. 6-70. Composite AP axial foot.

Congenital Clubfoot

The typical clubfoot, called talipes equinovarus, shows three deviations from the normal alignment of the foot in relation to the weight-bearing axis of the leg. These deviations are plantar flexion and inversion of the calcaneus (equinus), medial displacement of the forefoot (adduction), and elevation of the medial border of the foot (supination). There are numerous variations of the typical clubfoot and varying degrees of deformity in each of the typical abnormalities described above.

KITE METHODS

The classic Kite[1,2] methods—exactly placed AP and lateral projection—for radiography of the clubfoot are employed to demonstrate the anatomy of the foot and the bones or ossification centers of the tarsals and their relation to one another. *A primary objective makes it essential that no attempt be made to change the abnormal alignment of the foot when placing it on the cassette.* Davis and Hatt[3] state that even slight rotation of the foot can show marked alteration in the radiographically projected relation of the ossification centers.

AP PROJECTION

The AP projection demonstrates the degree of adduction of the forefoot and the degree of inversion of the calcaneus.

Film: 8 × 10 in (18 × 24 cm).

Position of patient

- Place the infant in the supine position, with the hips and knees flexed to permit the foot to rest flat on the cassette. Elevate the body on firm pillows to knee height to simplify both gonad shielding and leg adjustment.

Position of part

- Rest the feet flat on the cassette, with the ankles extended slightly to prevent superimposition of the leg shadow.
- Hold the knees together or in such a way that the legs are exactly vertical,

that is, so that they do not lean medially or laterally.
- Hold the toes by using a lead glove. When the adduction deformity is too great to permit correct placement of the legs and feet for bilateral images without overlap of the feet, they must be separately examined (Figs. 6-71 and 6-72).
- *Shield gonads.*

Central ray

- Direct the central ray perpendicular to the tarsals, midway between the tarsal areas for a bilateral projection.

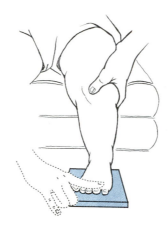

Fig. 6-71. AP foot for demonstration of clubfoot deformity.

- To be perpendicular to the tarsals, the central ray generally requires an approximate 15-degree posterior angle.
- Kite stresses the importance of directing the central ray vertically for the purpose of projecting the true relationship of the bones and ossification centers.

LATERAL PROJECTION
Mediolateral

The lateral radiograph demonstrates the anterior talar subluxation and the degree of plantar flexion (equinus).

Position of patient

- Place the infant on his or her side in as near the lateral position as possible.
- Flex the uppermost limb, draw forward, and hold in place.

Position of part

- After adjusting the cassette under the foot, place a support having the same thickness as the cassette under the knee to prevent angulation of the foot and to assure a lateral foot.
- Hold infant's toes in position with tape or a protected hand (Figs. 6-73 to 6-77).
- *Shield gonads.*

Central ray

- Direct the central ray perpendicular to the midtarsal area.

[1]Kite JH: Principles involved in the treatment of congenital clubfoot, J Bone Joint Surg 21:595-606, 1939.
[2]Kite JH: The clubfoot, New York, 1964, Grune & Stratton, Inc.
[3]Davis LA, and Hatt WS: Congenital abnormalities of the feet, Radiology 64:818-825, 1955.

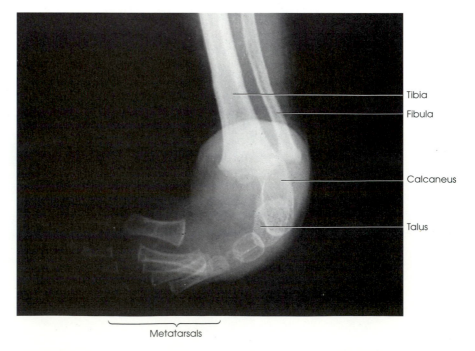

Tibia
Fibula
Calcaneus
Talus
Metatarsals

Fig. 6-72. AP projection showing near 90-degree adduction of forefoot.

□ Evaluation criteria

The following should be clearly demonstrated:

- No medial or lateral angulation of the leg.
- Fibula in lateral projection overlapping the posterior half of the tibia.
- The need for a repeat exam, should there be slight variations in rotation in either image when compared with previous radiographs.
- Sufficient density of the talus, calcaneus, and metatarsals to allow assessment of alignment variations.

NOTE: Freiberger, Hersh, and Harrison[1] recommend that dorsiflexion of infant feet be obtained by pressing a small plywood board against the sole of the foot. Older children and adults are placed in the upright position for a horizontal projection, with the patient leaning the leg forward to dorsiflex the foot.

NOTE: Conway and Cowell[2] recommend tomography for the demonstration of coalition at the middle facet and particularly for the hidden coalition involving the anterior facet.

[1]Freiberger RH, Hersh A, and Harrison MO: Roentgen examination of the deformed foot. Semin Roentgenol 5:341-353, 1970.
[2]Conway JJ, and Cowell HR: Tarsal coalition: clinical significance and roentgenographic demonstration, Radiology 92:799-811, 1969.

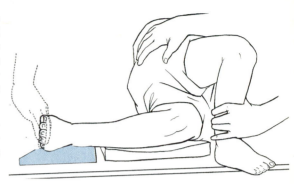

Fig. 6-73. Lateral foot.

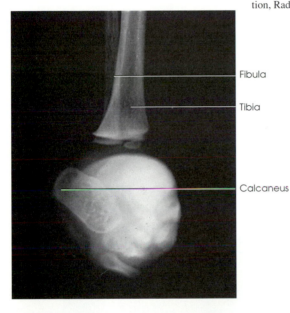

Fibula
Tibia

Calcaneus

Fig. 6-74. Lateral showing pitch of calcaneus, but other tarsals obscured by adducted forefoot.

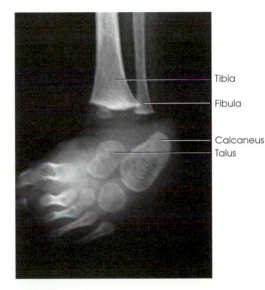

Tibia
Fibula
Calcaneus
Talus

Fig. 6-75. Nonroutine 45-degree medial rotation showing extent of talipes equinovarus.

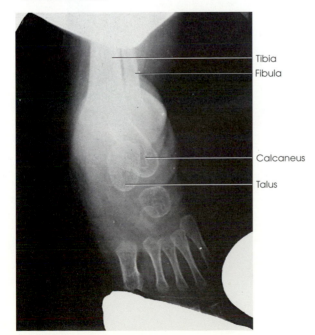

Tibia
Fibula
Calcaneus
Talus

Fig. 6-76. AP after treatment. (Same patient shown in Fig. 6-75.)

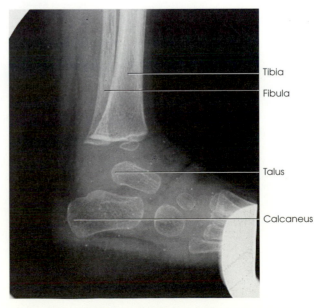

Tibia
Fibula
Talus
Calcaneus

Fig. 6-77. Lateral projection after treatment. (Same patient as in Fig. 6-74.)

Congenital Clubfoot

AXIAL PROJECTION
Dorsoplantar
Kandel Method

Kandel[1] recommends the inclusion of a dorsoplantar axial projection in the examination of clubfeet (Fig. 6-78).

For this method the infant is held in a vertical or a bending-forward position. The plantar surface of the foot should rest on the cassette, although a moderate elevation of the heel is acceptable when the equinus deformity is well marked. The central ray is directed 40 degrees anteriorly through the lower leg, as for the usual dorsoplantar projection of the calcaneus (Fig. 6-79).

Freiberger states that sustentaculum talar joint fusion cannot be assumed on one projection, since the central ray may not have been parallel with the articular surfaces. He recommends that three radiographs be obtained with varying central ray angulations (35, 45, and 55 degrees).

[1]Kandel B: The suroplantar projection in the congenital clubfoot of the infant, Acta Orthop Scand 22:161-173, 1952.

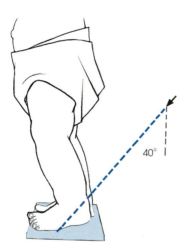

Fig. 6-78. Axial foot: (dorsoplantar) Kandel method.

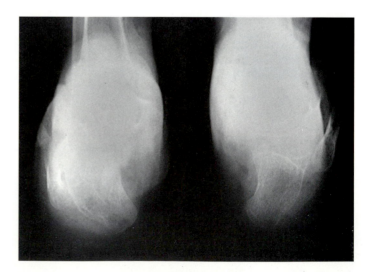

Fig. 6-79. Axial foot: (dorsoplantar) Kandel method.

Calcaneus

 AXIAL PROJECTION
Plantodorsal

Film: 8 × 10 in (18 × 24 cm).

Position of patient

- Place the patient in the supine or seated position with the legs fully extended.

Position of part

- Place the cassette under the ankle centered to the midline of the ankle (Figs. 6-80 and 6-81).
- Place a long strip of gauze around the ball of the foot. Have the patient grasp the gauze to hold the ankles in right-angle dorsiflexion.
- If the ankles cannot be flexed enough to place the plantar surface of the foot perpendicular to the cassette, elevate the leg on sandbags to obtain the correct position.
- *Shield gonads.*

Central ray

- Direct the central ray to the midpoint of the film at a cephalic angle of 40 degrees to the long axis of the foot. The central ray will enter the midline of the plantar surface of the foot at the level of the base of the fifth metatarsal and emerge just proximal to the ankle joint.

Structures shown

The resulting image will show an axial projection of the calcaneus from the tuberosity to the sustentaculum tali and trochlear process (Fig. 6-82).

☐ Evaluation criteria

The following should be clearly demonstrated:

- Calcaneus and the subtalar joint.
- No rotation of the calcaneus—the first or fifth metatarsals are not projected to the sides of the foot.
- Anterior portion of the calcaneus without excessive density over the posterior portion. Otherwise, two images may be needed for the two regions of thickness.

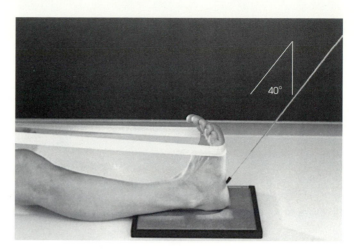

Fig. 6-80. Axial (plantodorsal) calcaneus.

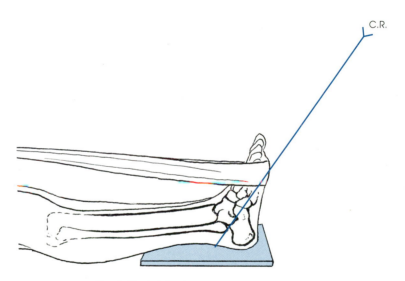

Fig. 6-81. Axial (plantodorsal) calcaneus.

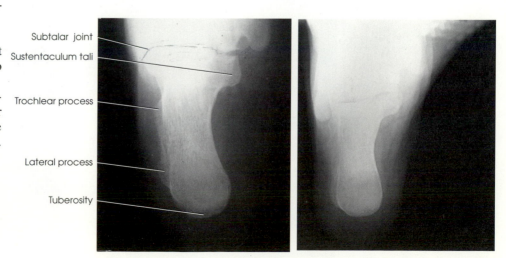

Subtalar joint

Sustentaculum tali

Trochlear process

Lateral process

Tuberosity

Fig. 6-82. Axial (plantodorsal) calcaneus.

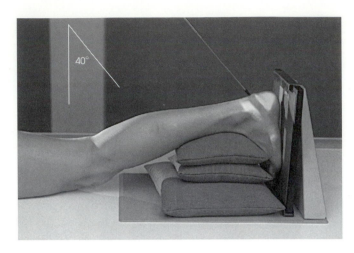

Fig. 6-83. Axial (dorsoplantar) calcaneus.

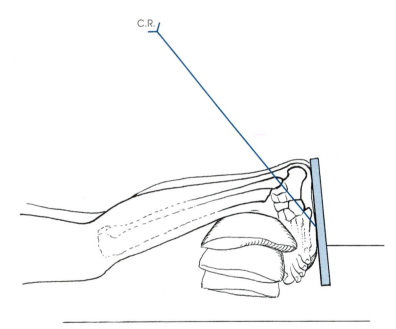

C.R.

Fig. 6-84. Axial (dorsoplantar) calcaneus.

Calcaneus
AXIAL PROJECTION
Dorsoplantar

Film: 8 × 10 in (18 × 24 cm).

Position of patient

- Place the patient in the prone position.

Position of part

- Elevate the ankle on sandbags.
- Adjust the height and position of the sandbags under the ankle in such a way that the patient can dorsiflex the ankle enough to place the long axis of the foot perpendicular to the tabletop.
- Place the cassette against the plantar surface of the foot, and support it in position with sandbags or a portable cassette holder (Figs. 6-83 and 6-84).
- *Shield gonads.*

Central ray

- Direct the central ray to the midpoint of the film at a caudal angle of 40 degrees to the long axis of the foot. The central ray will enter the dorsal surface of the ankle joint and emerge on the plantar surface at the level of the base of the fifth metatarsal.

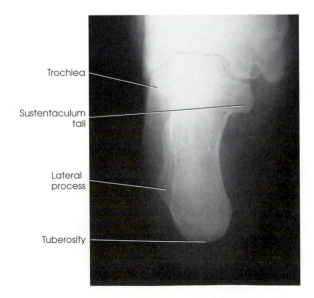

Trochlea

Sustentaculum tali

Lateral process

Tuberosity

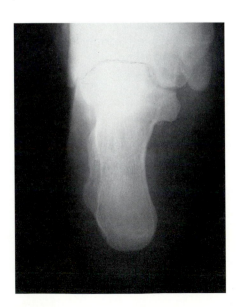

Fig. 6-85. Axial (dorsoplantar) calcaneus.

Structures shown

The resulting image will show an axial projection of the body of the calcaneus from the tuberosity to the sustentaculum tali and trochlear process (Fig. 6-85).

□Evaluation criteria

The following should be clearly demonstrated:
- Calcaneus and the subtalar joint.
- Sustentaculum tali.
- Calcaneus not rotated—the first or fifth metatarsals not projected to the sides of the foot.
- Anterior portion of the calcaneus, without excessive density over the posterior portion. (Otherwise, two images may be needed for the two regions of thickness.)

WEIGHT-BEARING "COALITION METHOD"

This method, described by Lilienfeld[1] (cit. Holzknecht), has come into use for the demonstration of calcaneotalar coalition.[2-4] For this reason, it has been called the "coalition position."

Position of patient

- Place the patient in the standing-upright position.

[1]Lilienfeld L: Anordnung der normalisierten Röntgenaufnahmen des menschlichen Körpers, ed 4, Berlin, 1927, Urban & Schwarzenberg, p 36.
[2]Harris RI, and Beath T: Etiology of peroneal spastic flat foot, J Bone Joint Surg 30B:624-634, 1948.
[3]Coventry MB: Flatfoot with special consideration of tarsal coalition, Minnesota Med 33:1091-1097, 1950.
[4]Vaughan WH, and Segal G: Tarsal coalition, with special reference to roentgenographic interpretation, Radiology 60:855-863, 1953.

Position of part

- Center the cassette to the long axis of the calcaneus with the posterior surface of the heel at the edge of the cassette.
- To prevent superimposition of the leg shadow, ask the patient to place the opposite foot one step forward (Fig. 6-86).
- With the central ray at an anterior angle of exactly 45 degrees, direct it through the posterior surface of the flexed ankle to a point on the plantar surface at the level of the base of the fifth metatarsal.

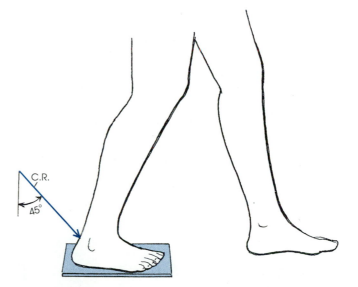

Fig. 6-86. Weight-bearing "coalition method."

Calcaneus

Calcaneus

LATERAL PROJECTION
Mediolateral

Film: 8 × 10 in (18 × 24 cm).

Position of patient

- Have the supine patient turn toward the affected side until the leg is approximately lateral. A support may be placed under the knee.

Position of part

- Adjust the calcaneus to the center of the film area, about 1 to 1½ inches (2.5 to 4 cm) distal to the medial malleolus.
- Adjust the cassette so the long axis is parallel to the plantar surface of the heel (Fig. 6-87).
- *Shield gonads*.

Central ray

- Direct the central ray perpendicular to the midportion of the calcaneus.

Structures shown

The resulting radiograph will show the ankle joint and the calcaneus in lateral profile (Fig. 6-88).

☐Evaluation criteria

The following should be clearly demonstrated:

- No rotation of the calcaneus.
- Density of the sustentaculum tali, lateral tuberosity and soft tissue.
- Sinus tarsi.
- Ankle joint and adjacent tarsals.

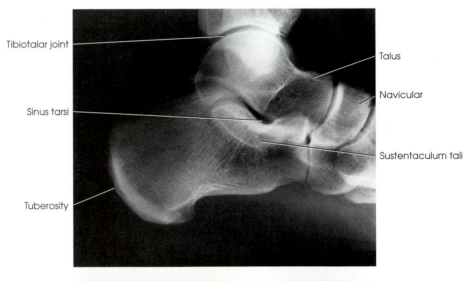

Tibiotalar joint

Sinus tarsi

Tuberosity

Talus

Navicular

Sustentaculum tali

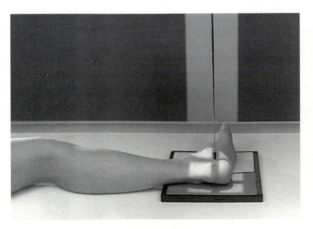

Fig. 6-87. Lateral calcaneus.

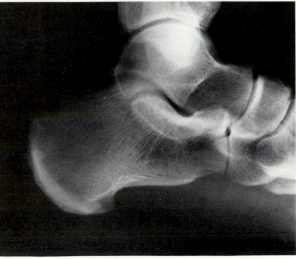

Fig. 6-88. Lateral calcaneus.

Calcaneus

LATEROMEDIAL OBLIQUE PROJECTION
WEIGHT-BEARING

Film: 8 × 10 in (18 × 24 cm).

Position of patient

- Have the patient stand with the affected heel centered toward the lateral border of the cassette (Fig. 6-89).
- The use of a mobile radiographic unit may assist in this examination.

Position of part

- Adjust the leg to ensure it is exactly perpendicular.
- Center the calcaneus so it will be projected to the center of the film.
- Center the lateral malleolus to the midline axis of the cassette.
- *Shield gonads.*

Central ray

- Direct the central ray medially at a caudal angle of 45 degrees to enter the lateral malleolus.

Structures shown

The resulting image will show the calcaneal tuberosity and is useful in diagnosing stress fractures of the calcaneus or tuberosity (Fig. 6-90).

Evaluation criteria

The following should be clearly demonstrated:
- Calcaneal tuberosity.
- Sinus tarsi.
- Cuboid.

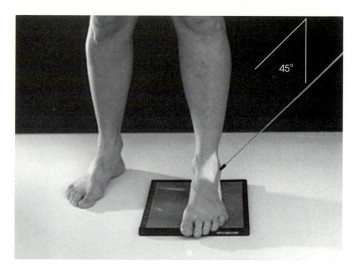

Fig. 6-89. Weight-bearing lateromedial oblique calcaneus.

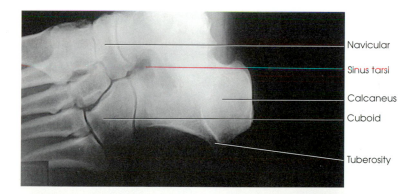

Navicular
Sinus tarsi
Calcaneus
Cuboid
Tuberosity

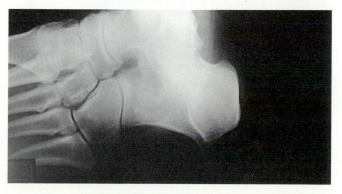

Fig. 6-90. Weight-bearing lateromedial oblique calcaneus.

(Courtesy Stephen Rusk, R.T.)

Subtalar Joint
PA AXIAL OBLIQUE PROJECTION
Lateral rotation

The calcaneus has three articular surfaces: anterior, middle, and posterior. These surfaces are located on the superior calcaneus and articulate with the inferior talus. The articulations form the subtalar (talocalcaneal) joint (see Fig. 6-11). This projection best demonstrates the anterior and posterior articulations.

Film: 8 × 10 in (18 × 24 cm).

Position of patient

- Have the patient lie on the affected side in the lateral position.
- Flex the uppermost knee to a comfortable position and support it on sandbags to prevent too much forward rotation of the body (Fig. 6-91).

Position of part

- Ask the patient to extend the affected limb.
- Roll the limb slightly forward from the lateral position.
- Center the cassette 1 to 1½ inches (2.5 to 4 cm) distal to the ankle joint and adjust it so that its midline is parallel with the long axis of the leg.

- Adjust the obliquity of the foot so that the heel is elevated about 1½ inches (4 cm) from the exact lateral position. The ball of the foot (the metatarsophalangeal area) will be angled forward approximately 25 degrees.
- *Shield gonads.*

Central ray

- Direct the central ray to the ankle joint with *a double angle* of 5 degrees anterior and 23 degrees caudal.

Structures shown

The resulting image will show the anterior and posterior articulations of the subtalar joint and gives an "end-on" image of the sinus tarsi and an unobstructed projection of the lateral malleolus (Fig. 6-92).

□ Evaluation criteria

The following should be clearly demonstrated:
- Open subtalar (talocalcaneal) joint articulations.
- Sinus tarsi.
- Lateral malleolus seen in profile.

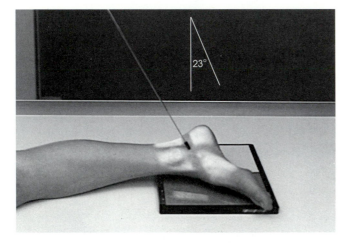

Fig. 6-91. PA axial oblique subtalar joint. Lateral rotation.

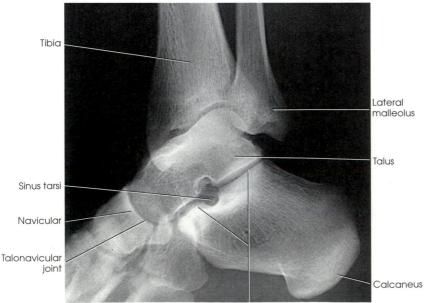

Subtalar (talocalcaneal) joint

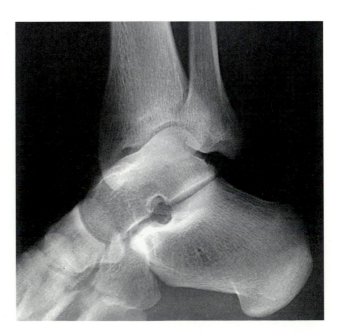

Fig. 6-92. PA axial oblique subtalar joint.

Subtalar Joint

AP AXIAL OBLIQUE PROJECTION
Medial rotation
BRODEN METHODS

Broden[1] recommends the lateromedial and mediolateral right-angle oblique projections for the demonstration of the *posterior articular surface* of the calcaneus to determine the presence of joint involvement in cases of comminuted fracture.

Film: 8 × 10 in (18 × 24 cm).

---

[1]Broden B: Roentgen examination of the subtaloid joint in fractures of the calcaneus, Acta Radiol 31:85-91, 1949.

Position of patient

- Place the patient in the supine position.
- Adjust a small sandbag under each knee.

Position of part

- Place the cassette under the lower leg and heel with its midline parallel with, and centered to, the leg.
- Adjust the film so that the lower edge will be about 1 inch distal to the plantar surface of the heel.
- Loop a strip of bandage around the ball

of the foot. Ask the patient to grasp the ends of the bandage and dorsiflex the foot enough to obtain right-angle flexion at the ankle joint. Ask the patient to maintain the flexion for the exposure.
- With patient's ankle joint maintained in right-angle flexion, rotate the leg and foot 45 degrees medially and rest the foot against a 45-degree foam wedge (Fig. 6-93).
- *Shield gonads.*

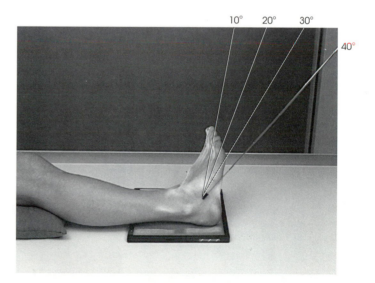

Fig. 6-93. AP axial oblique subtalar joint. Medial rotation.

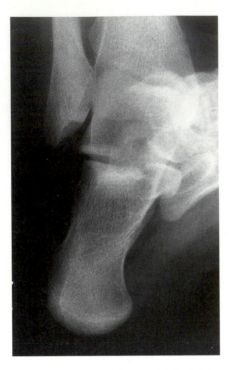

Fig. 6-94. AP axial oblique subtalar joint with angulation of 40 degrees.

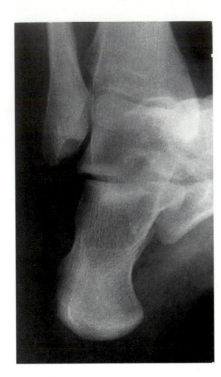

Fig. 6-95. AP axial oblique subtalar joint with angulation of 30 degrees.

Central ray

- Obtain four images with the central ray angled cephalad at 40, 30, 20, and 10 degrees, respectively.
- For each image, direct the central ray to a point 2 or 3 cm caudoanteriorly to the lateral malleolus, to the midpoint of an imaginary line extending between the most prominent point of the lateral malleolus and the base of the fifth metatarsal (Figs. 6-94 to 6-97).

Structures shown

The resulting images will show the anterior portion of the posterior facet to the best advantage. The 10-degree projection shows the posterior portion. The articulation between the talus and sustentaculum tali is usually shown best in one of the intermediate projections.

□ Evaluation criteria

The following should be clearly demonstrated:

■ Anterior and posterior portions of the subtalar joint.

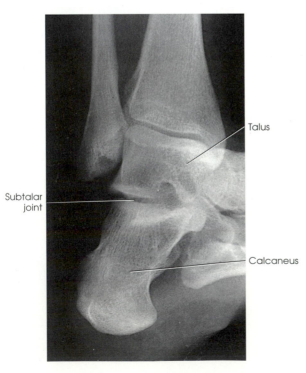

Talus

Subtalar joint

Calcaneus

Fig. 6-96. AP axial oblique subtalar joint with angulation of 20 degrees.

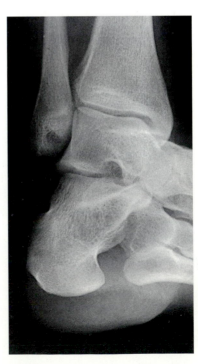

Fig. 6-97. AP axial oblique subtalar joint with angulation of 10 degrees.

Subtalar Joint

AP AXIAL OBLIQUE PROJECTION
Lateral rotation
BRODEN METHOD

Film: 8 × 10 in (18 × 24 cm).

Position of patient

- Place the patient in the supine position.
- Adjust a small sandbag under each knee.

Position of part

- With the ankle joint held in right-angle flexion, rotate the leg and foot 45 degrees laterally (Fig. 6-98).
- The foot may rest against a 45-degree foam wedge.
- *Shield gonads.*

Central ray

- Direct the central ray to a point 2 cm distal and 2 cm anterior to the medial malleolus, at a cephalic angulation of 15 degrees for the first exposure (Fig. 6-99).
- Two or three images may be made with a 3- or 4-degree difference in central ray angulation (Fig. 6-100).

Structures shown

The posterior talar articular surface of the calcaneus is shown in profile. The articulation between the talus and sustentaculum tali is usually shown.

☐ Evaluation criteria

The following should be clearly demonstrated:

- Posterior portion of the subtalar joint.

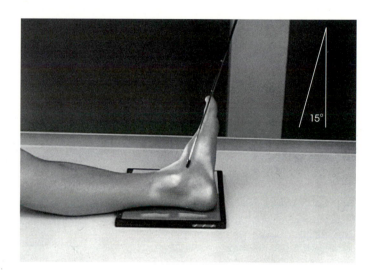

Fig. 6-98. AP axial oblique subtalar joint. Lateral rotation.

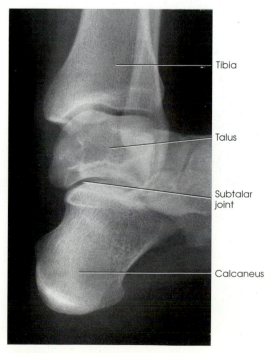

Tibia

Talus

Subtalar joint

Calcaneus

Fig. 6-99. AP axial oblique subtalar joint with angulation of 15 degrees.

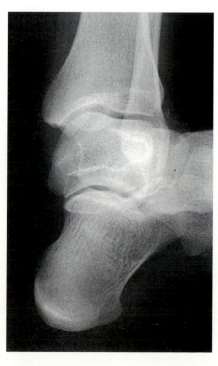

Fig. 6-100. AP axial oblique subtalar joint with angulation of 18 degrees.

Subtalar Joint
LATEROMEDIAL OBLIQUE PROJECTION
Medial rotation
ISHERWOOD METHOD

Isherwood[1] devised a method for each of the three separate articulations of the subtalar joint—an *oblique lateral* position for the demonstration of the anterior talar articular surface, a *medial oblique* for the middle talar articular surface for talus, and a *lateral oblique* for the posterior talar articular surface. Feist[2] later described a similar position.

Film: 8 × 10 in (18 × 24 cm) for each position.

Position of patient

- Place the patient in a semisupine or seated position, turned away from the side being examined.
- Ask the patient to flex the knee enough to place the ankle joint in near right-angle flexion and then to lean the leg and foot medially.

---

[1]Isherwood I: A radiological approach to the subtalar joint, J Bone Joint Surg 43B:566-574, 1961.
[2]Feist JH, and Mankin HJ: The tarsus: basic relationships and motions in the adult and definition of optimal recumbent oblique projection, Radiology 79:250-263, 1962.

Position of part

- With the medial border of the foot resting on the cassette, place a 45-degree foam wedge under the elevated leg.
- Adjust the leg so that its long axis is in the same plane as the central ray.
- Adjust the foot to be at a right angle.
- Place a support under the knee (Fig. 6-101).
- *Shield gonads*.

Central ray

- Direct the central ray perpendicular to a point 1 inch distal and 1 inch anterior to the lateral malleolus.

Structures shown

The resulting image will show the anterior subtalar articular surface and an oblique projection of the tarsals. The Feist-Mankin method produces a similar image representation (Fig. 6-102).

☐ Evaluation criteria

The following should be clearly demonstrated:
- Anterior talar articular surface.

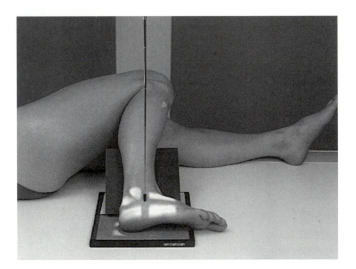

Fig. 6-101. Lateromedial oblique subtalar joint, medial rotation: Isherwood method.

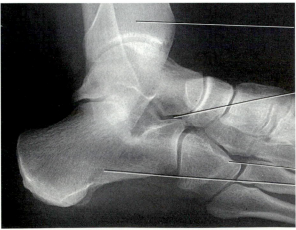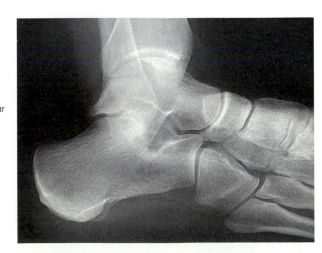

Tibia

Anterior talar articular surface

Cuboid

Calcaneus

Fig. 6-102. Lateromedial oblique subtalar joint demonstrating anterior talar articular surface: Isherwood method.

Subtalar Joint

AP AXIAL OBLIQUE PROJECTION
Medial rotation
ISHERWOOD METHOD

Film: 8 × 10 in (18 × 24 cm).

Position of patient

- Have the patient assume a seated position on the table and turn with his or her weight resting on the flexed hip and thigh of the unaffected side.
- If a semilateral recumbent position is more comfortable, adjust the patient accordingly.

Position of part

- Ask the patient to rotate the leg and foot medially, enough to rest the side of the foot and ankle on an optional 30-degree foam wedge (Fig. 6-103).
- Place a support under the knee and, if the patient is recumbent, place another under the greater trochanter.
- Dorsiflex the foot, invert it when possible, and have the patient maintain the position by pulling on a strip of 2- or 3-inch bandage looped around the ball of the foot if needed.
- *Shield gonads.*

Central ray

- Direct the central ray to a point 1 inch distal and 1 inch anterior to the lateral malleolus at an angle of 10 degrees cephalad.

Structures shown

The resulting image will show the middle articulation of the subtalar joint and an "end-on" projection of the sinus tarsi (Fig. 6-104).

□ Evaluation criteria

The following should be clearly demonstrated:

- Middle (subtalar) articulation.
- Open sinus tarsi.

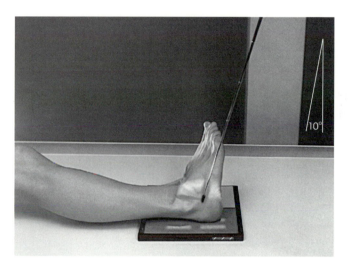

Fig. 6-103. AP axial oblique subtalar joint, medial rotation: Isherwood method.

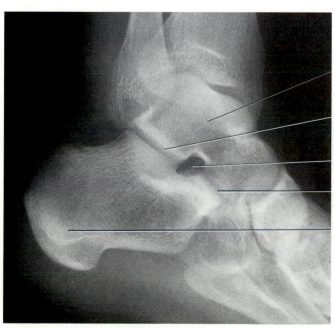
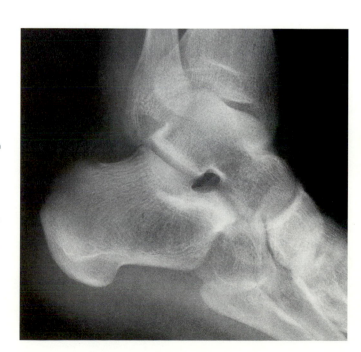

Talus

Posterior subtalar articulation

Sinus tarsi

Middle subtalar articulation

Calcaneus

Fig. 6-104. AP axial oblique subtalar joint. Isherwood method.

Subtalar Joint

AP AXIAL OBLIQUE PROJECTION
Lateral rotation
ISHERWOOD METHOD

Film: 8 × 10 in (18 × 24 cm).

Position of patient

- Place the patient in the supine or the seated position.

Position of part

- Ask the patient to rotate the leg and foot laterally until the side of the foot and ankle rests against an optional 30-degree foam wedge.
- Dorsiflex the foot, evert it when possible, and have the patient maintain the position by pulling on a broad bandage looped around the ball of the foot if needed (Fig. 6-105).
- *Shield gonads.*

Central ray

- Direct the central ray to a point 1 inch distal to the medial malleolus at an angle of 10 degrees cephalad.

Structures shown

The resulting image will show the subtalar joint in profile (Fig. 6-106).

□**Evaluation criteria**

The following should be clearly demonstrated:

- Posterior subtalar articulation.

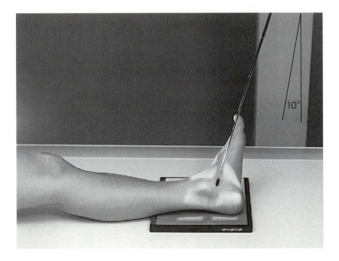

Fig. 6-105. AP axial oblique subtalar joint, lateral rotation: Isherwood method.

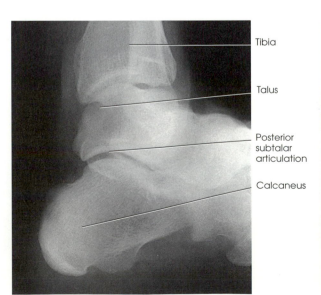
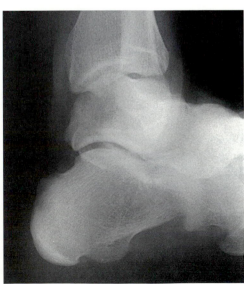

Tibia
Talus
Posterior subtalar articulation
Calcaneus

Fig. 6-106. AP oblique subtalar joint: Isherwood method.

Lower limb (extremity)

Ankle

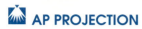

AP PROJECTION

Film: 8 × 10 in (18 × 24 cm) lengthwise; 10 × 12 in (24 × 30 cm) crosswise for two images on one film.

Position of patient

- Place the patient in the supine position with the affected limb fully extended.
- An optional sandbag may be placed under each knee to relieve strain.

Position of part

- Adjust the ankle joint for the AP projection by flexing the ankle and foot enough to place the long axis of the foot in the vertical position (Fig. 6-107).
- Ball and Egbert[1] state that the appearance of the ankle mortise will not be appreciably altered by moderate plantar flexion or dorsiflexion as long as the leg is rotated neither laterally nor medially.
- *Shield gonads.*

[1]Ball RP, and Egbert EW: Ruptured ligaments of the ankle, AJR 50:770-771, 1943.

Central ray

- Direct the central ray perpendicular to the ankle joint at a point midway between the malleoli.
- If a larger area of the leg is desired, use a larger cassette, and position the plantar surface of the heel to the lower edge of the film. However, if the joint is involved, *always* direct the central ray to the joint.

Structures shown

The resulting image will show an AP projection of the ankle joint, the distal ends of the tibia and fibula, and the proximal portion of the talus. Neither the inferior tibiofibular articulation nor the inferior portion of the lateral malleolus is well demonstrated in this projection (Fig. 6-108).

Evaluation criteria

The following should be clearly demonstrated:

- Tibiotalar joint space.
- Ankle joint centered to exposure area.
- Normal moderate overlapping at the tibiofibular articulation.
- Area from the distal tibia and fibula to the talus.
- No overlapping of the medial talomalleolar articulation.
- Medial and lateral malleoli.
- Talus with proper density.
- Soft tissue.

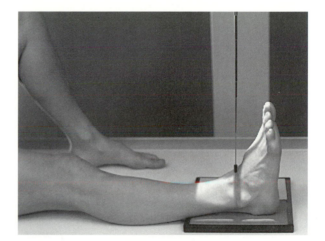

Fig. 6-107. AP ankle.

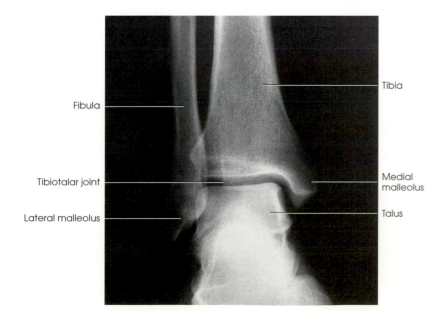

Fibula

Tibiotalar joint

Lateral malleolus

Tibia

Medial malleolus

Talus

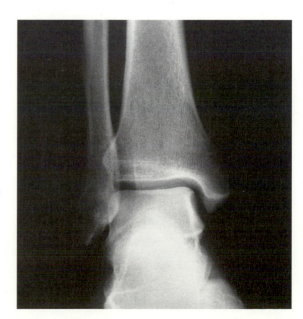

Fig. 6-108. AP ankle.

Ankle

 LATERAL PROJECTION
Mediolateral

Film: 8 × 10 in (18 × 24 cm).

Position of patient

- Have the supine patient turn toward the affected side until the leg is approximately lateral (Fig. 6-109).

Position of part

- With the midline of the cassette parallel to the long axis of the leg, center it to the ankle joint.
- Have the patient turn anteriorly or posteriorly as required to place the patella perpendicular to the horizontal plane and place a support under the knees.
- Dorsiflex the foot and adjust it in the lateral position; dorsiflexion is required to prevent lateral rotation of the ankle.
- *Shield gonads.*

Central ray

- Direct the central ray perpendicular to the ankle joint, entering the medial malleolus.

Structures shown

The resulting image will show a true lateral projection of the lower third of the tibia and fibula, of the ankle joint, and of the tarsals (Fig. 6-110).

□ **Evaluation criteria**

The following should be clearly demonstrated:

- Ankle joint centered to exposure area.
- Tibiotalar joint well visualized.
- Fibula over the posterior half of the tibia.
- Distal tibia and fibula, talus, and adjacent tarsals.
- Density of the ankle sufficient to see the outline of distal portion of the fibula.

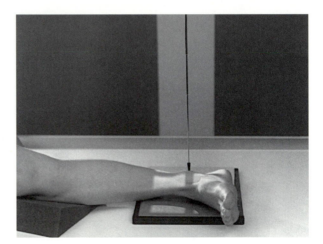

Fig. 6-109. Lateral ankle.

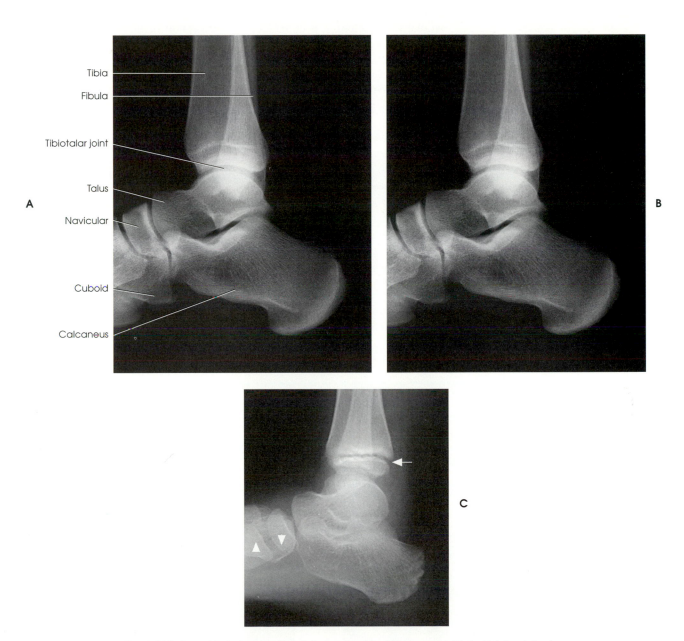

Tibia

Fibula

Tibiotalar joint

Talus

Navicular

Cuboid

Calcaneus

A

B

C

Fig. 6-110. A and **B,** Lateral ankle. **C,** Lateral ankle of 8-year-old. Note tibial epiphysis *(arrow)* and developing tarsals *(arrowheads)*.

(C, Courtesy Steve Bargiel, R.T.)

Ankle

LATERAL PROJECTION
Lateromedial

It is often recommended that the lateral projection of the ankle joint should be made with the medial side of the ankle in contact with the cassette. This position places the joint closer to the film and thus provides an improved image. A further advantage is that exact positioning of the ankle is more easily and more consistently obtained when the limb is rested on its comparatively flat medial surface.

Film: 8 × 10 in (18 × 24 cm).

Position of patient

- Have the supine patient turn away from the affected side until the extended leg is laterally placed.

Position of part

- Center the cassette to the ankle joint and adjust the cassette so that its midline is parallel with the long axis of the leg.
- Adjust the foot in the lateral position.
- Have the patient turn anteriorly or posteriorly as required to place the patella perpendicular to the horizontal (Fig. 6-111).
- If necessary, place a support under the knee.
- *Shield gonads.*

Central ray

- Direct the central ray perpendicular through the ankle joint entering one-half inch superior to the lateral malleolus.

Structures shown

The resulting image will show a lateral projection of the lower third of the tibia and fibula, of the ankle joint, and of the tarsals (Fig. 6-112).

□ Evaluation criteria

The following should be clearly demonstrated:
- Ankle joint centered to exposure area.
- Tibiotalar joint well visualized.
- Fibula over the posterior half of the tibia.
- Distal tibia and fibula, talus, and adjacent tarsals.
- Density of the ankle sufficient to see the outline of distal portion of the fibula.

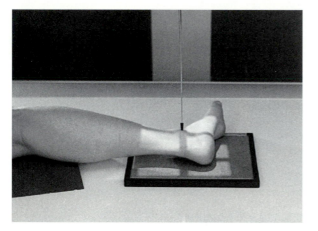

Fig. 6-111. Lateral ankle.

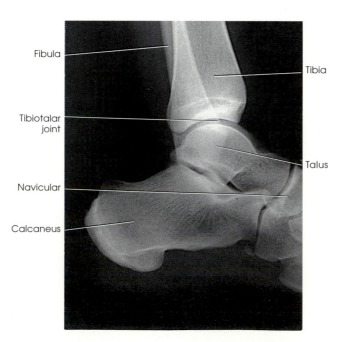
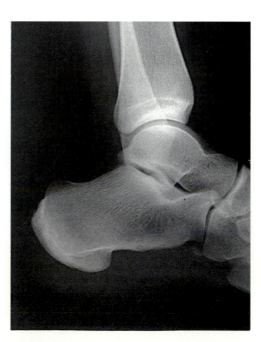

Fig. 6-112. Lateral ankle.

Ankle

 AP OBLIQUE PROJECTIONS
Medial rotations
INCLUDING ANKLE MORTISE

Film: 8 × 10 in (18 × 24 cm) lengthwise; 10 × 12 in (24 × 30 cm) crosswise for two images on one film.

Position of patient

• Place the patient in the recumbent position with the affected limb fully extended.

Position of part

• Rotate the *leg and foot* for all oblique projections of the ankle. Because the knee is a hinge joint, rotation of the limb can come only from the hip joint (Fig. 6-113).
• Center the cassette to the ankle joint midway between the malleoli, and adjust the cassette so its midline is parallel with the long axis of the leg.
• Dorsiflex the foot enough to place the ankle at near right-angle flexion. The ankle may be immobilized with sandbags placed against the sole of the foot or by having the patient hold the ends of a strip of bandage looped around the ball of the foot.
• Positioning the ankle for oblique projections requires that the leg and foot be medially rotated between 15 to 20 degrees, or 45 degrees, depending on the part to be demonstrated. Two medial oblique projections are possible; one to

demonstrate the ankle mortise; and a second to demonstrate the bones of the ankle in medial rotation.

Ankle mortise
• To demonstrate the mortise, medially rotate the leg and foot approximately 15 to 20 degrees. Adjust the degree of rotation until the *malleoli are parallel* with the cassette (Fig. 6-113).

Medial oblique for bony structure
• To demonstrate the distal tibia, fibula, and the talus, medially rotate the leg and foot 45 degrees and rest the foot against a foam wedge for support.
• *Shield gonads.*

Central ray

• For both projections, direct the central ray perpendicular to the ankle joint, entering midway between the malleoli.

Structures shown

Ankle mortise. The 15- to 20-degree medial oblique shows the ankle mortise in profile free of superimposition of the talus and the distal tibia or fibula. The open joint space represents the radiolucent articular cartilage between the talus and the malleoli (Fig. 6-114).

45-degree oblique. The 45-degree medial oblique demonstrates the distal ends of the tibia and fibula, parts of which are often superimposed over the talus (Fig. 6-115).

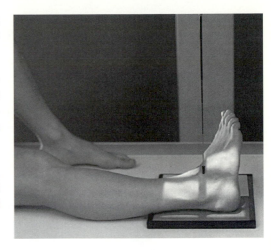

Fig. 6-113. AP oblique ankle, 15- to 20-degree medial rotation for demonstration of ankle mortise.

□ Evaluation criteria

The following should be clearly demonstrated:
   Ankle mortise
■ Ankle mortise in profile.
■ Talus and distal tibia and fibula adequately penetrated.
   45-degree oblique
■ Distal tibia and fibula may have some overlap of talus.
■ Distal tibia, fibula, and talus.
■ Talus and distal tibia and fibula adequately penetrated.

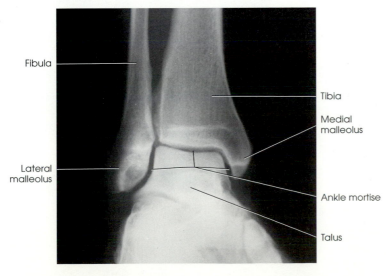

Fibula

Lateral malleolus

Tibia

Medial malleolus

Ankle mortise

Talus

Fig. 6-114. AP oblique ankle, 15- to 20-degree medial rotation, for demonstration of the ankle mortise.

(Courtesy Lois Baird, R.T.)

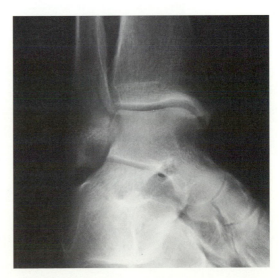

Fig. 6-115. AP oblique ankle, 45-degree medial rotation.

(Courtesy Eva M. James, R.T.)

Ankle

AP OBLIQUE PROJECTION
Lateral rotation

Film: 8 × 10 in (18 × 24 cm).

Position of patient

- Seat the patient on the radiographic table with the affected leg extended.

Position of part

- Place the plantar surface of the foot in the vertical position and laterally rotate the foot until an angle of 45 degrees is achieved.
- Rest the foot against a foam wedge for support, and center the ankle joint to the film (Fig. 6-116).
- *Shield gonads.*

Central ray

- Direct the central ray perpendicular through the ankle joint midway between the malleoli.

Structures shown

The lateral rotation oblique, is useful in determining fractures and to demonstrate the superior aspect of the calcaneus (Fig. 6-117).

□ Evaluation criteria

The following should be clearly demonstrated:

- The subtalar joint.
- The calcaneal sulcus (superior portion of calcaneus).

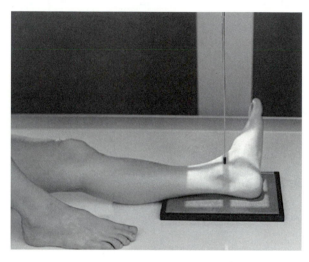

Fig. 6-116. AP oblique ankle. Lateral rotation.

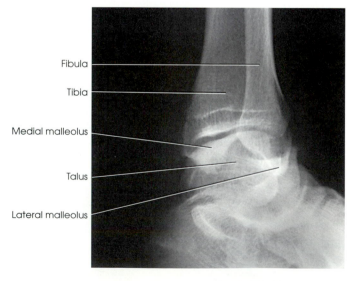

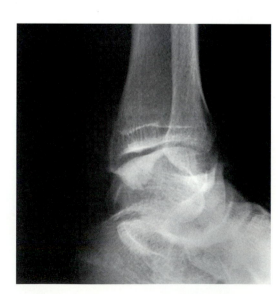

Fibula

Tibia

Medial malleolus

Talus

Lateral malleolus

Fig. 6-117. AP oblique ankle. Lateral rotation.

(Courtesy John Syring, R.T.)

Ankle

 ## AP PROJECTION

Stress studies

Stress studies of the ankle joint are usually obtained following an inversion or eversion injury, to verify the presence of a ligamentous tear. Rupture of a ligament is demonstrated by widening of the joint space on the side of the injury when, without moving or rotating the lower leg from the supine position, the foot is forcibly turned toward the opposite side.

When the injury is recent and the ankle is acutely sensitive to movement, the orthopedic surgeon may inject a local anesthetic into the sinus tarsi preceding the examination. The physician adjusts the foot when it must be turned into extreme stress and holds or straps it in position for the exposure. Under local anesthesia or when the ankle is not too painful, the patient can usually hold the foot in the stress position by asymmetrical pull on a strip of bandage looped around the ball of the foot (Figs. 6-118 to 6-121).

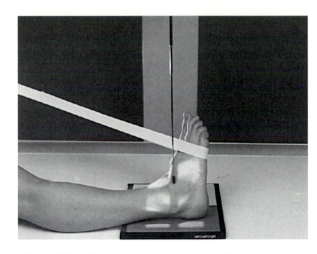

Fig. 6-118. AP ankle in neutral position. Use of lead glove and stress of the joint is required to obtain inversion and eversion radiographs (Figs. 6-120 and 6-121).

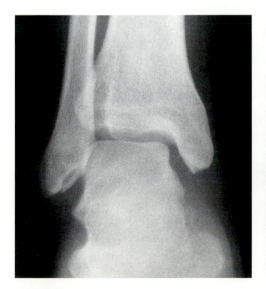

Fig. 6-119. AP ankle, neutral position.

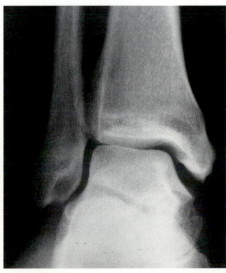

Fig. 6-120. Eversion stress—no damage to medial ligament indicated.

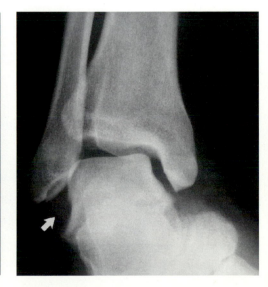

Fig. 6-121. Inversion stress—change in joint and rupture of lateral ligament (arrow).

(Courtesy Dr. William H. Shehadi).

Leg

 ### AP PROJECTION

For this projection, as well as the lateral and oblique projections that follow, the cassette is placed parallel with the long axis of the leg and centered to the midshaft. Unless the leg is unusually long, the film will extend beyond the knee and ankle joints enough to prevent their being projected off the film by the divergency of the x-ray beam. The film should extend from 1 to 1½ inches beyond the joints. When the leg is too long for these allowances and the site of the lesion is not known, two images should be made. Place the longer cassette high enough to include the knee joint and use a small cassette for the distal end of the leg. If the site of the lesion has been localized, adjust the cassette to include the closest joint. Diagonal use of a 14 × 17-inch cassette is also an option if the leg is too long to fit lengthwise and if permitted by the facility.

Film: 7 × 17 in (18 × 43 cm) or 14 × 17 in (35 × 43 cm) for two images on one film.

Position of patient

- Place the patient in the supine position.

Position of part

- With the patient supine, adjust the body so that there is no rotation of the pelvis.
- Adjust the leg so the femoral condyles are parallel to the cassette and the foot is vertical.
- Flex the ankle to a 90-degree angle.
- Place a sandbag against the plantar surface of the foot to immobilize it in the correct position if necessary (Fig. 6-122).
- *Shield gonads.*

Central ray

- Direct the central ray perpendicular to the center of the leg.

Structures shown

The resulting image shows the tibia, fibula, and adjacent joints (Fig. 6-123).

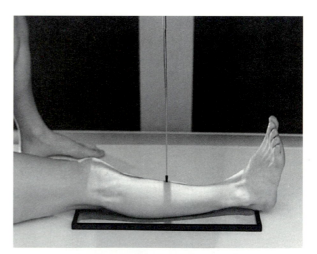

Fig. 6-122. AP tibia and fibula.

☐Evaluation criteria

The following should be clearly demonstrated:

■ Both the ankle and the knee joints on one or more AP projections.

■ Ankle and knee joints without rotation.

■ Proximal and distal articulations of tibia and fibula moderately overlapping.

■ Trabecular detail and soft tissue for the entire leg.

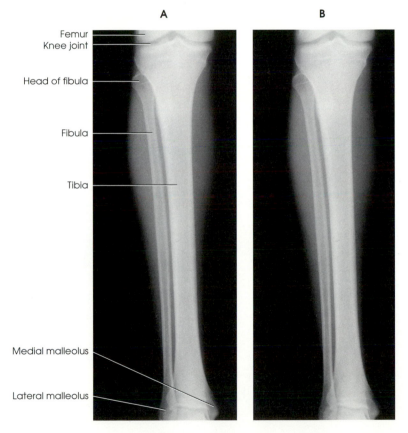

Femur
Knee joint
Head of fibula
Fibula
Tibia
Medial malleolus
Lateral malleolus

A   B

Fig. 6-123. A and **B,** AP tibia and fibula.

(**A** and **B,** courtesy Patti Chapman, R.T.)

Leg

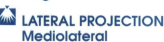

LATERAL PROJECTION
Mediolateral

Film: 7 × 17 in (18 × 43 cm) or 14 × 17 in (35 × 43 cm) for two images on one film.

Position of patient

• Place the patient in the supine position.

Position of part

• From the supine position, turn the patient toward the affected side with the leg on the cassette.
• Adjust the rotation of the body to place the patella perpendicular to the cassette, and ensure that a line drawn through the femoral condyles is perpendicular also. Place sandbag supports where needed for the patient's comfort and to stabilize the body position (Fig. 6-124).

Alternate method

• When the patient cannot be turned from the supine position, the lateral projection may be taken cross-table, utilizing a horizontal central ray.
• Lift the leg enough for an assistant to slide a rigid support under the leg.
• The film may be placed between the legs and the central ray directed from the lateral side.
• *Shield gonads.*

Central ray

• Direct the central ray perpendicular to the midpoint of the leg.

Structures shown

Resulting image will show the tibia, fibula, and adjacent joints (Fig. 6-125).

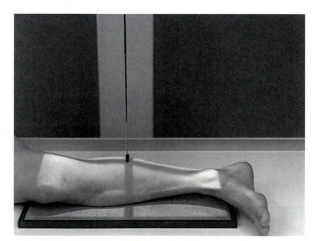

Fig. 6-124. Lateral tibia and fibula.

□Evaluation criteria

The following should be clearly demonstrated:

- Both the ankle and the knee joints on one or more images.
- Distal fibula lying over the posterior half of the tibia.
- Slight overlap of the tibia on the proximal fibular head.
- Ankle and knee joints not rotated.
- Possibly no superimposition of femoral condyles (because of the divergence of the beam).
- Moderate separation of the tibial and fibular bodies (shafts) seen except at their articular ends.
- Trabecular detail and soft tissue.

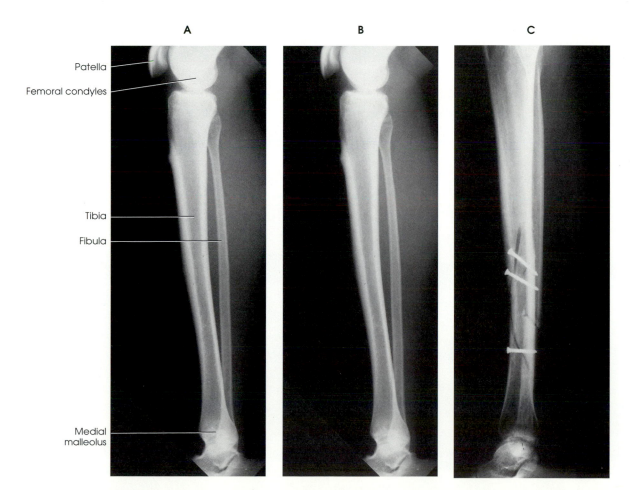

Fig. 6-125. A and **B,** Lateral tibia and fibula. **C,** Lateral postreduction tibia and fibula showing fixation device.

(**A** and **B,** courtesy Patti Chapman, R.T.; **C,** courtesy Dr. Hudson J. Wilson, Jr.)

Leg
AP OBLIQUE PROJECTIONS
Medial and lateral rotations

Film: 7 × 17 in (18 × 43 cm) or 14 × 17 in (35 × 43 cm) for two exposures on one film.

Position of patient

- Place the patient in the supine position on the radiographic table.

Position of part

- Oblique projections of the leg are taken by alternately rotating the limb 45 degrees medially (Fig. 6-126) or laterally (Fig. 6-127). Adjustment of the leg for the lateral oblique usually requires that the lateral side of the foot and ankle be rested against a 45-degree foam wedge.
- For the medial oblique, elevate the affected hip enough to rest the medial side of the foot and ankle against a 45-degree foam wedge and place a support under the greater trochanter.
- *Shield gonads.*

Central ray

- The central ray is directed perpendicular to the midpoint of the film.

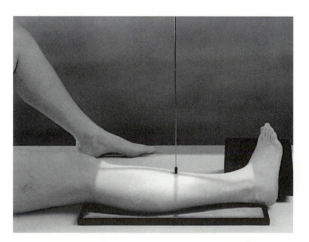

Fig. 6-126. AP oblique leg. Medial rotation.

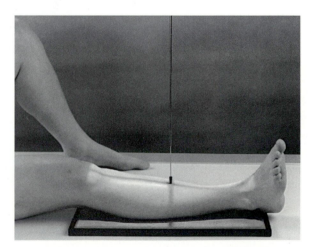

Fig. 6-127. AP oblique leg. Lateral rotation.

Structures shown

The resulting image will show a 45-degree oblique projection of the bones and soft tissues of the leg and one or both of the adjacent joints (Figs. 6-128 and 6-129).

□ Evaluation criteria

The following should be clearly demonstrated:

Medial rotation
- Proximal and distal tibiofibular articulations.
- Maximum interosseous space seen between the tibia and fibula.
- Ankle and knee joints.

Lateral rotation
- Fibula superimposed by lateral portion of tibia.
- Ankle and knee joints.

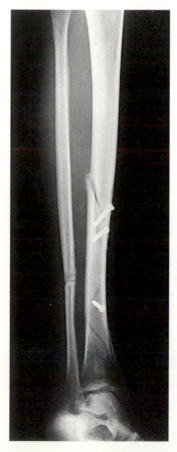

Fig. 6-128. AP oblique leg. Medial rotation showing fixation device.

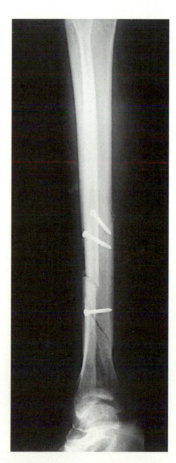

Fig. 6-129. AP oblique leg. Lateral rotation, with fixation device in place.

(Courtesy Dr. Hudson J. Wilson, Jr.)

Knee

 AP PROJECTION

Radiographs of the knee may be taken with or without the use of a grid. The size of the patient's knee and the preference of the radiographer and physician are the factors considered in reaching a decision. Most medical facilities establish a policy for the routine knee procedure, and, whether or not the policy is to use a grid or nongrid technique, the positioning of the body part remains the same.

Attention is again called to the need for gonad shielding in examinations of the lower limbs. (Not shown on illustrations of the patient model since the lead shielding would obstruct the demonstration of the body position.)

Film: 8 × 10 in (18 × 24 cm).

Position of patient

• Place the patient in the supine position, and adjust the body so that there is no rotation of the pelvis.

Position of part

• With the cassette under the patient's knee, flex the joint slightly, locate the apex of the patella, and as the patient extends the knee, center the cassette about ½ inch below the patellar apex. This will center the cassette to the joint space.
• Adjust the leg by placing the femoral epicondyles parallel with the cassette for a true AP projection (Fig. 6-130). The patella will lie slightly off center to the medial side. If the knee cannot be fully extended, a curved cassette may be used.
• *Shield gonads.*

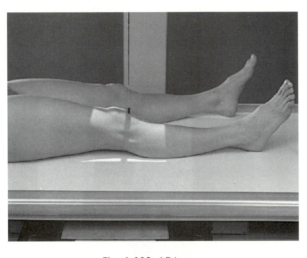

Fig. 6-130. AP knee.

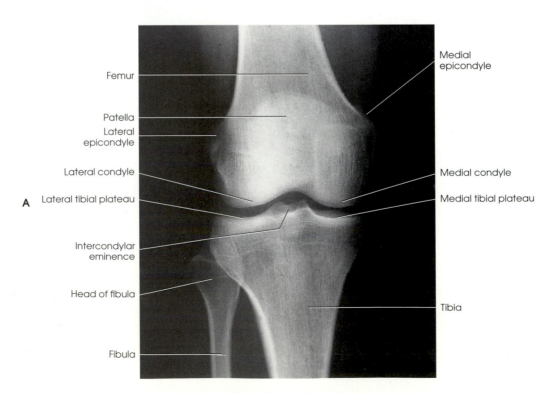

Fig. 6-131. A, AP knee.

Central ray

- When radiographing the joint space, the central ray is directed to a point ½ inch inferior to the patellar apex.
- Depending on the ASIS to tabletop measurement, direct the central ray as follows[1]:
  - Perpendicular for the sthenic patient when measurement is between 19 and 24 cm.
  - 5 degrees cephalad for hypersthenic patient when measurement is greater than 24 cm.
  - 5 degrees caudad for asthenic patient when measurement is less than 19 cm.
- When radiographing the distal end of the femur or the proximal ends of the tibia and fibula, the central ray may be directed perpendicularly to the joint.

Structures shown

The resulting image will show an AP projection of the knee structures (Figs. 6-131 to 6-132).

---

[1]Martensen KM: Alternate AP knee method assures open joint space. Radiol Technol 64(1): 19-23, 1992.

☐ Evaluation criteria

The following should be clearly demonstrated:

- Open femorotibial joint space.
- Knee fully extended if patient's condition permits.
- If the knee is normal, the interspaces should be equal in width on both sides.
- Patella completely superimposed on the femur.
- No rotation of the femur and tibia.
- Slight superimposition of the fibular head and the tibia is normal.
- Soft tissue around the knee joint.
- Bony detail surrounding the patella on the distal femur.

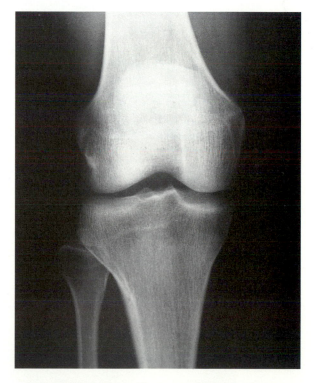

Fig. 6-132. AP knee with perpendicular central ray. (Same patient as Fig. 6-131.)

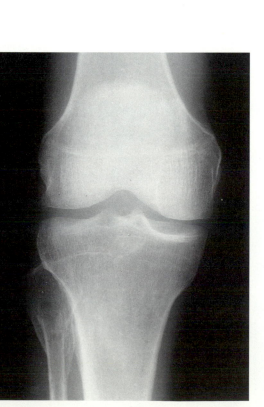

Fig. 6-131, cont'd. B, AP knee. CR angled 5 degrees cephalad.

(Courtesy Peter Degraaf, R.T.)

Knee

PA PROJECTION

Film: 8 × 10 in (18 × 24 cm).

Position of patient

- Place the patient in the prone position with the toes resting on the table, or place sandbags under the ankle for support.

Position of part

- Center a point ½ inch below the patellar apex to the center of the film, and adjust the leg so the femoral epicondyles are parallel to the tabletop. Because the knee is balanced on the medial side of the obliquely located patella, care must be used in adjusting the knee (Fig. 6-133).
- *Shield gonads.*

Central ray

- Direct the central ray perpendicular to exit a point ½ inch inferior to the patellar apex. Because the tibia and fibula are slightly inclined, the central ray will be parallel with the tibial plateau.

Structures shown

The resulting image will show a PA projection of the knee (Fig. 6-134).

□ Evaluation criteria

The following should be clearly demonstrated:

- Open femorotibial joint space.
- Knee fully extended if patient's condition permits.
- If the knee is normal, the interspaces should be equal in width on both sides.
- No rotation of femur and tibia is normal.
- Slight superimposition of the fibular head with the tibia.
- Soft tissue around the knee joint.
- Bony detail surrounding the patella.

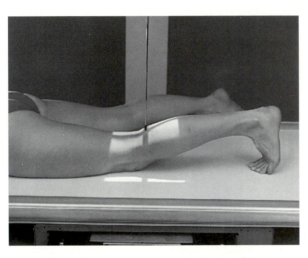

Fig. 6-133. PA knee.

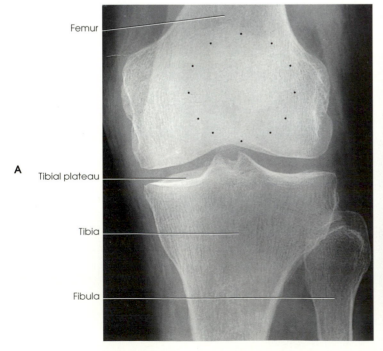
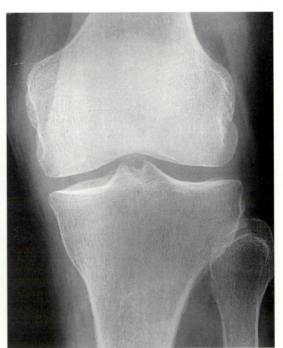

Femur

Tibial plateau

Tibia

Fibula

A

B

Fig. 6-134. A, PA knee (patella outlined by dots). **B,**.PA knee showing epiphyses of teenager.

Knee

LATERAL PROJECTION
Mediolateral

Film: 8 × 10 in (18 × 24 cm).

Position of patient

- Ask the patient to turn onto the affected side.
- When the knee is to be adjusted in right-angle flexion, have the patient bring it forward and extend the other limb behind, as shown (Fig. 6-135). When the knee is to be examined in extension or partial flexion, the opposite limb may be brought forward and the flexed knee supported to prevent forward rotation of the pelvis.
- A flexion of 20 to 30 degrees is usually preferred for survey studies because this position relaxes the muscles and shows the maximum volume of the joint cavity.
- To prevent fragment separation in new or unhealed patellar fractures, the knee should not be flexed more than 10 degrees.

Position of part

- Flex the knee to the desired angle (20 to 30 degrees recommended), and center the film to the knee joint. Locate the joint by palpating the depression between the femoral and tibial condyles on the medial side of the knee. The knee joint lies just below the level of the patellar apex. The knee joint is also located approximately 1 inch (2.5 cm) distal to the medial femoral condyle.
- A support may be placed under the ankle.
- Grasp the epicondyles and adjust so they are perpendicular to the cassette (condyles superimposed). The patella will be perpendicular to the plane of the film.
- *Shield gonads.*

Central ray

- Direct the central ray to the knee joint located 1 in (2 cm) distal to the medial epicondyle at an angle of 5 degrees cephalad. This slight angulation of the central ray will prevent the joint space from being obscured by the magnified shadow of the medial femoral condyle.

Structures shown

The resulting radiograph will show a lateral image of the distal end of the femur, the patella, the knee joint, the proximal ends of the tibia and fibula, and the adjacent soft tissue (Figs. 6-136 and 6-137).

□ Evaluation criteria

The following should be clearly demonstrated:

- Femoral condyles superimposed.
- Open joint space between femoral condyles and tibia.
- Patella in a lateral profile.
- Open patellofemoral space.
- Fibular head and tibia slightly superimposed.
- Knee flexed approximately 20 to 30 degrees.
- All soft tissue around the knee.
- Femoral condyles with proper density.

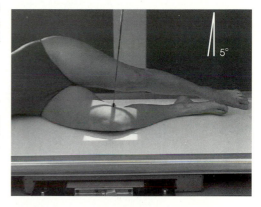

Fig. 6-135. Lateral knee showing 5 degree cephalad angulation of central ray.

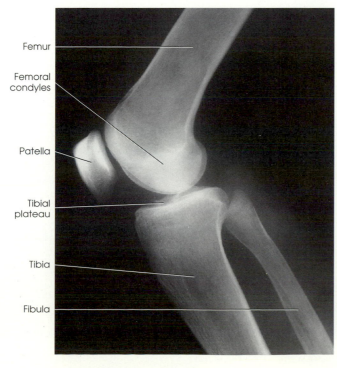

Fig. 6-136. Lateral knee flexed 55 degrees.

Femur

Femoral condyles

Patella

Tibial plateau

Tibia

Fibula

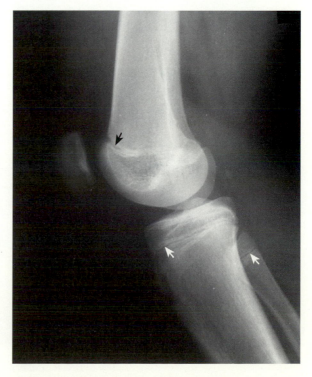

Fig. 6-137. Lateral knee of 15-year-old patient with knee in 25 degree flexion. Note epiphyses (*arrows*) of femur, tibia, and fibula.

(Courtesy Michael Desalu, R.T.)

Knees

 ## AP PROJECTION
WEIGHT-BEARING

Leach, Gregg, and Siber[1] recommend that a bilateral weight-bearing AP projection be routinely included in the radiographic examination of arthritic knees. They found that a weight-bearing study often reveals narrowing of a joint space that appears normal on the non–weight-bearing study.

Film: 10 × 12 in (24 × 30 cm) or 11 × 14 in (30 × 35 cm) crosswise for bilateral image.

---

[1]Leach, RE, Gregg, T, and Siber, FJ: Weight-bearing radiography in osteoarthritis of the knee. Radiology 97:265-268, 1970.

Position of patient

Place the patient in the upright position before, and with his or her back toward, a vertical grid device.

Position of part

- Have the patient adjust his or her position and center the knees to the film.
- Ask the patient to place the toes straight ahead, with the feet separated enough for good balance.
- Ask the patient to stand straight with his or her knees fully extended and weight equally distributed on the feet.
- Center the film at the level of the apices of the patellae (Fig. 6-138).
- *Shield gonads*.

Central ray

- Direct the central ray horizontal and center it midway between the knees at the level of the apices of the patellae.

Structures shown

The resulting image will show the joint spaces of the knees. Varus and valgus deformities can also be evaluated with this procedure (Fig. 6-139).

☐ Evaluation criteria

The following should be clearly demonstrated:
- No rotation of the knees.
- Both knees.
- Knee joint space centered to the exposure area.
- Adequate film size to demonstrate the longitudinal axis of the femoral and tibial bodies (shafts).

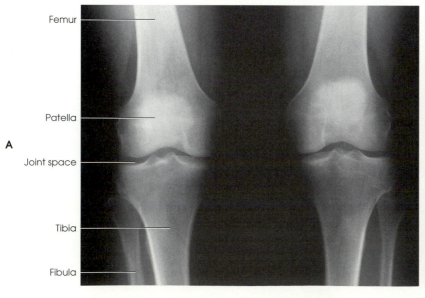

Fig. 6-138. AP bilateral weight-bearing knees.

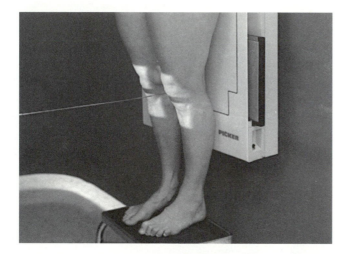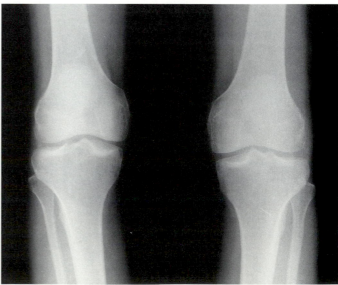

Femur

Patella

A

Joint space

Tibia

Fibula

B

Fig. 6-139. A and **B,** AP bilateral weight-bearing knees.

(**A,** courtesy John Syring, R.T.; **B,** courtesy Robbie F. Hockenberry, R.T.)

Knees

PA PROJECTION
WEIGHT-BEARING

Film: 10×12 in (24×30 cm) or 11×14 in (30×35 cm) crosswise for bilateral knees.

Position of patient

- Place the patient in the standing position with the anterior aspect of the knees centered to the vertical grid device.

Position of part

- With the knees in contact with the vertical grid device, have the patient stand upright for a direct PA projection.
- Center the film at the level of the apices of the patellae.
- A *modification* to better demonstrate the knee joints and the articular cartilage is to have the patient grasp the edges of the grid device and flex the knees to place the femurs at an angle ranging between 30 to 60 degrees (Fig. 6-140).
- *Shield gonads.*

Central ray

- Direct the central ray horizontally, and center it midway between the knees at the level of the patellar apices, or direct it 10 degrees caudad.

Structures shown

The PA weight-bearing knee projection is useful in evaluating joint space narrowing. When the knees are flexed between 30 to 60 degreees, the PA flexion projection is beneficial in demonstrating articular cartilage disease (Fig. 6-141). The image obtained when the knees are flexed is similar to the image obtained when radiographing the intercondylar fossa described on pages 250 to 255.

□Evaluation criteria

The following should be clearly demonstrated:

- No rotation of the knees.
- Both knees.
- Knee joint space centered to the exposure area.
- Adequate film to demonstrate the longitudinal axis of the femoral and tibial bodies (shafts).

NOTE: For a weight-bearing study of a single knee, have the patient put full weight on the affected side. The patient may balance with slight pressure on the toes of the unaffected side.

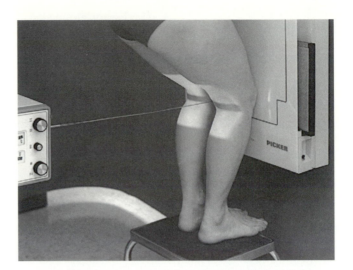

Fig. 6-140. PA with patient's knees flexed 30 degrees and a perpendicular central ray.

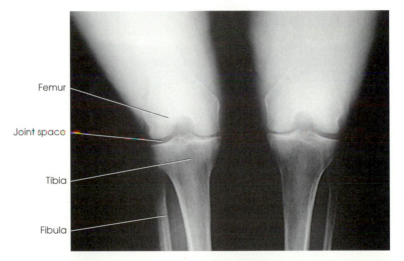

Femur

Joint space

Tibia

Fibula

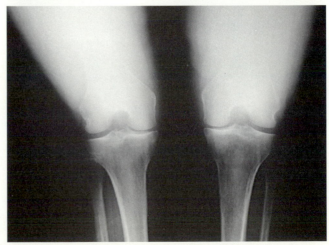

Fig. 6-141. PA with knees flexed 45 degrees and central ray directed 10 degrees caudad.

(Courtesy Betty Jo Mixon, R.T.)

Knee

AP OBLIQUE PROJECTION
Lateral rotation

Film: 8 × 10 in (18 × 24 cm) lengthwise.

Position of patient

- Place the patient on the table in the supine position, and support the ankles.

Position of part

- If necessary, elevate the hip of the *unaffected* side enough to rotate the affected limb.
- Support the elevated hip and knee of the unaffected side (Fig. 6-142).
- With the cassette parallel with the long axis of the knee, center the cassette ½ inch below the apex of the patella.
- *Shield gonads.*

Central ray

- Direct the central ray 5 degrees cephalad to the knee joint at a level just below the patellar apex.

Structures shown

The resulting image will show an AP oblique projection in lateral rotation of the femoral condyles, the patella, the tibial condyles, and the head of the fibula (Fig. 6-143).

□Evaluation criteria

The following should be clearly demonstrated:

- Medial femoral and tibial condyles.
- Tibial plateaus.
- Open knee joint.
- Fibula superimposed over the lateral half of the tibia.
- Margin of the patella projected slightly beyond the edge of the lateral femoral condyle.
- Soft tissue around the knee joint.
- Bony detail on the distal femur and proximal tibia.

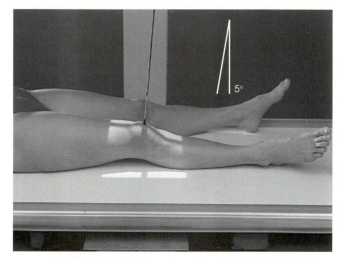

Fig. 6-142. AP oblique knee. Lateral rotation.

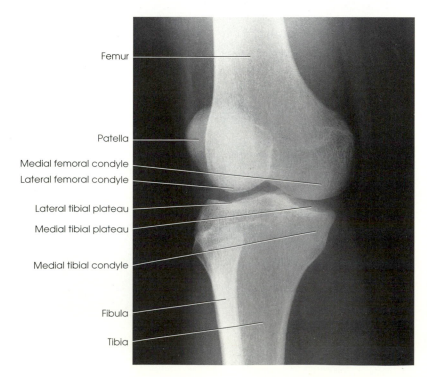
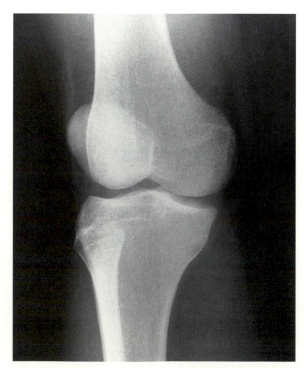

Femur

Patella

Medial femoral condyle
Lateral femoral condyle

Lateral tibial plateau
Medial tibial plateau

Medial tibial condyle

Fibula

Tibia

Fig. 6-143. AP oblique knee.

Knee

AP OBLIQUE PROJECTION
Medial rotation

Film: 8 × 10 in (18 × 24 cm) lengthwise.

Position of patient

- Place the patient on the table in the supine position and support the ankles.

Position of part

- Medially rotate the leg and foot and elevate the hip of the affected side enough to rotate the limb 45 degrees medially.
- Place a support under the hip if needed (Fig. 6-144).
- *Shield gonads.*

Central ray

- Direct the central ray 5 degrees cephalad to the knee joint at a level just below the patellar apex.

Structures shown

The resulting image will show an AP oblique projection in medial rotation of the femoral condyles, the patella, the tibial condyles, the proximal tibiofibular joint, and the head of the fibula (Fig. 6-145).

□Evaluation criteria

The following should be clearly demonstrated:
- Tibia and fibula separated at their proximal articulation.
- Posterior tibia.
- Lateral condyles of the femur and tibia.
- Both tibial plateaus.
- Open knee joint.
- Margin of the patella projecting slightly beyond the medial side of the femoral condyle.
- Soft tissue around the knee joint.
- Bony detail on the distal femur and proximal tibia.

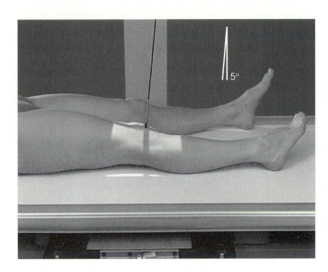

Fig. 6-144. AP oblique knee. Medial rotation.

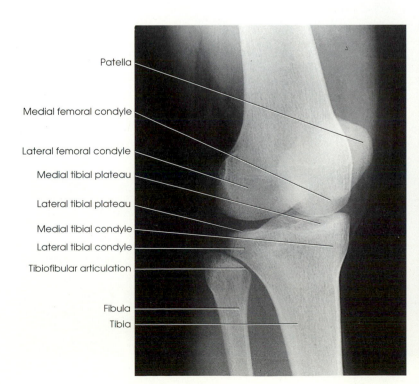
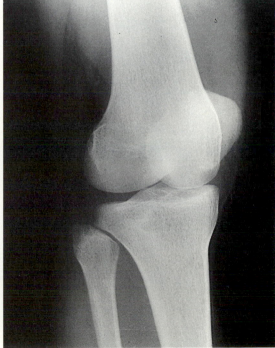

Patella
Medial femoral condyle
Lateral femoral condyle
Medial tibial plateau
Lateral tibial plateau
Medial tibial condyle
Lateral tibial condyle
Tibiofibular articulation
Fibula
Tibia

Fig. 6-145. AP oblique knee.

Knee

PA OBLIQUE PROJECTION
Lateral rotation

Film: 8 × 10 in (18 × 24 cm) lengthwise.

Position of patient

• Place the patient on the table in the prone position.

Position of part

• Elevate the hip of the affected side and laterally rotate the toes and knee to form a 45-degree angle.
• Support the hip (Fig. 6-146).
• *Shield gonads.*

Holmblad[1] recommends that the knee be flexed about 10 degrees.

Central ray

• Direct the central ray perpendicular through the knee joint at a level ½ inch below the patellar apex.

Structures shown

The resulting image will show a PA oblique projection in lateral rotation of the femoral condyles, patella, tibial condyles, and fibular head (Fig. 6-147).

□ Evaluation criteria

The following should be clearly demonstrated:
■ Medial femoral and tibial condyles.
■ Tibial plateaus.
■ Open knee joint.
■ Fibula superimposed over the lateral portion of the tibia.
■ Patellar margin projecting slightly beyond the side of the lateral femoral condyle.
■ Soft tissue around the knee joint.
■ Bony detail on the distal femur and proximal tibia.

[1]Holmblad EC: Improved x-ray technic in studying knee joints, South Med J 32:240-243, 1939.

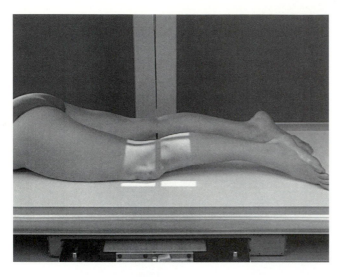

Fig. 6-146. PA oblique knee. Lateral rotation.

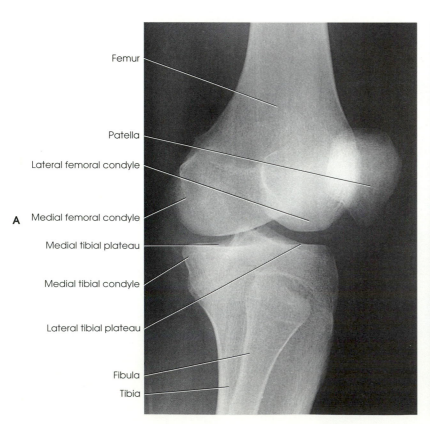

Femur
Patella
Lateral femoral condyle
A Medial femoral condyle
Medial tibial plateau
Medial tibial condyle
Lateral tibial plateau
Fibula
Tibia

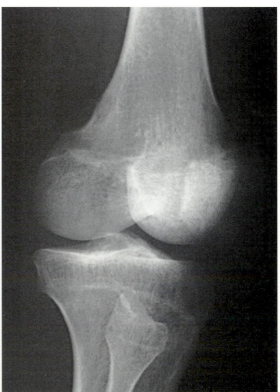

B

Fig. 6-147. A and **B**, PA oblique knee.

(**B**, Courtesy John Syring, R.T.)

Knee

PA OBLIQUE PROJECTION
Medial rotation

Film: 8 × 10 in (18 × 24 cm) lengthwise.

Position of patient

• Place the patient in the prone position.

Position of part

• From the prone position, medially rotate the leg and foot and elevate the hip of the unaffected side to rotate the limb 45 degrees medially.
• Place a support under the hip if needed (Fig. 6-148).
• *Shield gonads.*

Central ray

• Direct the central ray perpendicular through the knee joint at the level ½ inch below the apex of the patella.

Structures shown

The resulting image will show a PA oblique projection in medial rotation of the femoral condyles, patella, tibial condyles, proximal tibiofibular joint, and fibular head (Fig. 6-149).

□ Evaluation criteria

The following should be clearly demonstrated:
■ Tibia and fibula separated at their proximal articulation.
■ Posterior tibia.
■ Lateral condyles of the femur and tibia.
■ Both tibial plateaus.
■ Open knee joint.
■ Margin of the patella projecting slightly beyond the side of the medial femoral condyle.
■ Soft tissue around the knee joint.
■ Bony detail on the distal femur and proximal tibia.

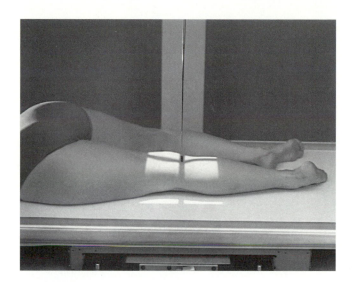

Fig. 6-148. PA oblique knee. Medial rotation.

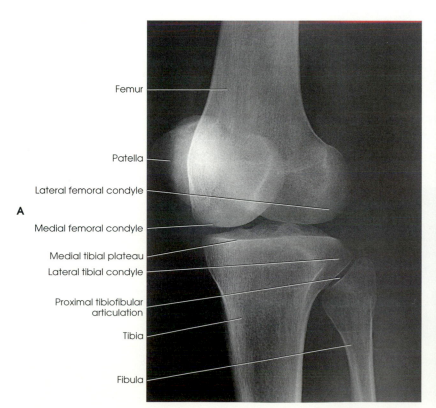
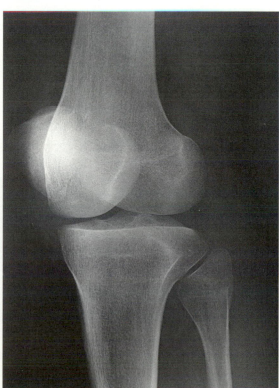

Femur

Patella

Lateral femoral condyle

Medial femoral condyle

Medial tibial plateau
Lateral tibial condyle

Proximal tibiofibular articulation

Tibia

Fibula

A

B

Fig. 6-149. A and **B,** PA oblique knee.

(**B,** Courtesy John Syring, R.T.)

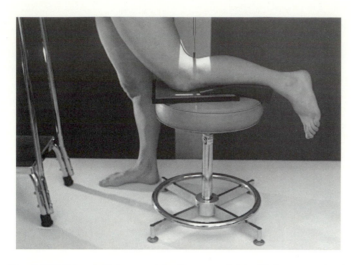

Fig. 6-150. PA axial intercondylar fossa: upright with knee on stool.

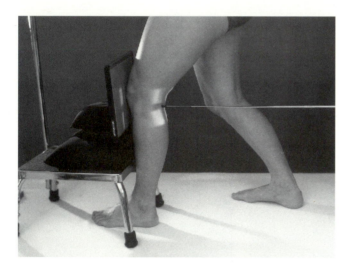

Fig. 6-151. PA axial intercondylar fossa: standing using horizontal central ray.

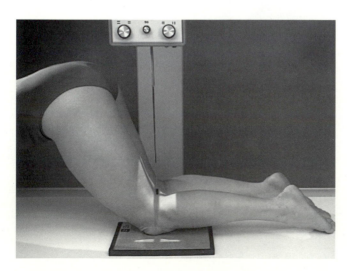

Fig. 6-152. PA axial intercondylar fossa: kneeling on radiographic table.

Intercondylar Fossa

 PA AXIAL PROJECTION
HOLMBLAD METHOD[1]

The PA axial, or "tunnel," projection, first described by Holmblad in 1937, required that the patient assume a kneeling position on the radiographic table. In 1983, the Holmblad method was modified so the patient could be radiographed in the upright position if the condition of the patient is such that he or she may safely be radiographed while in a standing or kneeling position.[2]

Film: 8 × 10 in (18 × 24 cm).

Position of patient

After consideration of the patient's safety, place the patient in any of three positions: (1) standing with the knee of interest flexed and resting on a stool at the side of the radiographic table (Fig. 6-150), (2) standing at the side of the radiographic table with the affected knee flexed and placed in contact with the front of the cassette (Fig. 6-151), and (3) kneeling on the radiographic table as originally described by Holmblad with the affected knee over the cassette (Fig. 6-152). In all three approaches, the patient leans on the radiographic table for support.

[1]Holmblad EC: Postero-anterior x-ray view of the knee in flexion, JAMA 109:1196-1197, 1937.
[2]Turner GW, Burns CB, and Previtte RG: Erect positions for "tunnel" views of the knee. Radiol Technol 55:640-642, 1983.

Position of part

- For all approaches, place the cassette against the anterior surface of the knee, and center to the apex of the patella. For all PA axial approaches, flex the knee 70 degrees from full extension (20-degree difference from the central ray as diagrammed in Fig. 6-153).
- *Shield gonads.*

Central ray

- Direct the central ray perpendicular to the lower leg entering the midpoint of the film.

Structures shown

The resulting image will show the intercondylar fossa of the femur and the medial and lateral intercondylar tubercles of the intercondylar eminence in profile (Fig. 6-154). Holmblad[1] states that the degree of flexion used in this position widens the joint space between the femur and tibia and gives an improved image of the joint and of the surfaces of the tibia and femur.

□ **Evaluation criteria**

The following should be clearly demonstrated:
- Open fossa.
- Posteroinferior surface of the femoral condyles.
- Intercondylar eminence and knee joint space.

- Apex of the patella not superimposing the fossa.
- No rotation, evident by seeing slight tibiofibular overlap.
- Soft tissue in the fossa and interspaces.
- Bony detail on the intercondylar eminence, distal femur, and proximal tibia.

NOTE: For a bilateral examination, see Figs. 6-140 and 6-141 described on page 245.

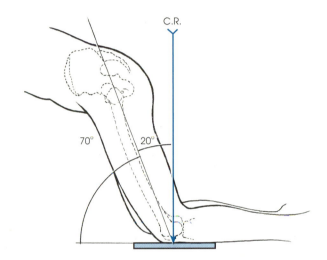

Fig. 6-153. Alignment relationship for any of three intercondylar fossa approaches.

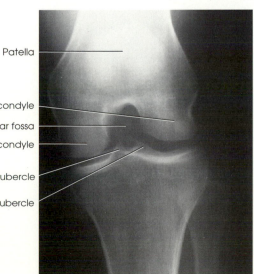

Patella

Lateral femoral condyle
Intercondylar fossa
A   Medial femoral condyle

Medial intercondylar tubercle

Lateral intercondylar tubercle

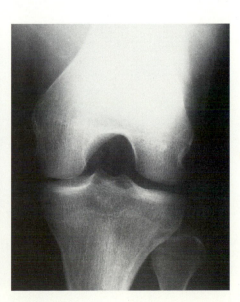

B

Fig. 6-154. A and **B,** PA axial ("tunnel") intercondylar fossa.

(**A,** Courtesy Michael Franklin.)

Intercondylar Fossa

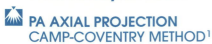

PA AXIAL PROJECTION
CAMP-COVENTRY METHOD[1]

Film: 8 × 10 in (18 × 24 cm) lengthwise.

Position of patient

• Place the patient in the prone position, and adjust the body so that there is no rotation.

Position of part

• Flex the knee to an approximate 40-degree angle and rest the foot on a suitable support.
• Center the proximal half of the cassette to the knee joint; the central ray angulation projects the joint to the center of the film (Figs. 6-155 and 6-156).
• According to the preferred angle, set the protractor arm at an angle of either 40 or 50 degrees from the horizontal and place it beside the leg.

[1]Camp, JD, and Coventry, MB: Use of special views in roentgenography of the knee joint, US Naval Med Bull 42:56-58, 1944.

• Adjust the position of the foot support to place the anterior surface of the leg parallel with the arm of the protractor.
• Adjust the leg so that there is no medial or lateral rotation of the knee.
• *Shield gonads.*

Central ray

• Direct the central ray perpendicular to the long axis of the leg and center to the knee joint; i.e., over the popliteal depression.
• The central ray will be angled 40 degrees when the knee is flexed 40 degrees, and 50 degrees when the knee is flexed 50 degrees.

Structures shown

This axial image demonstrates unobstructed projection of the intercondyloid fossa and the medial and lateral intercondylar tubercles of the intercondylar eminence (Figs. 6-157 and 6-158).

□ **Evaluation criteria**

The following should be clearly demonstrated:
■ Open fossa.
■ Posteroinferior surface of the femoral condyles.
■ Intercondylar eminence and knee joint space.
■ Apex of patella not superimposing the fossa.
■ No rotation, evident by seeing slight tibiofibular overlap.
■ Soft tissue in the fossa and interspaces.
■ Bony detail on the intercondylar eminence, distal femur, and proximal tibia.

NOTE: An intercondylar fossa projection is usually included in routine examinations of the knee joint for the detection of loose bodies (joint mice). The projection is also used in evaluating split and displaced cartilage in osteochondritis dissecans and flattening or underdevelopment of the lateral femoral condyle in congenital slipped patella.

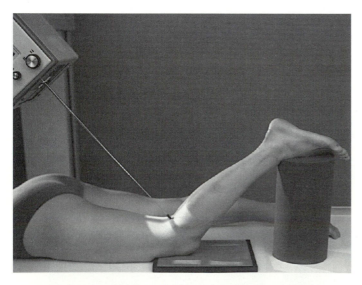

Fig. 6-155. PA axial ("tunnel") intercondylar fossa. Camp-Coventry method.

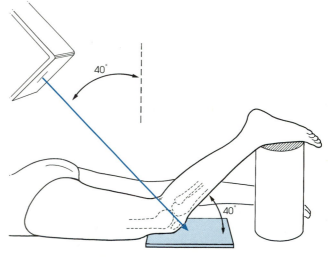

Fig. 6-156. PA axial ("tunnel") intercondylar fossa. Camp-Coventry method.

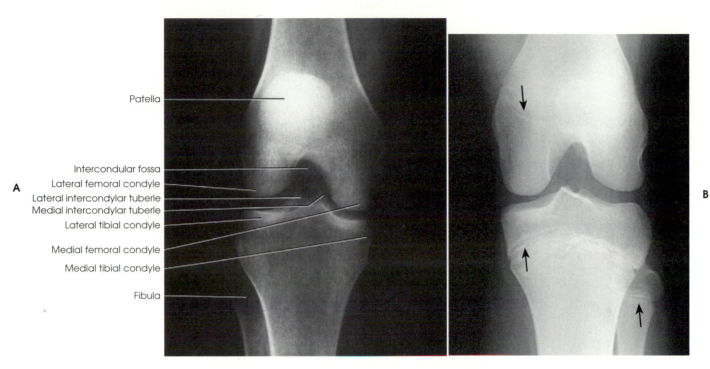

Patella

Intercondular fossa
Lateral femoral condyle
Lateral intercondylar tuberle
Medial intercondylar tuberle
Lateral tibial condyle

Medial femoral condyle
Medial tibial condyle

Fibula

A

B

Fig. 6-157. A, Flexion of knee at 40 degrees (same patient as Fig. 6-158). **B,** Flexion of knee at 40 degrees on 13-year-old patient. Note epiphyses *(arrows)*.

(**B,** Courtesy Ellen S. Titen, R.T.)

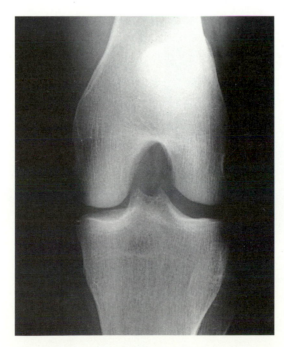

Fig. 6-158. Flexion of knee at 50 degrees (same patient as Fig. 6-157).

253

Intercondylar Fossa

AP AXIAL PROJECTION
BÉCLERÈ METHOD

Film: 8 × 10 in (18 × 24 cm).

A curved cassette is preferred to obtain a closer object-to-image receptor distance. An 8 × 10 in (18 × 24 cm) transverse cassette supported on sandbags may also be used.

Position of patient

- Place the patient in the supine position and adjust the body so that there is no rotation.

Position of part

Flex the affected knee enough to place the long axis of the femur at an angle of 60 degrees to the long axis of the tibia, open posteriorly.

- Support the knee on sandbags (Figs. 6-159 and 6-160).
- Place the cassette under the knee, and position it so that the center point will coincide with the central ray.
- Adjust the leg so the femoral condyles are equidistant from the film. Immobilize the foot with sandbags.
- *Shield gonads.*

Central ray

- Direct the central ray perpendicular to the long axis of the tibia entering the knee joint located ½ inch below the patellar apex.

Structures shown

The resulting image will show the intercondylar fossa, intercondylar eminence, and knee joint (Fig. 6-161).

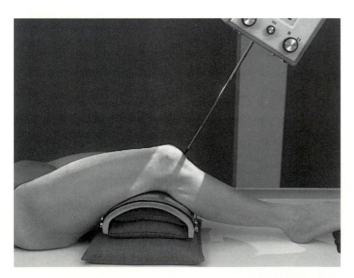

Fig. 6-159. AP axial intercondylar fossa with curved cassette.

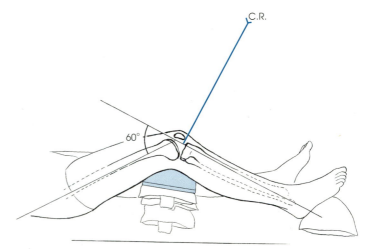

Fig. 6-160. AP axial intercondylar fossa with transverse cassette.

☐Evaluation criteria

The following should be clearly demonstrated:

- Open intercondylar fossa.
- Posteroinferior surface of the femoral condyles.
- Intercondylar eminence and knee joint space.
- No superimposition of the fossa by the apex of the patella.
- No rotation, evident by seeing slight tibiofibular overlap.
- Soft tissue in the fossa and interspaces.
- Bony detail on the intercondylar eminence, distal femur, and proximal tibia.

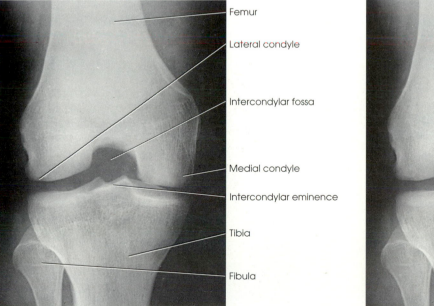 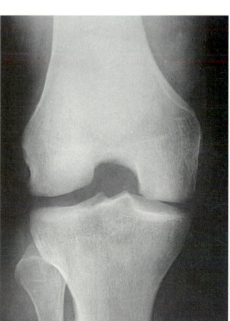

Femur

Lateral condyle

Intercondylar fossa

Medial condyle

Intercondylar eminence

Tibia

Fibula

Fig. 6-161. AP axial intercondylar fossa.

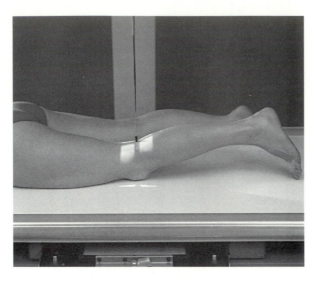

Fig. 6-162. PA patella.

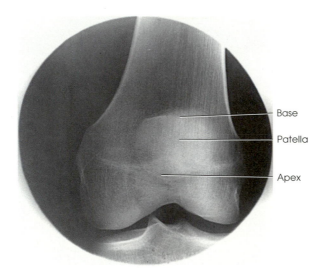

Base

Patella

Apex

Fig. 6-163. PA patella.

Patella

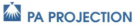 **PA PROJECTION**

Film: 8 × 10 in (18 × 24 cm) lengthwise.

Position of patient

- Place the patient in the prone position.
- If the knee is painful, place one sandbag under the thigh and another under the leg to relieve pressure on the patella.

Position of part

- Center the cassette to the patella.
- Adjust the position of the leg to place the patella parallel with the plane of the film. This usually requires that the heel be rotated 5 to 10 degrees laterally (Fig. 6-162).
- *Shield gonads.*

Central ray

- Direct the central ray perpendicular to the midpopliteal area exiting the patella.
- Collimate closely to the patellar area.

Structures shown

The PA projection of the patella provides sharper detail than can be obtained in the AP projection, because of a closer object-to-image receptor distance (Figs. 6-163 and 6-164).

☐ **Evaluation criteria**

The following should be clearly demonstrated:

- Patella completely superimposed by the femur.
- Adequate penetration present in order to see the patella clearly through the superimposing femur.
- No rotation.

Fig. 6-164. A, Conventional PA projection of the patella shows a vertical radiolucent line *(arrow)* passing through the junction of the lateral and middle third of the patella. **B,** On tomography this defect is seen to extend from the superior to the inferior margin of the patella. It is a bipartite patella and not a fracture.

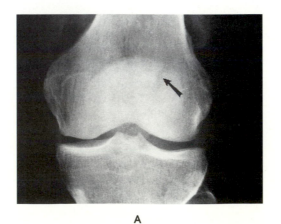

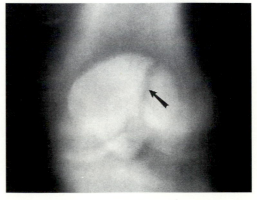

A

B

Patella

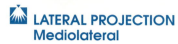

LATERAL PROJECTION
Mediolateral

Film: 8 × 10 in (18 × 24 cm) lengthwise.

Position of patient

- Place the patient in the supine position.

Position of part

- Ask the patient to turn onto the affected hip. A sandbag may be placed under the ankle for support.
- Have the patient flex the unaffected knee and hip, and place the unaffected foot in front of the affected limb for stability.
- Flex the affected knee approximately 5 to 10 degrees. (Increasing the flexion reduces the patellofemoral joint space.)
- Adjust the knee in the lateral position so the femoral epicondyles are superimposed and the patella is perpendicular to the film (Fig. 6-165).
- *Shield gonads.*

Central ray

- Direct the central ray perpendicular to the film, entering the knee at the anterior margin of the medial epicondyle.
- Collimate tightly to the patellar area.

Structures shown

The resulting image will show a lateral projection of the patella and the patellofemoral joint space (Fig. 6-166).

Evaluation criteria

The following should be clearly demonstrated:

- Knee flexed 5 to 10 degrees.
- Open patellofemoral joint space.
- Patella in lateral profile.
- Close collimation.

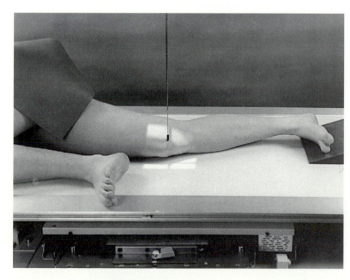

Fig. 6-165. Lateral patella.

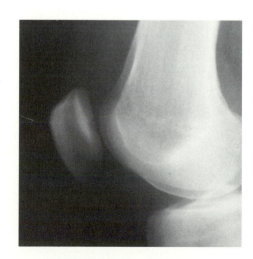

Fig. 6-166. Lateral patella.

Patella

PA OBLIQUE PROJECTION
Medial rotation

Film: 8 × 10 in (18 × 24 cm) lengthwise.

Position of patient

- Place the patient in the prone position.

Position of part

- Flex the knee approximately 5 to 10 degrees.
- Medially rotate the knee 45 to 55 degrees from the prone position.
- Center the medial portion of the patella to the film (Fig. 6-167).
- *Shield gonads.*

Central ray

- Direct the central ray perpendicular to the film exiting the palpated patella.

STRUCTURES SHOWN

A PA oblique image of the medial portion of the patella is demonstrated free of the femur (Fig. 6-168).

☐Evaluation criteria

The following should be clearly demonstrated:

- The majority of the medial patella free of superimposition of the femur.
- Lateral margin of patella superimposed over the femur.
- Closely collimated image.

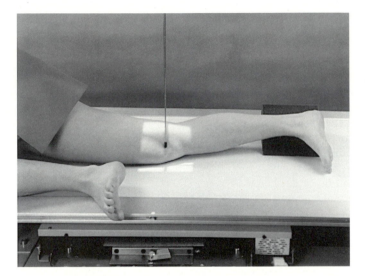

Fig. 6-167. PA oblique patella. Medial rotation.

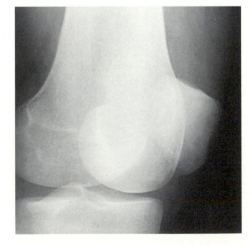

Fig. 6-168. PA oblique patella.

Patella

PA OBLIQUE PROJECTION
Lateral rotation

Film: 8 × 10 in (18 × 24 cm) lengthwise.

Position of patient

Place the patient in the prone position.

Position of part

- Flex the knee 5 to 10 degrees, and externally (laterally) rotate the knee 45 to 55 degrees from the prone position.
- Center the lateral portion of the patella to the film (Fig. 6-169).
- *Shield gonads.*

Central ray

- Direct the central ray perpendicular to the film exiting the palpated patella.

Structures shown

The resulting image will show an oblique projection of the lateral aspect of the patella free of the femur (Fig. 6-170).

□ Evaluation criteria

The following should be clearly demonstrated:
- The majority of the patella free of superimposition of the femur.
- Medial margin of patella superimposed over the femur.
- Closely collimated image.

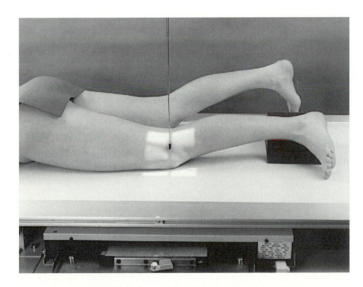

Fig. 6-169. PA oblique patella, lateral rotation.

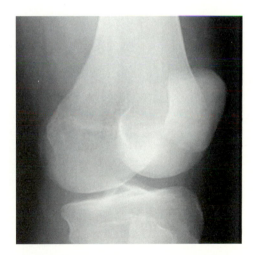

Fig. 6-170. PA oblique patella, lateral rotation.

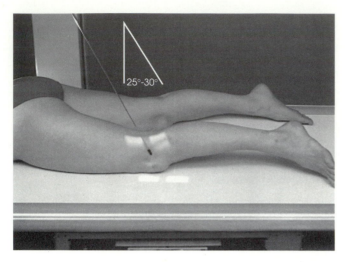

Fig. 6-171. PA axial oblique axial patella. Lateral rotation.

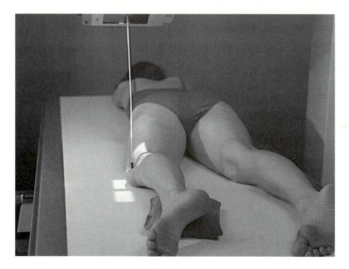

Fig. 6-172. PA axial oblique axial patella. Lateral rotation.

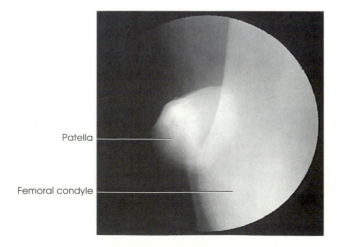

Patella

Femoral condyle

Fig. 6-173. PA axial oblique patella.

Patella
PA AXIAL OBLIQUE PROJECTION
Lateral rotation
KUCHENDORF METHOD

Film: 8 × 10 in (18 × 24 cm) lengthwise.

Position of patient

- Place the patient in the prone position.
- Elevate the hip of the affected side 2 or 3 inches.
- Place a sandbag under the ankle and foot, and adjust it so that the knee will be slightly flexed, approximately 10 degrees, to relax the muscles.

Position of part

- Center the cassette to the patella.
- Laterally rotate the knee approximately 35 to 40 degrees from the prone position.
- Place the index finger against the medial border of the patella, and press it laterally.
- Rest the knee on its anteromedial side to hold the patella in a position of lateral displacement (Figs. 6-171 and 6-172).
- *Shield gonads.*

Central ray

- Direct the central ray to the joint space between the patella and the femoral condyles at an angle of 25 to 30 degrees caudad. It enters the posterior surface of the patella.

Structures shown

Resulting image will show a slightly oblique PA projection of the patella, showing most of the patella free of superimposed structures (Fig. 6-173).

The body position is more comfortable for the patient than the direct prone, since no pressure is placed on the injured patella. The slight pressure required to displace the patella laterally is rarely objectionable to the patient.

□Evaluation criteria

The following should be clearly demonstrated:
- Majority of the patella free from the femur.
- Patella and its outline where it is superimposed by the femur.

Patella and Patellofemoral Joint

TANGENTIAL PROJECTION
HUGHSTON METHOD[1,2]

Radiography of the patella has been the topic of hundreds of articles. To obtain a tangential radiograph, the patient may be placed in any of the following body positions: prone, supine, lying on the side, seated on the table, seated on the table with the leg hanging over the edge, or standing.

Various authors have described the degree of flexion of the knee joint as being as little as 20 degrees to as great as 120 degrees. Laurin[3] reports that patellar subluxation is easier to demonstrate when the knee is flexed 20 degrees. Laurin also reports a limitation of using the small angle; modern radiographic equipment will often not permit such small angles because of the large size of the collimator.

Fodor, Malott, and Weinberg[4] and Merchant, et al.[5] recommend a 45-degree flexion of the knee, and Hughston[6] recommends an approximate 55-degree angle with the central ray angled 45 degrees.

Film: 8 × 10 in (18 × 24 cm) for unilateral; 10 × 12 in (24 × 30 cm) crosswise for bilateral examination.

Position of patient

- Place the patient in a prone position with the foot resting on the radiographic table.
- Adjust the body so that there is no rotation.

Position of part

- Place the cassette under the patient's knee, and slowly flex the affected knee so that the tibia and fibula form a 50- to 60-degree angle from the table.
- Rest the foot against the collimator or support in position (Fig. 6-174).

---

[1]Hughston JC: Subluxation of the patella, J Bone Joint Surg 50A:1003-1026, 1968.
[2]Kimberlin GE: Radiological assessment of the patellofemoral articulation and subluxation of the patella, Radiol Technol 45:129-137, 1973.
[3]Laurin CA: The abnormal lateral patellofemoral angle, J Bone Joint Surg 60A:55-60, 1968.
[4]Fodor J, Malott JC, and Weinberg, S: Accurate radiography of the patellofemoral joint, Radiol Technol 53:570-579, 1982.
[5]Merchant AC, Mercer RL, Jacobsen RH, and Cool CR: Roentgenographic analysis of patellofemoral congruence. J Bone Joint Surg 56A(7): 1391-1396, 1974.
[6]Hughston JC: Subluxation of the patella, J Bone Joint Surg 50A:1003-1026, 1968.

- Ensure the collimator surface is not hot, as this could burn the patient.
- Adjust the leg so that there is no medial or lateral rotation from the vertical.
- *Shield gonads.*

Central ray

- Angle the x-ray tube 45 degrees cephalad and direct through the patellofemoral joint.

Structures shown

The tangential image will show subluxation of the patella and patellar fractures and allows radiologic assessment of the femoral condyles. Hughston recommends that both knees be examined for comparison (Fig. 6-175).

□ Evaluation criteria

The following should be clearly demonstrated:

- Patella in profile.
- Open patellofemoral articulation.
- Surfaces of the femoral condyles.
- Soft tissue of the femoropatellar articulation.
- Bony detail on the patella and femoral condyles.

NOTE: Care must be taken to ensure that the foot does not come in contact with the hot collimator housing, which is heated by the light. It is also essential that the x-ray tube and support mechanism be properly grounded.

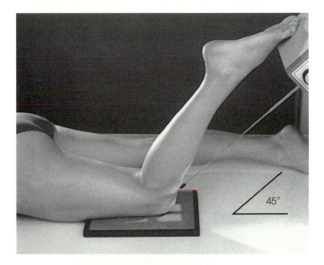

Fig. 6-174. Tangential patella and patellofemoral joint: Hughston method.

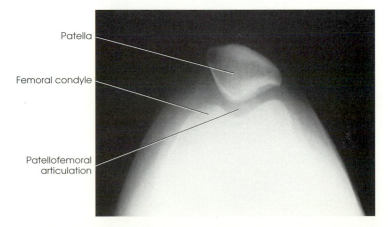

Patella

Femoral condyle

Patellofemoral articulation

Fig. 6-175. Tangential patella and patellofemoral joint: Hughston method.

(Courtesy Lois Baird, R.T.)

Patella and Patellofemoral Joint

TANGENTIAL PROJECTION
MERCHANT METHOD[1]

Film: 10 × 12 in (24 × 30 cm) crosswise for bilateral examination.

Position of patient

- Place the patient supine with both knees at the end of the radiographic table.
- Support the knees and lower legs by an adjustable cassette, holding device.[2]
- To increase comfort and relaxation of the quadriceps femoris, place pillows or a foam wedge under the patient's head and back.

[1]Merchant AC, Mercer RL, Jacobsen RH, and Cool CR: Roentgenographic analysis of patellofemoral congruence, J Bone Joint Surg 56A:1391-1396, 1974.
[2]Merchant AC: "The Axial Viewer" available from Orthopedic Products, 2500 Hospital Dr., Bldg. 7, Mountain View, CA 94040.

Position of part

- Elevate the knees to place the femora parallel with the table top (approximately 2 inches), using the "axial viewer" device (Figs. 6-176 and 6-177).
- Adjust the angle of knee flexion to 45 degrees. (Merchant reports the degree of angulation may be varied between 30 to 90 degrees to demonstrate various patellofemoral disorders.)
- Strap both legs together at the calf level to control leg rotation and allow patient relaxation.
- Place the cassette perpendicular to the central ray and resting on the patient's shins (a thin foam pad aids comfort) approximately 1 foot distal to the patellae.

- Ensure that the patient is able to relax. Relaxation of the quadriceps femoris is critical for an accurate diagnosis. If these muscles are not relaxed, a subluxed patella may be pulled back into the intercondylar sulcus, showing a false normal appearance.
- Record the angle of knee flexion for reproducibility during follow-up examinations, because the severity of patella subluxation frequently changes inversely with the angle of knee flexion.
- *Shield gonads.*

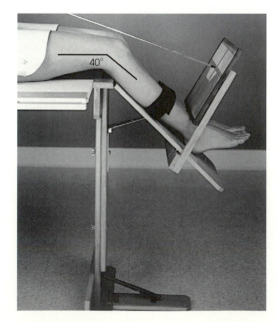

Fig. 6-176. Tangential patella and patellofemoral joint: Merchant method.

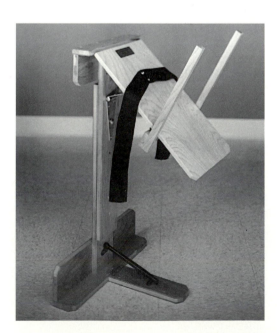

Fig. 6-177. "The axial viewer" device.

Central ray

- An approximate 6 ft (2 m) SID is recommended to reduce magnification.
- Direct the central ray perpendicular to the cassette.
- With 45-degree knee flexion, angle the central ray 30 degrees caudad to achieve a 30-degree central ray-to-femur angle. (The central ray is directed 15 degrees less than the angle of inclination of the leg.) The central ray enters midway between the patellae at the level of the patellofemoral joint.

Structures shown

The bilateral tangential image demonstrates an axial projection of the patellae and patellofemoral joints (Fig. 6-178). Because of right angle film-central ray alignment, the patellae are seen as nondistorted, albeit slightly magnified, images.

□Evaluation criteria

The following should be clearly demonstrated:
- Patellae in profile.
- Femoral condyles and intercondylar sulcus.
- Open patellofemoral articulations.

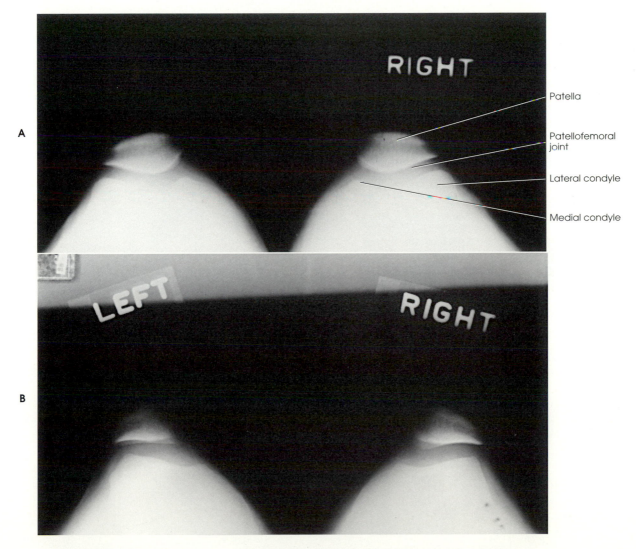

Fig. 6-178. A, Normal tangential radiograph of congruent patellofemoral joints showing the patellae to be well centered, with normal trabecular pattern. **B,** Abnormal tangential radiograph showing abnormally shallow intercondylar sulci *(arrow)*, misshapen and laterally subluxed patellae, and incongruent patellofemoral joints (left worse than right).

(**A,** Courtesy Alan C. Merchant, M.D.; **B,** Courtesy Alan J. Merchant, M.D.)

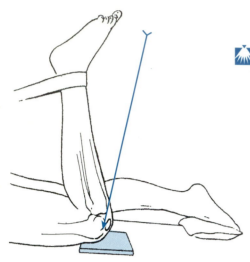

Fig. 6-179. Tangential patella: Settegast method.

Patella and Patellofemoral Joint

▨ TANGENTIAL PROJECTION

SETTEGAST METHOD

Because of the danger of fragment displacement by acute flexion of the knee required for this procedure, it should not be attempted until a transverse fracture of the patella has been ruled out with a lateral image.

Film: 8×10 in (18×24 cm).

Position of patient

- Place the patient in the supine (seated) or prone position. The latter is preferable, because the knee can usually be flexed to a greater degree and immobilization is easier (Figs. 6-179 and 6-180).

- If the patient is seated on the radiographic table, securely hold the cassette in place (Fig. 6-181). Alternative positions are shown in Figs. 6-182 and 6-183.

Position of part

- Place the patient in the prone position, and flex the knee slowly as much as possible or until the patella is perpendicular to the film. By *slow, even flexion*, the patient will be able to tolerate the position, whereas quick, uneven flexion may cause too much pain.

- If desired, loop a long strip of bandage around the ankle or foot. Have the patient grasp the ends over the shoulder to hold the leg in position. Adjust the leg so that its long axis is vertical.

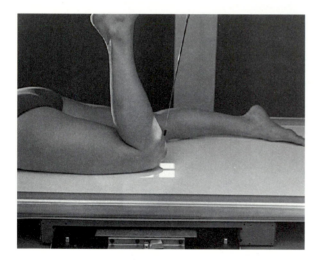

Fig. 6-180. Tangential: Settegast method.

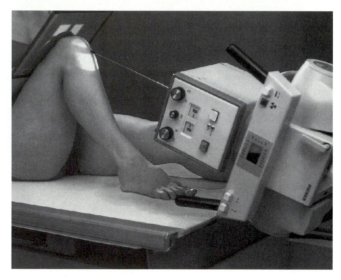

Fig. 6-181. Tangential patella: Settegast method.

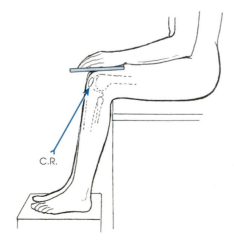

Fig. 6-182. Tangential patellal: (patient seated).

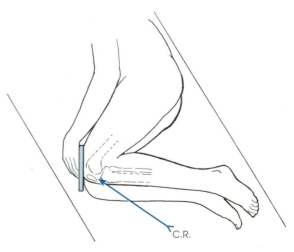

Fig. 6-183. Tangential patella (patient lateral).

- Place the cassette transversely under the knee, and center to the joint space between the patella and the femoral condyles.
- *Shield gonads.*
- By maintaining the same object-image receptor and tube-film relationships, this position can be obtained with the patient in the lateral or in a seated position, as illustrated.

NOTE: When the central ray is directed toward the patient's upper body (as in Figs. 6-181, 6-182, and 6-183), the thorax and thyroid should be shielded. Gonad shielding (not shown for illustration purposes) should be used in all instances.

Central ray

- Direct the central ray perpendicular to the joint space between the patella and the femoral condyles. The degree of central ray angulation will depend on the degree of flexion of the knee.
- Close collimation is recommended.

Structures shown

The resulting image will show vertical fractures of bone and the articulating surfaces of the patellofemoral articulation (Figs. 6-184 and 6-185).

□ Evaluation criteria

The following should be clearly demonstrated:
- Patella in profile.
- Open patellofemoral articulation.
- Surfaces of the femoral condyles.
- Soft tissue of the patellofemoral articulation.
- Bony detail on the patella and femoral condyles.

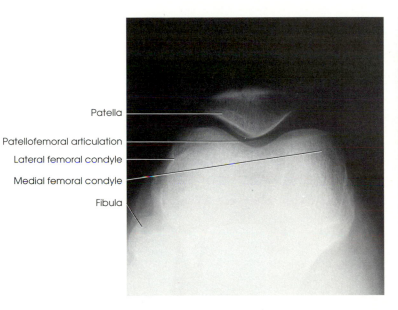
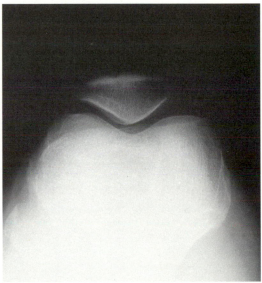

Patella
Patellofemoral articulation
Lateral femoral condyle
Medial femoral condyle
Fibula

Fig. 6-184. Tangential patella: Settegast method.

(Courtesy Randy Miller, R.T.)

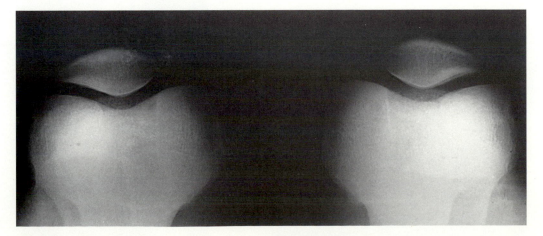

Fig. 6-185. Bilateral patella examination. For this examination it is recommended to strap the two legs together at the level of the calf using an appropriate binding. This helps control femoral rotation.

Femur

 AP PROJECTION

In this projection, if the femoral heads are separated by an unusually broad pelvis, the bodies (shafts) will be more strongly angled toward the midline.

Film: 7 × 17 in (18 × 43 cm); 14 × 17 in (35 × 43 cm).

Position of patient

- Place the patient in the supine position.
- Check the pelvis to ensure there is no rotation.

Position of part

- Center the affected thigh to the midline of the film.
- Internally rotate the limb approximately 15 degrees to overcome the anteversion of the femoral necks.
- Recall that the proximal and mid-femur are laterally located in the thigh. When the patient is too tall to include the entire femur, include the knee joint (or the joint closest to the area of interest) on one film (Fig. 6-186).
- Obtain second radiograph to include the proximal femur (or the knee) according to institutional policy.
- *Shield gonads.*

Central ray

- Direct the central ray perpendicular to the mid-femur and the center of the cassette.

Structures shown

The resulting image will show an AP projection of the femur, including the knee joint and/or hip (Figs. 6-187 and 6-188).

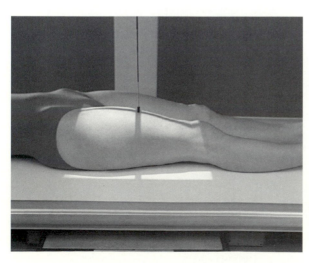

Fig. 6-186. AP distal femur.

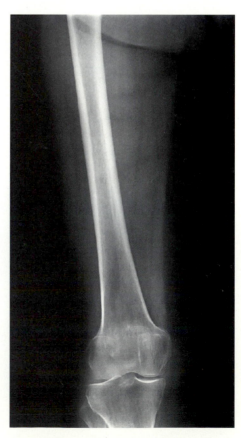

Fig. 6-187. AP distal femur.

□ Evaluation criteria

The following should be clearly demonstrated:

- Majority of the femur and the joint nearest to the pathology or injury. A second projection of the other joint is recommended.
- Femoral neck not foreshortened.
- Lesser trochanter either not seen beyond the medial border of the femur or only a very small portion seen.
- No knee rotation.
- Evident gonad shielding when indicated, but not covering proximal femur.
- Any orthopedic appliance in its entirety.
- Trabecular detail on the femoral shaft.

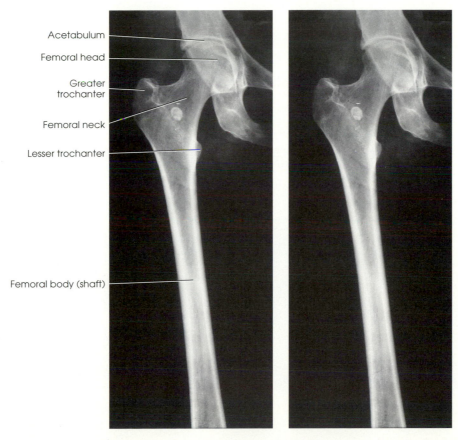

Acetabulum

Femoral head

Greater trochanter

Femoral neck

Lesser trochanter

Femoral body (shaft)

Fig. 6-188. AP proximal femur.

Femur

LATERAL PROJECTION
Mediolateral

Film: 7 × 17 in (18 × 43 cm) or 14 × 17 in (35 × 43 cm) lengthwise.

Position of patient

- Ask the patient to turn onto the affected side.
- Adjust the body position, and center the affected thigh to the midline of the grid.
- Have the patient grasp the side of the table with the upper hand to aid in maintaining the position.

Position of part

- If only the knee joint is to be included, draw the uppermost limb forward and support it at hip level on sandbags.
- Adjust the pelvis in a true lateral position (Fig. 6-189).
- Flex the affected knee somewhat, place a sandbag under the ankle, and adjust the body rotation to place the epicondyles perpendicular to the tabletop.
- Adjust the position of the Bucky tray so that the film will project approximately 2 inches beyond the knee to be included.

- If the hip joint is to be included, place the top of the film at the level of the anterior superior iliac spine.
- Draw the upper limb posteriorly and support it.
- Adjust the pelvis so that it is rolled posteriorly just enough to prevent superimposition; 10 to 15 degrees from the lateral position is sufficient (Fig. 6-190).
- *Shield gonads.*

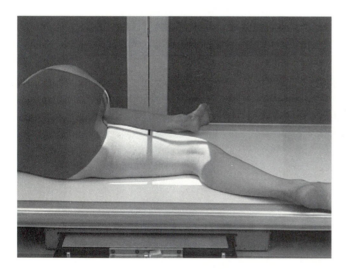

Fig. 6-189. Lateral distal femur.

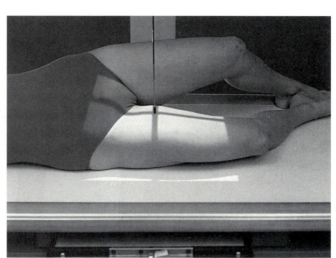

Fig. 6-190. Lateral proximal femur.

Central ray

- Direct the central ray perpendicular to the mid-femur and the center of the cassette.

Structures shown

The resulting image will show a lateral projection of about three-fourths of the femur and of the adjacent joint. Take two films if needed for the demonstration of the entire length of the adult femur (Figs. 6-191 and 6-192).

□ **Evaluation criteria**

The following should be clearly demonstrated:
- Majority of the femur and the joint nearest to the pathology or injury. A second radiograph of the other end of the femur is recommended.
- Any orthopedic appliance included in its entirety.
- Trabecular detail on the femoral body (shaft).
  With the knee included:
- Superimposed anterior surface of the femoral condyles.
- Patella in profile.
- Open patellofemoral space.
- Inferior surface of the femoral condyles not superimposed due to divergent rays.
  With the hip included:
- Opposite thigh not over area of interest.
- Greater and lesser trochanters not prominent.

NOTE: Because of the danger of fragment displacement, the above position is not recommended for fracture cases, nor should it be used if there is a question of destructive disease. These subjects should be examined in the supine position by placing the cassette vertically along the medial or lateral aspect of the thigh and knee and directing the central ray horizontally. A wafer grid or a grid-front cassette should be used to minimize secondary radiation.

Femur

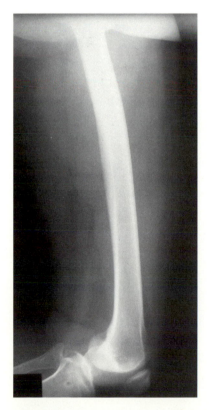

Fig. 6-191. Lateral distal femur.

(Courtesy Cheryl Stillberger, R.T.)

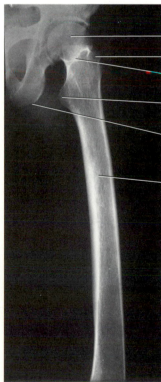

Femoral head

Greater trochanter

Femoral neck

Lesser trochanter

Ischial tuberosity

Femoral body (shaft)

Fig. 6-192. Lateral proximal femur.

Chapter 7

PELVIS AND UPPER FEMORA

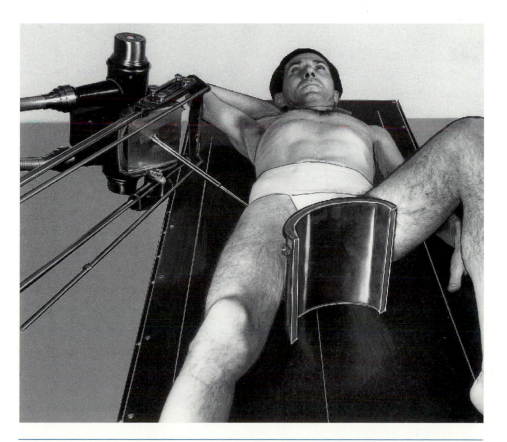

Patient positioned for a superoinferior projection of the femoral neck using the Leonard-George method; 1940s. The radiographic curved cassette reduces the distance from the film to the femoral neck.

The pelvis serves as a base for the trunk and a girdle for the attachment of the lower limbs. The pelvis is formed by the two hip bones anteriorly and laterally and by the sacrum and coccyx posteriorly.

Hip Bone

The hip bone (os coxae or innominatum) consists of three parts: the ilium, pubis, and ischium (Figs. 7-1 and 7-2). All three bones enter into the formation of the acetabulum, the cup-shaped socket that receives the head of the femur. The three bones are separated by cartilage in youth but become fused into one bone in adulthood.

ILIUM

The *ilium* consists of a body and a broad, curved, winglike portion called the ala. The *body* of the ilium forms approximately two fifths of the superior portion of the *acetabulum*. The *ala* projects superiorly from the body to form the prominence of the hip. The ala has three margins, or borders: the anterior, posterior, and superior. The anterior and posterior borders each present two prominent projections, the *superior* and *inferior spines,* respectively.

The anterior superior iliac spine (ASIS) is an important and frequently used radiographic positioning reference point. The superior margin extends from the anterior to the posterior superior iliac spine and is called the *crest of the ilium* (iliac crest). The medial surface of the ala is divided into anterior and posterior portions. The anterior portion is called the *iliac fossa* and is separated from the body of the bone by a smooth, arc-shaped ridge, the *arcuate line,* which forms a part of the circumference of the pelvic brim. The arcuate line passes obliquely, inferiorly, and medially to its junction with the pubis. The inferior and posterior portions of the ala present a large facet, the *auricular surface,* for articulation with the sacrum. Below the articular surface the ilium curves inward as the *greater sciatic notch.*

PUBIS

The *pubis* consists of a body and two rami: the superior (ascending) ramus and inferior (descending) ramus. The *body* of the pubis forms approximately one fifth of the lower anterior portion of the acetabulum. The *superior ramus* projects inferiorly and medially from the acetabulum to the midline of the body. Here the bone curves inferiorly and then posteriorly and laterally to join the ischium. The lower prong is termed the *inferior ramus.* The upper surface of the superior ramus presents a ridge, the *pecten* (pectineal line), which is continuous with the arcuate line of the ilium.

ISCHIUM

The *ischium* consists of a body and a ramus. The *body* of the ischium forms approximately two fifths of the lower posterior portion of the acetabulum. It projects posteriorly and inferiorly from the acetabulum to form an expanded portion called the *ischial tuberosity.* In the seated position, the weight of the body rests on the two ischial tuberosities. The *ischial ramus* projects anteriorly and medially from the tuberosity to its junction with the inferior ramus of the pubis. By this posterior union the rami of the pubis and ischium enclose the *obturator foramen.* At the superoposterior border of the body is a prominent projection called the *ischial spine.* Just below the ischial spine is an indentation, the *lesser sciatic notch.*

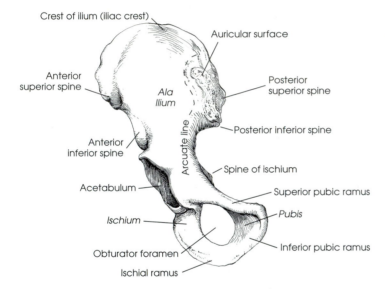

Fig. 7-1. Anterior aspect of right hip bone.

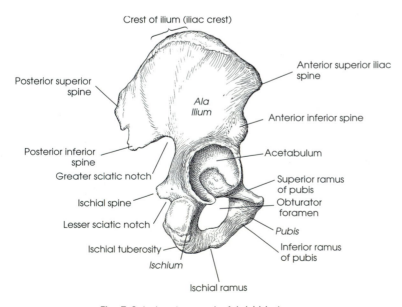

Fig. 7-2. Lateral aspect of right hip bone.

Femur

The proximal end of the femur consists of a head, a neck, and two large processes, the greater and lesser trochanters (Figs. 7-3 to 7-5). The smooth, rounded *head* is connected to the body (shaft) by a pyramid-shaped neck and is received into the acetabular cavity of the hip bone. A small depression at the center of the head, the *fovea capitis,* attaches to the ligamentum capitis femoris. The *neck* is constricted near the head but expands to a broad base at the *body* (shaft) of the bone. The neck projects medially, superiorly, and anteriorly from the body (shaft). The trochanters are situated at the junction of the shaft and the base of the neck. The *greater trochanter* is at the superolateral part of the femoral body, and the *lesser trochanter* is at the posteromedial part. The prominent ridge extending between the trochanters at the base of the neck on the posterior surface of the body (shaft) is called the *intertrochanteric crest.* The less prominent ridge connecting the trochanters anteriorly is called the *intertrochanteric line.* Two areas are common sites for fractures in the elderly. Those areas are the femoral neck and the intertrochanteric crest. The superior portion of the greater trochanter projects above the neck and curves slightly posteriorly and medially. The most prominent point of the lateral surface of the greater trochanter is always in direct line with the superior border of the neck of the femur. The angulation of the neck of the femur varies considerably with age, sex, and stature. In the adult of average form, the neck projects anteriorly from the body (shaft) at an angle of approximately 15 to 20 degrees and superiorly at an angle of approximately 120 to 130 degrees to the long axis of the femoral body (Figs. 7-6 and 7-7). In youth the latter angle is wider; that is, the neck is more vertical in position. In wide pelves the angle is narrower, placing the neck in a more horizontal position.

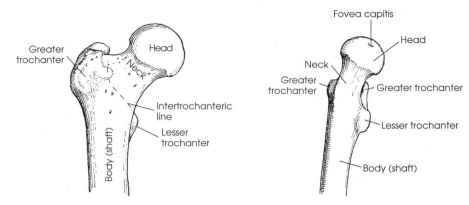

Fig. 7-3. Anterior aspect of proximal end of femur.

Fig. 7-4. Medial aspect of proximal end of femur.

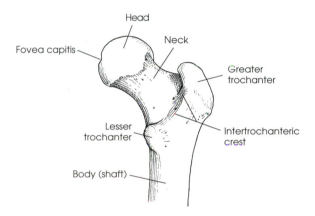

Fig. 7-5. Posterior aspect of proximal end of femur.

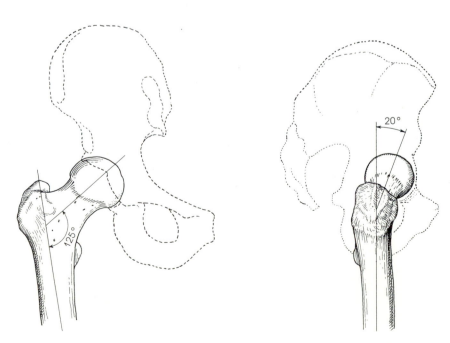

Fig. 7-6. Anterior aspect of femur.

Fig. 7-7. Lateral aspect of femur.

Articulations of the Pelvis

The articulation between the *acetabulum* and the head of the *femur* is a synovial (diarthrotic), spheroidal ball-and-socket joint, which permits free movement in all directions. The *knee* and *ankle* joints are synovial (diarthrotic) ginglymus or hinge joints; thus the wide range of movements of the lower limb depends on the spheroidal or ball-and-socket joint of the hip. Because the knee and ankle joints are ginglymus or hinge joints, medial (internal) and lateral (external) rotations of the foot cause rotation of the entire limb and, if carried far enough, of the pelvis. This makes the position of the feet important in radiography of the hip and pelvis; the feet must be immobilized in the correct position to avoid rotation, which would result in distortion of the proximal end of the femur.

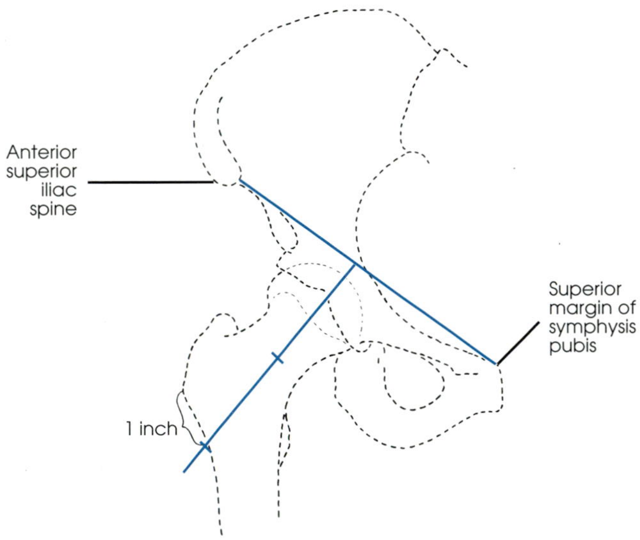

The two palpable bony points of *localization for the hip joint* are the anterior superior iliac spine (ASIS) and the superior margin of the symphysis pubis (Fig. 7-8). The midpoint of a line drawn between these two points will lie directly above the center of the dome of the acetabular cavity. A line drawn at right angles to the midpoint of the first line will lie parallel with the long axis of the femoral neck of an average adult in the anatomic position.

For *accurate localization of the femoral neck* in atypical subjects, or those in whom the limb is not in the anatomic position, (1) a line is drawn between the anterior superior iliac spine and the superior margin of the symphysis pubis, and (2) a line is drawn from a point 1 inch inferior to the greater trochanter to the midpoint of the previously marked line. The femoral head will lie in the same plane as this line (Fig. 7-8).

The *pubes* of the hip bones articulate with each other at the anterior midline of the body, forming a joint called the *symphysis pubis*. The symphysis pubis is a cartilaginous (amphiarthrotic) articulation.

The right and left *ilia* articulate with the sacrum posteriorly at the *sacroiliac joints*. The sacroiliac articulations are synovial (diarthrotic) plane or gliding joints. Because the bones of the sacroiliac joints interlock, movement is very limited or nonexistent. Because of this the sacroiliac joints tend to functionally resemble cartilaginous (amphiarthrotic) joints.

Fig. 7-8. Schematic drawing showing method of localizing long axis of femoral neck.

PELVIS

The female pelvis (Fig. 7-9) is lighter in structure than the male pelvis (Fig. 7-10). It is broader and shallower, and the inlet is larger and more rounded. The sacrum is wider, it curves more sharply posteriorly, and the sacral promontory is flatter. The width and depth of the pelvis vary with stature and gender.

The pelvis is divided into two portions by an oblique plane that extends from the upper anterior margin of the sacrum to the upper margin of the symphysis pubis. The boundary line of this plane is called the *brim of the pelvis*. The region above the brim is called the *greater* or *false pelvis*, and the region below the brim is called the *lesser* or *true pelvis*.

The brim forms the *superior aperture* (strait, or inlet) of the true pelvis and is measured in three directions in pelvimetry. Its anteroposterior, or conjugate, diameter is measured from the superoante-

rior margin of the sacrum to the superior margin of the symphysis pubis; its horizontal diameter, across the widest region; and its oblique diameter, from the iliopectineal eminence of one side to the sacroiliac joint of the opposite side. The *inferior aperture* (strait or outlet) of the true pelvis is measured from the tip of the coccyx to the inferior margin of the pubic symphysis in the anteroposterior direction and between the ischial tuberosities in the horizontal direction. The region between the inlet and the outlet is called the *pelvic cavity* (Fig. 7-11).

When the body is in the upright or seated position, the pelvic brim forms an angle of approximately 60 degrees to the horizontal plane. This angle varies with other body positions, the degree and direction of the variation depending on the lumbar and sacral curves.

The bony landmarks used in radiography of the pelvis and hips (Fig. 7-12) are

the crest of the ilium, the anterior superior iliac spine, the symphysis pubis, the greater trochanter of the femur, the ischial tuberosity, and the tip of the coccyx. Most of these points are easily palpable even in hypersthenic subjects. However, because of the heavy muscles immediately above the crest of ilium, care must be exercised in locating this structure to avoid centering too high. It is advisable to have the patient inhale deeply, and, while the muscles are relaxed during exhalation, palpate for the highest point of the crest of the ilium.

The highest point of the greater trochanter, which can be palpated immediately below the depression in the soft tissues of the lateral surface of the hip, is in the same horizontal plane as the midpoint of the hip joint and the coccyx. The most prominent point of the greater trochanter is in the same horizontal plane as the symphysis pubis.

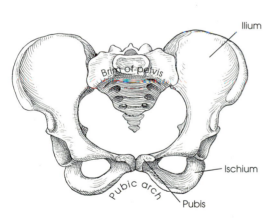

Fig. 7-9. Female pelvis.

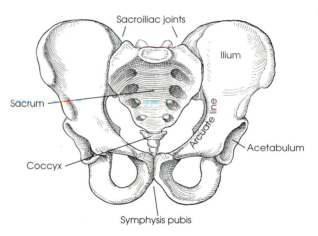

Fig. 7-10. Male pelvis.

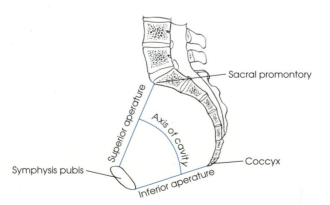

Fig. 7-11. Median sagittal section showing inlet and outlet of true pelvis.

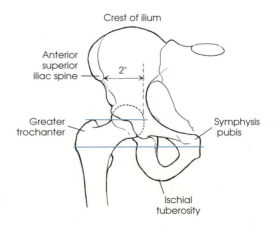

Fig. 7-12. Bony landmarks and localization planes of pelvis.

Articulations of the pelvis

275

Radiation Protection

Protection of the patient from unnecessary radiation is a professional responsibility of the radiographer. (See Chapter 1 for specific guidelines.) In this chapter, the *"Shield gonads"* statement at the end of the "Position of part" section indicates the patient is to be protected from unnecessary radiation by restricting the radiation beam using proper collimation. Additionally, placing lead shielding between the gonads and the radiation source is appropriate *when the clinical objectives of the examination are not compromised.*

Pelvis and Upper Femora

AP PROJECTION

Film: 14 × 17 in (35 × 43 cm) crosswise.

Position of patient

- Place the patient on the table in the supine position.

Position of part

- Center the median sagittal plane of the body to the midline of the grid, and adjust it in a true supine position.
- Adjust the shoulders to lie in the same horizontal plane, flex the elbows, and rest the hands on the upper chest.

- Unless contraindicated because of trauma or pathologic factors, internally rotate the feet and lower limbs about 15 degrees to overcome the anteversion of the femoral necks and thus place their long axes parallel with the plane of the film (Figs. 7-13 and 7-14). Note the appearance of the femoral head, femoral neck, and trochanters.
- Because the ankle and knee joints are synovial ginglymus or hinge joints, internal rotation of the foot causes rotation of the entire limb medially. Perform internal rotation of the foot by grasping the heel and turning the toes medially until the position of the longitudinal axis of the heel indicates that the desired degree of limb rotation has been obtained.
- Immobilize with a sandbag across the ankles, if needed.
- Measure the distance from the anterior superior iliac spine to the tabletop on each side to be sure that there is no rotation of the pelvis.
- If a soft tissue abnormality (swelling or atrophy) is causing rotation of the pelvis, elevate one side on a radiolucent pad to overcome the rotation.

- With the cassette in the Bucky tray, center at the level of the soft tissue depression just above the greater trochanter (approximately 2 inches). This centering will include the entire pelvic girdle and the upper fourth of the femora on pelves of average size and shape.
- If the pelvis is deep, palpate for the crest of the ilium, and adjust the position of the film so that its upper border will project 1 to 1½ inches above the crest of the ilium.
- *Shield gonads.* (See Figs. 7-15 and 7-16.)
- Ask patient to suspend respiration for the exposure.

Central ray

- Direct the central ray perpendicular to the midpoint of the film at a point approximately 2 inches (5 cm) superior to the symphysis pubis.

Structures shown

The resulting image will show an AP projection of the pelvis and of the head, neck, trochanters, and proximal third or fourth of the shaft of the femora (Figs. 7-17 and 7-18).

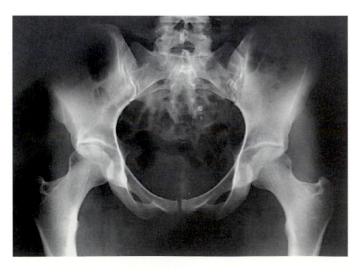

Fig. 7-13. AP pelvis with the feet and lower limbs correctly placed.

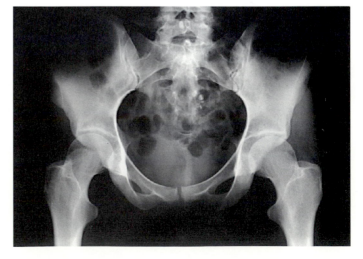

Fig. 7-14. AP pelvis with the feet and lower limbs incorrectly placed.

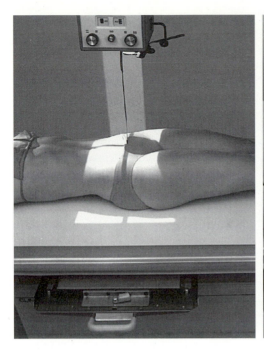

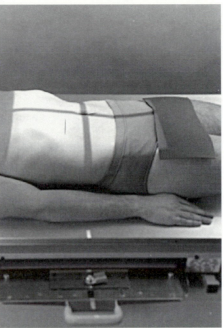

Fig. 7-15. Female AP pelvis with gonad (shadow) shield.

Fig. 7-16. Male AP abdomen with gonad (contact) shield.

□ Evaluation criteria

The following should be clearly demonstrated:

- Entire pelvis along with the proximal femora.
- Lesser trochanters, if seen, demonstrated on the medial border of the femora.
- Femoral necks in their full extent without anteversion.
- Greater trochanters in profile.
- Femoral heads through the underlying acetabula.
- Both ilia equidistant to the edge of the radiograph.
- Both greater trochanters equidistant to the edge of the radiograph.
- Lower vertebral column centered to the middle of the radiograph.
- No rotation of pelvis.
- Symmetrical obturator foramina.
- The ischial spines equally demonstrated.
- Symmetrical iliac alae.
- Sacrum and coccyx aligned with the symphysis pubis.

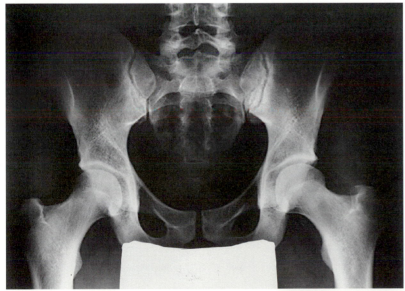

Fig. 7-17. Male AP pelvis.

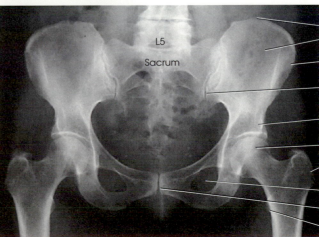

Fig. 7-18. Female AP pelvis.

(Courtesy Marilyn Knight, R.T.)

Crest of ilium
Ala of ilium
Anterior superior iliac spine
Sacroiliac articulation
Anterior inferior iliac spine
Femoral head
Greater trochanter
Obturator foramen
Symphysis pubis
Lesser trochanter

L5
Sacrum

277

Congenital dislocation of the hip

Martz and Taylor[1] recommend two AP projections of the pelvis for the demonstration of the relationship of the femoral head to the acetabulum in patients with congenital dislocation of the hip. The first projection is obtained with the central ray directed perpendicular to the symphysis pubis to detect any lateral or superior displacement of the femoral head. The second projection is obtained with the central ray directed to the symphysis pubis at a cephalic angulation of 45 degrees (Fig. 7-19). This angulation will cast the shadow of an anteriorly displaced femoral head above that of the acetabulum and the shadow of a posteriorly displaced head below that of the acetabulum.

[1]Martz CD and Taylor CC: The 45-degree angle roentgenographic study of the pelvis in congenital dislocation of the hip. J Bone Joint Surg 36A:528-532, 1954.

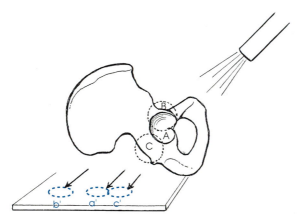

Fig. 7-19. Special projection taken for congenital dislocation of the hip.

Pelvis and Upper Femora
LATERAL PROJECTION
R or L position

Film: 14 × 17 in (35 × 43 cm) lengthwise.

Position of patient

- Place the patient in the recumbent or upright position. If the recumbent position is used, extend the thighs enough to prevent the femora from obscuring the shadow of the pubic arch.

Position of part

Recumbent position

- When the patient can be placed in the lateral position, center the median coronal plane of the body to the midline of the grid.
- Place a support under the lumbar spine, and adjust it to place the vertebral column parallel with the tabletop (Fig. 7-20). If the vertebral column is allowed to sag, it will tilt the pelvis in the longitudinal plane.
- Adjust the pelvis in a true lateral position, with the anterior superior iliac spines lying in the same vertical plane.
- Berkebile et al.[1] recommend a cross-table lateral projection of the pelvis for the demonstration of the gull-wing sign in cases of fracture dislocation of the acetabular rim and posterior dislocation of the femoral head.

[1]Berkebile RD, Fischer DL, and Albrecht LF: The gull-wing sign: value of the lateral view of the pelvis in fracture dislocation of the acetabular rim and posterior dislocation of the femoral head, Radiology 84:937-939, 1965.

Upright position

- Place the patient in the lateral position before a vertical grid device, and center the median coronal plane of the body to the midline of the grid.
- Have the patient stand straight, with the weight of the body equally distributed on the feet.
- Adjust the position of the body so the median sagittal plane is parallel with the plane of the film.

- If the limbs are of unequal length, place a support of suitable height under the foot of the short side.
- Have the patient grasp the side of the stand for support.
- *Shield gonads.*
- Ask patient to suspend respiration for the exposure.

Central ray

- With the cassette in the Bucky tray, direct the central ray perpendicular to a point centered at the level of the soft tissue depression just above the greater trochanter (approximately 2 inches).

Structures shown

The resulting image will show a lateral radiograph of the lumbosacral junction, the sacrum and coccyx, and the superimposed hip bones and upper femora (Fig. 7-21).

☐**Evaluation criteria**

The following should be clearly demonstrated:

- ■ Entire pelvis and the proximal femora.
- ■ Sacrum and coccyx.
- ■ Superimposed posterior margins of the ischium and ilium.
- ■ Superimposed femora.
- ■ Perfectly superimposed acetabular shadows. The larger circle of the fossa (farther from the film) will be equidistant from the smaller circle of the fossa nearer the film throughout their circumference.
- ■ Pubic arch unobscured by the femora.

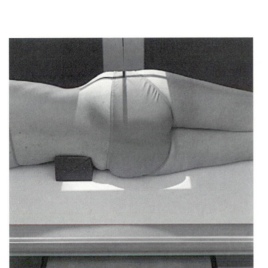

Fig. 7-20. Lateral pelvis.

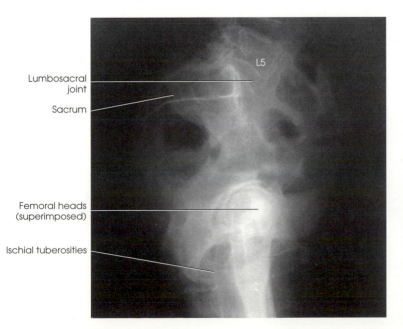
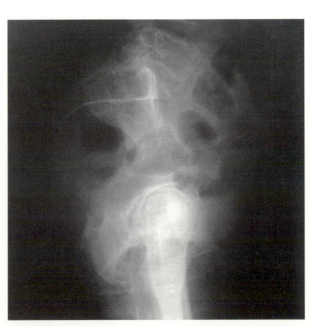

Lumbosacral joint

Sacrum

L5

Femoral heads (superimposed)

Ischial tuberosities

Fig. 7-21. Lateral pelvis.

Pelvis and upper femora

Pelvis and Hip Joints
AXIAL PROJECTION
CHASSARD-LAPINÉ METHOD

Chassard and Lapiné[1] devised this method for the purpose of measuring the horizontal, or biischial, diameter in pelvimetry. It is being used by some to determine the relationship of the femoral head to the acetabulum and by others for the demonstration of the opacified rectosigmoid portion of the colon.

NOTE: This examination is contraindicated for patients with suspected fracture or pathology.

Film: 14 × 17 in (35 × 43 cm) crosswise.

Position of patient

- Seat the patient well back on the end or side of the table so that the posterior surface of the knees is in contact with the edge of the table.

[1]Chassard and Lapiné: Ètude radiographique de l'arcade pubienne chez la femme enceinte; une nouvelle méthode d'appréciation du diamètre bi-ischiatique, J Radiol Electrol. 7:113-124, 1923.

Position of part

- Center the longitudinal axis of the film to the median sagittal plane of the body, or, if the patient is seated on the end of the table, center the median sagittal plane of the body to the midline of the grid. If needed, place a stool or other suitable support under the feet (Fig. 7-22).
- To prevent the thighs from limiting flexion of the body too greatly, have the patient abduct them as far as the end of the table permits.
- Instruct the patient to lean directly forward until the symphysis pubis is in close contact with the table; the vertical axis of the pelvis will be tilted forward approximately 45 degrees. The average patient can achieve this degree of flexion without strain.
- Have the patient grasp the ankles to aid in maintaining the position.
- The exposure factors required for this position are approximately the same as those required for a lateral position of the pelvis.
- *Shield gonads.*
- Ask patient to suspend respiration for the exposure.

Central ray

- Direct the central ray perpendicular through the lumbosacral region at the level of the greater trochanters.
- When flexion of the body is restricted, direct the central ray anteriorly, perpendicular to the coronal plane of the symphysis pubis.

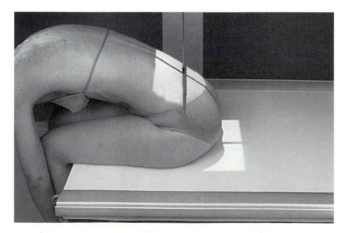

Fig. 7-22. Axial pelvis.

Structures shown

The resulting image will show an axial projection of the pelvis, demonstrating the relationship between the femoral heads and the acetabula, the pelvic bones, and any opacified structure within the pelvis (Fig. 7-23).

□ Evaluation criteria

The following should be clearly demonstrated:

- The femoral heads and acetabula.
- Entire pelvis along with the proximal femora.
- No rotation of the pelvis.
- Greater trochanters equidistant to the sacrum.

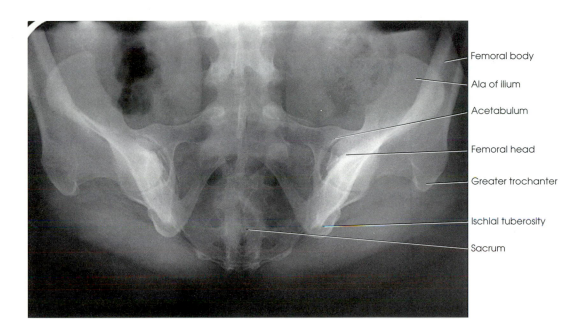

Femoral body

Ala of ilium

Acetabulum

Femoral head

Greater trochanter

Ischial tuberosity

Sacrum

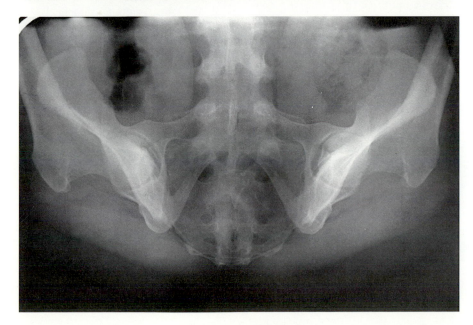

Fig. 7-23. Axial pelvis.

Femoral Necks

 AP OBLIQUE PROJECTION
MODIFIED CLEAVES METHOD

Film: 14 × 17 in (35 × 43 cm) crosswise.

This projection, often called the bilateral "frogleg" position, is contraindicated for the patient suspected of having a fracture or other pathologic disease of the hip area.

Position of patient

- Place the patient in the supine position.
- Adjust the shoulders to lie in the same horizontal plane, flex the elbows, and rest the hands on the upper chest.

Position of part

- Center the median sagittal plane of the body to the midline of the grid.
- Adjust the patient so there is no rotation of the pelvis by placing the anterior superior iliac spines (ASIS) equidistant from the table.

- If needed, place a compression band across the patient well above the hip joints for stability.

Step 1

- Have the patient flex the hips and knees and draw the feet up as much as possible—that is, enough to place the femora in a near vertical position if the affected side will permit.
- Instruct the patient to hold this position, which is relatively comfortable, while the x-ray tube and cassette are adjusted.

Step 2

- Adjust the x-ray tube to direct the central ray perpendicular to the film, and centered 1 inch (2.5 cm) superior to the symphysis pubis.

Step 3

- Abduct the thighs and have the patient turn the feet inward to brace the soles against each other for support.
- Center the feet to the midline of the grid (Fig. 7-24).
- Check the position of the thighs, being careful to abduct them to the same degree.
- If possible, abduct the thighs approximately 40 degrees from the vertical to place the long axis of the femoral necks parallel with the plane of the film.

Unilateral Projection

- This projection is adapted for a *unilateral examination* by adjusting the body position to center the anterior superior iliac spine of the affected side to the midline of the grid.
- Have the patient flex the hip and knee of the affected side and draw the foot up to the opposite knee.
- After adjusting the perpendicular central ray and positioning the cassette tray, have the patient brace the sole of the foot against the opposite knee and lean the thigh laterally approximately 40 degrees (Fig. 7-25).
- *Shield gonads.*
- Ask patient to suspend respiration for the exposure.

Option

- The patient may be rolled onto the affected hip with the knee in contact with the table to obtain a lateral hip projection on the non-injured patient, as shown in Fig. 7-34.

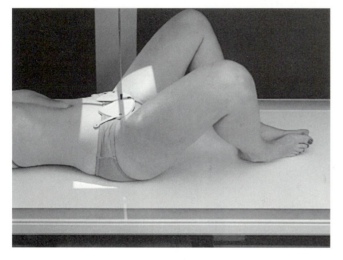

Fig. 7-24. AP oblique femoral necks with perpendicular central ray and gonad (contact) shielding: modified Cleaves method.

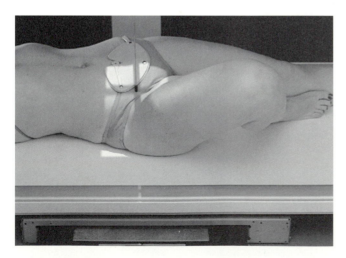

Fig. 7-25. Unilateral AP oblique femoral neck: modified Cleaves method.

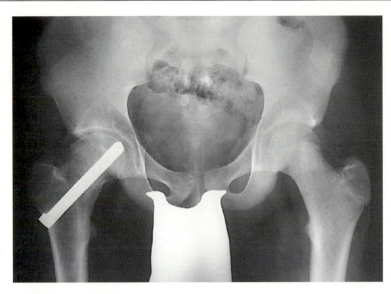

Fig. 7-26. AP oblique femoral necks. Note fixation device in right hip and gonad shield.

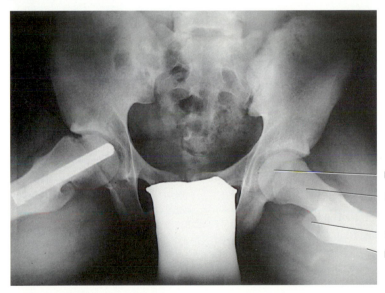

Femoral head

Femoral neck

Lesser trochanter

Femoral body (shaft)

Fig. 7-27. AP oblique femoral necks: modified Cleaves method. Same patient as Fig. 7-26.

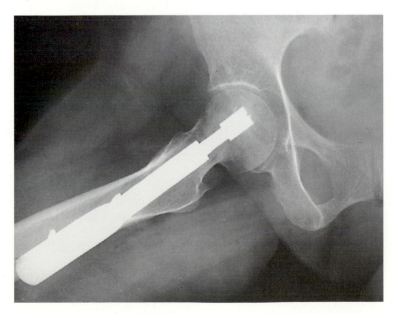

Fig. 7-28. AP oblique femoral neck: modified Cleaves method.

Central ray

- Direct the perpendicular central ray to enter the patient's median sagittal plane or affected hip at the level 1 inch superior to the symphysis pubis.

Structures shown

The resulting image will show an AP oblique projection of the femoral heads, necks, and trochanteric areas projected onto one radiograph for comparison (Figs. 7-26 to 7-28).

□ Evaluation criteria

The following should be clearly demonstrated:

- The acetabulum, femoral head, and lateral femoral neck.
- Lesser trochanter on the medial side of the femur.
- No rotation of the pelvis, as evidenced by a symmetrical appearance.

Femoral Necks

AXIOLATERAL PROJECTION
ORIGINAL CLEAVES METHOD

Film: 14 × 17 in (35 × 43 cm) crosswise.

Position of patient

- Position the patient as described in steps 1 and 2 on p. 282.

Position of part

- Before having the patient abduct the thighs (described in step 3 on p. 282), direct the x-ray tube parallel with the long axes of the femoral shafts as seen in Fig. 7-29.
- Adjust the film so the midpoint coincides with the central ray.
- *Shield gonads*. (Not shown for illustrative purposes.)
- Ask patient to suspend respiration for the exposure.

Central ray

- Direct the central ray to enter the symphysis pubis; angle the central ray approximately 40 degrees cephalad.

Structures shown

The resulting image will show an axial projection of the femoral heads, necks, and trochanteric areas.

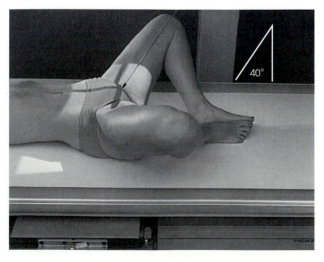

Fig. 7-29. Axiolateral femoral necks: Cleaves method.

□Evaluation criteria

The following should be clearly demonstrated:

- As much of the femoral necks, as possible without overlap from the greater trochanter.
- Only a small part of the lesser trochanters on the posterior surface of the femurs.
- Only a small amount of the greater trochanters on both the posterior and anterior surfaces of the femurs.
- Both sides equidistant from the edge of the radiograph.
- No rotation of pelvis.
- Femoral heads through the underlying acetabula.
- A greater amount of the proximal femur on a unilateral examination.

Congenital dislocation of the hip

Diagnosis of congenital dislocation of the hip in newborns has been the topic of numerous articles. Andren and von Rosén[1] described a method based on certain theoretical considerations. Their method requires the accurate and judicious application of the positioning technique to make an accurate diagnosis. The Andren-von Rosén approach involves taking a bilateral hip projection with both legs forcibly abducted to at least 45 degrees with appreciable inward rotation of the femora. Knake and Kuhns[2] described the construction of a device that controlled the degree of abduction and rotation of both limbs. They reported that the device essentially eliminated and greatly simplified the positioning difficulties while reducing the number of repeat examinations.

---

[1]Andren L and von Rosén S: The diagnosis of dislocation of the hip in newborns and the primary results of immediate treatment, Acta Radiol 49:89-96, 1958.
[2]Knake JE and Kuhns LR: A device to aid in positioning for the Andren-von Rosén hip view, Radiology 117:735-736, 1975.

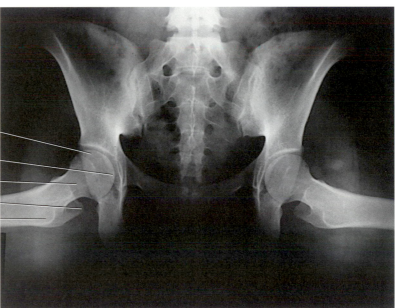

Femoral head
Femoral head within acetabulum
Femoral neck
Greater trochanter
Lesser trochanter

Fig. 7-30. Axiolateral, femoral necks: Cleaves method.

Hip

⬛ AP PROJECTION

Film: 10 × 12 in (24 × 30 cm) length-wise.

Position of patient

- Place the patient in the supine position.

Position of part

- Center the sagittal plane passing 2 inches medial to the anterior superior iliac spine to the midline of the grid.
- Adjust the pelvis so there is no rotation by placing the anterior superior iliac spines equidistant from the table.
- Place the arms in a comfortable position.
- Adjust the shoulders to lie in the same horizontal plane (Figs. 7-31 and 7-32).

- Unless contraindicated or otherwise instructed, internally rotate the feet and the lower limb approximately 15 degrees to overcome the anteversion of the femoral neck and thereby place its long axis parallel with the plane of the film.
- With the cassette in the Bucky tray, center at the level of the highest point of the greater trochanter.
- *Shield gonads.*
- Ask patient to suspend respiration for the exposure.

Central ray

- Direct the perpendicular central ray to the center of the cassette as positioned above. The central ray should enter approximately 2.5 inches (6 cm) distal on a line drawn perpendicular to the midpoint of a line between the ASIS and the symphysis pubis (see p. 274, Fig. 7-8).
  - Another localization technique is to direct the central ray to a sagittal plane 2 inches (5 cm) medial to the affected side ASIS at the level just superior to the greater trochanter.
  - In the groin, the femoral artery lies midway between the ASIS and the symphysis pubis. Just distal to the inguinal ligament, the femoral pulsations can be palpated where the artery overlies the hip joint.

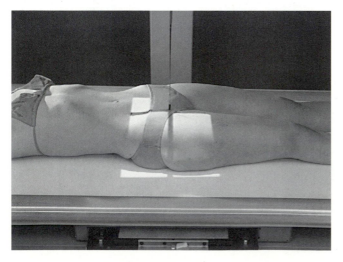

Fig. 7-31. AP hip.

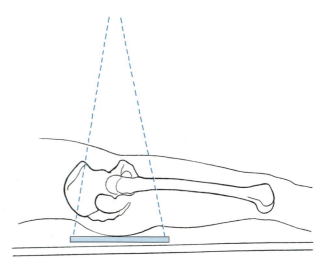

Fig. 7-32. AP hip.

Structures shown

The resulting image will show the head, neck, trochanters, and proximal third of the body (shaft) of the femur (Fig. 7-33).

In the initial examination of a hip lesion, whether traumatic or pathologic in origin, the AP projection is often made on a film large enough to include the entire pelvic girdle and upper femora. Progress studies may be restricted to the affected side.

Hip

□ Evaluation criteria

The following should be clearly demonstrated:
- The femoral head, penetrated and seen through the acetabulum.
- Adjoining region of the ilium and the pubic bones to the symphysis pubis.
- Any orthopedic appliance in its entirety.
- Hip joint.
- Greater trochanter in profile.
- Entire long axis of the femoral neck not foreshortened.
- Proximal third of the femur.
- The lesser trochanter is usually not projected beyond the medial border of the femur; or, only a very small amount of the trochanter is seen.

NOTE: Trauma patients who have sustained severe injury are not usually transferred to the radiographic table but rather radiographed on the stretcher or bed. After the localization point has been established and marked, one assistant should be on each side of the stretcher to grasp the sheet and lift the pelvis just enough for the placement of the cassette, while a third person supports the injured limb. Any necessary manipulation of the limb must be made by a physician.

Ilium

Acetabulum

Femoral head

Greater trochanter

Femoral neck

Symphysis pubis

Lesser trochanter

Femoral body

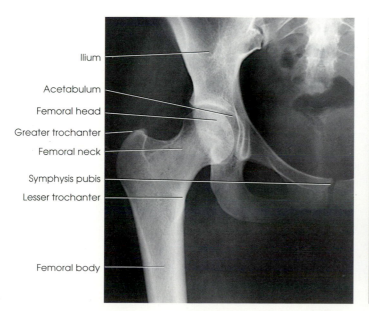 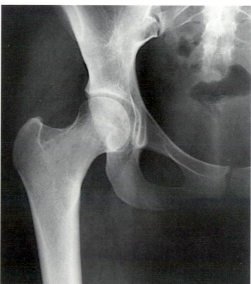

Fig. 7-33. AP hip.

Hip

 LATERAL PROJECTION
Mediolateral
LAUENSTEIN AND HICKEY METHODS

The Lauenstein and Hickey methods are used to demonstrate the hip joint and the relationship of the femoral head to the acetabulum. Because of the danger of fragment displacement or injury, this body position is not used in the presence of trauma, unhealed fracture, or destructive disease. This position, similar to the previously described Cleaves method, is also called the "frogleg" position.

Film: 10 × 12 in (24 × 30 cm) crosswise.

Position of patient

- Turn the patient slightly toward the affected side.

Position of part

- Adjust the body and center the affected hip to the midline of the grid.
- Ask the patient to flex the affected knee and draw the thigh up to a near right-angle position.
- The body (shaft) of the affected femur is parallel to the table.
- Extend the opposite limb and support it at hip level and under the knee.
- Adjust the position of the pelvis so that the upper side is rotated posteriorly enough to prevent its superimposition on the affected hip (Fig. 7-34).
- Position the Bucky tray so the midpoint of the film will coincide with the central ray.
- *Shield gonads.*
- Ask patient to suspend respiration for the exposure.

Central ray

- Direct the central ray through the hip joint, which is located midway between the anterior superior iliac spine and the symphysis pubis, (1) perpendicular for the Lauenstein method (Fig. 7-35) and (2) at a cephalic angle of 20 to 25 degrees for the Hickey method (Fig. 7-36).

Structures shown

The resulting image will show a lateral projection of the hip, showing the acetabulum, the proximal end of the femur, and the relationship of the femoral head to the acetabulum (Figs. 7-35 and 7-36).

□ Evaluation criteria

The following should be clearly demonstrated:

- Hip joint centered to the radiograph.
- Hip joint, acetabulum, and femoral head.
- Femoral neck overlapped by the greater trochanter in the Lauenstein projection.
- The cephalic angulation of the Hickey method will demonstrate the femoral neck free of superimposition.

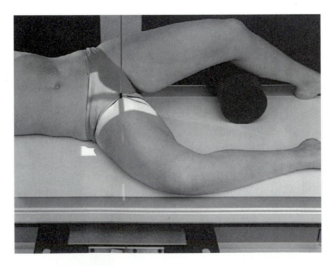

Fig. 7-34. Mediolateral hip using gonad (shadow) shield: Lauenstein method.

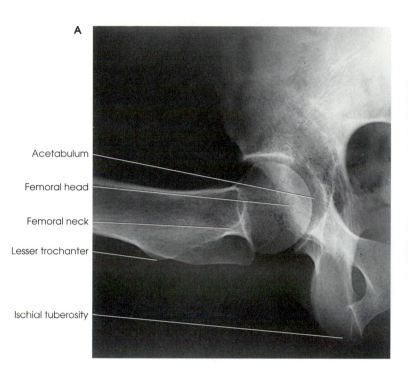

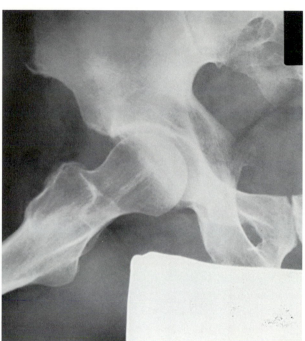

Acetabulum

Femoral head

Femoral neck

Lesser trochanter

Ischial tuberosity

Fig. 7-35. A, Mediolateral hip with perpendicular central ray: Lauenstein method. **B,** Mediolateral hip with perpendicular central ray using gonad (contact) shield.

(B, Courtesy Marek Anderson, R.T.)

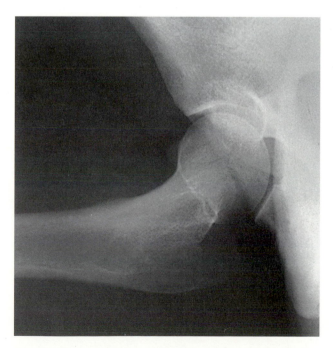

Fig. 7-36. Mediolateral hip with 20-degree cephalad angulation: Hickey method.

Hip

Hip

AXIOLATERAL PROJECTION
DANELIUS-MILLER MODIFICATION
OF LORENZ[1] METHOD

Film: 8 × 10 in (18 × 24 cm) lengthwise.

[1]Lorenz: Die röntgenographische Darstellung des subskapularen Raumes und des Schenkelhalses im Querschnitt. Fortschr Roentgenstr 25:342-343, 1917-1918.

Position of patient

- Adjust the patient in the supine position.
- When examining a subject who is thin or is lying on a soft bed, elevate the pelvis on a firm pillow or folded sheets enough to center the most prominent point of the greater trochanter to the midline of the film. The support must not extend beyond the lateral surface of the body; otherwise it will interfere with the placement of the cassette.
- Support the affected limb at hip level on sandbags or firm pillows when pelvis is elevated.

Position of part

- Flex the knee and hip of the unaffected side, and adjust the limb in a position that will not interfere with the central ray.
- Rest the unaffected leg on a suitable support. Special support devices are available.
- Place the unaffected thigh in a vertical position, and adjust the pelvis *so there is no rotation* (Figs. 7-37 and 7-38).
- Unless contraindicated, grasp the heel and internally rotate the foot and lower limb of the affected side about 15 or 20 degrees. A sandbag may be used to hold the leg and foot in this position. The manipulation of patients with unhealed fractures should be performed by a physician.

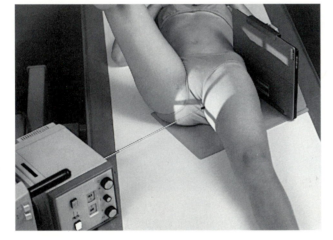

Fig. 7-37. Axiolateral hip: Danelius-Miller modification.

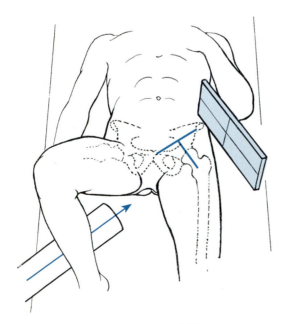

Fig. 7-38. Axiolateral hip: Danelius-Miller modification.

Position of film

- Place the cassette in the vertical position with its upper border in the crease above the crest of the ilium.
- Angle the lower border away from the body until the cassette is exactly parallel with the long axis of the femoral neck.
- The cassette is supported in position with sandbags, a vertical cassette holder, or the patient may support it.
- Be careful to place the grid so that the lead strips will be in the horizontal position.
- *Shield gonads* by using close collimation.
- Ask patient to suspend respiration for the exposure.

Central ray

- Direct the central ray perpendicular to the long axis of the femoral neck. Center about 2.5 inches (6 cm) below the point of intersection of the localization lines described previously.

Structures shown

The resulting image will show the head, neck, and trochanters of the femur (Fig. 7-39).

□Evaluation criteria

The following should be clearly demonstrated:

- As much of the femoral neck as possible without overlap from the greater trochanter.
- Only a small amount of the lesser trochanter on the posterior surface of the femur.
- A small amount of the greater trochanter on the anterior and posterior surfaces of the proximal femur when the femur is properly inverted.
- Soft tissue shadow of the unaffected thigh not overlapping the hip joint or proximal femur.
- Hip joint with the acetabulum.
- Any orthopedic appliance in its entirety.

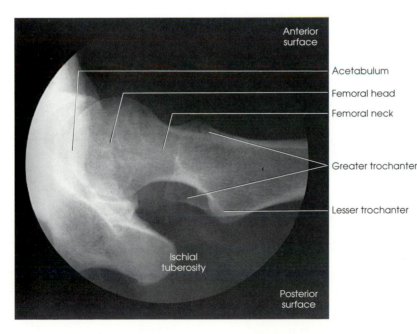

Anterior surface

Acetabulum

Femoral head

Femoral neck

Greater trochanter

Lesser trochanter

Ischial tuberosity

Posterior surface

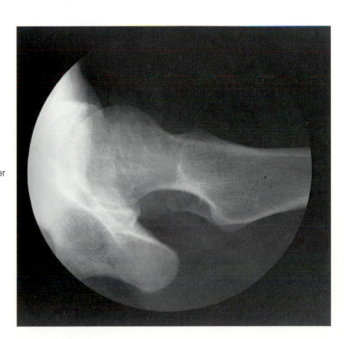

Fig. 7-39. Axiolateral hip: Danelius-Miller method.

Hip

Hip

AXIOLATERAL PROJECTION
CLEMENTS-NAKAYAMA
MODIFICATION

When the patient has bilateral hip fractures, bilateral hip arthroplasty (plastic surgery of hip joints), or limitation of movement of the unaffected leg, the previous approach cannot be used. Clements and Nakayama[1] describe a modification using a 15-degree posterior angulation of the central ray (Fig. 7-40).

Film: 10 × 12 in (24 × 30 cm).

---

[1]Clements RS and Nakayama HK: Radiographic methods in total hip arthroplasty, Radiol Technol 51:589-600, 1980.

Position of patient

• Position the patient supine on the table with the affected side near the edge of the radiographic table.

Position of part

• For this position the lower limb is *not* internally rotated but remains in the neutral or slightly externally rotated position.
• This leg position yields a lateral hip image because the central ray is angled 15 degrees posterior instead of the toes being internally rotated.

• Support a grid cassette on the Bucky tray; place the grid so the grid lines run parallel with the floor.
• Adjust the grid surface so it is perpendicular to the central ray. It must be tilted back 15°.
• *Shield gonads.*
• Ask patient to suspend respiration for the exposure.

Central ray

• Direct the central ray 15 degrees posteriorly and aligned perpendicular to the femoral neck.

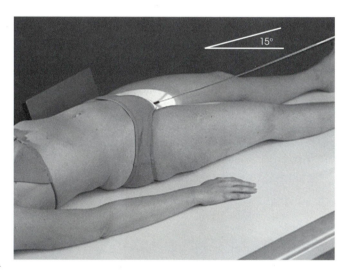

Fig. 7-40. Axiolateral hip: Clements and Nakayama method.

Structures shown

The resulting image will show the proximal femur including the head, neck, and trochanters in lateral profile. The Clements and Nakayama modification (Figs. 7-41 and 7-42) can be compared to the Danelius-Miller approach described previously.

□**Evaluation criteria**

The following should be clearly demonstrated:
- Hip joint with the acetabulum.
- Femoral head, neck, and trochanters.
- Soft tissue of the unaffected thigh not overlapping the hip joint or proximal femur.
- Any orthopedic appliance in its entirety.

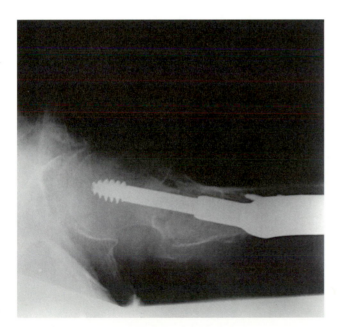

Fig. 7-41. Clements and Nakayama method with 15-degree central ray angulation.

(Courtesy Roland Clements, R.T., F.A.S.R.T.)

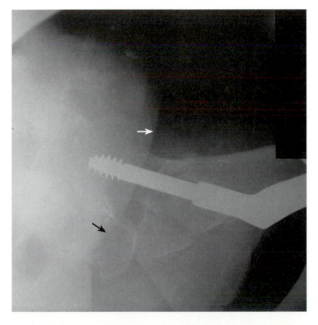

Fig. 7-42. Postoperative Danelius-Miller method on patient unable to flex unaffected hip. Contralateral thigh *(arrows)* is obscuring the femoral head and acetabular area.

(Courtesy Roland Clements, R.T., F.A.S.R.T.)

Hip

Hip

AXIOLATERAL PROJECTION
LEONARD-GEORGE METHOD

Film: 8 × 10 in (18 × 24 cm) (curved cassette preferred for reduced part-film distance).

Position of patient

- Place the patient in the supine position.
- If needed, elevate the pelvis on a small, firm pillow or folded sheets to place the greater trochanters 4 inches above the tabletop to center the hip to the vertically placed curved cassette.
- Support the affected limb at hip level on pillows or sandbags when pelvis is elevated.

Position of part

- Flex the hip and knee of the unaffected side, if they are not immobilized, and abduct the thigh to accommodate the position of the curved cassette.

- The affected limb is usually in abduction in a cast or a splint. If not, and if possible, abduct the leg enough to accurately place the curved cassette in the groin.
- Place the cassette in the vertical position well up between the thighs and center it to the crease of the groin of the affected side. With the leg in abduction, this center point will be perpendicular to the femoral neck (Figs. 7-43 and 7-44).
- If the limb can be safely moved, grasp the heel and internally rotate the foot and lower limb about 15 or 20 degrees to overcome the anteversion of the femoral neck and thus place its long axis parallel with the horizontal and its lateral aspect perpendicular to the plane of the film.
- *Shield gonads* by using close collimation.
- Ask patient to suspend respiration for the exposure.

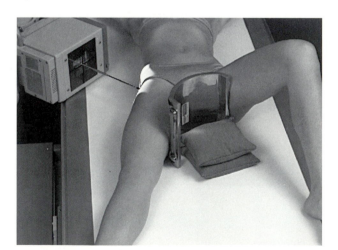

Fig. 7-43. Axiolateral hip with curved cassette: Leonard-George method.

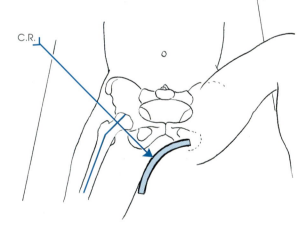

Fig. 7-44. Axiolateral hip with curved cassette: Leonard-George method.

Central ray

• Direct the central ray inferiorly and medially perpendicular to the long axis of the femoral neck. It enters the lateral surface of the hip above the soft tissue depression just above the greater trochanter.

Structures shown

The resulting image will show the head, neck, and trochanteric area of the femur (Fig. 7-45). Because of the convexity of the cassette, the femoral head and trochanteric areas are somewhat elongated.

□ Evaluation criteria

The following should be clearly demonstrated:

■ Most of the femoral neck without overlapping from the trochanters.
■ Only a small amount of the lesser trochanter on the posterior surface of the femur.
■ A small amount of the greater trochanter on the anterior and posterior surfaces of the proximal femur when the femur is properly placed.
■ Hip joint with the acetabulum.

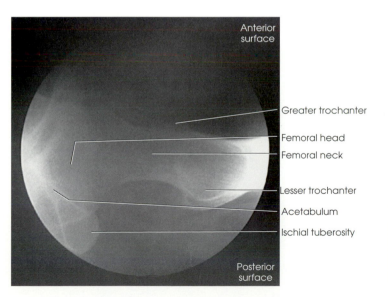

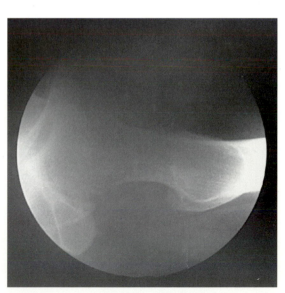

Anterior surface

Greater trochanter

Femoral head
Femoral neck

Lesser trochanter

Acetabulum

Ischial tuberosity

Posterior surface

Fig. 7-45. Axiolateral femoral neck: Leonard-George method.

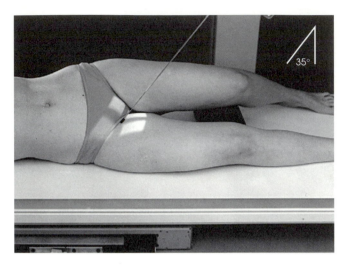

Fig. 7-46. Axiolateral hip with central ray angulation of 35 degrees: Friedman method

Hip

AXIOLATERAL PROJECTION
FRIEDMAN METHOD

NOTE: This examination is contraindicated for patients with suspected fracture or pathology.

Film: 10 × 12 in (24 × 30 cm) lengthwise.

Position of patient

- Have the patient lie in the lateral recumbent position on the affected side.
- Center the median coronal plane of the body to the midline of the table.

Position of part

- Extend the affected limb and adjust it in a lateral position. Roll the upper side gently posteriorly, approximately 10 degrees, and place a support under the knee to support it at hip level. The affected femur will not change position if it is properly immobilized; the pelvis will rotate from the femoral head (Fig. 7-46).

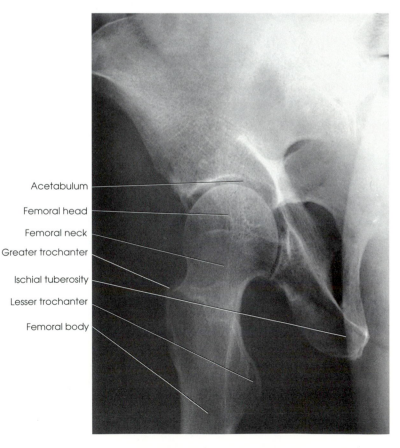

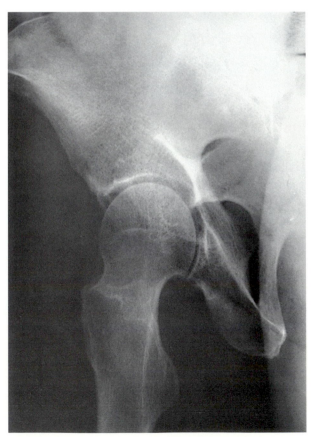

Acetabulum
Femoral head
Femoral neck
Greater trochanter
Ischial tuberosity
Lesser trochanter
Femoral body

Fig. 7-47. Axiolateral hip with central ray angulation of 35 degrees: Friedman method.

- With the cassette in the Bucky tray, adjust its position so that the midpoint of the film will coincide with the central ray.
- *Shield gonads* by using close collimation.
- Ask patient to suspend respiration for the exposure.

Central ray

- Direct the central ray to the femoral neck at an angle of 35 degrees cephalad (Fig. 7-47).
- Kisch[1] recommends that the central ray be angled 15 or 20 degrees cephalad for this position (Fig. 7-48).

---

[1]Kisch E: Eine neue Methode für röntgenolische Darstellung des Hüftgelenks in frontaler Ebene, Fortschr Roentgenstr 27:309, 1920.

Structures shown

The resulting image will show an axiolateral projection of the head, neck, trochanters, and proximal body (shaft) of the femur.

□ Evaluation criteria

The following should be clearly demonstrated:
- Distorted femoral head, neck, and trochanters because of the angulation of the x-ray beam.
- Hip joint.
- Prominent trochanters.

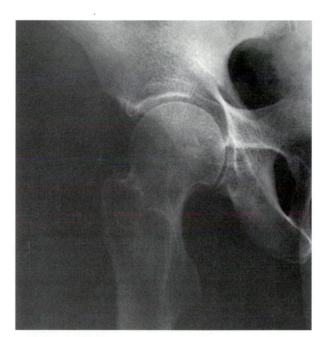

Fig. 7-48. Axiolateral hip with central ray angulation of 20 degrees: Friedman method.

Hip

PA OBLIQUE PROJECTION
RAO and LAO positions
HSIEH METHOD

Hsieh[1] recommends this projection for demonstrating posterior dislocations of the femoral head in cases other than acute fracture dislocations.

Film: 10 × 12 in (24 × 30 cm) lengthwise.

Position of patient

• Place the patient with a suspected posterior hip dislocation in the semiprone position and center the affected hip to the midline of the table.

[1]Hsieh CK: Posterior dislocation of the hip, Radiology 27:450-455, 1936.

Position of part

• Elevate the unaffected side approximately 40 to 45 degrees and have the patient support himself or herself on the flexed knee and forearm of the elevated side.
• Adjust the position of the body to place the posterior surface of the affected iliac bone over the midline of the grid (Fig. 7-49).
• With the cassette in the Bucky tray, adjust its position so that the center of the film will lie at the level of the superior border of the greater trochanter.
• *Shield gonads* by using close collimation.
• Ask patient to suspend respiration for the exposure.

Central ray

• Direct the central ray perpendicular to the midpoint of the film passing between the posterior surface of the iliac blade and the dislocated femoral head.

Structures shown

The resulting image will show a PA oblique projection of the ilium, the hip joint, and the proximal femur (Fig. 7-50).

Urist[1] has recommended a right or left posterior oblique position (AP projection) for the demonstration of the posterior rim of the acetabulum in acute fracture-dislocation injuries of the hip. For this, the patient is adjusted from the supine position. Elevate the injured hip 60 degrees to place the posterior rim of the acetabulum in profile, and adjust the body to center the sagittal plane passing through the anterior superior iliac spine to the midline of the table. Center the cassette at the level of the upper border of the greater trochanter. Direct the central ray perpendicular to the midpoint of the film (Fig. 7-51).

☐ Evaluation criteria

The following should be clearly demonstrated:
■ Hip joint near the center of the radiograph.
■ Hip joint and femoral head.
■ Superimposed soft tissue of buttock over the area of the femoral neck.

[1]Urist MR: Fracture-dislocation of the hip joint, J Bone Joint Surg 30A:699-727, 1948.

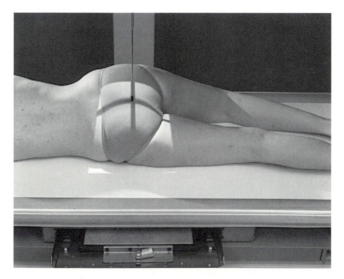

Fig. 7-49. PA oblique hip: Hsieh method. LAO.

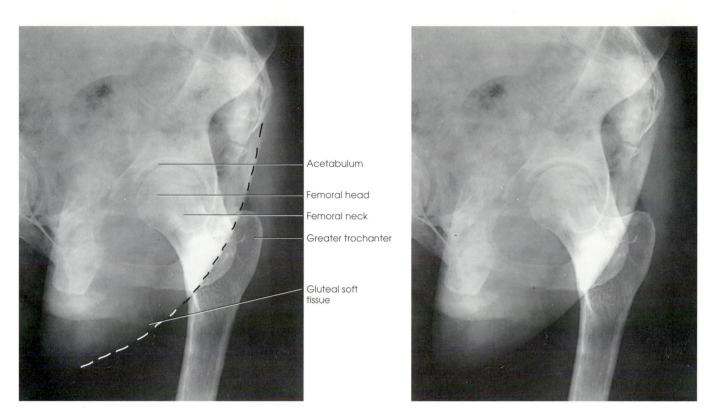

Acetabulum

Femoral head

Femoral neck

Greater trochanter

Gluteal soft
tissue

Fig. 7-50. PA oblique hip: Hsieh method.

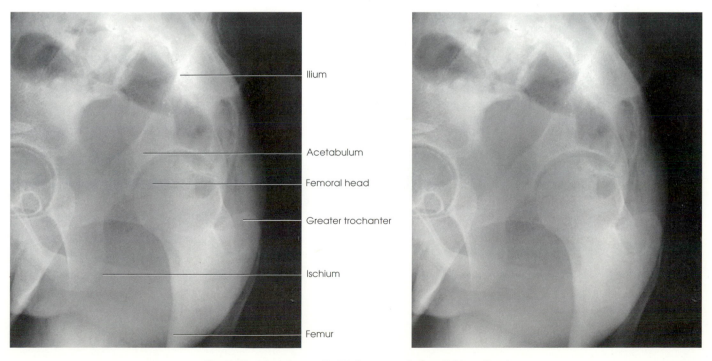

Ilium

Acetabulum

Femoral head

Greater trochanter

Ischium

Femur

Fig. 7-51. AP oblique with 60 degrees rotation. Urist method.

Hip
PA OBLIQUE PROJECTION
RAO or LAO position
LILIENFELD METHOD

NOTE: This examination is contraindicated for patients with suspected fracture or pathology.

Film: 10 × 12 in (24 × 30 cm) lengthwise.

Position of patient

- Have the patient lie in the lateral recumbent position on the affected side.

Position of part

- Center the median coronal plane of the body to the midline of the grid.
- Fully extend the affected thigh, adjust it in a true lateral position, and immobilize it with sandbags.
- Have the patient grasp the side of the table to aid in stabilizing the position.
- Roll the upper side gently forward approximately 15 degrees, or just enough to separate the two sides of the pelvis.
- Support the limb at hip level on sandbags.
- If the affected side is well immobilized and the upper side is gently rolled forward, the affected hip will not change position; the pelvis will rotate from the femoral head (Fig. 7-52).
- With the cassette in the Bucky tray, adjust its position so that the center point of the film will lie at the level of the greater trochanter.
- *Shield gonads* by using close collimation.
- Ask patient to suspend respiration for the exposure.

Central ray

- Direct the central ray perpendicular to the midpoint of the film, traversing the affected hip joint.

Structures shown

The resulting image will show a PA oblique projection of the ilium, the acetabulum, and the proximal femur (Fig. 7-53).

☐ Evaluation criteria

The following should be clearly demonstrated:

- Hip joint near the center of the radiograph.
- Hip joint and acetabulum.
- Unaffected hip and acetabulum not overlapping the same structures of the side of interest.

NOTE: Since the Lilienfeld projection is not used with patients who have an acute hip injury, these patients can be comfortably, safely, and satisfactorily examined in the position described by Colonna.[1] The patient is positioned in approximately the manner described for the Lilienfeld method, except that the patient is placed *on the unaffected* side and adjusted to center the uppermost hip to the midline of the table. Colonna recommends that the uppermost side, the affected side, be rotated about 17 degrees anteriorly from the true lateral position. He states that this degree of rotation separates the shadows of the hip joints and gives the optimum projection of the slope of the acetabular roof and the depth of the socket (Fig. 7-54).

[1]Colonna PC: A diagnostic roentgen view of the acetabulum, Surg Clin North Am 33:1565-1569, 1953.

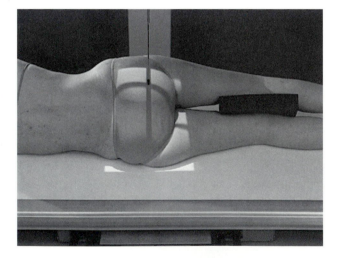

Fig. 7-52. PA oblique hip: Lilienfeld method. LAO.

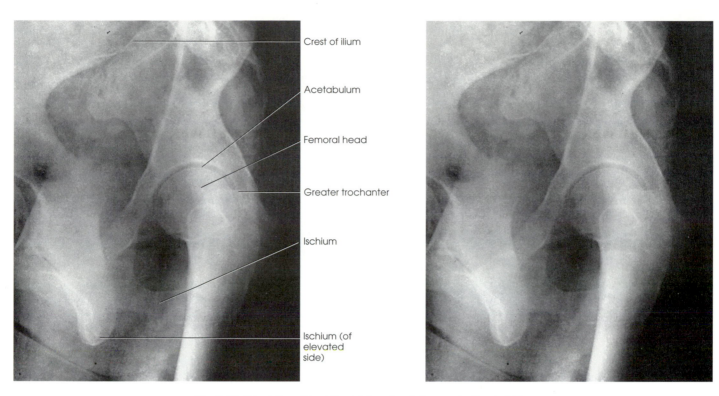

Crest of ilium

Acetabulum

Femoral head

Greater trochanter

Ischium

Ischium (of elevated side)

Fig. 7-53. PA oblique hip: Lilienfeld method demonstrating left hip.

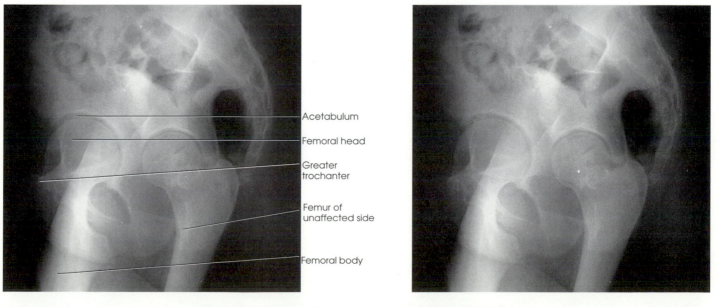

Acetabulum

Femoral head

Greater trochanter

Femur of unaffected side

Femoral body

Fig. 7-54. Colonna method demonstrating elevated right hip.

Acetabulum

PA AXIAL OBLIQUE PROJECTION
RAO or LAO position
TEUFEL METHOD

Film: 8 × 10 in (18 × 24 cm) lengthwise.

Position of patient

- Have the patient lie in a semiprone position on the affected side.
- Have the patient support himself or herself on the forearm and flexed knee of the elevated side.

Position of part

- Align the body, and center the hip being examined to the midline of the grid.
- Elevate the unaffected side so that the anterior surface of the body forms a 38-degree angle from the table (Fig. 7-55).
- With the cassette in the Bucky tray, adjust its position so that the midpoint of the film coincides with the central ray.
- *Shield gonads* by using close collimation.
- Ask patient to suspend respiration for the exposure.

Central ray

- Direct the central ray through the acetabulum at an angle of 12 degrees cephalad. The central ray enters the body at the inferior level of the coccyx and approximately 2 inches lateral to the median sagittal plane toward the side being examined.

Structures shown

The resulting image will show the fovea capitis and, particularly, the superoposterior wall of the acetabulum (Fig. 7-56).

□ Evaluation criteria

The following should be clearly demonstrated:

- Hip joint and acetabulum near the center of the radiograph.
- Femoral head in profile to demonstrate the concave area of the fovea capitis.

Acetabulum

JUDET METHOD

Judet et al.[1] described two posterior oblique positions useful to diagnose fractures of the acetabulum. Both obliques are 45-degree posterior oblique positions; internal oblique (affected side up) and ex-

[1]Judet R, Judet J, and Letournel E: Fractures of the acetabulum: Classification and surgical approaches for open reduction, J Bone Joint Surg 46A:1615-1646, 1964.

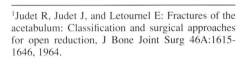

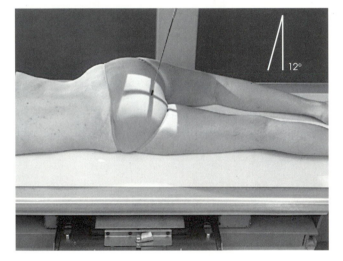

Fig. 7-55. PA axial oblique acetabulum: Teufel method.

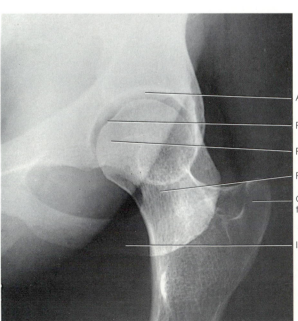

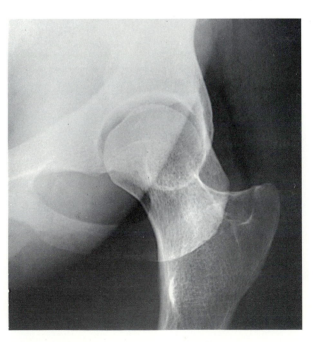

Acetabulum

Fovea capitis

Femoral head

Femoral neck

Greater trochanter

Ischium

Fig. 7-56. PA axial oblique acetabulum: Teufel method.

ternal oblique (affected side down). In both positions a perpendicular central ray is directed through the acetabulum.

Acetabulum

SUPEROINFERIOR OBLIQUE PROJECTION
DUNLAP, SWANSON, AND PENNER METHOD

Film: 7 × 17 in (18 × 43 cm) or 14 × 17 in (35 × 43 cm) crosswise for a bilateral examination of adults.

Close collimation is used to restrict the radiation to the adjacent half of the film.

Position of patient

- Place the patient in the seated-upright position on the side of the table.

Position of part

- Ask the patient to move back far enough to place the posterior surface of the knees in contact with the edge of the table (Fig. 7-57).
- Center the midline of the longitudinal half of the cassette opposite to the side being examined to the median sagittal plane of the body.
- Mark the position of the grid so that it can be moved back to this position for the second exposure without disturbing the patient's position; then center the

[1]Dunlap K, Swanson AB, and Penner RS: Studies of the hip joint by means of lateral acetabular roentgenograms, J Bone Joint Surg 38A:1218-1230, 1956.

opposite half of the film to the median sagittal plane of the body for the first exposure.

- Ask the patient to sit upright with the thighs together.
- Have the patient cross the arms over the chest so that they will be well away from the crests of the ilia.
- Instruct the patient to maintain the exact position when the x-ray tube is shifted for the second exposure.
- *Shield gonads* by using close collimation.
- Respiration need not be suspended for the exposures.

Central ray

- Direct the central ray to the crest of the ilium at a medial angle of 30 degrees, first from one side and then from the other.
- The originators[1] of this position have stated that the plane of the acetabulum forms an angle of 35 degrees with the sagittal plane in the average adult and 32 degrees in children, but they have found that a central ray angulation of 30 degrees results in the least superimposition of parts.

Structures shown

The resulting image will show the acetabula in profile projected from a plane at right angles to the frontal projection and the relationship of the femoral heads to the acetabula. The femoral heads, necks, and trochanters are seen from a near frontal plane, because there is little change in the position of the femora between the supine and the seated positions (Fig. 7-58).

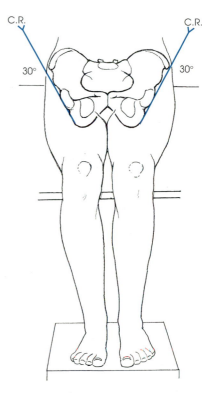

Fig. 7-57. Superoinferior oblique acetabulum.

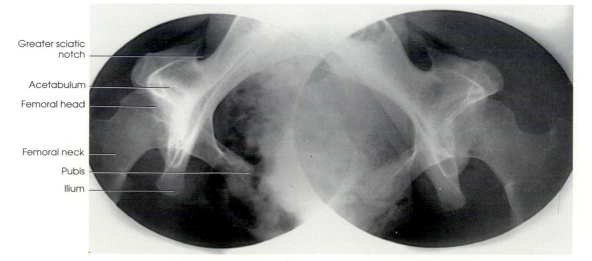

Greater sciatic notch

Acetabulum

Femoral head

Femoral neck

Pubis

Ilium

Fig. 7-58. Superoinferior oblique acetabulum.

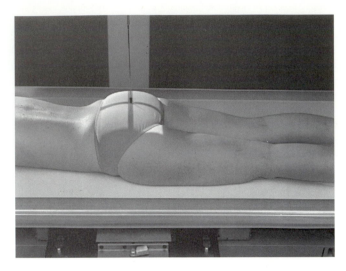

Fig. 7-59. PA pelvic bones.

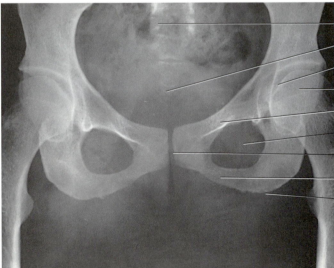

Sacrum
Coccyx
Acetabulum
Femoral head
Superior pubic ramus
Obturator foramen
Symphysis pubis
Inferior pubic ramus
Ischial tuberosity

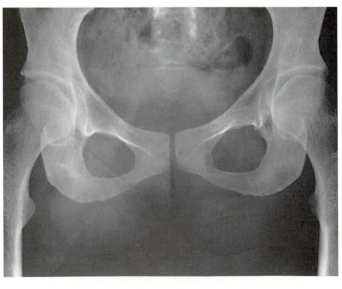

Fig. 7-60. PA pelvic bones.

□ **Evaluation criteria**

The following should be clearly demonstrated:

■ Acetabula in profile.
■ Ilium, ischium, or pubic bones not overlapping the acetabular region.
■ Acetabula and hip joints near the center of the image.

Anterior Pelvic Bones
PA PROJECTION

Film: 8 × 10 in (18 × 24 cm) crosswise.

Position of patient

• Place the patient in the prone position and center the median sagittal plane of the body to the midline of the grid.

Position of part

• Adjust the body in the *prone position* without any rotation.
• With the cassette in the Bucky tray, center at the level of the greater trochanters; this will center the film to the symphysis pubis (Fig. 7-59).
• *Shield gonads.*
• Ask patient to suspend respiration for the exposure.

Central ray

• Direct the central ray perpendicular to the midpoint of the film. It enters the distal coccyx and exits the symphysis pubis.

Structures shown

The resulting image will show a PA projection of the pubic and ischial bones, including the symphysis pubis and obturator foramina (Fig. 7-60).

□ **Evaluation criteria**

The following should be clearly demonstrated:

■ Pubic and ischial bones not magnified or superimposing the sacrum or coccyx.
■ No rotation.
■ Pubic and ischial bones near the center of the radiograph.
■ Hip joints.

Anterior Pelvic Bones

AP AXIAL PROJECTION
TAYLOR METHOD

Film: 10 × 12 in (24 × 30 cm) crosswise.

Position of patient

• Place the patient in the supine position.

Position of part

• Center the median sagittal plane of the body to the midline of the grid, and adjust the pelvis so there is no rotation by placing the anterior superior iliac spines equidistant from the table (Fig. 7-61).
• With the cassette in the Bucky tray, adjust its position so the midpoint of the film will coincide with the central ray.
• *Shield gonads.*
• Ask patient to suspend respiration for the exposure.

Central ray

Males
• Direct the central ray approximately 25 degrees (20 to 35 degrees) cephalad, and center to a point 2 inches distal to the superior border of the symphysis pubis.

Females
• Direct the central ray approximately 40 degrees (30 to 45 degrees) cephalad, and center to a point 2 inches distal to the upper border of the symphysis pubis. The entrance point may be established with sufficient accuracy from the most prominent lateral position of the greater trochanter.

Structures shown

The resulting image will show an elongated projection of the pubic and ischial rami (Figs. 7-62 and 7-63).

☐ Evaluation criteria

The following should be clearly demonstrated:
■ Pubic and ischial bones magnified with pubic bones superimposed over the sacrum and coccyx.
■ Symmetrical obturator foramina.
■ Pubic and ischial rami near the center of the radiograph.
■ Hip joints.

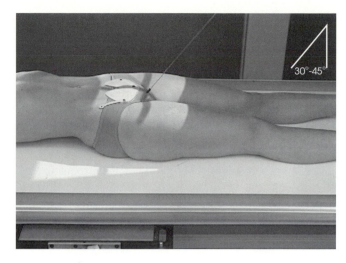

Fig. 7-61. AP axial pelvic bones: Taylor method.

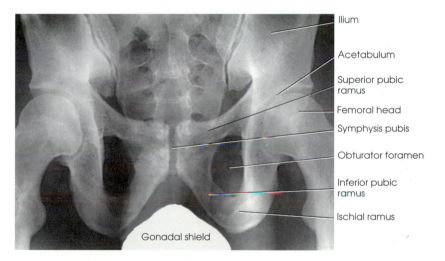

Ilium

Acetabulum

Superior pubic ramus

Femoral head

Symphysis pubis

Obturator foramen

Inferior pubic ramus

Ischial ramus

Gonadal shield

Fig. 7-62. Male AP axial pelvic bones: Taylor method.

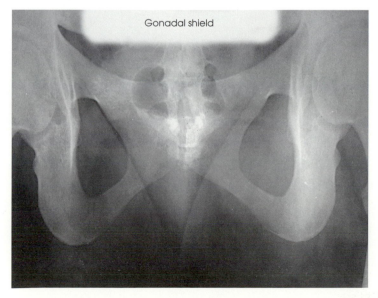

Gonadal shield

Fig. 7-63. Female AP axial pelvic bones: Taylor method.

Anterior Pelvic Bones
SUPEROINFERIOR AXIAL PROJECTION
LILIENFELD METHOD

Film: 8 × 10 in (18 × 24 cm) crosswise.

Position of patient

• Place the patient on the radiographic table in a seated-upright position.

Position of part

• Center the median sagittal plane of the body to the midline of the grid.

• To relieve strain, flex the knees slightly and support them. If the travel of the cassette tray is great enough to permit centering near the end of the table, the patient will be more comfortable seated, so that the legs can hang over and the feet can rest on a suitable support.

• Adjust the pelvis so the anterior superior iliac spines are equidistant from the table.

• Have the patient extend the arms for support, lean backward 45 or 50 degrees, and then arch the back, if possible, to place the pubic arch in a vertical position (Fig. 7-64).

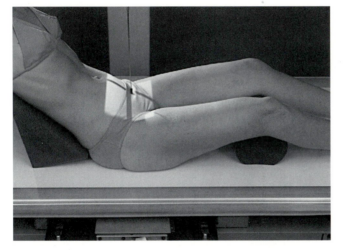

Fig. 7-64. Superoinferior axial pelvic bones: Lilienfeld method.

• With the cassette in the Bucky tray, center at the level of the greater trochanters.
• *Shield gonads.*
• Ask patient to suspend respiration for the exposure.

Central ray

• Direct the central ray perpendicular to a point 1½ inches superior to the symphysis pubis.

Structures shown

The resulting image will show a superoinferior projection of the anterior pubic and ischial bones and the symphysis pubis (Fig. 7-65).

□ Evaluation criteria

The following should be clearly demonstrated:
■ Medially superimposed superior and inferior rami of the pubic bones.
■ Nearly superimposed lateral two thirds of the pubic and ischial bones.
■ No rotation.
■ Pubic and ischial bones centered to the radiograph.
■ Hip joints.

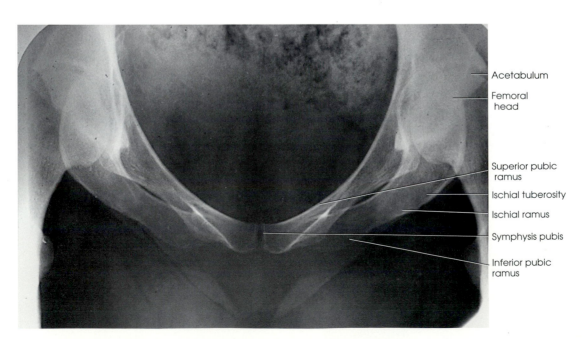

Acetabulum

Femoral head

Superior pubic ramus

Ischial tuberosity

Ischial ramus

Symphysis pubis

Inferior pubic ramus

Fig. 7-65. Superoinferior axial pelvic bones: Lilienfeld method.

Anterior Pelvic Bones

PA AXIAL PROJECTION
STAUNIG METHOD

Film: 8 × 10 in (18 × 24 cm) crosswise.

Position of patient

- Place the patient in the prone position.

Position of part

- Center the median sagittal plane of the body to the midline of the table.
- Adjust body so there is no rotation of the pelvis.
- With the cassette in the Bucky tray, adjust its position so that the midpoint of the film will coincide with the central ray (Fig. 7-66).
- *Shield gonads.*
- Ask patient to suspend respiration for the exposure.

Central ray

- Direct the central ray 35 degrees cephalad exiting the symphysis pubis, which lies in the median sagittal plane at the level of the greater trochanters.

Structures shown

The resulting image will show a projection of the pubic and ischial bones and of the symphysis pubis. The appearance of this radiograph will be nearly identical to the superoinferior axial projection discussed on the previous page.

The following should be clearly demonstrated:

- Medially superimposed superior and inferior rami of the pubic bones.
- Nearly superimposed lateral two thirds of the pubic and ischial bones.
- No rotation.
- Pubic and ischial bones centered to the radiograph.
- Hip joints.

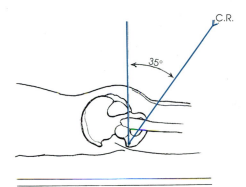

Fig. 7-66. PA axial anterior pelvic bones: Staunig method.

Anterior pelvic bones

Ilium

AP AND PA OBLIQUE PROJECTIONS

Film: 10 × 12 in (24 × 30 cm) length-wise.

RPO and LPO positions

Position of patient

- Place the patient in the supine position.

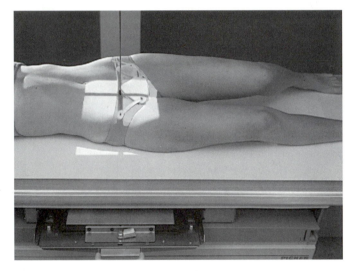

Fig. 7-67. AP oblique ilium. RPO.

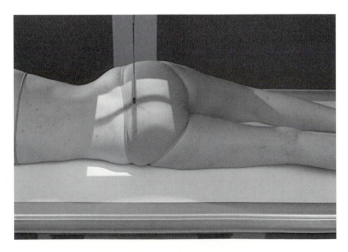

Fig. 7-68. PA oblique ilium. LAO.

Position of part

- Center the sagittal plane passing through the hip joint of the affected side to the midline of the grid.
- Elevate the *unaffected* side approximately 40 degrees to place the broad surface of the wing of the affected ilium parallel with the plane of the film.
- Support the elevated shoulder, hip, and knee on sandbags.
- Adjust the position of the uppermost limb to place the anterior superior iliac spines in the same transverse plane (Fig. 7-67).
- *Shield gonads.*
- Ask patient to suspend respiration for the exposure.

RAO and LAO positions

Position of patient

- Place the patient in the prone position.

Position of part

- Center the sagittal plane passing through the hip joint of the affected side to the midline of the grid.
- Elevate the *unaffected* side about 40 degrees to place the affected ilium perpendicular to the plane of the film.
- Have the patient rest on the forearm and flexed knee of the elevated side.
- Adjust the position of the uppermost thigh to place the anterior superior iliac spines in the same horizontal plane.
- Center the film at the level of the horizontal plane passing midway between the anterior superior iliac spines and the upper border of the greater trochanters (Fig. 7-68).
- *Shield gonads.*
- Ask patient to suspend respiration for the exposure.

Central ray

- Direct the central ray perpendicular to the midpoint of the film.

Structures shown

The AP oblique image will show an unobstructed projection of the iliac wing and sciatic notches and a profile image of the acetabulum (Fig. 7-69).

The PA oblique image shows the ilium and the proximal end of the femur (Fig. 7-70).

□Evaluation criteria

The following should be clearly demonstrated:

- Entire ilium.
- Hip joint, proximal femur, and sacroiliac joint.
  AP oblique projection
- The broad surface of the iliac wing without rotation.
  PA oblique projection
- The ilium in profile.

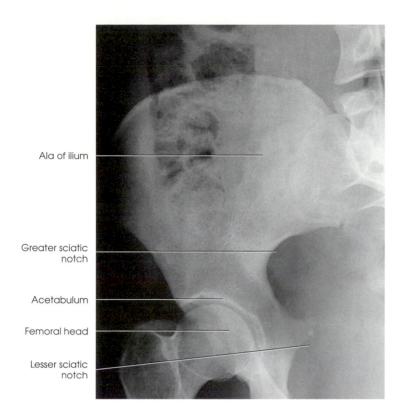

Ala of ilium

Greater sciatic
notch

Acetabulum

Femoral head

Lesser sciatic
notch

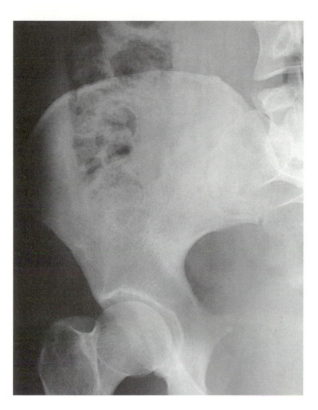

Fig. 7-69. AP oblique ilium.

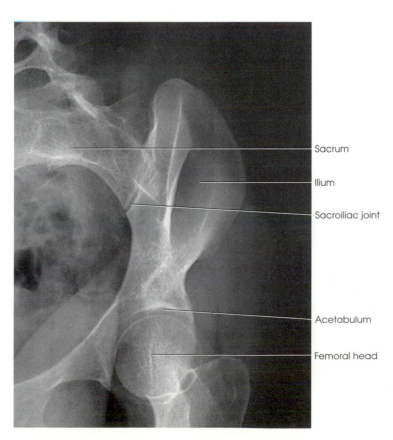

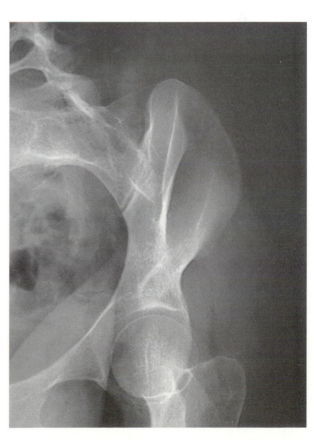

Sacrum

Ilium

Sacroiliac joint

Acetabulum

Femoral head

Fig. 7-70. PA oblique ilium.

Chapter 8

VERTEBRAL COLUMN

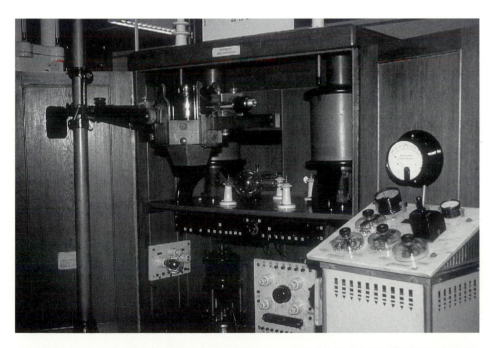

Self-contained radiographic unit from the 1920s. All x-ray generation equipment for this unit was stored inside the wooden cabinet.

Vertebral column

The vertebral column which forms the central axis of the skeleton, is centered in the median sagittal plane of the posterior part of the trunk. The vertebral column has many functions; it encloses and protects the spinal cord; acts as a support for the trunk; supports the skull superiorly; and affords attachment for the deep muscles of the back and the ribs laterally. The upper limbs are supported indirectly via the ribs which articulate with the sternum. The sternum in turn articulates with the shoulder girdle. The vertebral column articulates with each hip bone (os coxa) at the sacroiliac joints. This articulation supports the vertebral column and, through the hip joints, transmits the weight of the trunk to the lower limbs. The vertebral column is composed of small segments of bone (vertebrae) with disks of fibrocartilage interposed between the vertebrae which act as cushions. The vertebral column is held together by ligaments, jointed and curved so that it has considerable flexibility and resilience.

In early life the vertebral column normally consists of 33 small, irregular bones called *vertebrae*. The vertebrae are divided into five groups and named according to the regions they occupy (Figs. 8-1 and 8-2). The most superior seven vertebrae occupy the region of the neck and are termed *cervical* vertebrae. The succeeding twelve bones lie in the dorsal portion of the thorax and are called the *thoracic* vertebrae. The five vertebrae occupying the region of the loin, or lumbus, are termed *lumbar* vertebrae. The following five, located in the pelvic region, are termed *sacral* vertebrae. The terminal vertebrae, also in the pelvic region, vary from three to five in number and are called the *coccygeal* vertebrae.

The 24 vertebral segments in the upper three regions remain distinct throughout life and are termed the *true,* or movable vertebrae. The pelvic segments in the two lower regions are called *false,* or fixed, vertebrae because of the change they undergo in adults. The sacral segments usually fuse into one bone termed the *sacrum,* and the coccygeal segments, referred to as the *coccyx,* often fuse into one bone.

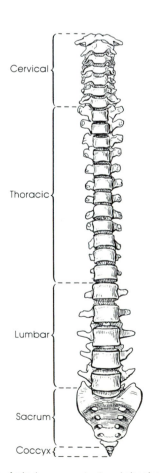

Cervical

Thoracic

Lumbar

Sacrum

Coccyx

Fig. 8-1. Anterior aspect of vertebral column.

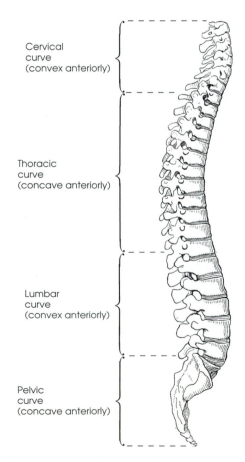

Cervical curve (convex anteriorly)

Thoracic curve (concave anteriorly)

Lumbar curve (convex anteriorly)

Pelvic curve (concave anteriorly)

Fig. 8-2. Lateral aspect of vertebral column showing regions (with vertebral curvature).

Vertebral Curvature

Viewed from the side the vertebral column presents four curves that arch anteriorly and posteriorly from the median coronal plane of the body. These curves are called cervical, thoracic, lumbar, and pelvic curves, for the regions they occupy. In this text, the vertebral curves are discussed in reference to the *anatomical position* and are referred to as convex, or concave, anteriorly. It must be realized that most physicians and surgeons prefer to evaluate the spine from the posterior aspect of the body and so the convex, concave terminology can be exact opposites. For example, when viewed from the posterior, the normal lumbar curve can also correctly be referred to as concave posteriorly. Whether the curve is described as convex anteriorly or concave posteriorly, the curvature of the patient's spine is the same. The cervical and lumbar curves, which are convex anteriorly, are called *lordotic* curves. The thoracic and pelvic curves are concave anteriorly, and are called *kyphotic* curves (Fig. 8-2). The cervical and thoracic curves merge smoothly. The lumbar and pelvic curves join at an obtuse angle termed the *lumbosacral,* or sacrovertebral, angle. The degree of angle in the lumbar and pelvic curve junction varies in different subjects. The thoracic and pelvic curves are called primary curves, because they are present at birth. The cervical and lumbar curves are called secondary, or compensatory, curves because they develop after birth. The cervical curve, which is the least pronounced of the curves, develops when the child begins to hold the head up at about 3 or 4 months of age and begins to sit alone at about 8 or 9 months of age. The lumbar curve develops when the child begins to walk at about 1 to 1½ years of age. The lumbar and pelvic curves are more pronounced in females, causing a more acute angle at the lumbosacral junction. Any abnormal increase in the anterior concavity, or posterior convexity, of the thoracic curve is termed *kyphosis,* whereas any abnormal increase in the anterior convexity, or posterior concavity, of the lumbar or cervical curve is termed *lordosis.*

Viewed from the front, the vertebral column is seen to vary in width in several regions (see Fig. 8-1). Generally the width gradually increases from the second cervical vertebra to the superior part of the sacrum, from which level it decreases sharply. There is sometimes a *slight* lateral curvature in the upper thoracic region. The increase of this curve is to the right in right-handed persons and to the left in left-handed persons; for this reason it is believed to be the result of muscle action and to be influenced by occupation. An abnormal lateral curvature of the spine is called *scoliosis.* This condition also causes the vertebrae to rotate toward the concavity. A second, or compensatory, curve in the opposite direction develops in the vertebral column to keep the head centered over the feet.

Viewed posteriorly, the spine exhibits deep depressions on both sides of the spinous processes. These bilateral depressions are called the *vertebral grooves,* and they contain the deep muscles of the back. The vertebral grooves are deeper in the thoracic region because of the sharp curve of the attached ribs.

TYPICAL VERTEBRA

A typical vertebra is composed of two main parts—an anterior mass of bone called the *body* and a posterior, ringlike portion called the *vertebral arch* (Figs. 8-3 and 8-4). The body and the vertebral arch enclose a space called the *vertebral foramen*. In the articulated column the vertebral foramina form the vertebral, or neural, canal.

The *body* of the vertebra, approximately cylindrical in shape, is composed largely of cancellous bony tissue covered by a layer of compact tissue. From the superior aspect the posterior surface is flattened, and from the lateral aspect, the anterior and lateral surfaces are concave. The superior and inferior surfaces of the bodies are flattened and covered by a plate of articular cartilage. In the articulated column the bodies are separated by cartilaginous disks. These disks consist of a central mass of soft, pulpy, semigelatinous material called the *nucleus pulposus,* surrounded by an outer fibrocartilaginous disk called the *annulus fibrosus.* It is fairly common for the nucleus pulposus to rupture or protrude into the vertebral canal causing impingement upon a spinal nerve. This condition is called *herniated nucleus pulposus* (HNP), or more commonly, "slipped disk." It most often occurs in the lumbar region resulting in considerable discomfort and pain.

The vertebral arch (see Figs. 8-3 and 8-4) is formed by two pedicles and two laminae that support four articular processes, two transverse processes, and one spinous process. The *pedicles* are short, thick processes that project posteriorly, one from each side, from the superior and lateral parts of the posterior surface of the vertebral body. The superior and inferior surfaces of the pedicles, or roots, are concave. These concavities are called *vertebral notches.* By articulation with the vertebrae above and below, the notches form *intervertebral foramina* for the transmission of the spinal nerves and blood vessels. The broad, flat *laminae* are directed posteriorly and medially from the pedicles.

The *transverse processes* project laterally and slightly posteriorly from the junction of the pedicles and laminae. The *spinous process* projects posteriorly and inferiorly from the junction of the laminae in the posterior midline.

The four articular processes (zygapophyses), two superior and two inferior, arise from the junction of the pedicles and laminae to articulate with the superjacent and subjacent vertebrae (see Fig. 8-4). In a typical vertebra, each superior articular process, *zygapophysis,* presents cartilaginous-covered articular facets on its posterior surface, whereas the inferior processes present cartilaginous-covered facets on their anterior surfaces. The planes of the facets vary in direction on the different regions and often in the same vertebra. The articulations between the articular processes of the vertebral arches are referred to as interarticular *zygapophyseal* (apophyseal) *joints,* or facet joints, to distinguish them from the articulations between the bodies of the vertebrae.

The movable vertebrae, with the exception of the first and second cervical, are similar in general structure; however, each group has certain distinguishing characteristics that must be considered in radiography of the vertebral column.

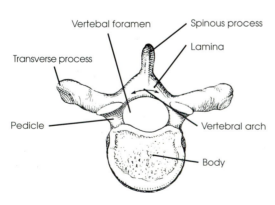

Fig. 8-3. Superior aspect of typical vertebra.

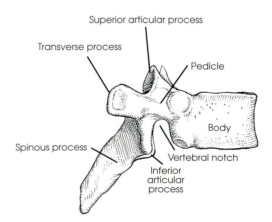

Fig. 8-4. Lateral aspect of typical vertebra.

Cervical Vertebrae

The *atlas,* the first cervical vertebra (Fig. 8-5), is a ringlike structure having no body and a very short, or vestigial, spinous process. The atlas consists of an anterior arch, a posterior arch, two lateral masses, and two transverse processes. The anterior and posterior arches extend between the lateral masses. The ring formed by the arches is divided into anterior and posterior portions by a ligament called the transverse atlantal ligament. The anterior portion of the ring receives the dens (odontoid process) of the axis, and the posterior portion transmits the proximal spinal cord.

The transverse processes are longer than those of the other cervical vertebrae, and they project laterally and slightly inferiorly from the lateral masses. Each lateral mass bears a superior and an inferior articular process. The superior processes lie in a horizontal plane, are large and deeply concave, and are shaped to receive the condyles of the occipital bone of the cranium.

The *axis,* the second cervical vertebra (Figs. 8-6 and 8-7), has a strong conical process arising from the upper surface of the body, which is called the *dens* (odontoid process). The dens (odontoid process) is received into the anterior portion of the atlantal ring to act as a pivot or body for the atlas. At each side of the dens (odontoid process) on the superior surface of the vertebral body are the superior articular processes, which are adapted to join with the inferior articular processes of the atlas. This pair of joints differs in position and direction from the other cervical zygapophyseal (apophyseal) joints. The inferior articular processes of the axis have the same direction as those of the succeeding cervical vertebrae. The laminae of the axis are broad and thick. The spinous process is horizontal in position.

The seventh cervical vertebra, which is termed the *vertebra prominens,* has a long, prominent spinous process that projects almost horizontally to the posterior. The spinous process of the vertebra prominens is easily palpable at the base of the neck posteriorly. It is convenient to use this process as a guide in localizing other vertebrae.

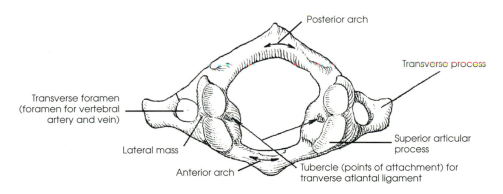

Fig. 8-5. Superior aspect of atlas.

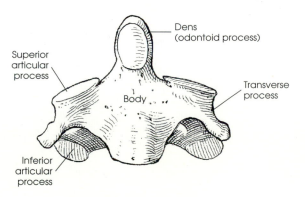

Fig. 8-6. Anterior aspect of axis.

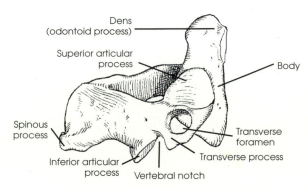

Fig. 8-7. Lateral aspect of axis.

The typical cervical vertebrae (Figs. 8-8 and 8-9) have small, transversely located oblong bodies with slightly prolonged anteroinferior borders. The result is anteroposterior overlapping of the bodies in the articulated column. The transverse processes of the cervical vertebrae arise partially from the side of the body and partially from the vertebral arch. They are short and wide, are perforated by the transverse foramina for the transmission of the vertebral artery and vein, and present a deep concavity on their upper surfaces for the passage of the spinal nerves.

The pedicles project laterally and posteriorly from the body, and their superior and inferior vertebral notches are nearly equal in depth. The laminae are narrow and thin. The spinous processes are short, have bifid tips, and are directed posteriorly and slightly inferiorly. Their palpable tips lie at the level of the interspace below the body of the vertebra from which they arise.

The *superior* and *inferior articular processes,* when covered with fibrocartilage, are called *articular facets* (Fig. 8-10). They are situated posterior to the transverse process, where, arising at the junction of the pedicle and the lamina, they form a short column of bone that is usually referred to as the *articular pillar.* The superior and inferior articulating surfaces of the pillars are directed obliquely, posteriorly, and inferiorly so that the zygapophyseal (apophyseal) joints are not radiographically demonstrated in conventional frontal plane projections. The inter-articular facet joints of the inferior six cervical vertebrae are situated at right angles to the median sagittal plane of the body so that they are clearly demonstrated in a lateral projection.

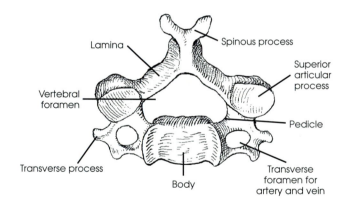

Fig. 8-8. Superior aspect of typical cervical vertebra.

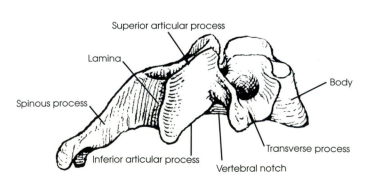

Fig. 8-9. Lateral aspect of typical cervical vertebra.

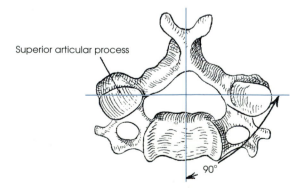

Fig. 8-10. Direction of cervical zygapophyseal (apophyseal) joints.

The *intervertebral foramina* of the cervical region (Figs. 8-11 and 8-12) are directed anteriorly at a 45-degree angle from the median sagittal plane of the body. The foramina are also directed at a 15-degree inferior angle to the horizontal plane of the body. Accurate radiographic demonstration of these foramina requires a 15-degree longitudinal angulation of the central ray as well as a 45-degree medial rotation of the patient (or a 45-degree medial angulation of the central ray). Table 8-1 summarizes the intervertebral foramina and zygapophyseal joints of the cervical spine, relating to degrees of positioning rotation needed for radiographic demonstration of each part.

Table 8-1. Spine foramina and zygapophyseal joint location relating to degree of positioning rotation needed for demonstration of the part.

	Intervertebral foramina placement	Zygapophyseal joint placement
Cervical spine	45 degree oblique AP—side up PA—side down	Lateral
Thoracic spine	Lateral	70 degrees* AP—side up PA—side down
Lumbar spine	Lateral	30 to 50 degrees* AP—side down PA—side up

*From the anatomical position.

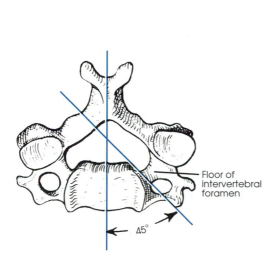

Fig. 8-11. Direction of cervical intervertebral foramina.

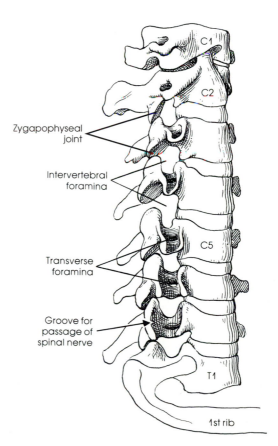

Fig. 8-12. Anterolateral oblique of cervical vertebrae showing intervertebral and transverse foramina.

Thoracic Vertebrae

The *bodies* of the thoracic segments increase in size from the first to the twelfth vertebra and vary in form from those resembling the cervical bodies in the superior part of the region to those resembling the lumbar bodies in the inferior part of the region. The bodies of the typical thoracic vertebrae (Figs. 8-13 and 8-14) from the third to the ninth are approximately triangular in form. The thoracic bodies are deeper posteriorly than anteriorly, and their posterior surface is concave from side to side. On each side of the bodies, at both the superior and inferior posterior borders, are *demifacets* that form, with the demifacet of the vertebrae above and below, the articular surfaces for the heads of the ribs. The body of the first thoracic vertebra presents a whole facet above for the first rib and a demifacet below for the second rib; the tenth, eleventh, and twelfth bodies present whole facets above and none below.

The *transverse processes* of the thoracic vertebrae project obliquely, laterally, and posteriorly. With the exception of the eleventh and twelfth pairs, each process has on the anterior surface of its extremity a small concave *facet* for articulation with the tubercle of a rib. The *laminae* are broad and thick and overlap the subjacent lamina. The spinous processes are long. From the fifth to the ninth vertebrae they project sharply inferiorly and overlap each other but are less vertical in direction above and below this region. The palpable tips of the *spinous processes* of the fifth to the ninth vertebrae correspond in position with the body of the subjacent vertebrae. The superior and inferior facets correspond in position with the interspace below the body from which they spring.

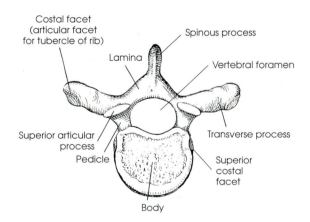

Fig. 8-13. Superior aspect of thoracic vertebra.

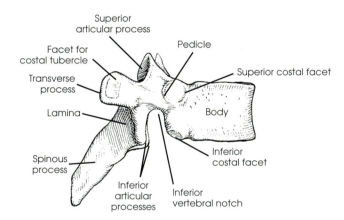

Fig. 8-14. Lateral aspect of thoracic vertebra.

The *zygapophyseal* (apophyseal) *joints* of the thoracic region (Figs. 8-15 and 8-16), except the inferior articular processes of the twelfth vertebra, angle anteriorly approximately 15 to 20 degrees to form an angle of 70 to 75 degrees, open anteriorly, to the median sagittal plane of the body. For the radiographic demonstration of the zygapophyseal (apophyseal) joints of the thoracic region, the body must be rotated 15 to 20 degrees from the lateral position. Anterior rotation is used to demonstrate the joints nearer the film, and posterior rotation is used to demonstrate those farther from the film.

The *intervertebral foramina* of the thoracic region (Figs. 8-15 and 8-17) are perpendicular to the median sagittal plane of the body. They are clearly demonstrated radiographically in a true lateral position. During inspiration the ribs are elevated. The arms must also be raised enough to elevate the ribs, which otherwise cross the intervertebral foramina. See Table 8-1 summarizing the radiographic demonstration of the intervertebral foramina and zygapophyseal joints of the thoracic spine.

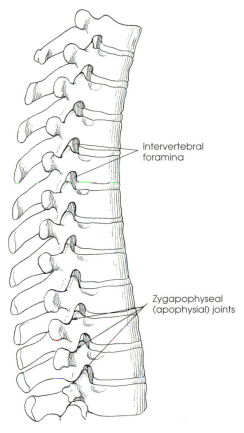

Intervertebral foramina

Zygapophyseal (apophysial) joints

Fig. 8-15. Posterolateral aspect of thoracic vertebrae showing zygapophyseal joints.

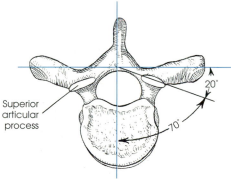

Superior articular process

20°

70°

Fig. 8-16. Direction of thoracic zygapophyseal joints.

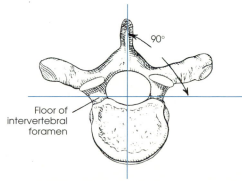

90°

Floor of intervertebral foramen

Fig. 8-17. Direction of thoracic intervertebral foramina.

Lumbar Vertebrae

The lumbar segments (Figs. 8-18 and 8-19) have large, bean-shaped bodies that increase in size from the first to the fifth vertebra. The bodies are deeper anteriorly than posteriorly, and their superior and inferior surfaces are flattened or slightly concave. The lumbar body, at its posterior surface, is flattened anteriorly to posteriorly and is transversely concave. The anterior and lateral surfaces are concave from the top to the bottom.

The *transverse processes* are smaller than those of the thoracic region. The superior three pairs are directed almost exactly laterally, whereas the inferior two pairs are inclined slightly superiorly. The *spinous processes* are large, thick, and blunt and project almost horizontally posteriorly. Their palpable tips correspond in position with the interspace below the vertebra from which they project. The *mammillary process* is a smoothly rounded projection on the back of each superior articular process. The *accessory process* is at the back of the root of the transverse process. Together with the posterior part of the root of the transverse process, these processes correspond to the transverse processes of the thoracic vertebrae.

The body of the fifth lumbar segment is considerably deeper in front than behind, which gives it a wedge shape that adapts it for articulation with the sacrum. The articular disk of this joint is also more wedge shaped than are those in the interspaces above. The spinous process of the fifth lumbar vertebra is smaller and shorter, and the transverse processes are much thicker than are those of the upper lumbar vertebrae.

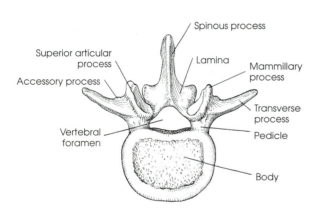

Fig. 8-18. Superior aspect of lumbar vertebra.

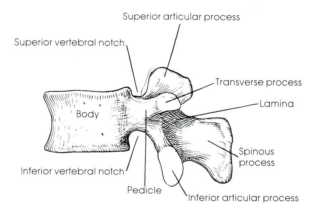

Fig. 8-19. Lateral aspect of lumbar vertebra.

The *zygapophyseal* (apophyseal) *joints* of the lumbar region (Figs. 8-20 and 8-21) are inclined posteriorly from the coronal plane, forming an angle, open posteriorly, of 30 to 50 degrees to the median sagittal plane of the body. These joints can be demonstrated radiographically by rotating the body from the supine or prone position.

The *intervertebral foramina* (Fig. 8-22) of the lumbar region are situated at right angles to the median sagittal plane of the body, except the fifth, which turns slightly anteriorly. The superior four pairs of foramina are demonstrated in a true lateral position; the last pair requires a slight obliquity of the body. See Table 8-1 summarizing the radiographic demonstration of the intervertebral foramina and zygapophyseal joints of the lumbar spine.

Spondylolysis is an acquired bony defect occurring in the *pars interarticularis* (or isthmus), the area of the lamina between the two articular processes. The defect may occur on either, or both, sides of the vertebra resulting in *spondylolisthesis*. Spondylolisthesis is the condition resulting in the anterior displacement of one vertebra over another, generally the fifth lumbar vertebra being anteriorly displaced over the sacrum. It almost exclusively involves the lumbar spine.

Spondylolisthesis is of radiological importance since oblique position radiographs demonstrate the "neck" area of the "Scotty dog," (i.e., the pars interarticularis). (See descriptions of oblique positions involving the lumbar spine, and Scotty dog illustrations, starting with Fig. 8-104, later in this chapter.)

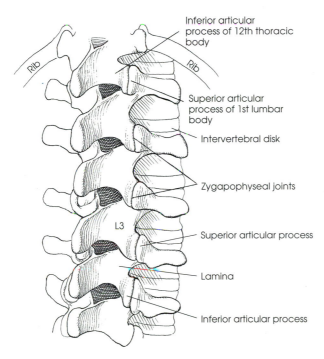

Fig. 8-20. Posterolateral oblique of lumbar vertebrae showing zygapophyseal (apophyseal) joints.

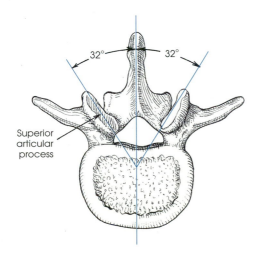

Fig. 8-21. Direction of lumbar zygapophyseal (apophyseal) joints.

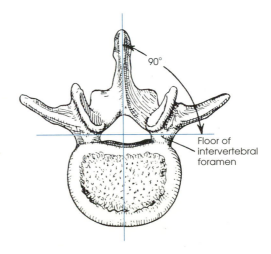

Fig. 8-22. Superior aspect showing direction of lumbar intervertebral foramina.

Sacrum and Coccyx

The *sacrum* (Figs. 8-23 to 8-25) is formed by the fusion of the five sacral segments into a curved, triangular bone. The sacrum is wedged between the iliac bones of the pelvis, its broad base directed obliquely, superiorly, and anteriorly, and its apex directed posteriorly and inferiorly. Although there is considerable variation in the size and degree of curvature of the sacrum in different subjects, the bone is normally longer, narrower, more evenly curved, and more vertical in position in male subjects than in female subjects. The female sacrum is more acutely curved on itself, the greatest curvature being in the lower half of the bone, and it lies in a more oblique plane, which results in a sharper angle at the junction of the lumbar and pelvic curves.

The superior portion of the first sacral segment (Fig. 8-25) remains distinct and resembles the vertebrae of the lumbar region. The superior surface of the base of the sacrum corresponds in size and shape to the inferior surface of the last lumbar segment, with which it articulates to form the lumbosacral (sacrovertebral) junction. The concavities on the upper surface of the pedicles of the first sacral segment, with the corresponding concavities on the lower surface of the pedicles of the last lumbar segment, form the last pair of intervertebral foramina. The superior articular processes of the first sacral segment articulate with the inferior articular processes of the last lumbar vertebra to form the last pair of zygapophyseal (apophyseal) joints.

The base of the sacrum has a prominent ridge at its upper anterior margin that is termed the *sacral promontory.* Directly behind the bodies of the sacral segments is the sacral canal, the continuation of the vertebral (spinal) canal, which is contained within the bone and transmits the sacral nerves. The anterior and posterior walls of the sacral canal are each perforated by four pairs of foramina for the passage of the sacral nerves and blood vessels.

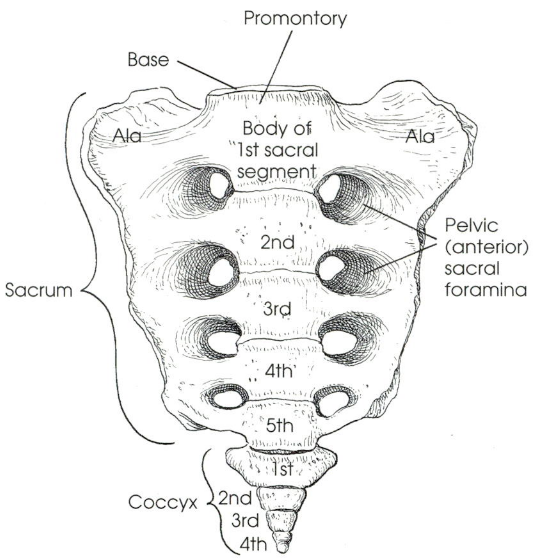

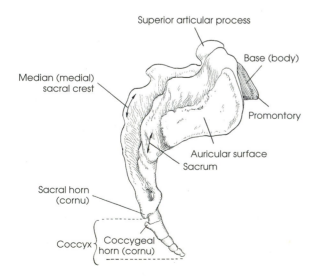

Fig. 8-23. Anterior aspect of sacrum and coccyx.

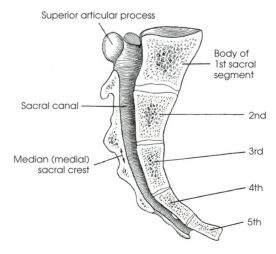

Fig. 8-24. Lateral aspect of sacrum and coccyx.

Fig. 8-25. Sagittal section of sacrum.

On each side of the sacral base is a large, winglike lateral mass, or *ala* (Fig. 8-26). At the superoanterior part of the lateral surface of each ala is a large articular process, the auricular surface, for articulation with similarly shaped processes on the iliac bones of the pelvis.

The inferior surface of the apex of the sacrum (Fig. 8-27) has an oval facet for articulation with the coccyx and two processes, the sacral horns (cornua), which project inferiorly from the posterolateral aspect of the last sacral segment to join the horns (cornua) of the coccyx.

The *coccyx* is composed of three to five (usually four) rudimentary vertebrae (see Figs. 8-23 and 8-24) that have a tendency to fuse into one bone in the adult. The coccyx diminishes in size from its base inferiorly to its apex. From its articulation with the sacrum it curves inferiorly and anteriorly, often deviating from the midline of the body. Two processes, the coccygeal horns (cornua), project superiorly from the posterolateral aspect of the first coccygeal segment to join the sacral horns (cornua).

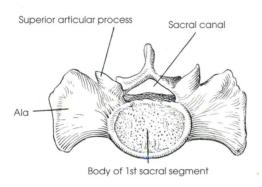

Superior articular process

Sacral canal

Ala

Body of 1st sacral segment

Fig. 8-26. Base of sacrum.

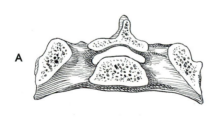

A

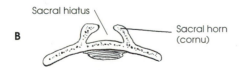

Sacral hiatus

B

Sacral horn (cornu)

Fig. 8-27. Transverse sections of sacrum. **A,** Through superior sacral portion. **B,** Through inferior sacral portion.

Vertebral Articulations

The vertebral articulations consist of two types of joints: (1) cartilaginous (amphiarthrotic) joints, which are between the two vertebral bodies and permit only slight movement to individual vertebrae but considerable motility for the column as a whole, and (2) synovial (diarthrotic) joints, which are between the articulation processes of the vertebral arches and are plane joints which permit gliding movements. The movements permitted in the vertebral column by the combined action of the joints are flexion, extension, lateral flexion, and rotation.

The articulations between the *atlas* and the occipital bone are synovial (diarthrotic) plane (gliding) joints and are called the atlanto-occipital (occipitocervical) articulations. The anterior arch of the atlas rotates about the dens of the axis to form the atlantoaxial joint, which is a synovial (diarthrotic) trochoidal, or pivot-type, articulation.

In the *thoracic region,* the heads of the ribs articulate with the bodies of the vertebrae to form the *costovertebral* joints, which are synovial (diarthrotic) plane or gliding articulations. The tubercles of the ribs and the transverse processes of the thoracic vertebrae articulate to form *costotransverse* joints, which are also synovial (diarthrotic) plane, or gliding, articulations.

The articulations between the sacrum and the two ilia, the *sacroiliac* joints, slant obliquely, posteriorly, and medially at an angle of 25 to 30 degrees and open anteriorly to the median sagittal plane of the body. Although these joints are synovial by classification, they permit very little movement and function like cartilaginous joints.

Radiation Protection

Protection of the patient from unnecessary radiation is a professional responsibility of the radiographer. (See Chapter 1 for specific guidelines.) In this chapter, the *"Shield gonads"* statement at the end of the "Position of part" section indicates the patient is to be protected from unnecessary radiation by restricting the radiation beam using proper collimation. Additionally, placing lead shielding between the gonads and the radiation source is appropriate when the clinical objectives of the examination are not compromised.

Contact gonad shields can be used for male patients when performing any procedure in this chapter. Female gonad shields can only be used when the ovaries do not lie within the area of interest.

Atlanto-occipital Articulations

AP OBLIQUE PROJECTION
R and L head rotations

Film: 8 × 10 in (18 × 24 cm).

Position of patient

- Place the patient in the supine position.
- Center the median sagittal plane of the body to the midline of the grid, and adjust the shoulders to lie in the same horizontal plane.

Position of part

- Place the cassette in the Bucky tray and adjust the patient's head so the midpoint of the cassette is 1 inch lateral to the median sagittal plane of the head at the level of the external acoustic meatus (Fig. 8-28).
- Rotate the head 45 to 60 degrees *away* from the side being examined.
- Adjust the flexion of the neck to place the infraorbitomeatal line perpendicular to the film.
- *Shield gonads.*
- Ask the patient to suspend respiration for the exposure.

Central ray

- Direct the central ray perpendicular to the midpoint of the film. It enters 1 inch anteriorly to the external acoustic (auditory) meatus and emerges at the atlanto-occipital articulation.

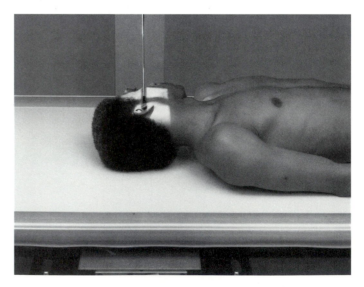

Fig. 8-28. AP oblique atlanto-occipital joint.

Structures shown

The resulting image will show a slightly oblique AP projection of the atlanto-occipital articulation with the joint being projected between the orbit and the vertical ramus of the mandible. Examine both sides for comparison (Fig. 8-29).

The dens (odontoid process) of the axis is also well demonstrated in this position; therefore, it can be used for this purpose when a patient cannot be adjusted in the open-mouth position.

[1]Buetti, C: Zur Darstellung der Atlanto-epistropheal-Gelenke bzw. der Procc. transversi atlantis und epistrophei, Radiol Clin North Am 20:168-172, 1951.

□ Evaluation criteria

The following should be clearly demonstrated:
- Open atlanto-occipital articulation.
- Dens (odontoid process).

NOTE: Buetti[1] recommends a position for the atlanto-occipital articulations wherein the head is turned 45 to 50 degrees to one side, and with the mouth wide open the chin is drawn down as much as the open mouth will allow. The central ray is then directed vertically through the open mouth to the dependent mastoid tip.

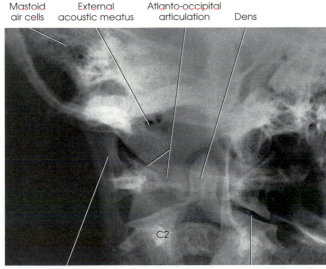

Mastoid air cells   External acoustic meatus   Atlanto-occipital articulation   Dens

C2

Ramus of mandible

C1-C2 articulation

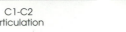

Fig. 8-29. AP oblique atlanto-occipital joint.

Atlanto-occipital Articulations
PA PROJECTION

Film: 8 × 10 in (18 × 24 cm) crosswise.

Position of patient

- Place the patient in the prone position.
- Center the median sagittal plane of the body to the midline of the grid.
- If the patient is thin, place a small, firm pillow under the chest to relieve strain in holding the position.
- Flex the patient's elbows, place the arms in a comfortable position, and adjust the shoulders to lie in the same horizontal plane.

Position of part

- Rest the patient's forehead and nose on the table and adjust it so that the median sagittal plane is perpendicular to the midline of the grid (Fig. 8-30).
- Adjust the flexion of the neck to place the orbitomeatal line perpendicular to the plane of the film; center the film at or slightly below the level of the infraorbital margins.
- *Shield gonads.*
- Ask the patient to suspend respiration for the exposure.

Central ray

- Direct the central ray perpendicular to the midpoint of the film. It enters the back of the neck at the level of the infraorbital margins.

Structures shown

The resulting image will show a PA projection of the atlanto-occipital (occipitoatlantal) joints projected through the maxillary sinuses (Fig. 8-31).

□ **Evaluation criteria**

The following should be clearly demonstrated:

- Open bilateral atlanto-occipital (occipitoatlantal) articulations.
- Mandibular condyles equidistant from the midline.

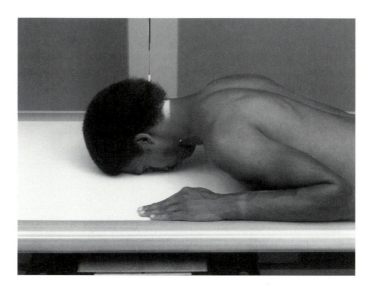

Fig. 8-30. PA atlanto-occipital articulations.

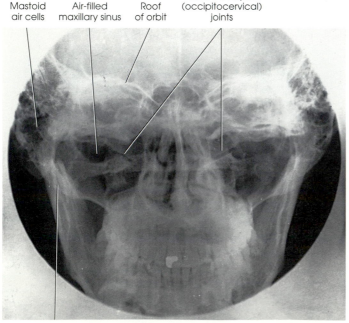
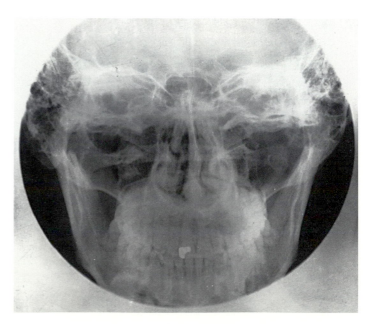

Mastoid air cells   Air-filled maxillary sinus   Roof of orbit   Atlanto-occipital (occipitocervical) joints

Mandibular ramus

Fig. 8-31. PA atlanto-occipital articulations.

Atlas and Axis

 ### AP PROJECTION
Open mouth

The open-mouth technique was described by Albers-Schönberg[1] in 1910 and by George[2] in 1919.

Film: 8 × 10 in (18 × 24 cm).

Position of patient

- Place the patient in the supine position.
- Center the median sagittal plane of the body to the midline of the grid.
- Place the patient's arms along the sides of the body and adjust the shoulders to lie in the same horizontal plane.

Position of part

- Place the cassette in the Bucky tray and center it at the level of the second cervical vertebra.
- Adjust the patient's head so that the median sagittal plane is perpendicular to the plane of the table (Figs. 8-32 and 8-33).
- Select the exposure factors, and move the x-ray tube into position so that any minor change can be made quickly after the final adjustment of the patient's head. This position is not easy to hold; however, the patient is usually able to cooperate fully, unless he or she is kept in the final, strained position too long.
- Have the patient open the mouth as wide as possible, and then adjust the head so that a line from the lower edge

[1]Albers-Schönberg, HE: Die Röntgentechnik, ed 3, Hamburg, 1910, Gräfe & Sillem.
[2]George, AW: Method for more accurate study of injuries to the atlas and axis, Boston Med Surg J 181:395-398, 1919.

of the upper incisors to the tip of the mastoid process is perpendicular to the film.
- *Shield gonads.*
- Respiration: Instruct the patient to keep the mouth wide open and to softly phonate "ah" during the exposure. This will affix the tongue in the floor of the mouth so that its shadow will not be projected on that of the atlas and axis and will prevent movement of the mandible.

Central ray

- Direct the central ray perpendicular to the midpoint of the open mouth.

Structures shown

The resulting image will show an AP projection of the atlas and axis through the open mouth (Fig. 8-34).

If the patient has a deep head or a long mandible, the entire atlas will not be demonstrated. When the exactly superimposed shadows of the occlusal surface of the upper central incisors and the base of the skull are in line with those of the tips of the mastoid processes, the position cannot be improved.

☐ Evaluation criteria

The following should be clearly demonstrated:
- Dens, atlas, axis, and articulations between C1 and C2.
- Superimposed occlusal surface of the upper central incisors and the base of the skull.
- Wide open mouth.
- The shadow of the tongue not projected over the atlas and axis.
- Mandibular rami equidistant from dens.

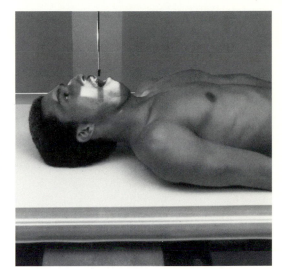

Fig. 8-32. AP atlas and axis.

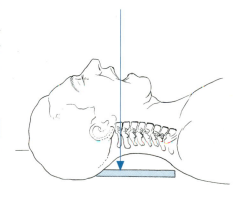

Fig. 8-33. Open-mouth spine alignment.

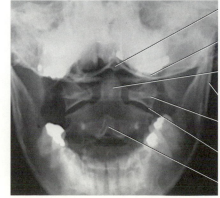

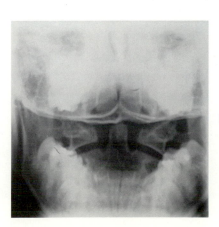

Occipital base

Occlusal surface of teeth

Dens (odontoid process)

Mandibular ramus

Lateral mass of atlas

Inferior articular process of atlas

Spinous process of axis

A

B

Fig. 8-34. A and **B,** Open-mouth atlas and axis.

(**A,** courtesy Patti Chapman, R.T.; **B,** courtesy Martha Montalvo, R.T.)

Dens

 ### AP PROJECTION
FUCHS METHOD

Fuchs[1] has recommended this projection for the demonstration of the dens (odontoid process) when its upper half is not clearly shown in the open-mouth position. This patient position must not be attempted if there is a suspected fracture or degenerative disease of the upper cervical region.

Film: 8 × 10 in (18 × 24 cm) crosswise.

[1]Fuch AW: Cervical vertebrae (part 1), Radiogr Clin Photogr 16:2-17, 1940.

Position of patient

- Place the patient in the supine position.
- Center the median sagittal plane of the body to the midline of the grid.
- Place the arms along the sides of the body, and adjust the shoulders to lie in the same horizontal plane.

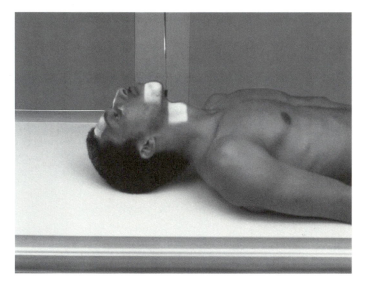

Fig. 8-35. AP dens: Fuchs method.

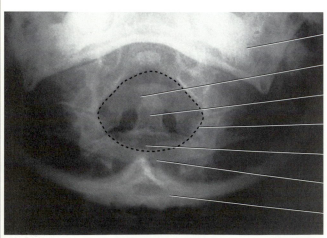

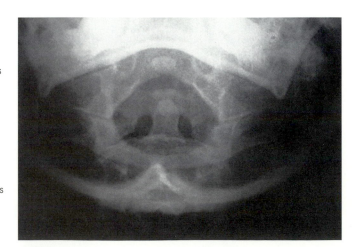

Mandible

Anterior arch of atlas

Dens

Foramen magnum

Body of axis

Posterior arch of atlas

Occipital bone

Fig. 8-36. AP dens: Fuchs method.

Vertebral column

Position of part

- Place the cassette in the Bucky tray and center it to the level of the tips of the mastoid processes.
- Extend the chin until the tip of the chin and the tip of the mastoid process are vertical (Fig. 8-35).
- Adjust the head so that the median sagittal plane is perpendicular to the plane of the grid.
- *Shield gonads.*
- Ask the patient to suspend respiration for the exposure.

Central ray

- Direct the central ray perpendicular to the midpoint of the film; it enters the neck just distal to the tip of the chin.

Structures shown

The resulting image will show an AP projection of the dens (odontoid process) lying within the shadow of the foramen magnum (Figs. 8-36 and 8-37).

□Evaluation criteria

The following should be clearly demonstrated:
- Entire dens (odontoid process) within the foramen magnum.
- No rotation of the head or neck.

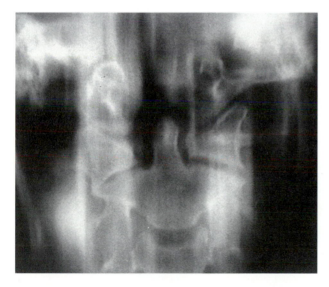

Fig. 8-37. Linear tomogram of superior cervical vertebrae.

Atlas and Dens
PA PROJECTION
JUDD METHOD

The radiographer must not attempt this position with a patient who has an unhealed fracture or with a patient who has a degenerative disease or suspected fracture of the upper cervical region.

Film: 8 × 10 in (18 × 24 cm) crosswise.

Position of patient

- Place the patient in the prone position.
- Center the median sagittal plane of the body to the midline of the grid.
- Flex the patient's elbows, place the arms in a comfortable position, and adjust the shoulders to lie in the same horizontal plane.

Position of part

- Have the patient extend the neck and rest the chin on the table.
- Place the cassette in the Bucky tray and adjust it so that the midpoint is centered to the throat at the level of the upper margin of the thyroid cartilage (Fig. 8-38).
- Adjust the head so that the tip of the nose is about 1 inch from the tabletop, that is, the orbitomeatal line is approximately 37 degrees to the plane of the film (Fig. 8-39).
- Adjust the median sagittal plane to be perpendicular to the table.
- *Shield gonads.*
- Ask the patient to suspend respiration for the exposure.

Central ray

- Direct the central ray perpendicular to the midpoint of the film. It enters the occiput just posterior to the level of the mastoid tips.

Structures shown

The resulting image will show a PA projection of the dens (odontoid process) and atlas, as seen through the foramen magnum (Fig. 8-40).

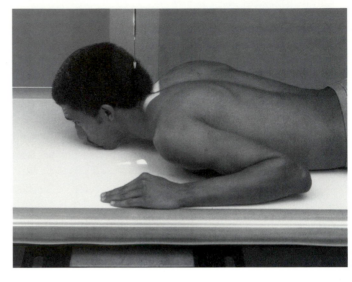

Fig. 8-38. PA atlas and dens: Judd method.

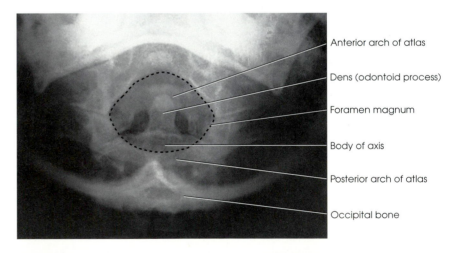

Anterior arch of atlas

Dens (odontoid process)

Foramen magnum

Body of axis

Posterior arch of atlas

Occipital bone

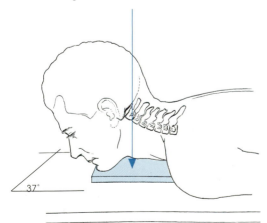

Fig. 8-39. PA dens.

☐ **Evaluation criteria**

The following should be clearly demonstrated:
- Entire dens within foramen magnum.
- Anterior and posterior arches of atlas.
- No rotation of the head or neck.

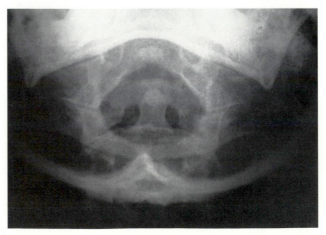

Fig. 8-40. PA atlas and dens: Judd method.

Dens

AP AXIAL OBLIQUE PROJECTION
R or L head rotation
KASABACH METHOD

NOTE: The head of a patient who has a possible fracture or degenerative disease must *not* be rotated. Kasabach[1] has recommended that the entire body, rather than only the head, be rotated.

Film: 8×10 in (18×24 cm).

Position of patient

- Place the patient in the supine position.
- Center the median sagittal plane of the body to the midline of the grid.
- Place the arms along the sides of the body, and adjust the shoulders to lie in the same horizontal plane.

Position of part

- Place the cassette in the Bucky tray, and center it to the median sagittal plane at the level of the mastoid tip.
- Rotate the head either right or left approximately 40 to 45 degrees. Adjust the head so that the infraorbitomeatal line is perpendicular to the plane of the table (Fig. 8-41).
- For right-angle images of the dens make one exposure with the head turned to the right and one with the head turned to the left.
- *Shield gonads.*
- Ask the patient to suspend respiration for the exposure.

Central ray

- Angle the central ray 10 to 15 degrees caudad.
- Center to a point midway between the outer canthus and the external acoustic meatus.

Structures shown

The resulting image will show an axial oblique of the dens (odontoid process) and is recommended by Kasabach[1] for use in conjunction with the AP and lateral projections (Fig. 8-42).

☐ Evaluation criteria

- The radiograph should clearly demonstrate the dens.

[1]Kasabach HH: A roentgenographic method for the study of the second cervical vertebra, AJR 42:782-785, 1939.

NOTE: Herrmann and Stender[2] have described a position for the demonstration of the atlanto-occipital-dens relationship, wherein the head is adjusted as for the Kasabach method. The central ray is then directed vertically midway between the mastoid processes at the level of the atlanto-occipital joints.

[2]Herrmann, E, and Stender, H: Ein einfache Aufnahmetechnik zur Darstellung der Dens axis, Fortschr Roentgenstr 96:115-119, 1962.

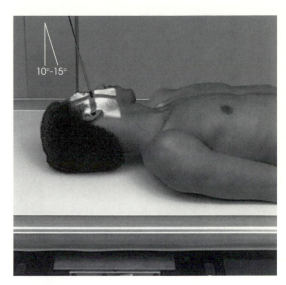

Fig. 8-41. AP axial oblique dens: Kasabach method.

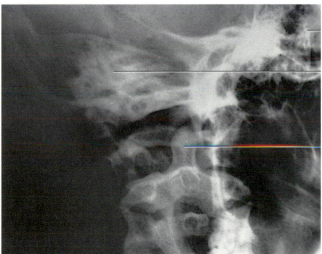

Mastoid air cells (side down)

Mastoid air cells (side up)

Dens

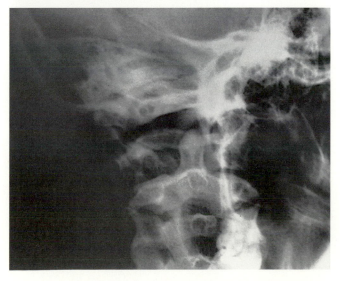

Fig. 8-42. AP axial oblique dens: Kasabach method.

Dens

Atlas and Axis
LATERAL PROJECTION
R or L position

Film: 8 × 10 in (18 × 24 cm).

Position of patient

- Place the patient in the supine position.
- Place the arms along the sides of the body, and adjust the shoulders to lie in the same horizontal plane.
- Place a sponge or pad under the patient's head unless there is traumatic injury in which the neck should not be moved.

Position of part

- With the cassette in the vertical position and in contact with the upper neck, center at the level of the atlantoaxial articulation (1 inch distal to the tip of the mastoid process).
- Adjust the cassette so that it is parallel with the median sagittal plane of the neck and then support it in position (Fig. 8-43).
- Extend the neck slightly so that the shadow of the mandibular rami will not overlap that of the spine.
- Adjust the head so that the median sagittal plane is perpendicular to the table.
- *Shield gonads.*
- Ask the patient to suspend respiration for the exposure.

Central ray

- Direct the central ray perpendicular to a point 1 inch distal to the adjacent mastoid tip. A grid and close collimation should be used to minimize secondary radiation.

Structures shown

The resulting image will show a lateral projection of the atlas and axis. The atlanto-occipital articulations are also demonstrated (Fig. 8-44). Because of the short OID, better definition is obtained with this technique than with the customary method of performing the lateral examination of the cervical vertebrae.

□ Evaluation criteria

The following should be clearly demonstrated:
- The upper cervical vertebrae.
- The neck extended so the rami of the mandible will not overlap C1 or C2.
- Nearly superimposed rami of the mandible.

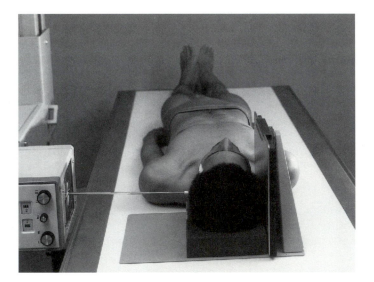

Fig. 8-43. Lateral atlas and axis.

NOTE: Pancoast, Pendergrass, and Schaeffer[1] recommend that the head be rotated slightly to prevent superimposition of the laminae of the atlas. They further recommend a slight horizontal tilt of the head for the demonstration of the arches of the atlas.

Smith and Abel[2] describe a method for the demonstration of the laminae and articular facets of the upper cervical vertebrae. They slightly extend the patient's neck, and the mouth is opened wide. The central ray is directed 35 degrees caudad and centered to the third cervical vertebra. The exposure is made with the head passively rotated 10 degrees to the side, thus removing the mandible from the overlying areas of interest.

[1]Pancoast HK, Pendergrass EP, and Schaeffer JP: The head and neck in roentgen diagnosis, Springfield, Ill, 1940, Charles C Thomas, Publisher.

[2]Smith G, and Abel M: Visualization of the posterolateral elements of the upper cervical vertebrae in the anteroposterior projection, Radiology 115:219-220, 1975.

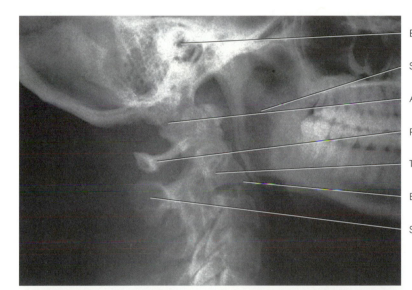

External acoustic meatus

Superimposed mandibular rami

Atlanto-occipital articulation

Posterior arch, atlas

Transverse process, axis

Body of axis

Spinous process, axis

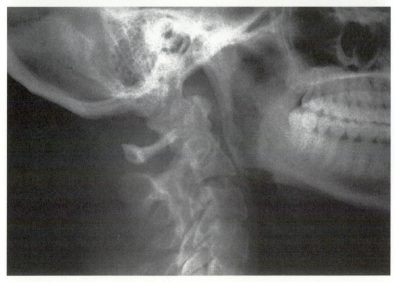

Fig. 8-44. Lateral atlas and axis.

Cervical Vertebrae

 AP AXIAL PROJECTION

Film: 8 × 10 in (18 × 24 cm) lengthwise.

Position of patient

- Place patient in the supine or upright position with the back against the film holder.
- Adjust the shoulders to lie in the same horizontal plane to prevent rotation.

Position of part

- Center the median sagittal plane of the patient's body to the midline of the table or vertical grid device.
- Extend the chin enough so that a line from the upper occlusal plane to the mastoid tips is perpendicular to the tabletop. This will prevent superimposition of the mandible and midcervical vertabrae (Figs. 8-45 and 8-46).
- Center the cassette at the level of the fourth cervical vertebra.
- *Shield gonads.*
- Ask the patient to suspend respiration for the exposure.

Central ray

- To compensate for the lordotic curve of the cervical spine, direct the central ray through the fourth cervical body at an angle of 15 to 20 degrees cephalad. It enters at or slightly inferior to the most prominent point of the thyroid cartilage.

Structures shown

The resulting image will show the lower five cervical bodies and the upper two or three thoracic bodies, the interpediculate spaces, the superimposed transverse and articular processes, and the intervertebral disk spaces (Fig. 8-47).

This projection is also used to demonstrate the presence or absence of cervical ribs.

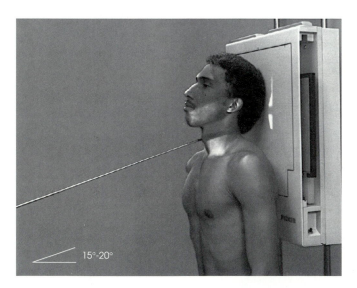

Fig. 8-45. AP axial cervical vertebrae, upright.

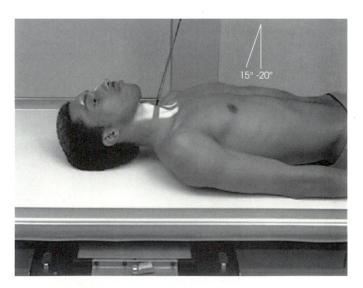

Fig. 8-46. AP axial cervical vertebrae, recumbent.

□ Evaluation criteria

The following should be clearly demonstrated:

- Area from C3 to T2.
- Shadows of the mandible and occiput superimposed over C1 and most of C2.
- Open intervertebral disk spaces.
- Spinous processes equidistant to the pedicles.
- Mandibular angles equidistant to the vertebrae.

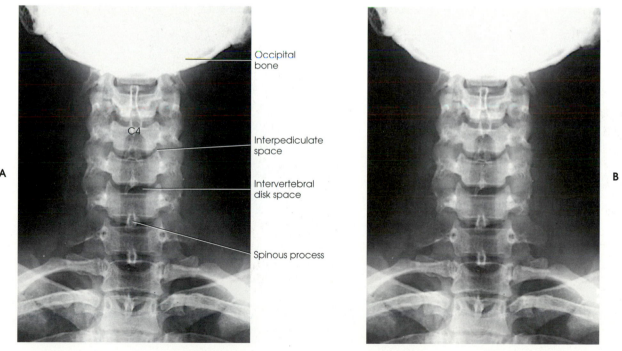

Occipital bone

Interpediculate space

Intervertebral disk space

Spinous process

C4

A

B

Fig. 8-47. A and **B,** AP axial cervical vertebrae.

Cervical Vertebrae

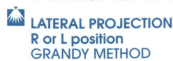

LATERAL PROJECTION
R or L position
GRANDY METHOD

Film: 8 × 10 in (18 × 24 cm) lengthwise.

Position of patient

- Place the patient in a lateral position, either seated or standing, before a vertical grid device.
- Have the patient sit or stand straight, and adjust the height of the cassette so that it is centered at the level of the fourth cervical vertebra.

---

[1]Grandy CC: A new method for making radiographs of the cervical vertebrae in the lateral position, Radiology 4:128-129, 1925.

Position of part

- Center the coronal plane that passes through the mastoid tips to the midline of the film.
- Move the patient close enough to the cassette to permit the adjacent shoulder to rest against the casette for support (Fig. 8-48).
- Rotate the shoulders anteriorly or posteriorly, according to the natural kyphosis of the back: if the subject is round shouldered, rotate them anteriorly; otherwise, rotate them posteriorly.
- Adjust the shoulders to lie in the same horizontal plane, depress them as much as possible, and immobilize them by attaching one small sandbag to each wrist. The sandbags should be of equal weight.
- Another strategy sometimes used is placing a long strip of gauze bandage under the patient's feet, or, if the patient is seated, under the rungs of the stool. Have him or her grasp one end of the gauze in each hand and pull. This will allow the shoulders to be depressed, according to the needs of the patient.

- Care must be taken to ensure that the patient does not elevate the shoulder.
- Adjust the body in a true lateral position, with the long axis of the cervical vertebrae parallel with the plane of the film.
- Elevate the chin slightly and/or have the patient protrude the mandible to prevent superimposition of the mandibular rami and the spine. At the same time, with the median sagittal plane of the head vertical, ask the patient to look steadily at one spot on the wall to aid in maintaining the position of the head. The fraction of a second needed for the exposure time of this image makes elaborate immobilization measures unnecessary in a majority of cases.
- *Shield gonads.*
- Ask the patient to suspend respiration at the end of full exhalation to obtain maximum depression of the shoulders.

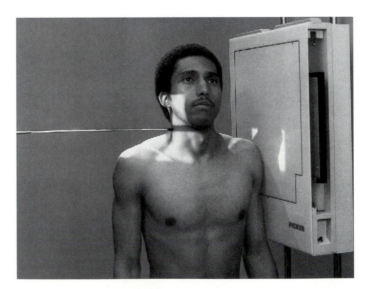

Fig. 8-48. Lateral cervical vertebrae: Grandy method.

Central ray

- Direct the central ray horizontal to the fourth cervical vertebra. With such centering, the magnified shadow of the shoulder *farthest from the film* will be projected below the lower cervical vertebrae.
- Because of the great OID, use an SID of 60 to 72 inches to obtain optimum recorded detail.

Structures shown

The resulting image will show a lateral projection of the cervical bodies and their interspaces, the articular pillars, the lower five zygapophyseal joints, and the spinous processes (Fig. 8-49). Depending on how well the shoulders can be depressed, the seventh cervical vertebra and sometimes the upper one or two thoracic vertebrae also can be seen.

□ Evaluation criteria

The following should be clearly demonstrated:

- All seven cervical vertebrae or else a separate radiograph of the cervicothoracic region is recommended.
- Neck extended so that the rami of the mandible is not overlapping C1 or C2.
- Superimposed, or nearly superimposed, rami of the mandible.
- Fourth cervical vertebrae in the center of the radiograph.
- Bone detail and soft tissues.

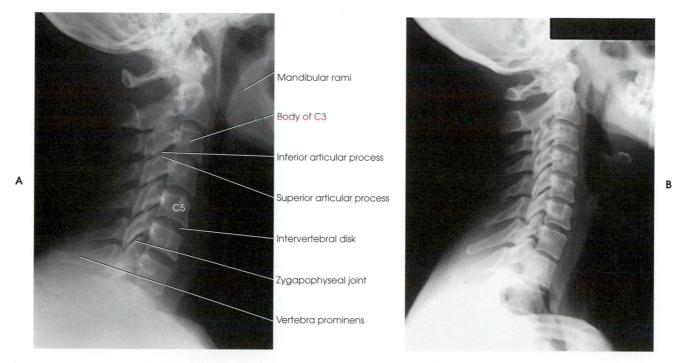

A

Mandibular rami

Body of C3

Inferior articular process

Superior articular process

Intervertebral disk

Zygapophyseal joint

Vertebra prominens

C5

B

Fig. 8-49. A and **B,** Lateral cervical vertebrae: Grandy method.

(**A,** courtesy Karen Cubler, R.T.; **B,** courtesy Annette Wendt, R.T.)

Cervical Vertebrae

**LATERAL PROJECTION
R or L position
Hyperflexion and
hyperextension**

NOTE: This procedure must not be attempted until cervical spine pathology or fracture has been ruled out.

Functional studies of the cervical vertebrae in the lateral position are made for the purpose of demonstrating normal anteroposterior movement or, as a result of trauma or disease, an absence of movement. The spinous processes are elevated and widely separated in the hyperflexion position and are depressed in close approximation in the hyperextension position.

Film: 8 × 10 in (18 × 24 cm) lengthwise.

Position of patient

- Place the patient in a lateral position, either seated or standing, before a vertical grid device.
- Have the patient sit or stand straight, and adjust the height of the cassette so that it is centered at the level of the fourth cervical vertebra.

Position of part

- Move the patient close enough to the Bucky to permit the adjacent shoulder to rest against it for support.
- While keeping the median sagittal plane of the patient's head and neck parallel with the plane of the film:

Hyperflexion.
- Ask the patient to drop the head forward and then to draw the chin as close as possible to the chest to place the cervical vertebrae in a position of *hyperflexion* (forced flexion) for the first exposure (Fig. 8-50).

Hyperextension.
- Ask the patient to elevate the chin as much as possible to place the cervical vertebrae in a position of *hyperextension* (forced extension) for the second exposure (Fig. 8-51).
- *Shield gonads.*
- Ask the patient to suspend respiration for the exposure.

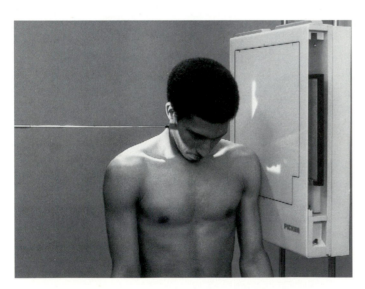

Fig. 8-50. Lateral cervical vertebrae. Hyperflexion.

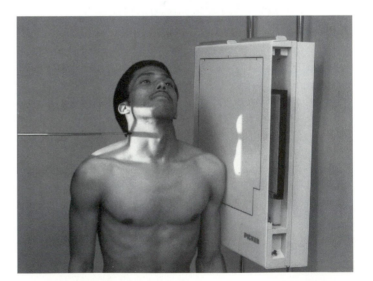

Fig. 8-51. Lateral cervical vertebrae. Hyperextension.

Central ray

- Direct the perpendicular central ray to the fourth cervical vertebra. Because of increased OID, an SID of 60 to 72 inches is recommended.

Structure shown

The resulting image will show the motility of the cervical spine when hyperflexed (Fig. 8-52) and hyperextended (Fig. 8-53). The intervertebral disks and the zygapophyseal joints are also shown.

□ Evaluation criteria

The following should be clearly demonstrated:

Hyperflexion.

- The body of the mandible almost perpendicular to the lower border of the film for hyperflexion on the normal patient.
- All seven spinous processes.

Hyperextension.

- The body of the mandible almost parallel to the lower border of the film for the normal patient.
- All seven cervical vertebrae.

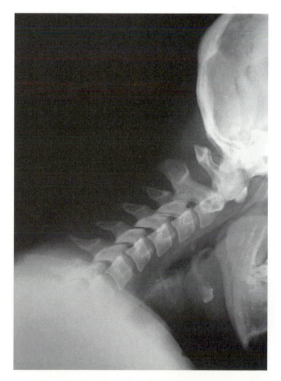

Fig. 8-52. Hyperflexion lateral cervical spine.

(Courtesy Michael Franklin, R.T.)

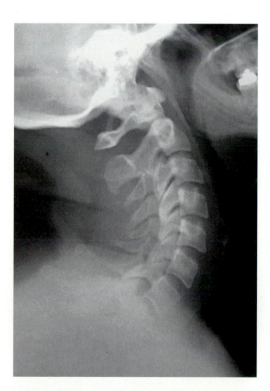

Fig. 8-53. Hyperextension lateral cervical spine.

(Courtesy Michael Franklin, R.T.)

Cervical Intervertebral Foramina

AP AXIAL OBLIQUE PROJECTION
RPO and LPO positions

Oblique projections for the demonstration of the cervical intervertebral foramina were first described by Barsóny and Koppenstein.[1,2] Both sides are examined for comparison.

Film: 8 × 10 in (18 × 24 cm) lengthwise.

---

[1]Barsóny T, and Koppenstein E: Eine neue Method zur Röntgenuntersuchung der Halswirbelsäule, Fortschr Roentgenstr 35:593-594, 1926.
[2]Barsóny T, and Koppenstein E: Beitrag zur Aufnahmetechnik der Halswirbelsäule; Darstellung der Foramina intervertebralia, Röntgenpraxis 1:245-249, 1929.

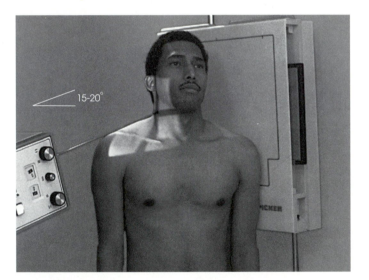

Fig. 8-54. Upright AP axial oblique right intervertebral foramina: LPO.

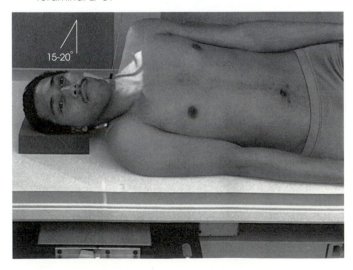

Fig. 8-55. Recumbent AP axial oblique left intervertebral foramina: RPO.

Position of patient

- Place patient supine or upright facing the x-ray tube. The upright position, standing or seated, is preferable for the patient's comfort and for greater ease of positioning.

Position of part

- Adjust the body (including the head) at a 45-degree angle and center the cervical spine to the midline of the cassette.
- To compensate for the cephalic angulation of the central ray, center the cassette to the third cervical body (1 inch superior to the most prominent point of the thyroid cartilage). The foramina *farthest* from the cassette are demonstrated.

Upright position

- Ask the patient to sit or stand straight without strain and to rest the adjacent shoulder firmly against the vertical film holder for support.
- Ensure that the degree of body rotation is 45 degrees.
- While the patient looks straight ahead, elevate and, if needed, protrude the chin so the mandible will not overlap the spine (Fig. 8-54). Turning the chin to the side causes slight rotation of the superior vertebrae and should be avoided.

Semisupine position

- Rotate the patient's head and body approximately 45 degrees.
- Center the cervical spine to the midline of the grid.
- Place suitable supports under the lower thorax and the elevated hip.
- Place a support under the head, and adjust it so the cervical column is horizontal.
- Check and adjust the 45-degree body rotation.
- Elevate the patient's chin and protrude the jaw as for the upright study (Fig. 8-55). Turning the chin to the side causes slight rotation of the superior vertebrae and should be avoided.
- *Shield gonads*.
- For either approach, ask the patient to suspend respiration for the exposure.

Central ray

- Direct the central ray to the fourth cervical vertebra at a cephalic angle of 15 to 20 degrees so that the central ray coincides with the angle of the foramina.
- Due to the increased object-image receptor distance, an SID of 60 to 72 inches is recommended.

Structures shown

The resulting image will show the intervertebral foramina and pedicles *farthest* from the film and an oblique projection of the bodies and other parts of the cervical vertebrae (Fig. 8-56).

□Evaluation criteria

The following should be clearly demonstrated:

- "Open" intervertebral foramina *farthest* from the film.
- "Open" intervertebral disk spaces.
- Elevated chin so that it does not overlap C1 and C2.
- Occipital bone not overlapping C1.
- All seven cervical and the first thoracic vertebrae.

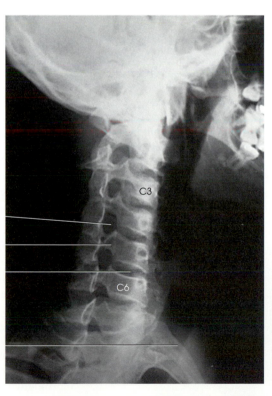
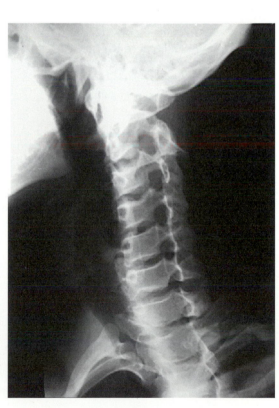

A

Intervertebral foramen C4-C5

Pedicle C5

C5-C6 Intervertebral disk space

1st rib

C3

C6

B

Fig. 8-56. AP axial oblique intervertebral foramina. **A,** LPO position demonstrating right side. **B,** RPO position demonstrating left side.

(Courtesy Ellen S. Titen, R.T.)

Cervical Intervertebral Foramina

PA AXIAL OBLIQUE PROJECTION
RAO and LAO positions

Oblique positions for the demonstration of the cervical intervertebral foramina were first described by Barsóny and Koppenstein.[1,2] Both sides are examined for comparison.

Film: 8 × 10 in (18 × 24 cm) lengthwise.

Position of patient

- Place the patient prone or upright with the back toward the x-ray tube.
- For the patient's comfort and to facilitate accurate adjustment of the part, the standing or seated upright position is preferred.

Position of part

- Keeping one shoulder adjacent to the film, rotate the patient's entire body to a 45-degree angle to place the foramina parallel with the film. Center the cervical spine to the midline of the grid device. The foramina *closest* to the cassette are demonstrated.
- To allow for the caudal angulation of

[1]Barsóny T, and Koppenstein E: Eine neue Method zur Röntgenuntersuchung der Halswirbelsäule, Fortschr Roentgenstr 35:593-594, 1926.
[2]Barsóny T, and Koppenstein E: Beitrag zur Aufnahmetechnik der Halswirbelsäule; Darstellung der Foramina intervertebralia, Röntgenpraxis 1:245-249, 1929.

the central ray, center the cassette at the level of the fifth cervical vertebra (1 inch caudal to the most prominent point of the thyroid cartilage).

Upright position

- Ask the patient to sit or stand straight without strain and, with the arm hanging free, rest the adjacent shoulder against the grid device (Fig. 8-57).
- Using a protractor, ensure that the degree of body rotation is 45 degrees.
- With the median sagittal plane of the head aligned with that of the spine, elevate and protrude the chin slightly to prevent superimposition of the shadows of the mandibular rami and the foramina. Turning the chin to the side causes slight rotation of the superior vertebrae and should be avoided.

Semiprone position

- With the patient's body at an angle of 45 degrees and the cervical spine centered to the midline of the grid, have the patient support himself or herself on the forearm and flexed knee of the elevated side.
- Adjust a suitable support under the head to place the long axis of the cervical column parallel with the film.
- Check and adjust the degree of body rotation (Figs. 8-58 and 8-59).
- Adjust the position of the patient's head so that the median sagittal plane is aligned with that of the spine.
- Elevate and protrude the chin just enough to prevent superimposition of the shadows of the mandibular rami and the intervertebral foramina. Turning the chin to the side causes slight rotation of

the superior vertebrae and should be avoided.

- *Shield gonads.*
- For either approach, ask the patient to suspend respiration for the exposure.

Central ray

- Direct the central ray to the fourth cervical vertebra at an angle of 15 to 20 degrees caudad so that it will coincide with the angle of the foramina.
- Because of the increased object-to-image receptor distance, an SID of 60 to 72 inches (150 to 180 cm) is recommended.

Structures shown

The resulting image will show the intervertebral foramina and pedicles *closest* to the film and an oblique projection of the bodies and other parts of the cervical column (Fig. 8-60).

□Evaluation criteria

The following should be clearly demonstrated:

- ■ "Open" intervertebral foramina *closest* to the film.
- ■ "Open" intervertebral disk spaces.
- ■ Elevated chin and protruded jaw so the angle of the mandible does not overlap C1 and C2.
- ■ Occipital bone not overlapping C1.
- ■ All seven cervical and the first thoracic vertebrae.

OBLIQUE HYPERFLEXION-EXTENSION PROJECTIONS

Boylston[1] has suggested functional studies of the cervical vertebrae in the oblique position for the demonstration of fractures of the articular processes and of obscure dislocations and subluxations. The manipulation of the patient's head must be performed by a physician when acute injury has been sustained.

The patient is placed in a direct frontal body position facing the x-ray tube with the shoulders held firmly against the grid device. The head is carefully rotated maximally to one side and kept so, while the neck is flexed for the first exposure and extended for the second exposure. Both sides are examined for comparison.

[1]Boylston, BF Oblique roentgenographic views of the cervical spine in flexion and extension: An aid in the diagnosis of cervical subluxations and obscure dislocations, J Bone Joint Surg 39A:1302-1309, 1957.

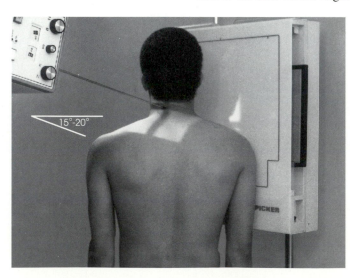

Fig. 8-57. PA axial oblique right intervertebral foramina RAO.

15°-20°

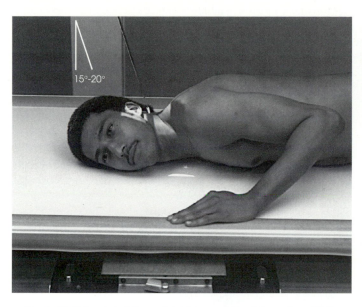

Fig. 8-58. PA axial oblique right intervertebral foramina. RAO.

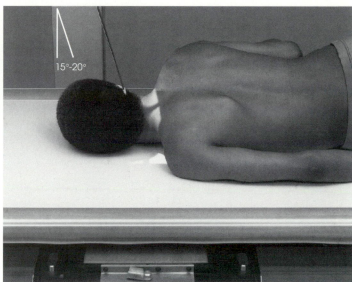

Fig. 8-59. PA axial oblique left intervertebral foramina. LAO.

A

B

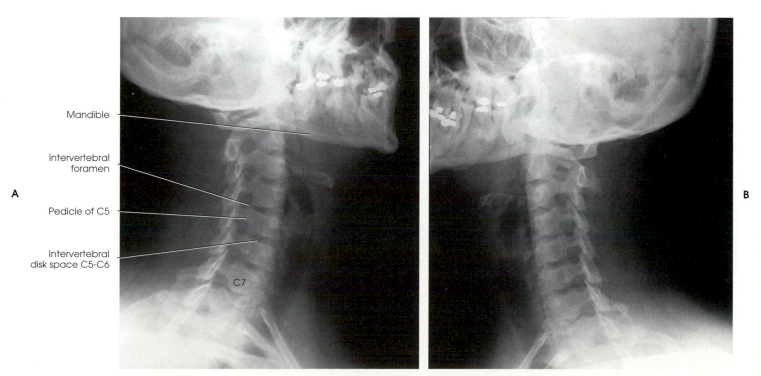

Mandible

Intervertebral foramen

Pedicle of C5

Intervertebral disk space C5-C6

C7

Fig. 8-60. PA axial oblique intervertebral foramina. **A,** RAO position demonstrating right side. **B,** LAO position demonstrating left side.

(**A,** courtesy Michael Franklin, R.T.)

Cervical Vertebrae

AP PROJECTION
OTTONELLO METHOD

With the Ottonello method, the mandibular shadow is blurred, if not obliterated, by utilizing an even chewing motion of the mandible during the exposure. The head must be rigidly immobilized to prevent movement of the vertebrae. The exposure time must be long enough to cover several complete excursions of the mandible.

Film: 8 × 10 in (18 × 24 cm) lengthwise.

Position of patient

- Place the patient in the supine position.
- Center the median sagittal plane of the body to the midline of the grid.
- Place the arms along the sides of the body, and adjust the shoulders to lie in the same horizontal plane.
- Place a long sandbag under the knees for the patient's comfort.

Position of part

- Adjust the head so that the median sagittal plane is perpendicular to the table.
- Elevate the chin enough to place the occlusal surface of the upper incisors and the mastoid tips in the same vertical plane.
- Immobilize the head, and have the patient practice opening and closing the mouth until he or she can move the mandible smoothly without striking the teeth together (Fig. 8-61).
- With the cassette in the Bucky tray, center it at the level of the fourth cervical vertebra.
- *Shield gonads.*
- Ask the patient to suspend respiration for the exposure.

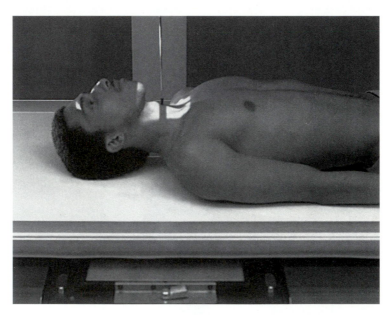

Fig. 8-61. AP cervical vertebrae: Ottonello method.

Central ray

- Direct the central ray perpendicular to the fourth cervical vertebra using low mA and long exposure time (at least one second).

Structures shown

The resulting image will show an AP projection of the entire cervical column with the mandible being blurred if not obliterated (Figs. 8-62 and 8-63).

☐ Evaluation criteria

The following should be clearly demonstrated:

- All seven cervical vertebrae.
- Mandible blurred with resultant visualization of the underlying first and second cervical vertebrae.

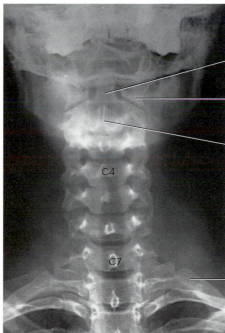

Dens

C1 lateral mass

Spinous process of C2

C4

C7

1st rib

Fig. 8-62. AP cervical spine Ottonello method with chewing motion of the mandible and perpendicular central ray.

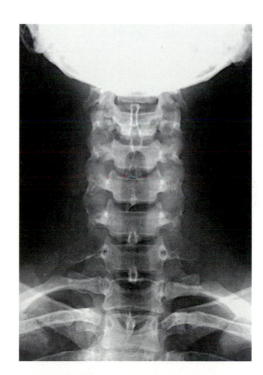

Fig. 8-63. Conventional AP axial cervical spine with stationary mandible and 15-20° cephalic angulation of the central ray.

Cervical and Upper Thoracic Vertebrae

Vertebral Arch
AP AXIAL PROJECTION[1]

The vertebral arch projections, sometimes referred to as *pillar* or *lateral mass* projections, are employed for the demonstration of the posterior elements of the cervical and upper three or four thoracic vertebrae, the articular processes and their facets, the laminae, and the spinous processes. The central ray angulations employed project the vertebral arch elements free of the anteriorly situated vertebral bodies and transverse processes so that when the central ray angulation is correct the resultant film resembles a hemisection of the vertebrae. In addition to frontal plane delineation of the articular pillars and facets, these positions are especially useful for the demonstration of the cervicothoracic spinous processes in patients with a whiplash injury.[2]

Film: 8 × 10 in (18 × 24 cm) or 10 × 12 in (24 × 30 cm) lengthwise.

---

[1]Dorland P, and Frémont J: Aspect radiologique normal du rachis postérieur cervicodorsal (vue postérieure ascendante), Semaine Hop, pp 1457-1464, 1957.
[2]Abel MS: Moderately severe whiplash injuries of the cervical spine and their roentgenologic diagnosis, Clin Orthop 12:189-208, 1958.

Position of patient

- Adjust the patient in the supine position, with the median sagittal plane of the body centered to the midline of the grid.
- Depress the shoulders, and adjust them to lie in the same horizontal plane.
- If necessary, place a long strip of bandage around the patient's feet, and with the knees slightly flexed, have the patient grasp the ends of the bandage and then extend the knees to depress the shoulders.

Position of part

- With the median sagittal plane of the head perpendicular to the table, *hyperextend* the neck; the success of this projection depends on the hyperextension (Figs. 8-64 and 8-65).
- When the patient cannot tolerate hyperextension without undue discomfort, an oblique projection is recommended.
- *Shield gonads.*
- Ask the patient to suspend respiration for the exposure.

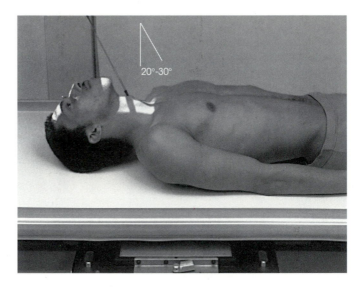

Fig. 8-64. AP axial vertebral arch.

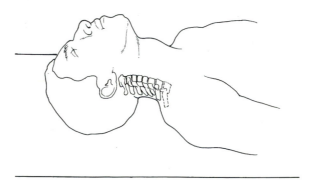

Fig. 8-65. AP axial vertebral arch.

Central ray

- Direct the central ray to the seventh cervical vertebra at an average angle of 25 (20 to 30) degrees caudad. It enters the neck in the region of the thyroid cartilage.
- The degree of the central ray angulation is determined by the cervical lordosis. The goal is to have the central ray coincide with the plane of the articular facets, so that a greater angle is required when the cervical curve is accentuated and a lesser angle is required when the curve is diminished.
- To reduce an accentuated cervical curve and thus place the third to seventh cervical vertebrae in the same plane as the first to fourth thoracic vertebrae, the originators[1] have suggested that a radiolucent wedge be placed under the neck and shoulders, with the head extended somewhat over the edge of the wedge.

[1]Dorland P, et al: Techniques d'examen radiologique de l'arc postérieur des vertebres cervicodorsales, J Radiol 39:509-519, 1958.

Structures shown

The resulting image will show the posterior portion of the cervical and upper thoracic vertebrae, including the articular and the spinous processes (Fig. 8-66).

□Evaluation criteria

The following should be clearly demonstrated:
- Vertebral arch structures, especially the superior and inferior articulating processes, without overlapping of the vertebral bodies and transverse processes.
- Articular processes.
- Open zygapophyseal joints between the articular processes.

NOTE: For a PA axial projection showing both sides on one film, rest the patient's head on his or her fully extended neck with the median sagittal plane of the head perpendicular to the table. Direct the central ray at an average angle of 40 (35 to 45) degrees cephalad.

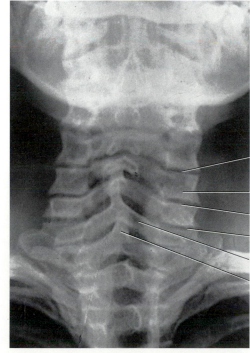

Zygapophyseal joint

Pillar or lateral mass

Inferior articular process

Superior articular process

Lamina

Spinous process

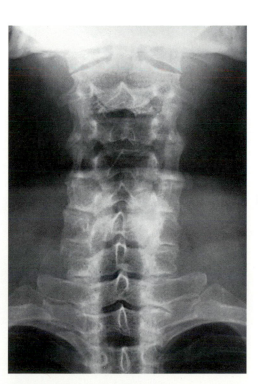

Fig. 8-66. AP axial. **A,** Central ray parallel with plateau of articular processes. **B,** Head fully extended but inadequate central ray angulation. Central ray not parallel with zygapophyseal joints.

Cervical and Upper Thoracic Vertebrae

Vertebral Arch
AP AXIAL OBLIQUE PROJECTION
R and L head rotation[1]

These radiographic projections are used to demonstrate the vertebral arches or pillars when the patient cannot hyperextend the head for the AP or PA axial projection. Both sides are examined for comparison.

Film: 8 × 10 in (18 × 24 cm).

Position of patient

• Place the patient in the supine position.

[1]Dorland P, et al: Techniques d'examen radiologique de l'arc postérieur des vertebres cervicodorsales, J Radiol 39:509-519, 1958.

Position of part

• Rotate the head 45 to 50 degrees toward the *unaffected* side. A 45- to 50-degree rotation of the head usually demonstrates the articular processes of the second to seventh cervical vertebrae and of the first thoracic vertebra. A rotation of as much as 60 to 70 degrees is sometimes required for the demonstration of the processes of the sixth and seventh cervical vertebrae and of the first to fourth thoracic vertebrae (Fig. 8-67).
• Position the cassette so the top edge is at the level of the mastoid tip.
• *Shield gonads.*
• Ask the patient to suspend respiration for the exposure.

Central ray

• Direct the central ray to exit the spinous process of the seventh cervical vertebra at an average angle of 35 (30 to 40) degrees caudad.

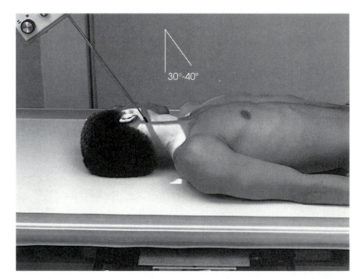

Fig. 8-67. AP axial oblique demonstrating right vertebral arches.

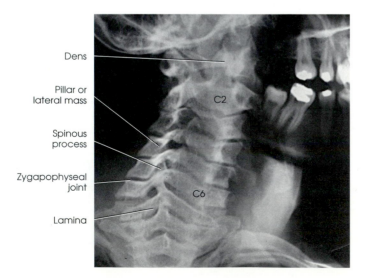
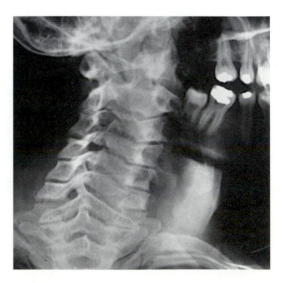

Fig. 8-68. AP axial oblique demonstrating right vertebral arches.

PA AXIAL OBLIQUE PROJECTIONS
R and L head rotations

Film: 8 × 10 in (18 × 24 cm).

Position of patient

- Unless contraindicated, place the patient in the prone position, which seems to be more comfortable for injured patients than the supine position.
- Center the median sagittal plane of the body to the midline of the grid.
- When the patient is thin, place a pillow under his or her chest to obviate accentuation of the cervical curve.
- Depress the shoulders and adjust them to lie in the same horizontal plane.

Position of part

- Rest the patient's head on one cheek (both sides are examined for comparison), and adjust the head so that the median sagittal plane is at an angle of 45 degrees.
- For demonstration of the second to fifth cervical vertebrae, flex the neck somewhat to reduce the cervical curve.
- For the fifth to seventh cervical vertebrae and the first to fourth thoracic vertebrae, adjust the head in moderate extension.
- Position the cassette so the bottom edge is at the level of the tip of the seventh cervical spinous process (Fig. 8-69).
- *Shield gonads.*
- Ask the patient to suspend respiration for the exposure.

Central ray

- Direct the central ray to the seventh cervical vertebra at an average angle of 35 (30 to 40) degrees cephalad exiting at the level of the mandibular symphysis.

Structures shown, AP and PA projections

The resulting images will show the dependent posterior arch of the cervical and upper thoracic vertebrae with open zygapophyseal articulations (Figs. 8-68 and 8-70).

☐ Evaluation criteria

The following should be clearly demonstrated:

- Vertebral arch structures, especially the superior and inferior articular processes, free of overlap of the vertebral bodies and transverse processes.
- Articular processes and facets on the side of interest.
- Open joints between the articular facets on the side of interest.

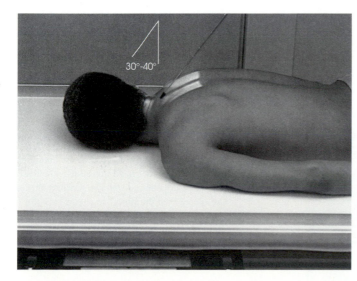

Fig. 8-69. PA axial oblique demonstrating left vertebral arches.

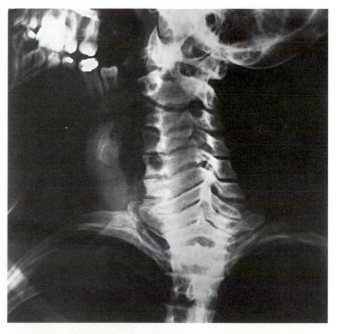

Fig. 8-70. PA axial oblique demonstrating left vertebral arches.

Cervical Vertebrae: Trauma

 ADAPTATION OF POSITIONS TO THE SEVERELY INJURED PATIENT

When a patient who has sustained a severe injury of the cervical spine arrives by stretcher or bed, he or she should not be transferred to the radiographic table and must not be rotated. Unless removed by a physician, any cervical collar should always be left in place for the initial radiographs. To preclude the possibility of damaging the spinal cord by the sharp edge of a bone fragment or by a subluxed vertebra as a result of movement, any necessary manipulation of the patient's head must be performed by a physician.

If there is not a specially equipped emergency room, the initial examination is performed with a mobile unit or in an examining room that is large enough to accommodate the placement of a stretcher or bed where the x-ray tube can be brought into position for the required images.

Grid-front cassettes or a stationary grid are recommended for the AP and oblique projections.

Shield gonads: Place a lead shield over the patient's pelvis. (Not shown for illustration purposes.)

Ask the patient to suspend respiration for all exposures.

 LATERAL PROJECTION

The lateral projection, using a horizontal central ray, presents no problem because it requires little or no adjustment of the patient's head and neck.

The cassette is placed in the vertical position, with its lower portion in contact with the lateral aspect of the shoulder, centered to the fourth cervical vertebra and then immobilized. The central ray is directed horizontal to the fourth cervical vertebra (Figs. 8-71 and 8-72). Because of the increased OID, an SID of 60 to 72 inches is recommended.

This radiograph must be reviewed by a physician before any further positioning is attempted.

For the demonstration of the seventh cervical vertebra, the shoulders must be fully depressed. Depending on the patient's condition, this can be done by looping a long strip of bandage around the patient's feet, and, with his or her knees slightly flexed, attach the other end of the bandage to each wrist, and then extend the knees to pull the shoulders down. If the patient's condition will not permit this maneuver, an assistant can depress the shoulders by applying symmetrical traction on the arms. To prevent additional injury to the patient, any body adjustments must be made only by qualified personnel.

NOTE: Although a grid is used in the lateral position photographs, it need not be used because of the increased object-to-image receptor distance. The increase in the object-to-image receptor distance creates an air gap, which reduces the amount of scatter radiation reaching the film.

Fig. 8-71. Cross-table lateral cervical vertebrae.

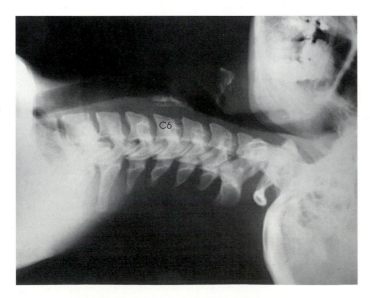

Fig. 8-72. Cross-table lateral cervical vertebrae.

350

AP AXIAL PROJECTION

For an AP axial projection, the patient's head must be held (to prevent it from turning) and lifted enough for the cassette to be slipped into position without appreciable movement of the patient's head and neck. If the patient comes into the radiographic room on a backboard, the cassette may be placed under the backboard for the initial radiograph so the patient's head is not moved.

Two AP projections may be obtained: (1) a 15- to 20-degree cephalic angulation of the central ray for the demonstration of the vertebral bodies and their interspaces (Fig. 8-73) and (2) a 20- to 30-degree caudal angulation of the central ray for the demonstration of the posterior vertebral elements, the articular pillars and facets, the laminae, and the spinous processes. The latter study should be made on a 10 × 12 in (24 × 30 cm) film to include the upper three or four thoracic vertebrae.

AP AXIAL OBLIQUE PROJECTION

For the demonstration of the pedicles and the intervertebral foramina the cassette must be positioned near the side *opposite* the one being examined so that its midpoint will coincide with the 45-degree lateromedial angulation of the central ray.

The cassette may be placed directly under the patient or under a backboard. Lift the backboard or the patient's head slightly. With the cassette held so that its midpoint is at the level of the fourth cervical body, gently slide it under the head just far enough to center it under the adjacent mastoid process. This centering places the midline of the film approximately 3 inches lateral to the median sagittal plane of the neck.

From the opposite side, the side being projected, the central ray is directed to the fourth cervical vertebra at a compound angle of 45 degrees medial and 15 to 20 degrees cephalad (Figs. 8-74 to 8-76).

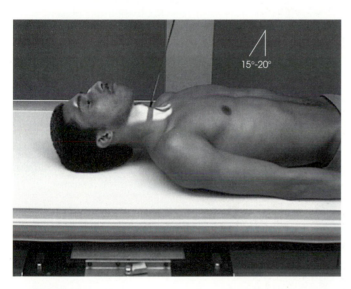

Fig. 8-73. AP axial cervical vertebrae, 15-degree grid technique.

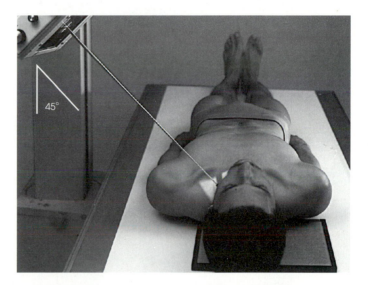

Fig. 8-74. AP axial oblique cervical vertebrae showing 45-degree medial central ray angulation and 20-degree cephalad angulation. Non-grid technique.

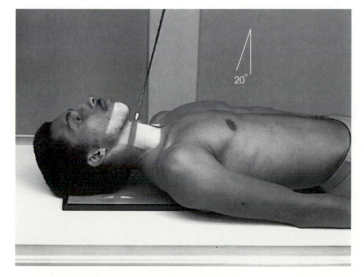

Fig. 8-75. AP axial oblique cervical vertebrae showing 20-degree cephalad central ray angulation and 45-degree medial central ray angulation. Non-grid technique.

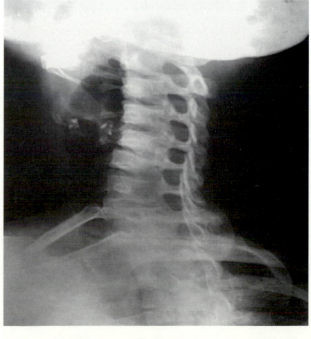

Fig. 8-76. Resultant non-grid AP axial oblique cervical vertebrae demonstrating left structures.

Cervicothoracic Region

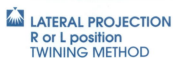

LATERAL PROJECTION
R or L position
TWINING METHOD

This projection is often called the "swimmer's lateral."

Film: 10 × 12 in (24 × 30 cm) lengthwise.

Position of patient

- Place the patient in a lateral position, either seated or standing, against a vertical grid device.

Position of part

- Center the median coronal plane of the body to the midline of the grid.
- Elevate the arm that is adjacent to the Bucky to a vertical position, flex the elbow, and rest the forearm on the patient's head.
- Move the shoulder adjacent to the Bucky posteriorly or anteriorly, according to what seems better for the individual patient.
- Move the patient close enough to the stand so that he or she can rest the shoulder firmly against it for support.
- Adjust the head so that the median sagittal plane is parallel with the film (Fig. 8-77).

- Adjust the height of the cassette so that the film is centered at the level of the second thoracic vertebra (¾ inch or 2 cm superior to the jugular notch).
- Adjust the body in a true lateral position, with the median sagittal plane parallel with the plane of the film.
- Depress the shoulder that is farthest from the film as much as possible, and move it anterior or posterior, according to the placement of the opposite side. Immobilize it by having the patient hold a sandbag or an anchored strip of gauze.
- The goal is to have one shoulder placed slightly anterior and the other slightly posterior, and simultaneously elevating one shoulder while depressing the opposite one. Such shoulder placement is just enough to prevent the humeral heads from being superimposed over the vertebrae.
- *Shield gonads.*
- Ask the patient to suspend respiration for the exposure.
- If the patient can cooperate and be immobilized, a long exposure time (low mA) should be utilized while the patient takes shallow breaths. Shallow breathing blurs the lung anatomy.

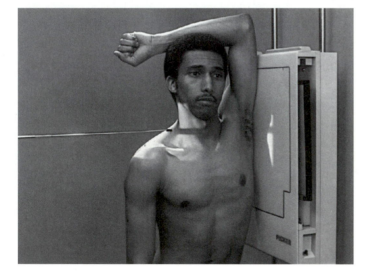

Fig. 8-77. Upright lateral cervicothoracic region: Twining method.

Central ray

- Direct the central ray to the second thoracic vertebra (1) perpendicular if the shoulder is well depressed or (2) at a caudal angle of 5 degrees when the shoulder cannot be well depressed.

Structures shown

The resulting image will show a lateral projection of the lower cervical and upper thoracic vertebrae projected between the two shoulders (Fig. 8-78).

□ Evaluation criteria

The following should be clearly demonstrated:

- Lateral vertebrae, not appreciably rotated.
- Shoulders separated from each other.
- Area from approximately C5 to T5.
- Exposure penetration of the shoulder region.

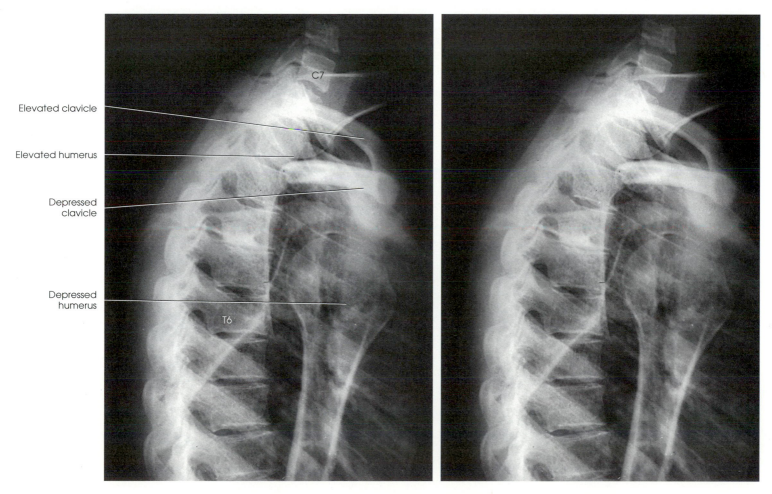

Fig. 8-78. Lateral cervicothoracic region: Twining method.

Elevated clavicle

Elevated humerus

Depressed clavicle

Depressed humerus

C7

T6

353

Cervicothoracic Region

 LATERAL PROJECTION
R or L position
PAWLOW METHOD

Film: 10 × 12 in (24 × 30 cm) length-wise.

Position of patient

- Place the patient in a lateral recumbent position with the head elevated on the patient's arm, sandbags, or a small, firm pillow.

Position of part

- Center the median coronal plane of the body to the midline of the grid.
- Adjust the support under the head, and place another support under the lower thorax so that the long axis of the cervicothoracic vertebrae is horizontal.
- Extend the arm which the patient is lying on above the head. Move the humeral head anteriorly or posteriorly.
- Place the top arm at the patient's side, and immobilize it by having the patient grab the posterior thigh. Move the humeral head *opposite* that of the bottom arm.
- Adjust the body in an exact lateral position (Fig. 8-79).
- Center the cassette at the level of the jugular notch.
- *Shield gonads.*
- Ask the patient to suspend respiration for the exposure.

Central ray

- Direct the central ray to the cervicothoracic area at an angle of 3 to 5 degrees caudad.

Structures shown

The resulting image will show a lateral projection of the cervicothoracic vertebrae between the shoulders (Fig. 8-80).

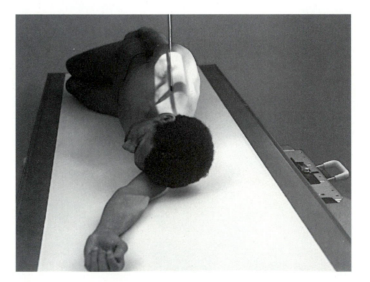

Fig. 8-79. Recumbent lateral cervicothoracic region: Pawlow method.

□Evaluation criteria

The following should be clearly demonstrated:

- Lateral vertebrae not appreciably rotated.
- Shoulders separated from each other.
- Area from approximately C5 to T5.
- Exposure penetrating the shoulder region.

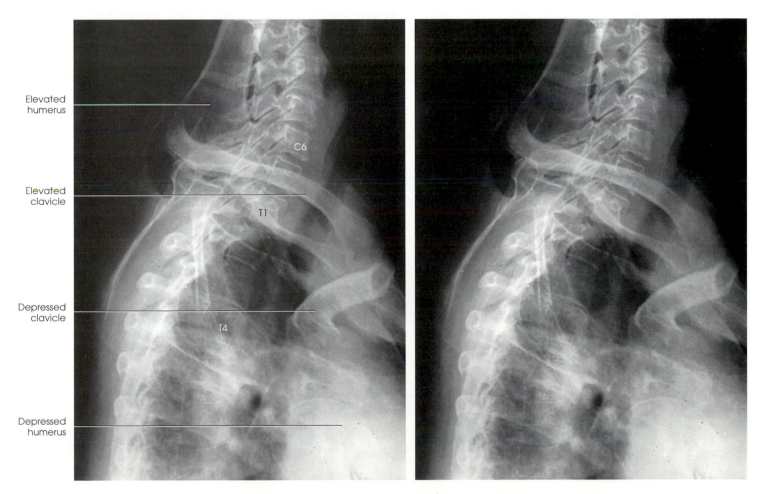

Elevated humerus

Elevated clavicle

Depressed clavicle

Depressed humerus

C6

T1

T4

Fig. 8-80. Lateral cervicothoracic region: Pawlow method.

Thoracic Vertebrae

 AP PROJECTION

Film: 14 × 17 in (35 × 43 cm) or 7 × 17 in (18 × 43 cm) lengthwise.

Position of patient

- Place the patient in the supine or upright body position.
- If the patient is supine, let the head rest directly on the table or on a thin pillow to avoid accentuating the dorsal kyphosis.

Position of part

- Center the median sagittal plane of the body to the midline grid.
- Place the patient's arms along the sides of the body, and adjust the shoulders to lie in the same horizontal plane.
- If the supine position is being used, further reduce the dorsal kyphosis by flexing the hips and knees enough to place the back in contact with the table (Fig. 8-81).
- Adjust the thighs in a vertical position, and immobilize the feet with sandbags.
- If the limbs cannot be flexed, support the knees to relieve strain and invert the feet slightly.
- When the upright position is used, have the patient stand so his or her weight is equally distributed on the feet to prevent rotation of the vertebral column.
- If the lower limbs are of unequal length, place a support of correct height under the foot of the shorter side.
- Center the film at the level of the seventh thoracic vertebra. Depending on the stature of the patient, the anterior localization point will lie 3 to 4 inches (7.5 to 10 cm) distal to the jugular notch; as a quick check, the superior edge of the film should lie 1½ to 2 inches (4 to 5 cm) above the shoulders.
- *Shield gonads.*
- Respiration: The patient may be allowed to take shallow breaths during the exposure unless breathing is labored. In this case, respiration is suspended at the end of full exhalation to obtain a more uniform density.

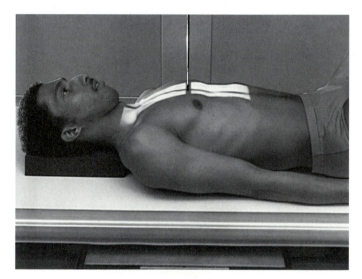

Fig. 8-81. AP thoracic vertebrae.

Central ray

- Direct the central ray perpendicular to T7 (approximately 3 to 4 inches distal to the jugular notch).
- As suggested by Fuchs,[1] a more uniform density of the thoracic vertebrae will be obtained if the "heel effect" of the tube is used. This is done by positioning the tube with the cathode end toward the feet. With the tube in this position, the greatest percentage of radiation will go through the thickest part of the thorax. Compare the radiographs shown in Fig. 8-82.

---

[1]Fuchs AW: Thoracic vertebrae, Radiogr Clin Photogr 17:2-13, 1941.

Structures shown

The resulting image will show an AP projection of the thoracic bodies, their interpediculate spaces, and the surrounding structures (Fig. 8-82).

The intervertebral spaces are not well demonstrated unless the SID is adjusted to the center of the radius of the thoracic curve to place the spaces parallel with the divergent rays. This is not desirable as a preliminary procedure, because it necessitates changing the SID for different patients and results in varying degrees of magnification. It should be employed only when an AP projection of the spaces is indicated and in conjunction with a radiograph made at the preliminary SID. A more practical way to demonstrate the disk spaces of a localized area is to angulate the central ray so that it is perpendicular to the long axis of the particular vertebral area. The degree of central ray angulation required can be estimated with reasonable accuracy by noting the angle of the dorsal curve at the area under investigation. Abnormal accentuation of the dorsal kyphosis requires that the patient be placed in the seated upright or recumbent position before a vertical grid device so that localized areas can be placed as nearly parallel with the film as possible.

□ Evaluation criteria

The following should be clearly demonstrated:

- All twelve vertebrae.
- Wide latitude of exposure (or two radiographs can be taken for the upper and lower vertebrae).
- X-ray beam collimated to the thoracic spine as shown in Fig. 8-82.
- Spinous processes at the midline of the patient.
- Vertebral column aligned to the middle of the radiograph.

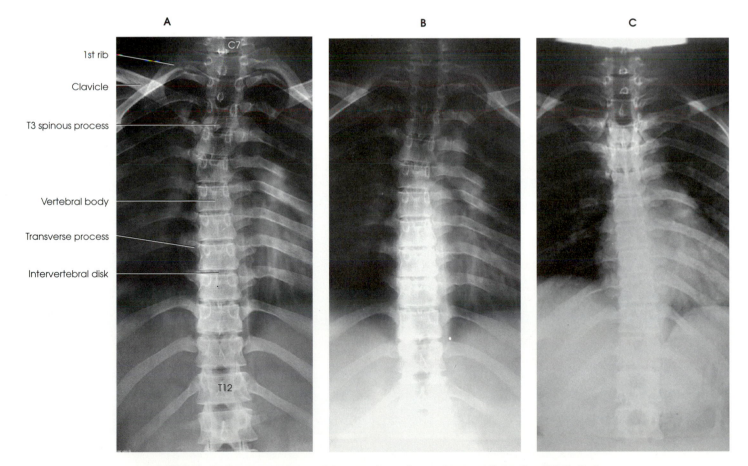

Fig. 8-82. A, Cathode end of x-ray tube over lower thorax (more uniform density). **B,** Cathode end of x-ray tube over upper thorax (nonuniform density). **C,** AP thoracic spine showing mild scoliosis.

(**C,** courtesy Karen Cubler, R.T.)

Thoracic Vertebrae

LATERAL PROJECTION
R or L position

Film: 14 × 17 in (35 × 43 cm) or 7 × 17 in (18 × 43 cm) lengthwise.

Position of patient

- Place the patient in a lateral position, either recumbent or upright.
- If possible, use the left lateral position to place the heart closer to the film; this will minimize its overlapping the vertebrae.
- Oppenheimer[1] recommends the use of the orthostatic (upright) position to reproduce the physiologic conditions and reports that the subject should be allowed to stand in a normal position—no attempt should be made to force the patient into an unwanted position, especially straightening of the vertebral column.
- Have the patient dressed in an open-backed gown so that the vertebral column can be exposed for the adjustment of the position.

[1]Oppenheimer A: The apophyseal intervertebral articulations roentgenologically considered, Radiology 30:724-740, 1938.

Recumbent position

- Place a firm pillow under the patient's head to elevate the median sagittal plane to the level of the long axis of the vertebral column.
- Flex the hips and knees to a comfortable position.
- Center the median coronal plane of the body to the midline of the grid at the level of the seventh thoracic vertebra.
- Elevate the lower knee to hip level and support it.
- With the knees exactly superimposed to prevent rotation of the pelvis, place a small sandbag between them.
- Adjust the arms at right angles to the long axis of the body to elevate the ribs enough to clear the intervertebral foramina. This placement of the arms gives a clear projection of the vertebrae distal to the level of the scapulohumeral joints. Drawing the arms forward or extending them to more than a right-angle position carries the scapulae forward where they will superimpose over the upper thoracic vertebrae.

- Place a radiolucent support under the lower thoracic region, and adjust the position of the support so that the long axis of the vertebral column is horizontal, as illustrated in Fig. 8-83, A.
- If support is not placed under the lower thoracic region, the central ray may have to be directed perpendicular to the long axis of the vertebral column. This will require a cephalic angulation as seen in Fig. 8-83, B.
- The degree of angulation required is approximately 10 to 15 degrees.
- Adjust the body in a true lateral position.
- When necessary, apply a compression band across the trochanteric area of the pelvis. This does not interfere with the alignment of the body, as does a band placed higher.
- *Shield gonads.*
- Ask the patient to suspend respiration at the end of exhalation unless the exposure is to be made during quiet breathing.

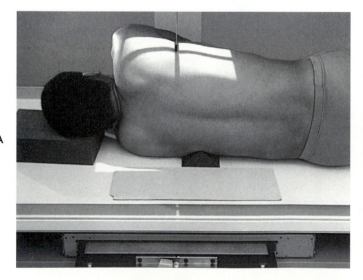
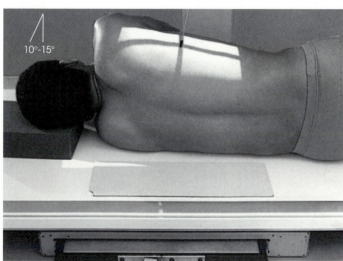

A   10°-15°   B

Fig. 8-83. Recumbent lateral thoracic spine **A,** Support placed under lower thoracic region, perpendicular central ray. **B,** No support under lower thoracic spine, central ray angled 10 to 15 degrees cephalad.

Vertebral column

Upright position

- Have the patient stand straight without strain, and adjust the height of the vertical grid device so that the midpoint of the film is at the level of the seventh thoracic vertebra.
- Center the median coronal plane of the body to the midline of the grid, and move the patient close enough to the grid to allow him or her to rest the adjacent shoulder firmly against the grid front for support.
- The weight of the body must be equally distributed on the feet.
- If the limbs are of unequal length, place a support of correct height under the foot of the shorter side.
- Adjust the body so that the long axis of the vertebral column is parallel with the plane of the film.

- Elevate the ribs by raising the arms to a position at right angles to the long axis of the body, and support them in this position. An IV stand is very useful for this purpose. Place it in front of the patient, immobilize it with sandbags, and, placing one of the patient's hands on the other for correct alignment of the arms, have him or her grasp the standard at the correct height (Fig. 8-84).
- The support of the upper limbs usually furnishes sufficient immobilization.
- *Shield gonads.*
- Respiration: To obliterate, or at least diffuse, the vascular markings and ribs, it is often desirable to make the exposure during quiet breathing.

Central ray

- Direct the central ray perpendicularly to the median coronal plane at the level of T7 located approximately 3 to 4 inches (7.5 cm) below the jugular notch.
- If the vertebral column is not elevated to a horizontal plane when the patient is in a recumbent position, angle the tube to direct the central ray perpendicular to the long axis of the thoracic column and then center it at the level of the seventh thoracic vertebra. An average angle of 10 degrees cephalad on female patients and, because of greater shoulder width, an average angle of 15 degrees on male patients is satisfactory for a majority of patients.

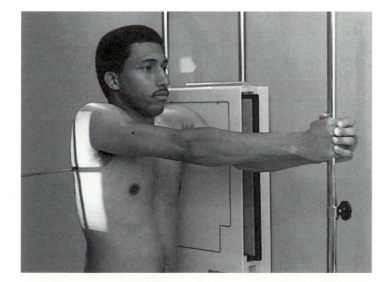

Fig. 8-84. Upright lateral thoracic spine.

Thoracic vertebrae

359

Improving radiographic quality

- The quality of the radiographic image can be improved if a sheet of leaded rubber is placed on the table behind the patient, as shown in Fig. 8-83. The lead will absorb the scatter radiation coming from the patient; scatter radiation serves only to decrease the quality of the radiograph. More important perhaps is that with automatic exposure control (AEC), the scatter radiation coming from the patient is often sufficient to prematurely terminate the exposure. The resultant image may be underexposed because of the effect of the scatter radiation on the AEC device. For the same reason, close collimation is necessary for lateral spine radiographs.

Structures shown

The resulting image will show a lateral projection of the thoracic bodies showing their interspaces, the intervertebral foramina, and the lower spinous processes. Because of the overlapping shoulders, the upper three or four segments are not demonstrated in this position (Fig. 8-85).

□ Evaluation criteria

The following should be clearly demonstrated:

- Vertebrae clearly seen through rib and lung shadows.
- Twelve thoracic vertebra. Because the upper thoracic vertebrae are usually not demonstrated, the film can be centered low enough to include L1 and L2. The absence of any rib on L1 usually confirms that T12 has been included.
- Ribs superimposed posteriorly to indicate that the patient was not rotated.
- A wide latitude of exposure.
- X-ray beam tightly collimated to reduce scatter radiation.

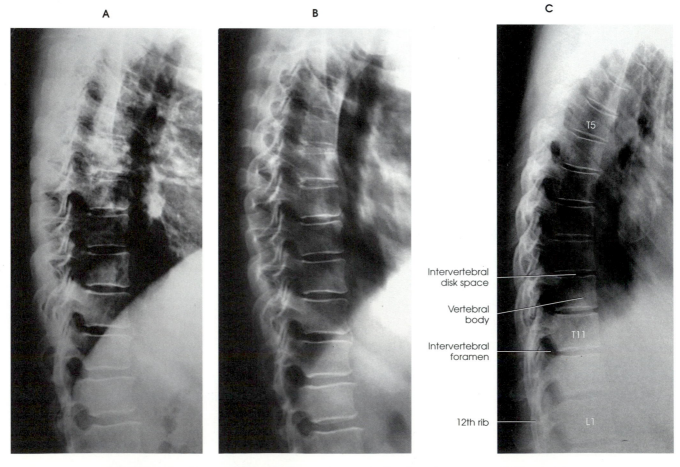

Fig. 8-85. Lateral thoracic spine. **A,** Suspended respiration for an exposure of 0.75 second. **B,** Quiet breathing for an exposure of 7.5 seconds (same patient as in **A**). **C,** Lateral thoracic spine with breathing technique.

(**C,** courtesy Barbara Davis, R.T.)

Zygapophyseal Joints

AP OR PA OBLIQUE PROJECTIONS
RAO and LAO, or
RPO and LPO positions
Upright

The thoracic zygapophyseal joints are examined using PA oblique projections as recommended by Oppenheimer,[1] or AP oblique projections as recommended by Fuchs.[2] The joints are well demonstrated with either projection. The AP obliques demonstrate the joints *farthest* from the film, and the PA obliques demonstrate the joints *closest* to the film. Although the difference in OID between the two projections is not great, the same technique of rotation is used bilaterally.

Film: 14 × 17 in (35 × 43 cm) lengthwise.

---

[1]Oppenheimer A: The apophyseal intervertebral articulations roentgenologically considered, Radiology 30:724-740, 1938.
[2]Fuchs AW: Thoracic vertebrae (part 2), Radiogr Clin Photogr 17:42-51, 1941.

AP or PA oblique

Position of patient

- Place the patient in a lateral position before a vertical grid device.

Position of part

- Rotate the body slightly anterior (PA oblique) or posterior (AP oblique) so the coronal plane forms an angle of 70 degrees from the plane of the film (the median sagittal plane forming an angle of 20 degrees with the film).
- Center the vertebral column to the midline of the grid, and have the patient rest the adjacent shoulder firmly against it for support.
- Adjust the height of the grid to center the film to the seventh thoracic vertebra.
- Flex the elbow of the arm adjacent to the grid, and rest the hand on the hip.
- If rotated anteriorly, have the patient grasp the side of the grid device for support (Figs. 8-86 and 8-87); if rotated posteriorly, place both hands on the hips.

- Adjust the shoulders to lie in the same horizontal plane.
- Have the patient stand straight to place the long axis of the vertebral column parallel with the film.
- The weight of the body must be equally distributed on the feet, and the head must not be turned laterally.
- Having the shoulder rest against the vertical Bucky usually furnishes sufficient support.
- *Shield gonads.*
- Ask the patient to suspend respiration at the end of exhalation.

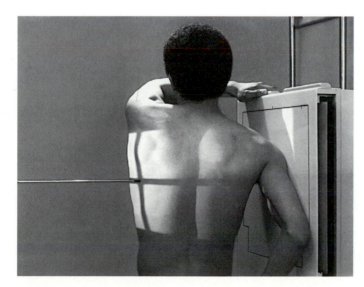

Fig. 8-86. PA oblique zygapophyseal joints, RAO for joints closest to film.

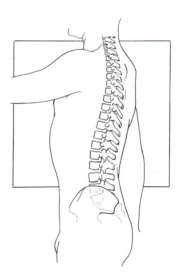

Fig. 8-87. PA oblique zygapophyseal joints, RAO for joints closest to film.

Zygapophyseal Joints

AP OBLIQUE PROJECTION
RPO and LPO positions

PA OBLIQUE PROJECTION
RAO and LAO positions
Recumbent

Film: 14 × 17 in (35 × 43 cm) or 7 × 17 in (18 × 43 cm).

Position of patient

- Place the patient in a lateral recumbent position.
- Elevate the head on a firm pillow so that its median sagittal plane is continuous with that of the vertebral column.
- Flex the patient's hips and knees to a comfortable position.

AP or PA oblique
Position of part

- For anterior (PA oblique) rotation, place the lower arm behind the back (Fig. 8-88).
- For posterior (AP oblique) rotation, adjust the lower arm at right angles to the long axis of the body, flex the elbow, and place the hand under or beside the head (Fig. 8-89).
- For the PA oblique, place the upper arm forward with the hand on the table (Fig. 8-88). For the AP oblique, place the upper arm posteriorly and support it (Fig. 8-89).
- Rotate the body slightly, either anteriorly or posteriorly as preferred, so that the coronal plane forms an angle of 70 degrees with the horizontal (20 degrees with the vertical).

- Center the vertebral column to the midline of the grid; then check and adjust the body rotation.
- With the cassette in the Bucky tray, center at the level of the seventh thoracic vertebra.
- If needed, apply a compression band across the hips, but be careful not to change the position.
- *Shield gonads.*
- Ask the patient to suspend respiration for the exposure.

Central ray

- Direct the central ray perpendicular to the film exiting T7.

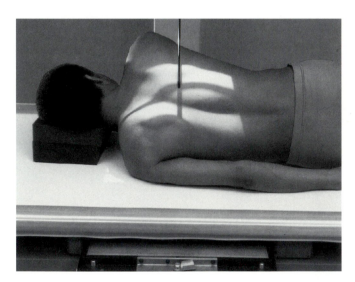

Fig. 8-88. PA oblique zygapophyseal joints, LAO for joints closest to film.

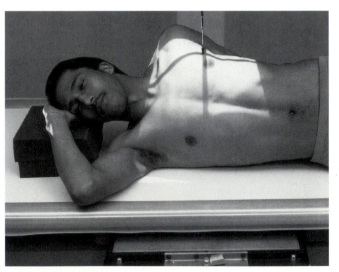

Fig. 8-89. AP oblique zygapophyseal joints, RPO for joints farthest from film.

Structures shown

The resulting images will show oblique projections of the zygapophyseal joints (*arrow* on radiograph) (Figs. 8-90 and 8-91). The number of joints shown depends on the thoracic curve. A greater degree of rotation from the lateral position is required to show the joints at the proximal and distal ends of the region on patients who have an accentuated dorsal kyphosis. The inferior articular processes of the twelfth thoracic vertebra, having an inclination of about 45 degrees, are not shown in this projection.

The following should be clearly demonstrated:
- All twelve thoracic vertebrae.
- Zygapophyseal joints closest to the film on PA obliques, and joints farthest from the film on AP obliques.
- Wide exposure latitude.

NOTE: The posterior rotation position gives an excellent demonstration of the cervicothoracic spinous processes and is used for this purpose when the patient cannot be satisfactorily positioned for a direct lateral position.

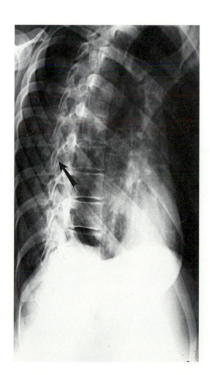

Fig. 8-90. *Upright* PA oblique zygapophyseal joints, LAO. *Arrow* indicates articulation closest to film.

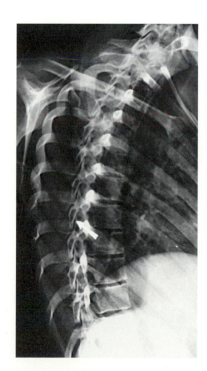

Fig. 8-91. *Recumbent* AP oblique zygapophyseal joints, RPO. *Arrow* indicates articulation farthest from film.

Lumbar-Lumbosacral Vertebrae

 AP PROJECTION
PA PROJECTION

It is desirable to have the intestinal tract free of gas and fecal material for examinations of the bones lying within the abdominal and pelvic regions. The urinary bladder should be emptied just before the examination to eliminate the superimposition cast by the secondary radiation generated within the filled bladder. This is especially important in examinations of older men, in whom it is frequently possible to detect prostatic enlargement, as shown by urinary retention.

Of the two projections, it is the AP projection that is considered the essential step to master.

> **Film:** 14 × 17 in (35 × 43 cm) or 11 × 14 in (30 × 35 cm) for general survey examinations.

Position of patient

- Examine the lumbar-lumbosacral spine either AP or PA, with the patient recumbent or upright.
- Acute back disorders are excruciatingly painful. For the ambulatory patient, it is less painful when the examination is performed in the upright position whenever possible.

- In addition, for patients having *severe* back pain, place the footboard on the radiographic table before beginning the examination.
- The patient may stand on the upright footboard and assume the radiographic position.
- The table can then be turned to the horizontal position for the exposure and returned to the upright position for the next projection.
- This procedure takes a few minutes, but the patient will appreciate its ability to minimize pain.

PA projection

Because the PA projection presents the concave side of the lordotic curve toward the x-ray tube, it places the intervertebral disk spaces at an angle closely paralleling the divergence of the beam of radiation (Figs. 8-92 and 8-93). For this reason the PA projection is sometimes used for upright studies of the lumbar-lumbosacral spine. The position does not increase the OID, except with subjects who have a large abdomen. When used in the recumbent position, it has the advantage of being more comfortable for the patient with a painful back and is especially more comfortable for the emaciated patient. An additional advantage of performing the PA projection is that the gonad dose can be significantly reduced compared with the AP projection.

AP projection

The AP projection is generally used for recumbent examinations and, unfortunately, with the back fully arched by extension of the lower limbs. The extended limb position accentuates the lordotic curve, which in turn increases the angle between the vertebral bodies and the divergent rays, with resultant distortion of the bodies as well as poor delineation of the intervertebral disk spaces (Figs. 8-94 and 8-95). The lordotic curve can be reduced and the intervertebral disk spaces clearly delineated in the AP projection simply by flexing the hips and knees enough to place the back in firm contact with the table (see Figs. 8-96 and 8-97 on the following page).

Comparison of the images in Figs. 8-93 and 8-95 shows that when the patient is correctly adjusted in the supine position there is little difference between the PA and AP projections. The only consideration left is the patient's comfort.

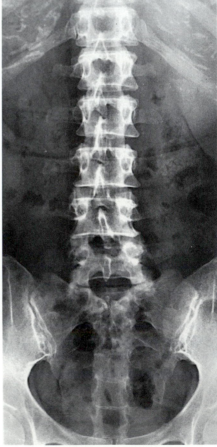

Fig. 8-93. PA lumbar spine. Same patient as in Fig. 8-95.

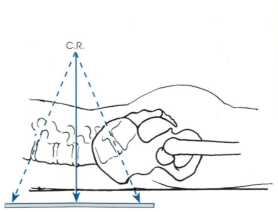

Fig. 8-92. Lumbar spine showing intervertebral disk spaces nearly parallel with divergent PA x-ray beam.

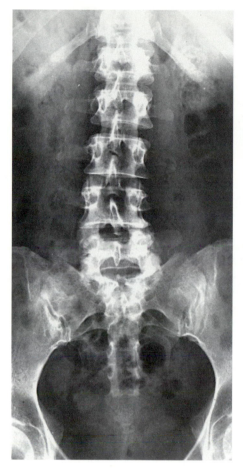

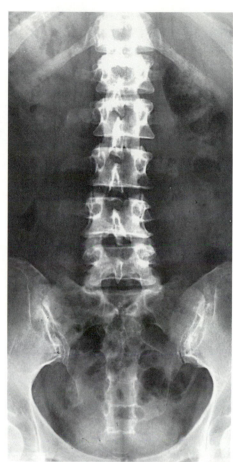

Fig. 8-94. Lumbar spine demonstrating intervertebral disk spaces and diverging central ray are not parallel.

Fig. 8-95. AP lumbar spine. **A,** Limbs extended. **B,** Limbs flexed.

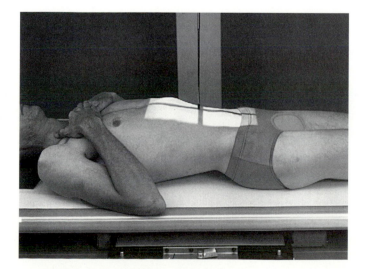

Fig. 8-96. AP lumbar spine with limbs extended, creating increased lordotic curve.

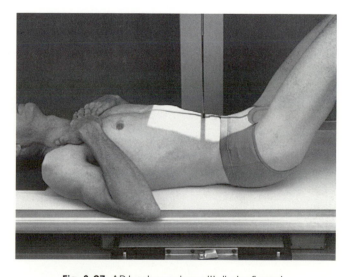

Fig. 8-97. AP lumbar spine with limbs flexed, decreasing lordotic curve.

Lumbar-Lumbosacral Vertebrae
Continued

Position of part

Supine position, AP projection

- Center the median sagittal plane of the body to the midline of the grid.
- To prevent rotation of the spine, adjust the shoulders and hips to lie in the same horizontal plane, and adjust the head so that its median sagittal plane is aligned in the same plane with that of the spine.
- Flex the patient's elbows and place the hands on the upper chest so that the forearms will not lie within the exposure field.
- When a soft tissue abnormality (atrophy or swelling) is causing rotation of the pelvis, adjust a radiolucent support under the lower side.
- Reduce the lumbar lordosis by flexing the hips and knees enough to place the back in firm contact with the table.
- Have the patient lean the knees together for support (Figs. 8-96 and 8-97).

Prone position, PA projection

- Center the median sagittal plane of the body to the midline of the grid.
- With elbows flexed, adjust the arms and forearms in a comfortable, bilaterally symmetrical position.
- Adjust the shoulders and hips to lie in the same horizontal plane, and have the patient rest the head on the chin to prevent rotation of the spine.

Film centering

- Center the 14×17 in (35×43 cm) film at the level of the crests of the ilia (L4).
- Care must be used to palpate for the crest of the bone to avoid being misled by the contour of the heavy muscles and fatty tissue lying above it.
- When an 11×14 in (30×35 cm) film is used, center to the third lumbar vertebra (at the level of the inferior median coronal costal margin).
- When two 10×12 in (24×30 cm) films are used, center the first the same as for an 11×14 in film.
- Center the second film to coincide with the cranially or caudally angulated central ray, which is directed through the lumbosacral joint.
- *Shield gonads.*
- Ask the patient to suspend respiration for the exposure.

Central ray

- Direct the central ray perpendicular to the midline at the level of the crests of the ilia (L4-L5 interspace) to the center of the cassette.

Structures shown

The resulting image will show the lumbar bodies, the intervertebral disk spaces, the interpediculate spaces, the laminae, and the spinous and transverse processes (Fig. 8-98). When the larger film is used, one or two of the lower thoracic vertebrae, the sacrum, and the pelvic bones are included. Because of the angle at which the last lumbar segment joins the sacrum, the lumbosacral disk space is not well shown in the AP projection. The positions used for this purpose are described on the following pages.

□ Evaluation criteria

The following should be clearly demonstrated:

- Area from the lower thoracic vertebrae to the sacrum.
- X-ray beam collimated to the lateral margin of the psoas muscles.
- No artifact across the midabdomen from any elastic in the patient's underclothing.
- Exposure penetrating all the vertebral structures.
- Open intervertebral joints.
- Sacroiliac joints equidistant from the vertebral column.

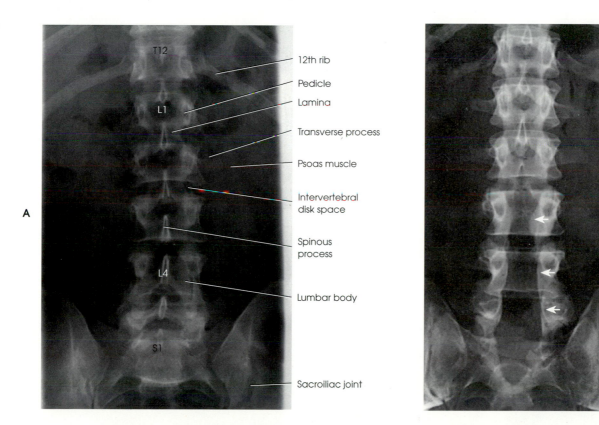

Fig. 8-98. **A,** AP lumbar spine. **B,** AP lumbar spine demonstrating spina bifida *(arrows).*

(**A,** courtesy Thomas White, R.T.; **B,** Courtesy David M. Jones, R.T.)

Lumbar-Lumbosacral Vertebrae

LATERAL PROJECTION
R or L position

Film: 14 × 17 in (35 × 43 cm) or 11 × 14 in (30 × 35 cm) for general survey examinations.

Position of patient

- The overall body position (recumbent or upright) used for the AP or PA projection is maintained for the lateral position.
- Have the patient dressed in an open-back gown so that the spine can be exposed for final adjustment of the position.

Recumbent position

Position of part

- Ask the patient to turn onto the indicated side (usually the left) and flex the hips and knees to a comfortable position.
- When examining a thin patient, adjust a suitable pad under the dependent hip to relieve pressure.
- Align the median coronal plane of the body to the midline of the grid. Remember that no matter how large the patient, the long axis of the spine is situated in the median coronal plane.

- Adjust the pillow to place the median sagittal plane of the head in alignment with that of the spine.
- With the patient's elbow flexed, adjust the dependent arm at right angles to the body.
- To prevent rotation, exactly superimpose the knees and place a small sandbag between them.
- Unless central ray angulation is to be used, place a suitable radiolucent support under the lower thorax, and adjust it so that the long axis of the spine is horizontal (Fig. 8-99).
- Recheck the position for rotation.
- Detect rotation and correct it by looking down the back while adjusting the position.
- When using a large film, center at the level of the crest of the ilium.
- The central ray is not moved from the median coronal plane of the body.
- *Shield gonads.*
- Ask the patient to suspend respiration at the end of exhalation.

Central ray

- After the spine has been adjusted so it is horizontal, direct the perpendicular central ray at the level of the crest of the ilium entering the median coronal plane (Fig. 8-99).
- When the spine cannot be adjusted so it is horizontal, angle the central ray caudad so it is perpendicular to the long axis (Fig. 8-100). The degree of central ray angulation depends on the angulation of the lumbar column and the breadth of the pelvis. An average caudal angle of 5 degrees for men and 8 degrees for women with a wide pelvis is satisfactory in a majority of cases (Fig. 8-100).

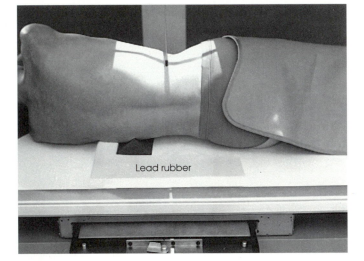

Fig. 8-99. Lateral lumbar spine. Horizontal spine and perpendicular central ray.

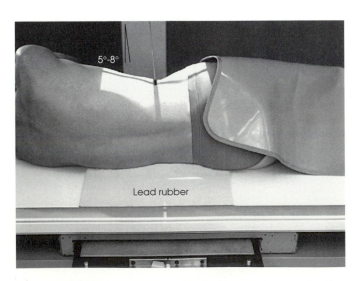

Fig. 8-100. Lateral lumbar spine. Central ray angled caudad to be perpendicular to long axis of spine.

Upright position

Position of part

- From the upright position assumed for the PA projection, ask the patient to turn to the side and center the median coronal plane of the body to the midline of the grid.
- Immobilize the patient by placing an IV stand in front of the patient, and having him or her grasp it with both hands at shoulder height.
- Ensure that the patient stands straight. Subjects who have severe low back pain tend to relieve the discomfort by tilting the pelvis anteriorly and superiorly. The movement reduces the lumbosacral angle and thus defeats the aim to demonstrate it in the orthostatic (upright) position.
- The weight of the body must be equally distributed on the feet.
- *Shield gonads.*
- Ask the patient to suspend respiration at the end of exhalation.

Central ray

- Direct the central ray perpendicular to the median coronal plane at the level of the crest of the ilium.

Structures shown

The resulting image will show the lumbar bodies and their interspaces, the spinous processes, and the lumbosacral junction (Fig. 8-101). This projection gives a profile image of the superior four lumbar intervertebral foramina. The fifth lumbar intervertebral foramina (right and left) are not usually well visualized in this projection because of their oblique direction. Oblique projections are used for these foramina.

□ Evaluation criteria

The following should be clearly demonstrated:

- Area from the lower thoracic vertebrae to the sacrum.
- Open intervertebral disk spaces.
- Superimposed posterior margins of each vertebral body.
- Vertebrae aligned down the middle of the radiograph.
- Nearly superimposed crests of the ilia when x-ray beam is not angled.
- Spinous processes.

Improving radiographic quality

The quality of the radiographic image can be improved if a sheet of leaded rubber is placed on the table behind the patient, as shown in Figs. 8-99 and 8-100. The lead will absorb the scatter radiation coming from the patient; scatter radiation serves only to decrease the quality of the radiograph. More important perhaps is that with automatic exposure control (AEC), the scatter radiation coming from the patient is often sufficient to prematurely terminate the exposure. The resultant image may be underexposed because of the effect of the scatter radiation on the AEC device. For the same reason, close collimation is necessary for lateral spine radiographs.

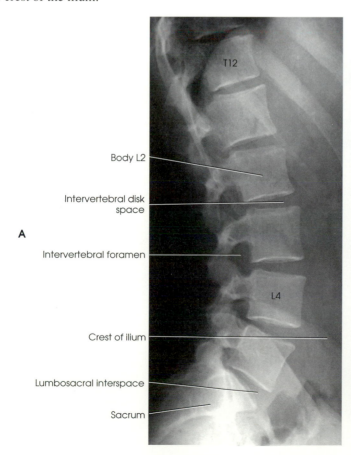
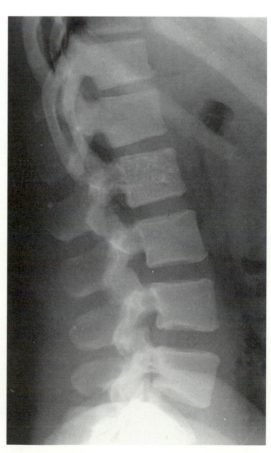

Fig. 8-101. A and **B,** Lateral lumbar spine.

(**A,** courtesy John Syring, R.T.; **B,** courtesy Holly Simmons, R.T.)

L5-S1 Lumbosacral Junction

 LATERAL PROJECTION
R or L position

Film: 8 × 10 in (18 × 24 cm) lengthwise.

Position of patient

- Examine the L5-S1 lumbosacral region in the recumbent position, because patients who have low back pain tend, when upright, to assume a protective position that reduces the lumbosacral angle. It is further recommended that questionable cases be checked with a lateral position made in the upright position as well as in the usual recumbent position.

Position of part

- To center the laterally positioned lumbosacral joint to the film, align the patient's body so that a plane passing 1½ inches (4 cm) posterior to the median coronal plane is centered to the midline of the grid.
- With the patient in the recumbent position, adjust the pillow to place the median sagittal plane of the head in the same plane with that of the spine.
- With the patient's elbow flexed, adjust the dependent arm in a position at right angles to the body (Fig. 8-102).
- It is desirable to have the hips fully extended for this study. When this cannot be done, extend them as much as possible, and support the dependent knee at hip level on sandbags.

- Place sandbags under—and sponges between—the ankles and knees.
- Francis[1] identified a technique to demonstrate the open L5-S1 interspace: With the patient in the lateral position, locate both crests of the ilia.
  - Draw an imaginary line between the two points (the interiliac line).
  - Adjust central ray angulation to be parallel with interiliac line.
- *Shield gonads.*
- Ask the patient to suspend respiration for the exposure.

---

[1]Francis C: Method improves consistency in L5-S1 joint space films. Radiol. Technol. 63(5):302-305, 1992.

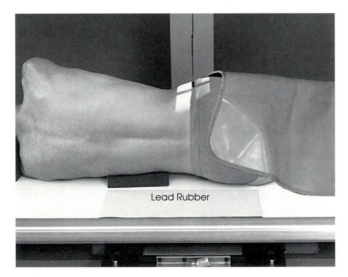

Lead Rubber

Fig. 8-102. Lateral L5-S1.

Central ray

- Direct the central ray parallel with the interiliac line entering the patient 1½ inches (4 cm) anterior to the palpated spinous process of L5, and 1½ inches (4 cm) inferior to the crest of the ilium.
- When the spine is not in the true horizontal position, the central ray is angled caudally, 5 degrees for male patients and 8 degrees for female patients.

Structures shown

The resulting image will show a lateral projection of the lumbosacral joint, the lower one or two lumbar vertebrae, and the upper sacrum (Fig. 8-103).

□ Evaluation criteria

The following should be clearly demonstrated:

- Open lumbosacral joint.
- Collimated x-ray beam including all of the fifth lumbar vertebra and the upper sacrum.
- Lumbosacral joint in the center of the exposure area.
- The crests of the ilia closely superimposing each other when x-ray beam is not angled.
- The lumbosacral joint.

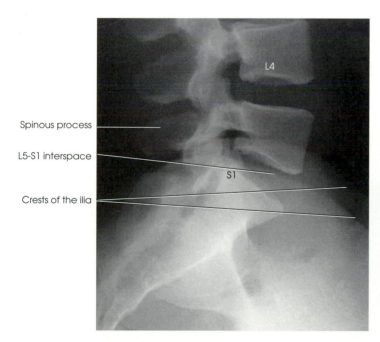
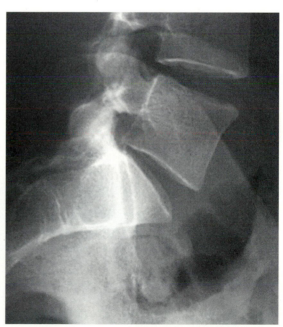

Spinous process

L5-S1 interspace

Crests of the ilia

L4

S1

Fig. 8-103. A and **B,** Lateral L5-Sl.

(**A,** courtesy Holly Simmons, R.T.; **B,** courtesy John Syring, R.T.)

Zygapophyseal Joints

AP OBLIQUE PROJECTION
RPO and LPO positions

The articular processes of the lumbar vertebrae form an angle of 30 to 50 degrees, and those between the last lumbar vertebra and the sacrum form an angle of 30 degrees to the median sagittal plane in a majority of patients. The angulation does vary, however, not only from patient to patient but from side to side in the same patient. Exact adjustment of the part on the first examination makes it possible to determine any necessary change in rotation for further studies. Both sides are generally radiographed for comparison.

Film: 14 × 17 in (35 × 43 cm) or 11 × 14 in (30 × 35 cm) lengthwise; 8 × 10 in (18 × 24 cm) for last zygapophyseal joint.

Position of patient

- Oblique projections are, when indicated, generally taken immediately following the AP projection and in the same body position—recumbent or upright. The recumbent position is described because it is more frequently used, but the directions can be easily adapted to the upright position.

Position of part

- Have the patient turn from the supine position toward the affected side approximately 45 degrees to demonstrate the joints *closest* to the film (opposite the thoracic zygapophyseal joints).
- Center the spine to the midline of the grid. In the oblique position the lumbar spine lies in the longitudinal plane that passes 2 inches (5 cm) medial to the elevated ASIS.

- Ask the patient to place the arms in a comfortable position. A support may be placed under the elevated shoulder, hip, and knee (Figs. 8-104 and 8-105).
- Check and adjust the degree of body rotation. Adjust at an angle of 45 degrees for the demonstration of the articular processes in the lumbar region and at an angle of 30 degrees from the horizontal plane for the demonstration of the lumbosacral processes.
- For the lumbar region, center the cassette at the level of the third lumbar vertebra.
- For the fifth zygapophyseal joint, center the cassette at the level of the horizontal plane passing midway between the crests of the ilia and the anterior superior iliac spines.
- *Shield gonads.*
- Ask the patient to suspend respiration for the exposure.

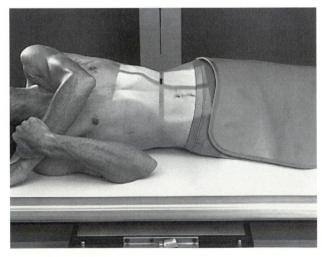

Fig. 8-104. AP oblique lumbar spine. RPO for right zygapophyseal joints.

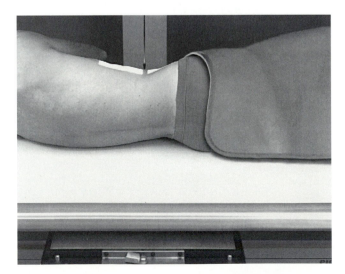

Fig. 8-105. AP oblique lumbar spine. LPO for left zygapophyseal joints.

Central ray

- Direct the central ray perpendicular to the third lumbar vertebra (1 to 1½ inches above the crest of the ilium), entering the elevated side approximately 2 inches laterally from the patient's midline.

Structures shown

The resulting image will show an oblique projection of the lumbar and/or the lumbosacral spine, demonstrating the articular processes of the side *closest* to the film. Both sides are examined for comparison (Figs. 8-106 to 8-108).

When the body is placed in a 30- to 45-degree oblique position and the lumbar spine radiographed, the articular processes and the zygapophyseal joints are demonstrated. When the patient has been properly positioned, images of the lumbar vertebrae have the appearance of "Scotty dogs." Fig. 8-106 identifies the different structures that comprise the "Scotty dog."

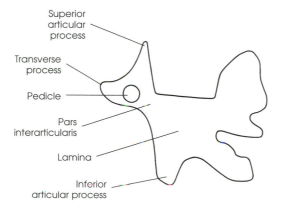

Superior articular process

Transverse process

Pedicle

Pars interarticularis

Lamina

Inferior articular process

Fig. 8-106. Parts of "Scotty dog."

□ Evaluation criteria

The following should be clearly demonstrated:

- Area from the lower thoracic vertebrae to the sacrum.
- Zygapophyseal joints closest to the film.
  - □ When the joint is not well demonstrated and the pedicle is quite anterior on the vertebral body, the patient is not obliqued enough.
  - □ When the joint is not well demonstrated and the pedicle is quite posterior on the vertebral body, the patient is obliqued too much.
- Vertebral column parallel with the tabletop so the T12-L1 and L1-L2 joint spaces remain open.

Zygapophyseal joints

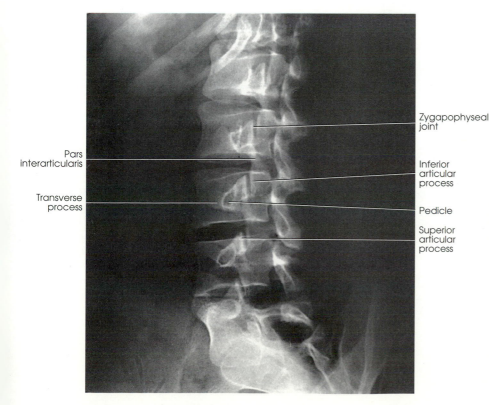

Pars interarticularis

Transverse process

Zygapophyseal joint

Inferior articular process

Pedicle

Superior articular process

Fig. 8-107. AP oblique lumbar spine. RPO for right zygapophyseal joints. (Note "Scotty dogs.")

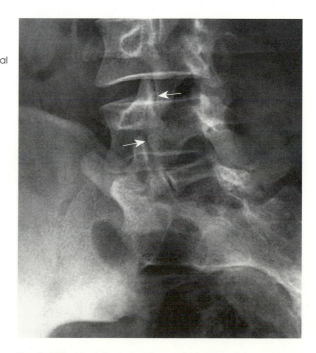

Fig. 8-108. AP oblique lumbar spine. RPO demonstrating L5 zygapophyseal joint *(arrows)* using a 30-degree position.

Zygapophyseal Joints
PA OBLIQUE PROJECTION
RAO and LAO positions

Film: 14 × 17 in (35 × 43 cm) or 11 × 14 in (30 × 35 cm) lengthwise; 8 × 10 in (18 × 24 cm) for the last zygapophyseal joint.

Position of patient

- Examine the patient in the upright or the recumbent position. The recumbent position is generally used because it facilitates immobilization.
- Greater ease in positioning the patient and a resultant higher percentage of success in duplicating results make the semiprone position preferable to the semisupine position.

Position of part

- The joints *farthest* from the film are demonstrated with the PA oblique projection (opposite the thoracic zygapophyseal joints).
- Have the patient turn to a semiprone position and support the body on the forearm and flexed knee.
- Align the body to center the third lumbar vertebra of the elevated side to the midline of the grid (Fig. 8-109).
- Check and, if necessary, adjust the degree of body rotation to an angle of 45 degrees for the lumbar region and 30 degrees from the horizontal for the lumbosacral zygapophyseal joint.
- Center the film at the level of the third lumbar vertebra.
- To demonstrate the fifth intervertebral foramen, position the patient as described above but center to the zygapophyseal joint of the fifth lumbar vertebra.
- *Shield gonads.*
- Ask the patient to suspend respiration for the exposure.

Central ray

- Direct the central ray perpendicularly to enter the third lumbar vertebra (1 to 1½ inches above the crest of the ilium). The central ray enters the elevated side approximately 2 inches (5 cm) lateral to the median sagittal plane.

Structures shown

The resulting image will show an oblique projection of the lumbar and/or lumbosacral vertebrae, demonstrating the articular processes of the side *farther* from the film (Figs. 8-110 to 8-112). The articulation between the twelfth thoracic and first lumbar vertebrae, having the same direction as those in the lumbar region, is shown on the larger film.

The fifth intervertebral foramen is usually well shown in oblique positions (Fig. 8-112).

When the body is placed in a 30- to 45-degree oblique position and the lumbar spine radiographed, the articular processes and the zygapophyseal joints are demonstrated. When the patient has been properly positioned, images of the lumbar vertebrae have the appearance of "Scotty dogs." Fig. 8-110 identifies the different structures that comprise the "Scotty dog."

☐ Evaluation criteria

The following should be clearly demonstrated:
- Area from the lower thoracic vertebrae to the sacrum.
- Zygapophyseal joints *farthest* from the film:
  - ☐ When the joint is not well demonstrated and the pedicle is quite anterior on the vertebral body, the patient is not obliqued enough.
  - ☐ When the joint is not well demonstrated and the pedicle is quite posterior on the vertebral body, the patient is obliqued too much.
- Vertebral column parallel with the tabletop so the T12-L1 and L1-L2 joint spaces remain open.

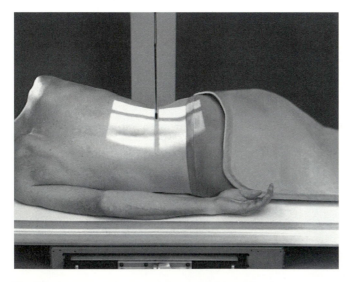

Fig. 8-109. PA oblique lumbar spine. LAO for right zygapophyseal joint.

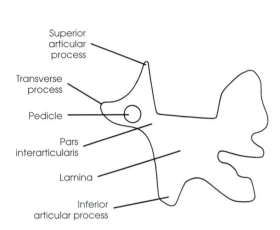

Fig. 8-110. Parts of "Scotty dog."

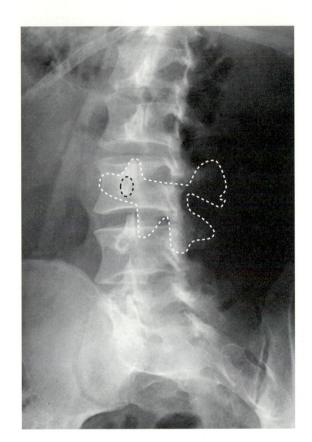

Fig. 8-111. PA oblique lumbar spine. LAO for right zygapophyseal joints. (Note "Scotty dogs.")

(Courtesy Thomas White, R.T.)

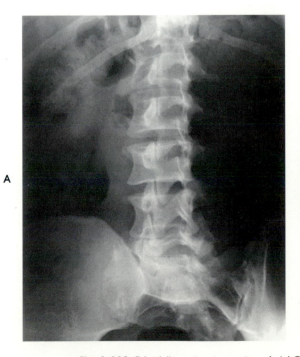

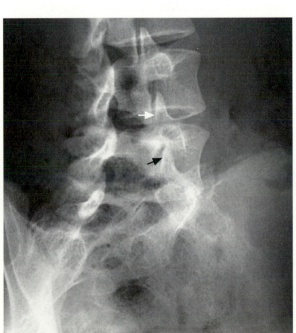

Fig. 8-112. PA oblique lumbar spine. **A,** LAO for right zygapophyseal joints. **B,** RAO for left L5 zygapophyseal joint *(arrows).*

(**A,** courtesy Thomas White, R.T.)

Intervertebral Foramen Fifth Lumbar

PA AXIAL OBLIQUE PROJECTION
RAO and LAO positions
KOVACS METHOD[1]

Film: 8 × 10 in (18 × 24 cm) lengthwise.

Position of patient

- Place the patient in the lateral recumbent position lying on the side being examined.

---

[1]Kovács, A: X-ray examination of the exit of the lowermost lumbar root, Radiol Clin North Am 19:6-13, 1950.

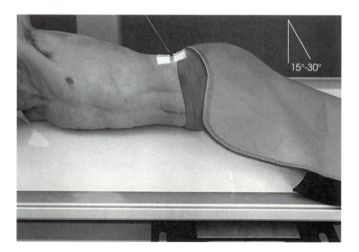

Fig. 8-113. PA axial oblique intervertebral foramen, fifth lumbar vertebrae, RAO: Kovacs method.

Position of part

- With the patient in the lateral position, align the body so a plane that passes 1½ inches (4 cm) posterior to the median coronal plane is centered to the midline of the grid.
- Have the patient extend the upper arm and grasp the end of the table to maintain the thorax in the lateral position when the pelvis is rotated.
- Keeping the patient's thorax exactly lateral, rotate the pelvis 30 degrees anteriorly from the lateral position.
- Place a sandbag support under the flexed uppermost knee to prevent too much rotation of the hips (Fig. 8-113).
- Adjust the position of the cassette so that its midpoint will coincide with the central ray.
- *Shield gonads.*
- Ask the patient to suspend respiration for the exposure.

Central ray

- Direct the central ray along a straight line extending from the superior edge of the crest of the uppermost ilium through the fifth lumbar vertebra to the inguinal region of the dependent side. According to the alignment of the spine, the central ray angulation will vary from 15 to 30 degrees caudad.

Structures shown

The resulting image will show the fifth lumbar intervertebral foramen. Both sides are examined for comparison.

The Kovács method (Figs. 8-114 and 8-115) is shown beside the lateral L5 to S1 (Fig. 8-115, *B*) for comparison purposes.

□Evaluation criteria

The following should be clearly demonstrated:

- Open fifth lumbar intervertebral foramen.
- Fifth lumbar intervertebral foramen in the center of the radiograph.

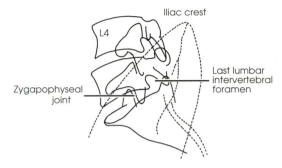

Fig. 8-114. PA axial oblique, intervertebral foramen, fifth lumbar vertebrae.

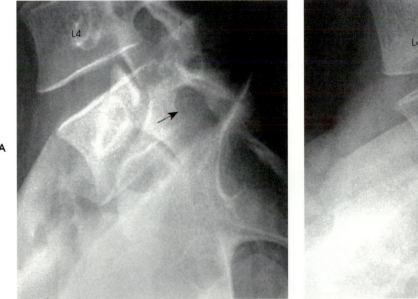
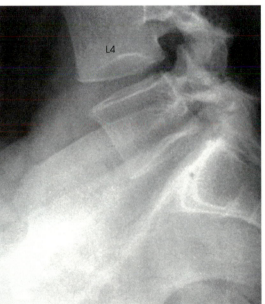

Fig. 8-115. A, PA axial oblique intervertebral foramen, fifth lumbar vertebrae, RAO: Kovacs method. Intervertebral foramen *(arrow).* **B,** Lateral L5-S1. Same patient as **A.**

Lumbosacral Junction and Sacroiliac Joints

AP AXIAL PROJECTION

Film: 8 × 10 in (18 × 24 cm) or 10 × 12 in (24 × 30 cm) lengthwise.

Position of patient

• The AP axial projection of the lumbosacral and sacroiliac joints, is made with the patient in the supine position immediately following the AP projection of the lumbar vertebrae.

Position of part

• With the patient supine, extend the lower limbs or abduct the thighs and adjust in the vertical position (Figs. 8-116 and 8-117).
• *Shield gonads.*
• Ask the patient to suspend respiration for the exposure.

Central ray

• Direct the central ray through the lumbosacral joint at an average angle of 30 to 35 degrees cephalad. The central ray enters about 1.5 inches superior to the symphysis pubis.
• An angulation of 30 degrees for the male patient and 35 degrees for the female patient is satisfactory in a majority of patients. By noting the contour of the lower back, unusual accentuation or diminution of the lumbosacral angle can be estimated and the central ray angulation varied accordingly.

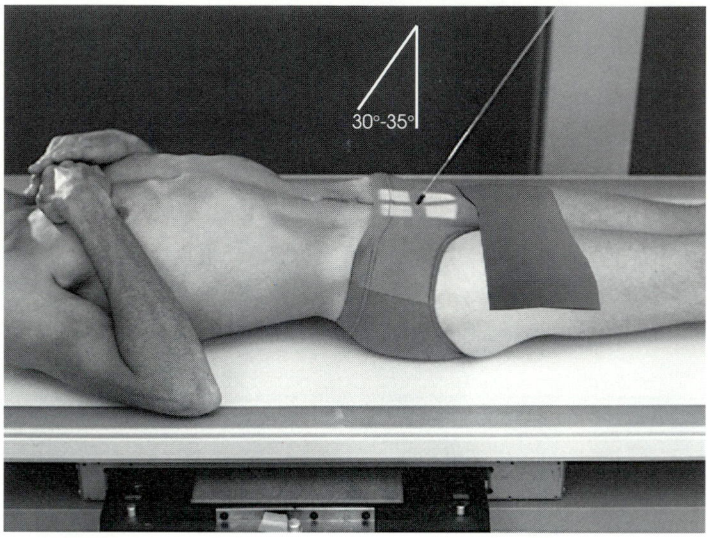

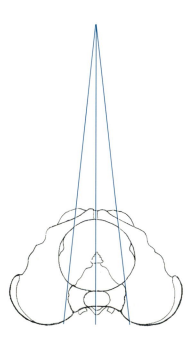

Fig. 8-116. AP axial lumbosacral junction and sacroiliac joints.

Fig. 8-117. AP axial sacroiliac joints.

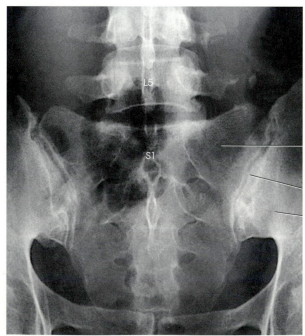

Fig. 8-118. AP axial lumbosacral junction and sacroiliac joints.

Structures shown

The resulting image will show the lumbosacral joint and a symmetrical image of both sacroiliac joints free of superimposition (Fig. 8-118).

☐ **Evaluation criteria**

The following should be clearly demonstrated:
- Fifth lumbosacral junction and sacrum.
- Both sacroiliac joints adequately penetrated.

NOTE: The PA axial projection for the lumbosacral junction can be modified after the AP axial projection just described. With the patient in the prone position, direct the central ray through the lumbosacral joint to the midpoint of the film at an average angle of 35 degrees caudad. The central ray enters the spinous process of the fourth lumbar vertebra (Figs. 8-119 and 8-120).

Meese[1] recommends the prone position for examinations of the sacroiliac joints because their obliquity places them in a position more nearly parallel with the divergence of the beam of radiation. Direct the central ray perpendicular; center at the level of the anterior superior iliac spines. It will enter the midline of the patient about 2 inches (5 cm) distal to the spinous process of the fifth lumbar vertebra (Fig. 8-21).

---

[1]Meese T: Die dorso-ventrale Aufnahme der Sacroiliacalgelenke, Fortschr Roentgenstr 85:601-603, 1956.

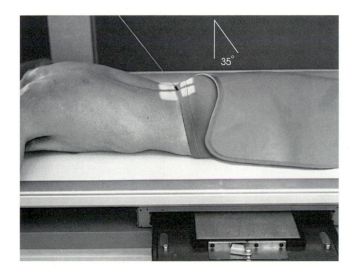

Fig. 8-119. PA axial lumbosacral junction and sacroiliac joints.

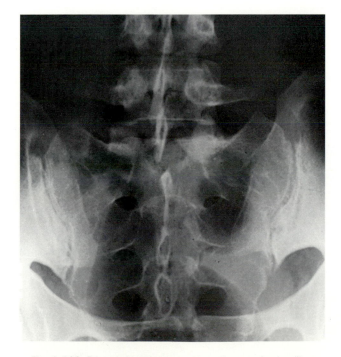

Fig. 8-120. PA axial lumbosacral junction and sacroiliac joints.

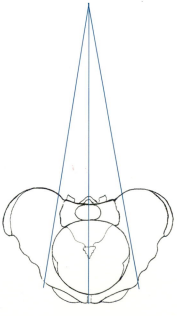

Fig. 8-121. PA bilateral sacroiliac joints.

Sacroiliac Joints

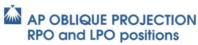 AP OBLIQUE PROJECTION
RPO and LPO positions

Film: 8 × 10 in (18 × 24 cm) or 10 × 12 in (24 × 30 cm) lengthwise. Both obliques are usually obtained for comparison.

Position of patient

- Place the patient in the supine position and elevate the head on a firm pillow.

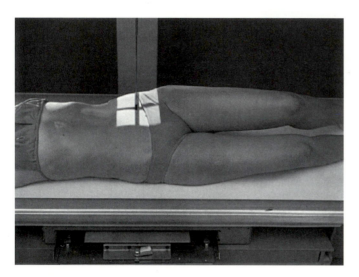

Fig. 8-122. AP oblique sacroiliac joint. RPO demonstrates left joint.

Position of part

- The LPO position will demonstrate the right joint and the RPO position the left joint. The side being examined is *farthest* from the film.
- Elevate the side being examined approximately 25 to 30 degrees and support the shoulder, lower thorax, and upper thigh.
- Align the body so that a sagittal plane passing 1 inch (2.5 cm) medial to the ASIS of the elevated side is centered to the midline of the grid.
- Place the arms in a comfortable position, and adjust the shoulders to lie in the same horizontal plane (Fig. 8-122).
- Adjust the position of the elevated thigh to place each ASIS in the same transverse plane as the other.
- Place supports under the knee to elevate it to hip level if needed.
- Adjust the degree of rotation so that the posterior surface of the body forms a 25- to 30-degree angle from the table (Fig. 8-123).
- Check the rotation at several points along the back.
- Center the cassette at the level of the ASIS.
- *Shield gonads.* Collimating close to the joint may shield the gonads on males. It may be difficult to use contact shielding on females.
- Ask the patient to suspend respiration for the exposure.

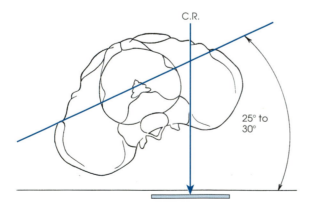

Fig. 8-123. Degree of obliquity required to demonstrate sacroiliac joint for an AP projection.

Central ray

- Direct the central ray perpendicular, so it enters 1 inch medial to the elevated ASIS.

Structures shown

The resulting image will show the sacroiliac joint *farthest* from the film and an oblique projection of the adjacent structures. Both sides are examined for comparison (Fig. 8-124).

■Evaluation criteria

The following should be clearly demonstrated:
- Open joint space with minimal overlapping of the ilium and sacrum.
- Joint centered on the radiograph.

NOTE: An AP axial oblique can be obtained by positioning the patient as described above. For the AP axial oblique, direct the central ray at an angle of 20 to 25 degrees cephalad, entering 1 inch medial and 1½ inches distal to the elevated anterior superior iliac spine (Fig. 8-125).

NOTE: Brower and Kransdorf[1] summarized difficulties in imaging the sacroiliac joints due to positioning and patient variability.

[1]Brower AC, and Kransdorf MJ: Evaluation of disorders of the sacroiliac joint, Applied Radiol 21(2):31-43, 1992.

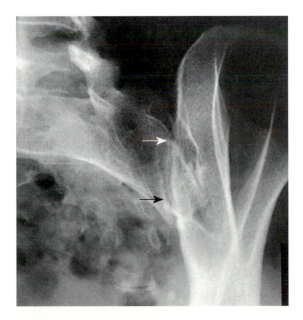

Fig. 8-124. AP oblique sacroiliac joint. RPO demonstrates left joint *(arrows)*.

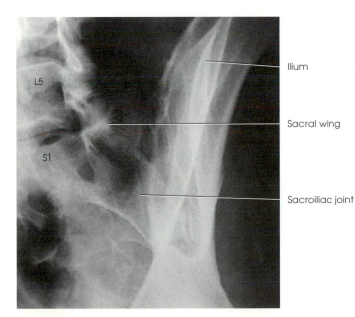

Fig. 8-125. AP axial oblique sacroiliac joint. RPO with 20-degree cephalad angulation demonstrates left joint.

Sacroiliac Joints
PA OBLIQUE PROJECTION
RAO and LAO positions

Film: 8 × 10 in (18 × 24 cm) or 10 × 12 in (24 × 30 cm) lengthwise. Both obliques are usually obtained for comparison.

Position of patient

- Place the patient in a semiprone position.
- The RAO position will demonstrate the right joint and the LAO position, the left joint. The side being examined is *closest* to the film
- Have the patient rest on the forearm and flexed knee of the elevated side.
- Place a small, firm pillow under the head.

Position of part

- Adjust the patient by rotating the side of interest toward the table until a body rotation of 25 to 30 degrees is achieved.
- Check the degree of rotation at several points along the anterior surface of the body.
- Center the body so a point 1 inch (2.5 cm) medial to the ASIS closest to the film is centered to the grid.
- Adjust the shoulders to lie in the same transverse plane.
- Place supports under the ankles and under the flexed knee.

- Adjust the position of the elevated thigh to place the ASIS in the same plane (Figs. 8-126 and 8-127).
- The forearm and flexed knee usually furnish sufficient support for this position.
- Center the cassette at the level of the ASIS.
- *Shield gonads.* Collimating close to the joint may shield the gonads in males. It may be difficult to use contact shielding on females.
- Ask the patient to suspend respiration for the exposure.

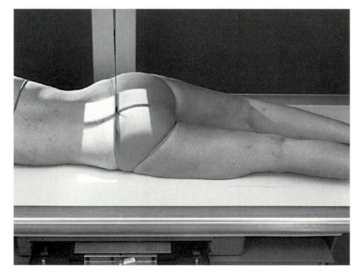

Fig. 8-126. PA oblique sacroiliac joint. LAO demonstrates left joint.

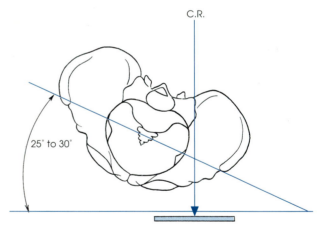

Fig. 8-127. Degree of obliquity required to demonstrate sacroiliac joint for a PA projection.

Central ray

- Direct the central ray perpendicular to the film, centered 1 inch (2.5 cm) medial to the lower ASIS.
- Use close collimation.

Structures shown

The resulting image will show the sacroiliac joint *closest* to the film (Fig. 8-128).

☐Evaluation criteria

The following should be clearly demonstrated:

- Open joint space closest to the film or minimal overlapping of the ilium and sacrum.
- Joint centered on the radiograph.

NOTE: A PA axial oblique can be obtained by positioning the patient as described above. For the PA axial oblique, direct the central ray 20 to 25 degrees caudad to enter the patient at the level of the transverse plane passing 1½ inches (4 cm) distal to the fifth lumbar spinous process; it will exit at the level of the anterior superior iliac spine (Fig. 8-129).

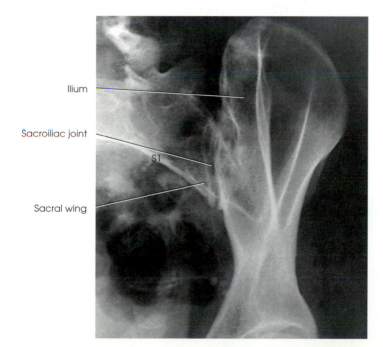

Ilium

Sacroiliac joint

S1

Sacral wing

Fig. 8-128. PA oblique sacroiliac joint. LAO demonstrates left joint.

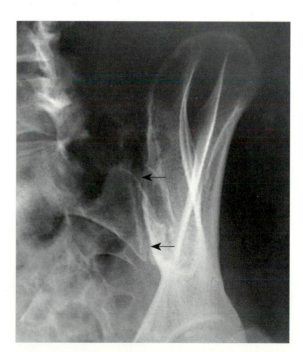

Fig. 8-129. PA axial oblique sacroiliac joint. LAO with 20-degree caudal central ray demonstrates left joint (*arrows*).

Symphysis Pubis
PA PROJECTION
CHAMBERLAIN METHOD FOR ABNORMAL SACROILIAC MOTION

Chamberlain[1] recommends the following upright projections in cases of sacroiliac slippage or relaxation:

1. A conventional lateral projection centered to the lumbosacral junction. Chamberlain prefers to have this image made with the patient upright.
2. Two PA projections of the pubic bones, with the patient in the upright position and with weight bearing on the alternate limbs to demonstrate symphysis pubis reaction by a change in the normal relation of the pubic bones in cases of sacroiliac slippage or relaxation.

This examination requires two blocks or supports approximately 6 inches high, the blocks being alternately removed to allow one leg to hang free.

Film: 8 × 10 in (18 × 24 cm) lengthwise for each exposure.

---

[1]Chamberlain WE: The symphysis pubis in the roentgen examination of the sacroiliac joint, AJR 24:621-625, 1930.

Position of patient

- Place the patient upright, facing the vertical grid device, standing on the two blocks.
- Adjust the height of the grid, and center the film to the symphysis pubis.

Position of part

- Center the median sagittal plane of the body to the midline of the grid, and adjust the ASISs equidistant from the film.
- The patient should grasp the sides of the device to steady himself or herself but must not be allowed to aid in supporting his or her weight in this way.
- If needed, place a compression band across the pelvis to immobilize the patient but not to aid in supporting the weight of the body.
- For the first exposure, remove one of the blocks so that one leg hangs free.
- The patient should be instructed to "let the leg hang like a dead weight," so there is no muscular resistance.
- For the second exposure, replace the first support and remove the opposite one permitting the second leg to hang free. Chamberlain suggests that the identification marker be placed on the weight-bearing side (Fig. 8-130).
- *Shield gonads.*
- Ask the patient to suspend respiration for the exposures.

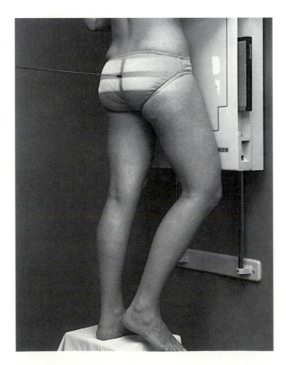

Fig. 8-130. PA symphysis pubis for demonstration of sacroiliac slippage.

Central ray

- Direct the central ray perpendicular and center to the symphysis pubis.
- Use close collimation.

Structures shown

The two images will show PA projections of the symphysis pubis. Abnormal motion of the sacroiliac joints will be demonstrated by a change in the normal relation of the pubic bones to each other when the body weight is borne on one leg (Figs. 8-131 and 8-132).

□ Evaluation criteria

The following should be clearly demonstrated:

- Symphysis pubis in the center of the radiograph.
- No rotation of the patient.
- Identification marker placed on the weight-bearing side.

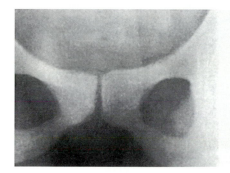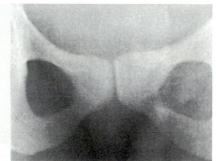

Fig. 8-131. PA symphysis pubis in a normal female patient.

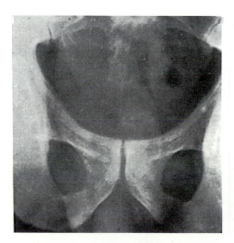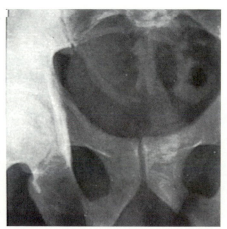

Fig. 8-132. PA symphysis in a normal male patient.

Sacrum and Coccyx

AP PROJECTION
PA AXIAL PROJECTION

Because bowel content may interfere with the image, it is particularly desirable to have the colon free of gas and fecal material for examinations of the sacrum and coccyx. A physician's order for a bowel preparation may be needed. The urinary bladder should be emptied before the examination.

Film: 10 × 12 in (24 × 30 cm) for sacrum; 8 × 10 in (18 × 24 cm) for coccyx.

Position of patient

- The patient is usually placed in the supine position for the AP axial projection of the sacrum and coccyx so the bones are as close as possible to the film. The prone position can be used without appreciable loss of detail and should be used with patients who have a painful injury or destructive disease.

Position of part

- With the patient either supine or prone, center the median sagittal plane of the body to the midline of the table grid.
- Adjust the patient so both anterior superior iliac spines are equidistant from the grid.

- Have the patient flex the elbows and place the arms in a comfortable, bilaterally symmetrical position.
- Adjust the shoulders to lie in the same horizontal plane.
- When the pelvis is rotated by a soft tissue abnormality (swelling or atrophy), adjust a radiolucent support under the low side.

- When the patient is supine, a support should be placed under the knees.
- Center the cassette to the central ray.
- *Shield gonads* on men. Women cannot be shielded for this projection.
- Ask the patient to suspend respiration for the exposure.

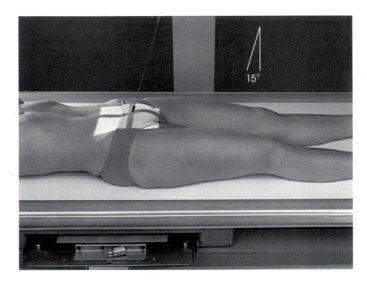

Fig. 8-133. AP axial sacrum.

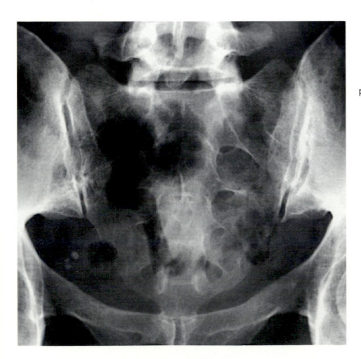

Fig. 8-134. AP axial sacrum.

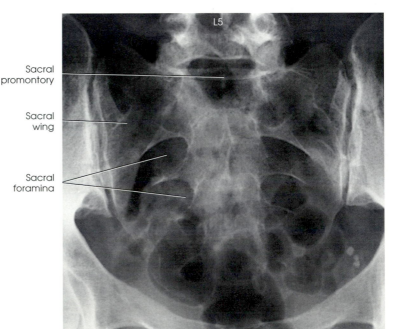

Fig. 8-135. PA axial sacrum.

Central ray

Sacrum

- With the patient supine, direct the central ray 15 degrees cephalad, and center to a point 2 inches superior to the symphysis pubis (Figs. 8-133 and 8-134).
- With the patient prone, angle the central ray 15 degrees caudad and center it to the clearly visible sacral curve (Fig. 8-135).

Coccyx

- With the patient supine, direct the central ray 10 degrees caudad and center to a point about 2 inches superior to the symphysis pubis (Figs. 8-136 and 8-137).
- With the patient prone, angle the central ray 10 degrees cephalad and center it to the easily palpable coccyx.

Structures shown

The resulting image will show a projection of the sacrum or coccyx, free of superimposition (Figs. 8-134, 8-135, and 8-137).

□ **Evaluation criteria**

The following should be clearly demonstrated:

Sacrum

- Sacrum free of foreshortening with the sacral curvature straightened.
- Pubic bones not overlapping the sacrum.
- Short scale contrast.
- No rotation of the sacrum.
- Sacrum centered and seen in its entirety.
- Tight collimation evident to improve the radiographic contrast.
- Fecal material not overlapping the sacrum.

Coccyx

- Coccygeal segments not superimposed.
- Short scale contrast on the radiograph.
- No rotation.
- Coccyx centered and seen in its entirety.
- Tight collimation evident to improve the visibility.

Radiation protection

- Because the ovaries lie within the exposure area, close collimation for the female patient should be used to limit the irradiated area and the amount of scatter radiation.
- For male patients, use the gonad shielding in addition to close collimation.

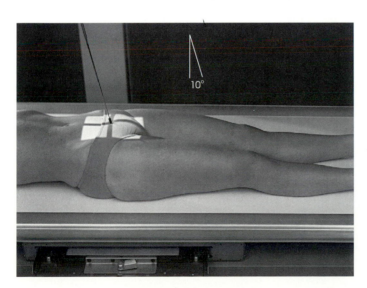

Fig. 8-136. AP coccyx.

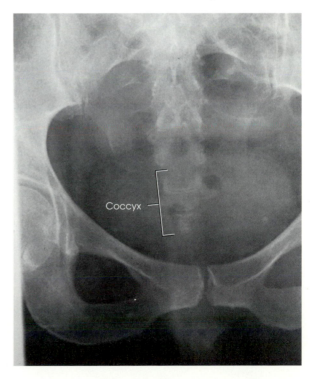

Fig. 8-137. AP coccyx.

Sacrum and Coccyx

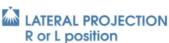

LATERAL PROJECTION
R or L position

Film: 10 × 12 in (24 × 30 cm) for sacrum; 8 × 10 in (18 × 24 cm) for coccyx.

Position of patient

- Ask the patient to turn onto the indicated side and flex the hips and knees to a comfortable position.

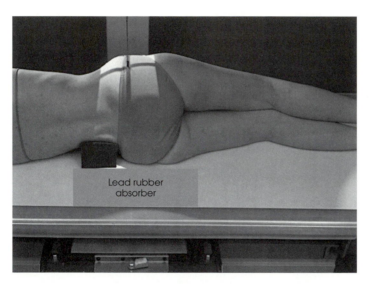

Fig. 8-138. Lateral sacrum.

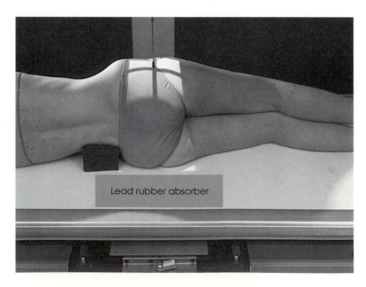

Fig. 8-139. Lateral coccyx.

Position of part

- For the sacrum, position the body so that a plane passing 3 inches posterior to the median coronal plane is centered to the midline of the grid (Fig. 8-138).
- A radiolucent sponge/support may be placed under the lumbar region to place the vertebral column parallel with the table.
- The coccyx lies approximately 5 inches posterior to the median coronal plane; its exact position depends on the pelvic curve. It can be easily palpated between the buttocks at the base of the spine, and the body can then be aligned to place the coccyx over the center line of the grid (Fig. 8-139).
- Adjust the arms in a position at right angles to the body, and have the patient grasp the side of the table with the upper hand to aid in maintaining the position.
- Superimpose the knees, and elevate the lower knee to hip level and support it on sandbags.
- If needed, place positioning sponges under and between the ankles and between the knees.
- Adjust a support under the body to place the long axis of the spine horizontal.
- Adjust the pelvis so that there is no rotation from the exact lateral position.
- Position the film so that its midpoint is at the level of the ASIS for the sacrum or at the level of the center of the coccyx.
- *Shield gonads.*
- Ask the patient to suspend respiration for the exposure.

Central ray

- *Sacrum:* Direct the central ray perpendicular to the film at the level of the ASIS and a plane 3 in (7.5 cm) posterior to the median coronal plane.
- *Coccyx:* Direct the central ray perpendicular through the coccyx at the level of the center of the coccyx and a plane 5 in (13 cm) posterior to the median coronal plane.
- Use close collimation.

Structures shown

The resulting image will show a lateral projection of the sacrum or coccyx (Figs. 8-140 and 8-141).

☐ Evaluation criteria

The following should be clearly demonstrated:

- Sacrum and coccyx seen clearly with short scale contrast.
- Use of tight collimation and a lead rubber absorber.
- Closely superimposed posterior margins of the ischia and ilia.
- Sacrum and coccyx.

Improving radiographic quality

The quality of the radiograph can be improved if a sheet of leaded rubber is placed on the table behind the patient, as shown in the photographs. The lead will absorb the scatter radiation coming from the patient; scatter radiation serves only to decrease the quality of the radiograph. More important perhaps is that with automatic exposure control (AEC), the scatter radiation coming from the patient is often sufficient to prematurely terminate the exposure. The resultant radiograph may be underexposed because of the effect of the scatter radiation on the AEC device. For the same reason, close collimation is necessary for lateral sacrum and coccyx images.

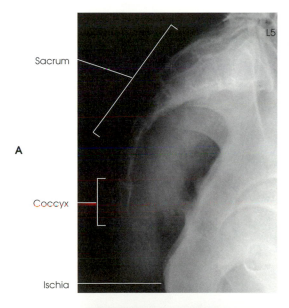

A

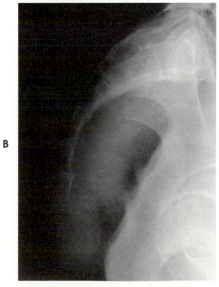

B

Fig. 8-140. A and **B,** Lateral sacrum.

(**B,** courtesy John Syring, R.T.)

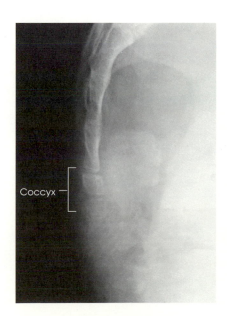

Fig. 8-141. Lateral coccyx.

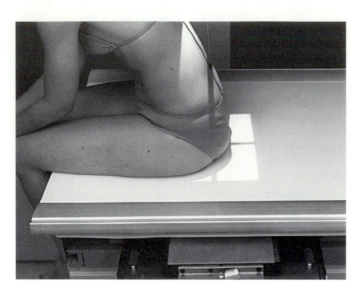

Fig. 8-142. Slight flexion.

Sacral Vertebral Canal and Sacroiliac Joints

AXIAL PROJECTION
NÖLKE METHOD

Film: 8 × 10 in (18 × 24 cm) or 10 × 12 in (24 × 30 cm) crosswise.

Position of patient

- In the examination of the sacral vertebral canal, seat the patient on the end of the table and flex the spine in different degrees for the several regions of the canal. The exact degree of flexion depends on the curvature of the sacrum.
- Seat the patient far enough back on the table to center the median coronal plane of the body to the horizontal axis of the Bucky tray.
- If the patient is too short to be comfortably seated so far back, the cassette can be shifted off center in the Bucky tray so that its midpoint will coincide with the region of the canal being projected (unless contraindicated by using automatic exposure control or automatic collimation.)
- Support the feet on a chair or a stool.

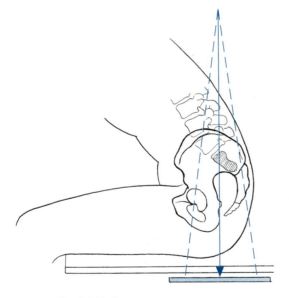

Fig. 8-143. Slight flexion alignment.

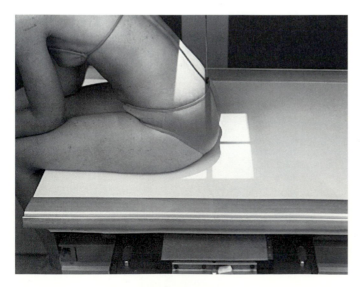

Fig. 8-144. Moderate flexion.

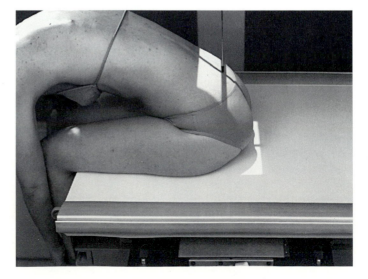

Fig. 8-145. Hyperflexion.

Position of part

- Adjust the position of the body so that the median sagittal plane is perpendicular to the midline of the grid.
- Have the patient lean forward enough so that the upper, middle, or lower portion of the sacral vertebral canal is vertical.
- The patient should not lean laterally.
- Have the patient grasp the sides of the table, or his or her legs or ankles, depending on the degree of leaning, to maintain the position.
- With the cassette in the Bucky tray, center to the vertically placed portion of the sacrum (Figs. 8-142 to 8-145).
- Respiration need not be suspended for the exposure unless the patient's breathing is labored.

Central ray

- Direct the central ray perpendicular to the long axis of the sacrum.
- Use close collimation.

Structures shown

The resulting image with the spine slightly flexed will show the lower sacral vertebral canal, the junction of the sacrum and coccyx, and the last lumbar vertebra (Fig. 8-146).

With the patient leaning forward in a position of moderate flexion, as illustrated in Fig. 8-144, the resultant image shows a cross section of the upper and lower sacral vertebral canal. The sacroiliac joints are also demonstrated in this position (Fig. 8-147).

With the patient leaning forward in a position of acute flexion, as illustrated in Fig. 8-145, the resultant image (Fig. 8-148) shows the upper sacral vertebral canal projected into the angle formed by the ascending rami of the ischial bones just posterior to the symphysis pubis. The spinous process of the last lumbar segment is projected across the shadow of the canal.

☐ Evaluation criteria

The following should be clearly demonstrated:

- Sacral vertebral canal in the center of the exposure area.
- No lateral rotation of the patient.

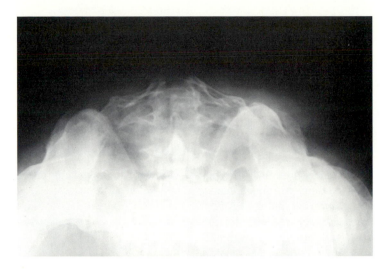

Fig. 8-146. Slight flexion.

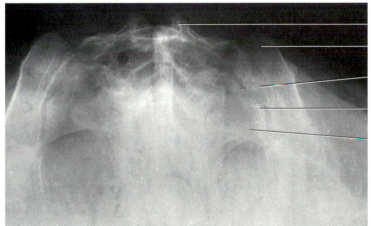

Sacral horn (cornu)

Ischial tuberosity

Obturator foramen

Sacroiliac joint

Inferior pubic ramus

Fig. 8-147. Moderate flexion.

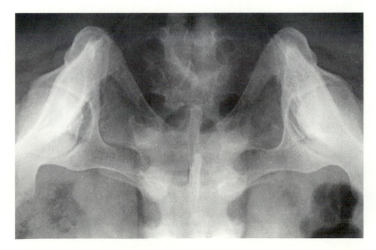

Fig. 8-148. Hyperflexion.

Lumbar Intervertebral Disks

PA PROJECTION
R and L bending
WEIGHT-BEARING

Film: 14 × 17 in (35 × 43 cm) lengthwise.

Position of patient

• This examination is done with the patient in the standing position. Duncan and Hoen[1] recommend that the PA projection be used, because in this direction the divergent rays are more nearly parallel with the intervertebral disk spaces.

Position of part

• With the patient facing the vertical grid device, adjust the height of the grid to be at the level of the third lumbar vertebra.
• Adjust the pelvis for rotation by ensuring that the anterior superior iliac spines are equidistant from the film.
• Center the median sagittal plane of the patient's body to the midline of the vertical grid device.

[1]Duncan W, and Hoen T: A new approach to the diagnosis of herniation of the intervertebral disc, Surg Gynecol Obstet 75:257-267, 1942.

• Adjust the shoulders to lie in the same horizontal plane and let the arms hang unsupported by the sides.
• Make one radiograph with the patient *bending* to the right and one with the patient *bending* to the left (Fig. 8-149).
• Have the patient lean directly lateral as far as possible without rotation and without lifting the foot.
• The degree of bending must not be forced, and the patient must not be supported in position.
• *Shield gonads.*
• Ask the patient to suspend respiration for the exposure.

Central ray

• Direct the central ray to the third lumbar vertebra at an angle of 15 to 20 degrees caudad, or direct it perpendicular to L3.
• Use close collimation.

Structures shown

The resulting image will show bending PA projections of the lower thoracic region and the lumbar region for demonstration of the mobility of the intervertebral joints. This type of examination is used in cases of disk protrusion to localize the involved joint as shown by limitation of motion at the site of the lesion (Fig. 8-150).

□ **Evaluation criteria**

The following should be clearly demonstrated:
■ Area from the lower thoracic interspaces to all of the sacrum.
■ No rotation of the patient in the bending position.
■ Bending direction must be correctly identified on the image with appropriate lead markers.

Radiation protection

The PA projection is recommended over the AP projection whenever the clinical information provided by the examination is not compromised. In the PA projection, the amount of radiation received by the gonad area and breast tissue of the patient is significantly reduced compared to the AP projection. Proper collimation will also reduce the radiation dose to the patient. In addition to proper collimation, lead shielding material should be placed between the x-ray tube and the male patient's gonads to further protect the patient from unnecessary radiation.

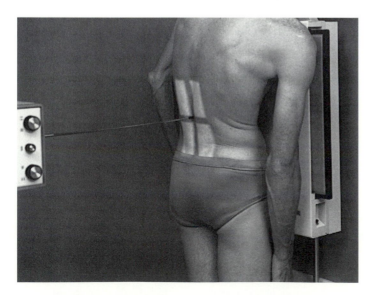

Fig. 8-149. PA lumbar intervertebral disks with right bending.

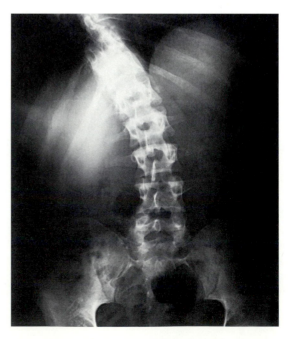

Fig. 8-150. PA lumbar intervertebral disks with right bending.

Scoliosis Radiography

Scoliosis is an abnormal lateral curvature of the vertebral column with some associated rotation of the vertebral bodies at the curve. This condition may be caused by disease, surgery, or trauma, but it is frequently idiopathic. Scoliosis is commonly detected in the adolescent years, and if not detected and treated, it may progress to the point of debilitation.

Diagnosis and monitoring of scoliosis requires a series of radiographs which may include upright, supine, and bending studies. A typical scoliosis study might include the following projections:

- PA[1] (or AP) upright
- PA (or AP) upright with lateral bending
- Lateral upright (with or without bending)
- PA (or AP) prone or supine

---

[1]Frank ED, et al: Use of the posteroanterior projection: a method of reducing x-ray exposure to specific radiosensitive organs. Radiol Technol 54(5), 343-347, 1983.

The AP or PA and lateral upright projections demonstrate the amount/degree of curvature with the force of gravity acting upon the body. Spinal fixation devices, such as Harrington rods, may also be evaluated. Bending studies are often used to differentiate primary from compensatory curves. Primary curves will not change when the patient bends; secondary curves will.

Since scoliosis is generally diagnosed and evaluated during the teenage years, proper radiographic techniques are important. Ideally, large film-screen systems and grids, such as 14×36 inches, are used to demonstrate the entire spine with one exposure. Due to the wide range of body part thickness and specific gravities in the thoracic and abdominal areas, compensating filters are used.

Radiation protection is crucial. Collimation must be closely limited to irradiate only the thoracic and lumbar spine. The gonads should be shielded by placing a lead apron at the level of the anterior superior iliac spines between the patient and the x-ray tube. The breasts should be shielded with leaded rubber or leaded acrylic,[1,2] or the breast exposure decreased by performing PA projections. Rare earth screens and high kVp techniques will also decrease the radiation dose.

---

[1]Frank ED and Kuntz JI: A simple method of protecting the breasts during upright lateral radiography for spine deformities. Radiol Technol, 55(1), 532-535, 1983.
[2]Butler PF et al: Simple methods to reduce patient exposure during scoliosis radiography. Radiol Technol 57(5):411-417, 1986.

Scoliosis Series

THORACIC AND LUMBAR SPINE

 ### AP, PA, OR LATERAL PROJECTIONS
FERGUSON METHOD[1]

The patient should be positioned to obtain a PA projection, in lieu of the AP, to reduce the radiation exposure[2] to selected radiosensitive organs. The decision whether to take a PA or AP projection is often determined by the physician and/or institutional policy.

Film: 14×36 in (35×90 cm) or 14×17 in (35×43 cm) placed lengthwise for each exposure.

Position of patient

- Place the patient in position, preferably for a PA projection, either seated or standing, before a vertical grid device.
- Have the patient sit or stand straight,

[1]Ferguson AB: Roentgen diagnosis of the extremities and spine, New York, 1939, Harper & Row, Publishers.
[2]Frank ED, et al: Use of the posteroanterior projection: a method of reducing x-ray exposure to specific radiosensitive organs. Radiol Technol 54(5), 343-347, 1983.

and then adjust the height of the cassette to include about 1 inch of the crests of the ilia (Fig. 8-151).

Position of part

- *For the first radiograph,* adjust the patient in a normally seated or standing position to check the spinal curvature.
- Center the median sagittal plane of the body to the midline of the grid.
- Allow the arms to hang relaxed at the sides; if the patient is seated, flex the elbows and rest the hands on the lap (Fig. 8-152).
- Do not support the patient or use a compression band.
- *Shield gonads.*
- *For the second radiograph,* elevate the hip or foot of the convex side of the primary curve approximately 3 or 4 inches (7.5 to 10 cm) by placing a block, a book, or sandbags under the buttock or the foot (Fig. 8-153). Ferguson[1] specifies that the elevation

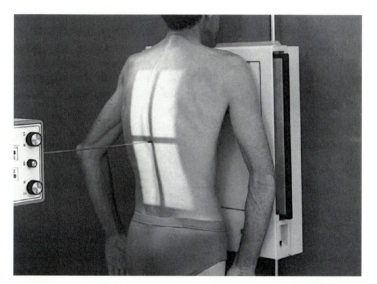

Fig. 8-151. PA thoracic and lumbar spine for scoliosis, upright.

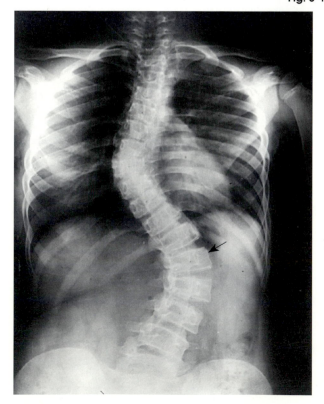

Fig. 8-152. PA thoracic and lumbar spine for scoliosis, upright, demonstrating structural (major or primary) curve (arrow).

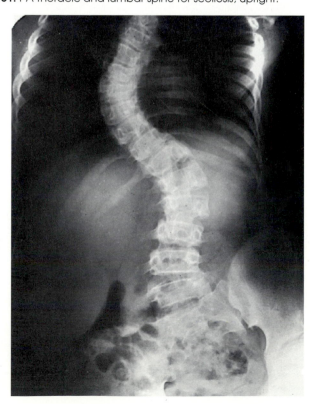

Fig. 8-153. PA thoracic and lumbar spine with left hip elevated.

must be sufficient to make the patient expend some effort in maintaining the position.

- Do not support the patient in these positions.
- Do not employ a compression band.
- *Shield gonads.*
- Ask the patient to suspend respiration for the exposures.
- Additional radiographs may be obtained by elevating the hip of the side *opposite* the major or primary curve (Fig. 8-154) and/or with the patient recumbent (Fig. 8-155).

Central ray

- Direct the central ray perpendicular to the midpoint of the film.

Structures shown

The resulting images will show PA or AP projections of the thoracic and lumbar vertebrae used for comparison to distinguish the deforming, or primary, curve from the compensatory curve in cases of scoliosis (Figs. 8-152 to 8-156).

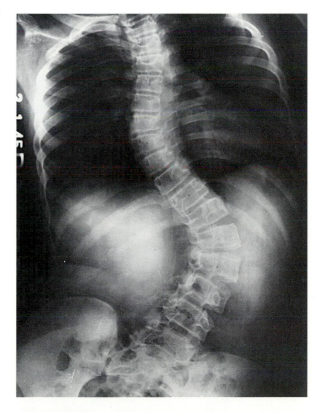

Fig. 8-154. PA thoracic and lumbar spine with right hip elevated.

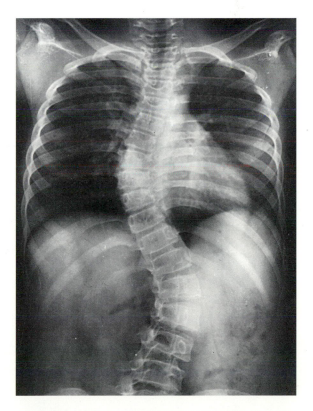

Fig. 8-155. PA thoracic and lumbar spine for scoliosis, prone.

□ Evaluation criteria

The following should be clearly demonstrated:

- Thoracic and lumbar vertebrae to include about 1 inch of the iliac crests.
- Vertebral column aligned down the center of the radiograph.
- Correct identification marker.

Lateral scoliosis radiography

Lateral scoliosis radiographs are obtained with the same considerations as above. The patient is placed in the lateral position with a radiograph obtained as shown in Fig. 8-157.

NOTE: Another widely used scoliosis series consists of four images of the thoracic and lumbar spine: (1) a direct PA projection with the patient standing, (2) a direct PA projection with the patient prone, and (3) and (4) PA projections with alternate right and left lateral flexion in the prone position. The right and left bending positions are described on the following page. For the scoliosis series, however, 14 × 17 inch (35 × 43 cm) films are used and are placed to include about 1 inch of the crests of ilia.

Young, Oestreich, and Goldstein[1] have described their application of this scoliosis procedure in detail. They recommend the addition of a lateral position made with the patient standing upright to show spondylolisthesis or to demonstrate exaggerated degrees of kyphosis or lordosis.

Kittleson and Lim[2] have described both the Ferguson and the Cobb methods of measurement of scoliosis.

[1]Young LW, Oestreich AE, and Goldstein LA: Roentgenology in scoliosis: contribution to evaluation and management, Radiology 97:778-795, 1970.
[2]Kittleson AC, and Lim LW: Measurement of scoliosis, AJR 108:775-777, 1970.

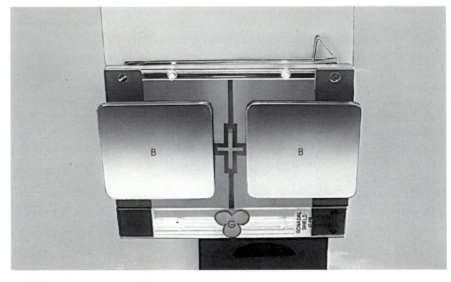

Fig. 8-156. AP thoracic and lumbar spine for scoliosis. **A,** Collimator face showing magnetically held breast shields (B) and gonad shield.(G) **B,** AP projection showing well protected breasts and gonads.

(Courtesy Nuclear Associates.)

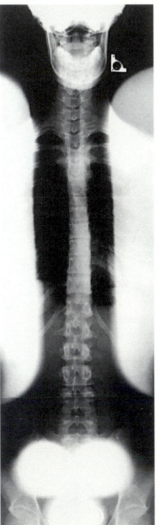

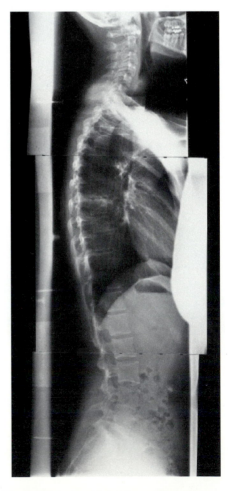

Fig. 8-157. Lateral full spine radiograph demonstrating value of thoracic and cervical filter. Breasts also shielded, with shadow shield.

(Courtesy Eugene D. Frank, R.T.)

Spinal Fusion Series

Lumbar Spine
AP PROJECTION
R and L bending

Film: 10 × 12 in (24 × 30 cm) or 14 × 17 in (35 × 43 cm) placed lengthwise for each exposure.

Position of patient

- Place the patient in the supine position, and center the median sagittal plane of the body to the midline of the grid.

Position of part

- Make the first radiograph with maximum right bending and the second with maximum left bending.
- To obtain equal bending force throughout the spine, cross the patient's leg on the opposite side to be flexed over the other leg. For example, a right bending requires the left leg to be crossed over the right.
- Both heels should be drawn toward the side flexed and immobilized with the sandbags.
- Next, draw the shoulders directly lateral as far as possible without rotating the pelvis (Fig. 8-158).
- After the patient is in position a compression band may be applied to prevent movement.
- *Shield gonads.*
- Ask the patient to suspend respiration for the exposure.

Central ray

- Direct the central ray perpendicular to the level of the third lumbar vertebra.

Structures shown

The resulting images show AP projections of the lumbar vertebrae, made in maximum right and left lateral flexion (Figs. 8-159 and 8-160). These studies are employed (1) in cases of early scoliosis to determine the presence of structural change when bending to the right and left, (2) to localize a herniated disk as shown by limitation of motion at the site of the lesion, and (3) to demonstrate whether there is motion in the area of a spinal fusion. The latter examination is usually performed 6 months after the fusion operation.

□ **Evaluation criteria**

The following should be clearly demonstrated:

- Site of the spinal fusion centered and including superior and inferior vertebrae.
- No rotation of the pelvis.
- Bending directions correctly identified with appropriate lead markers.
- Sufficient radiographic density to demonstrate the degree of movement when they are superimposed.

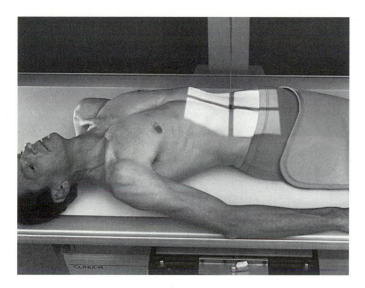

Fig. 8-158. AP lumbar spine, right bending.

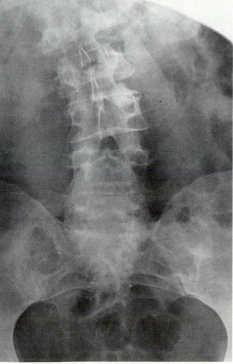

Fig. 8-159. AP lumbar spine, right bending fusion series.

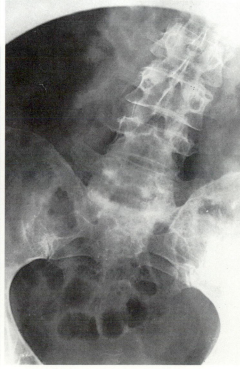

Fig. 8-160. AP lumbar spine, left bending fusion series.

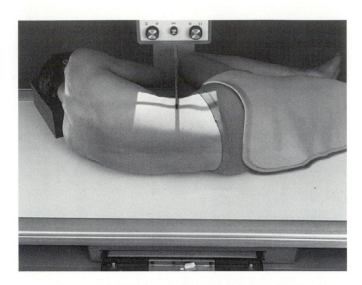

Fig. 8-161. Hyperflexion position.

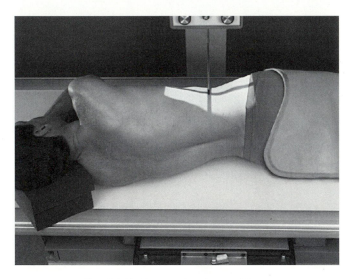

Fig. 8-162. Hyperextension position.

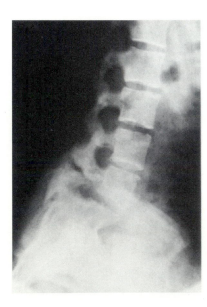

Fig. 8-163. Lateral with hyperextension.

(Courtesy Dr. Lawson E. Miller, Jr.)

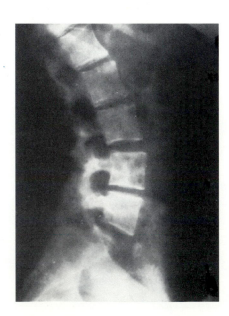

Fig. 8-164. Lateral with hyperflexion.

Spinal Fusion Series
Lumbar Spine
LATERAL PROJECTION
R or L position
Hyperflexion and hyperextension

Film: 14 × 17 in (35 × 43 cm) placed lengthwise for each exposure.

Position of patient

- Adjust the patient in a lateral recumbent position.
- Center the median coronal plane to the midline of the grid.

Position of part

- *For the first radiograph,* have the patient lean forward and draw the thighs up to forcibly flex the spine as much as possible (Fig. 8-161).
- *For the second radiograph,* have the patient lean the thorax backward and posteriorly extend the thighs and limbs as much as possible (Fig. 8-162).
- After the patient is in position, a compression band may be applied across the pelvis to prevent movement.
- Center the cassette at the level of the spinal fusion.
- *Shield gonads.*
- Ask the patient to suspend respiration for the exposures.

Central ray

- Direct the central ray perpendicular to the spinal fusion area or to the third lumbar vertebra.

Structures shown

The resulting images will show two lateral projections of the spine made in hyperflexion (Fig. 8-163) and hyperextension (Fig. 8-164) for the purpose of determining whether there is motion in the area of a spinal fusion or to localize a herniated disk as shown by limitation of motion at the site of the lesion.

☐ Evaluation criteria

The following should be clearly demonstrated:

- Site of the spinal fusion in the center of the radiograph.
- No rotation of the vertebral column.
- Hyperflexion and hyperextension identification markers correctly used for each respective projection.
- Density of the radiographs sufficient to demonstrate the degree of movement when the two images are superimposed.

Chapter 9

BONY THORAX

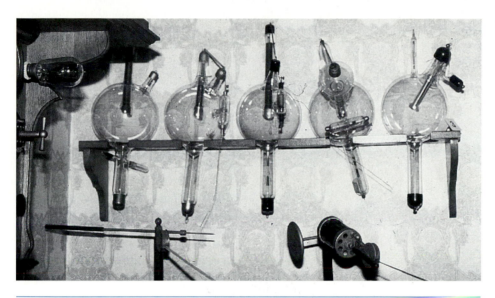

As voltages changed during the radiography of different body parts, it was the operator's responsibility to change the x-ray tubes. X-ray tubes shown were used with x-ray unit from 1901 that is shown at the beginning of Chapter 1.

The bony thorax is formed by the sternum, the 12 pairs of ribs, and the 12 thoracic vertebrae. The bony thorax protects the heart and lungs. Conical in shape, the bony thorax is narrower above than it is below, wider than it is deep, and longer posteriorly than it is anteriorly.

Sternum

The *sternum* (breastbone) (Figs. 9-1 to 9-3) is directed anteriorly and inferiorly, centered over the midline of the anterior thorax. A narrow, flat bone about 6 inches in length, the sternum consists of three parts: the manubrium sterni, body (corpus, gladiolus), and xiphoid process (ensiform). The sternum supports the clavicles at the superior manubrial angles and provides attachment to the costal cartilages of the first seven pairs of ribs at the lateral borders.

The *manubrium sterni,* the superior portion of the sternum, is quadrilateral in shape and the widest portion of the sternum. The superior border of the manubrium has an easily palpable concavity at its center, termed the *jugular* (manubrial or suprasternal) *notch*. In the upright position, the jugular notch of the average subject lies anterior to the interspace between the second and third thoracic vertebrae. On each side of the jugular notch the manubrium slants laterally and posteriorly and bears an articular surface for the reception of the sternal extremity of the clavicle. On the lateral borders, immediately below the articular notches for the clavicles, are shallow depressions for the attachment of the cartilages of the first pair of ribs.

The *body* (corpus, gladiolus), the longest part of the sternum, is joined to the manubrium at the *sternal angle*. This obtuse angle lies at the level of the junction of the second costal cartilage. Both the manubrium and body contribute to the attachment of the second costal cartilage. The succeeding five pairs of costal cartilages are attached to the lateral borders of the body. The sternal angle is palpable and, in the normally formed thorax, lies anterior to the interspace between the fourth and fifth thoracic vertebrae when the body is upright.

The *xiphoid* (ensiform) *process,* the distal and smallest part of the sternum, is cartilaginous in early life and partially or completely ossifies, particularly the superior portion, in later life. The xiphoid process is variable in shape and often deviates from the midline of the body. In the normal thorax, the xiphoid process lies over the tenth thoracic vertebra and is a useful bony landmark for locating the superior portion of the liver and the inferior border of the heart.

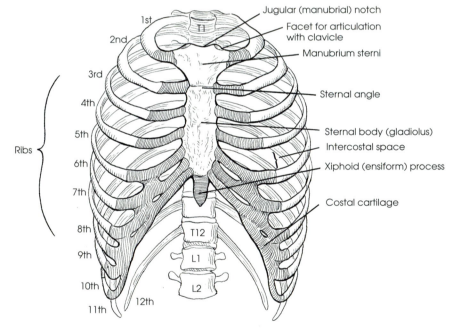

1st
2nd
3rd
4th
5th
6th
7th
8th
9th
10th
11th
12th
Ribs
T1
T12
L1
L2

Jugular (manubrial) notch
Facet for articulation with clavicle
Manubrium sterni
Sternal angle
Sternal body (gladiolus)
Intercostal space
Xiphoid (ensiform) process
Costal cartilage

Fig. 9-1. Anterior aspect of bony thorax.

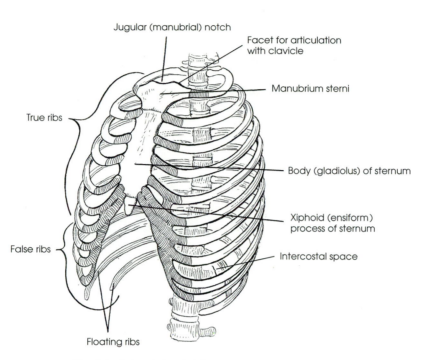

Fig. 9-2. Anterolateral oblique aspect of bony thorax.

Jugular (manubrial) notch

Facet for articulation with clavicle

Manubrium sterni

True ribs

Body (gladiolus) of sternum

Xiphoid (ensiform) process of sternum

Intercostal space

False ribs

Floating ribs

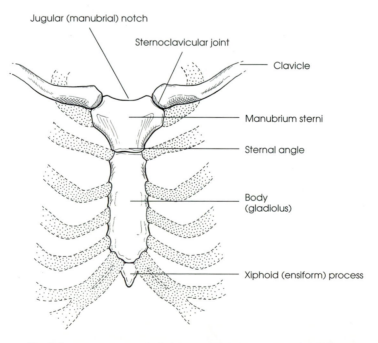

Fig. 9-3. Anterior aspect of sternum and sternoclavicular joints.

Jugular (manubrial) notch

Sternoclavicular joint

Clavicle

Manubrium sterni

Sternal angle

Body (gladiolus)

Xiphoid (ensiform) process

Ribs

There are 12 pairs of ribs numbered consecutively from the top inferiorly (Figs. 9-1, 9-2, and 9-4). Each rib is a long narrow curved bone with an anteriorly attached piece of hyaline cartilage, the *costal cartilage*. The ribs are situated in an oblique plane slanting anteriorly and inferiorly so that their anterior ends lie 3 to 5 inches below the level of their vertebral ends. The degree of obliquity gradually increases from the first to the ninth rib and then decreases to the twelfth rib. The spaces between the ribs are referred to as the *intercostal spaces*. The ribs vary in breadth and length. The first rib is the shortest and broadest; the breadth gradually decreases to the twelfth rib, the narrowest rib. The length increases from the first to the seventh rib and then gradually decreases to the twelfth rib.

A typical rib (Figs. 9-5 and 9-6) consists of a *head,* a flattened *neck,* a *tubercle,* and a *shaft.* The eleventh rib has a small tubercle and no facet on the head. The twelfth rib has no facet on the head, with a tubercle that is poorly marked or completely absent. From the point of articulation with the vertebral body, the rib projects posteriorly at an oblique angle to the point of articulation with the transverse process. The rib turns laterally to the angle of the shaft, where the bone arches anteriorly, medially, and inferiorly in an oblique plane. Located along the inferior and internal border of each rib are costal arteries, veins, and nerves. Trauma to the ribs can damage these neurovascular structures, causing pain and hemorrhage.

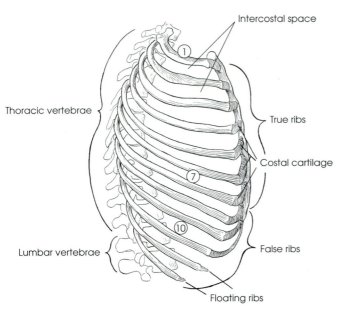

Fig. 9-4. Lateral aspect of bony thorax.

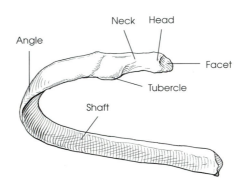

Fig. 9-5. A typical rib viewed from the back.

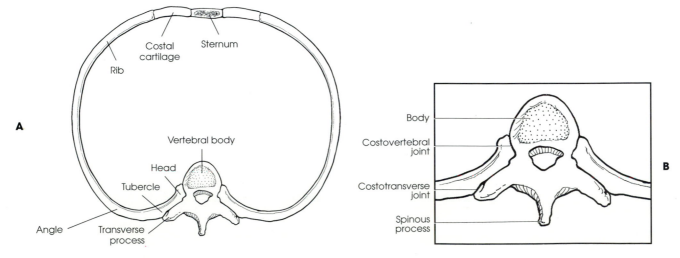

Fig. 9-6. A, Superior aspect of rib articulating with thoracic vertebra and sternum.
B, Enlarged image of costovertebral articulations.

Bony Thorax Articulations

The *sternoclavicular joints* (Fig. 9-3) are the only points of articulation between the upper limbs and the trunk. Formed by the articulation between the sternal extremity of the clavicles and the clavicular notches of the manubrium, these synovial (diarthrotic) plane or gliding joints permit limited movement that consists of the gliding of one surface on the other. A circular disk of fibrocartilage is interposed in each joint between the articular ends of the bones, and the joints are enclosed in articular capsules.

Posteriorly, the *head* of a rib is closely bound to the demifacets of two adjacent *vertebral bodies,* to form a synovial (diarthrotic) plane or gliding articulation called the *costovertebral joint* (Figs. 9-6 and 9-7). The first, tenth, eleventh, and twelfth ribs each articulate with only one vertebral body.

The *tubercle* of a rib articulates with the anterior surface of the *transverse process* of the lower vertebra at the *costotransverse joint,* and the head of the rib articulates at the costovertebral joint. The head of the rib also articulates with the body of the same vertebra and articulates with the vertebra directly above. The costotransverse articulation is also a synovial (diarthrotic) plane or gliding articulation. The articulations between the tubercles of the ribs and the transverse processes of the vertebrae permit only slight superior and inferior movements of the first six pairs. Greater freedom of movement is permitted in the succeeding four pairs.

Anteriorly, the cartilages of the first seven pairs of ribs are attached directly to the sternum, and these ribs are called *true* (vertebrosternal) *ribs* (Fig. 9-4). The cartilage of the succeeding three pairs of ribs are attached to superjacent cartilage, and these ribs are called *false* (vertebrochondral) *ribs*. The last two pairs, also considered false ribs, have their cartilage ending in the musculature and are called *floating* (vertebral) *ribs*.

Costochondral articulations are found between the anterior extremities of the ribs and the costal cartilages. These articulations are fibrous and allow no movement. The articulations between the costal cartilages of the true ribs and the sternum are called *sternocostal joints*. The first pair of ribs, rigidly attached to the sternum, forms the first *sternocostal joint*. This is a synarthrosis type of joint, allowing no movement. The second through seventh sternocostal joints are considered synovial (diarthrotic) plane or gliding joints. *Interchondral joints* are found between the costal cartilages of the sixth, seventh, eighth, ninth, and tenth ribs. The interchondral joints are synovial (diarthrotic) plane or gliding articulations.

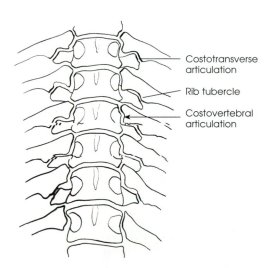

Fig. 9-7. Anterior aspect of costovertebral articulations.

- Costotransverse articulation
- Rib tubercle
- Costovertebral articulation

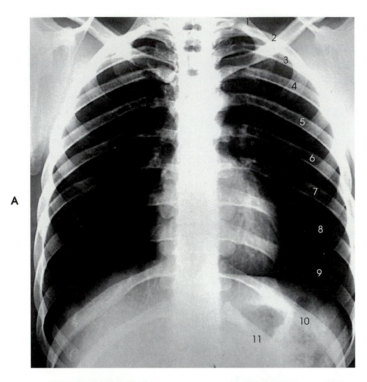

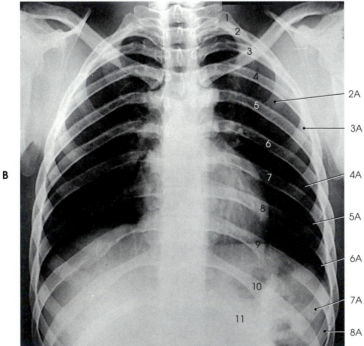

Fig. 9-8. Respiratory lung movement. **A,** Full inhalation showing posterior ribs numbered. **B,** Full exhalation with ribs numbered. Anterior ribs with *A* suffix.

RESPIRATORY EXCURSION

The normal oblique orientation of the ribs changes very little during quiet respiratory movements; however, *the degree of obliquity decreases with deep inhalation and increases with deep exhalation.* The first pair of ribs, which are rigidly attached to the manubrium, rotate at their vertebral ends and move with the sternum as one structure during respiratory movements.

On deep *inhalation* the anterior ends of the ribs are carried anteriorly, superiorly, and laterally, while their necks are rotated inferiorly (Fig. 9-8, *A*). On deep *exhalation* the anterior ends are carried inferiorly, posteriorly, and medially, while the necks are rotated superiorly (Fig. 9-8, *B*). The last two pairs of ribs are depressed and held in position by the action of the diaphragm when the anterior ends of the upper ribs are elevated during respiration.

DIAPHRAGM

The ribs situated above the diaphragm are best radiographically examined through the air-filled lungs, whereas those situated below the diaphragm must be examined through the upper abdomen. Because of the difference in penetration required for the two regions, the position and respiratory excursion of the diaphragm play a large part in radiography of the ribs.

The position of the diaphragm varies with body habitus, being at a higher level in hypersthenic subjects (see Figs. 3-7 to 3-10) and at a lower level in hyposthenic subjects. In sthenic subjects of average size and shape, the right side of the diaphragm arches posteriorly from the level of about the sixth or seventh costal cartilage to the level of the ninth or tenth thoracic vertebra when the body is in the upright position. The left side of the diaphragm will lie at a slightly lower level. Because of the oblique location of both the ribs and the diaphragm, several pairs of ribs appear, on radiographs, to lie partially above and partially below the diaphragm.

The position of the diaphragm changes considerably with the body position, reaching its lowest level when the body is upright and its highest level when the body is supine. For this reason it is desirable to place the patient in the upright position when examining the ribs above the diaphragm and in a recumbent position when examining the ribs below the diaphragm. When the body is in a lateral recumbent position, the diaphragm lies in an oblique plane, the side against the table being higher in position than the upper half.

The respiratory excursion of the diaphragm averages about 1½ inches between deep inhalation and deep exhalation. The excursion will be less in hypersthenic subjects and more in hyposthenic subjects. Deeper inhalation or exhalation, and therefore greater depression or elevation of the diaphragm, is achieved on the second respiratory movement than on the first. This point should be used when the ribs that lie at the diaphragmatic level are examined.

When the body is placed in the supine position, the anterior ends of the ribs are displaced superiorly, laterally, and posteriorly. For this reason the anterior ends of the ribs are less sharply visualized when the patient is radiographed in the supine position.

BODY POSITION

Although it is desirable in rib examinations to take advantage of the effect that body position has on the position of the diaphragm, the effect is not of sufficient importance to justify subjecting a patient to a painful change in position from the upright to the recumbent or vice versa. Rib injuries, minor as well as extensive, are painful, and even slight movement frequently causes the patient considerable distress. Therefore, unless the change can be effected with a tilting radiographic table, patients with recent injury should be examined in the position in which they arrive in the department. The ambulatory patient can be positioned for recumbent images with a minimum of discomfort by bringing the tilt table to the vertical position for each positioning change. The patient standing on the footboard can be comfortably adjusted and then lowered to the horizontal position.

TRAUMA PATIENTS

The first and usually the only requirement in the initial radiographic examination of a patient who has sustained severe trauma to the rib cage is to take an AP and lateral projection of the chest. These projections are obtained not only to demonstrate the site and extent of rib injury but also to investigate the possibility of injury to the underlying structures by depressed rib fractures. The patient is examined in the position in which he or she arrives, usually recumbent on a stretcher. This body position requires a recumbent position to demonstrate the presence of air and/or fluid levels using the decubitus technique.

Radiation Protection

Protection of the patient from unnecessary radiation is a professional responsibility of the radiographer. (See Chapter 1 for specific guidelines.) In this chapter, the "*Shield gonads*" statement indicates that the patient is to be protected from unnecessary radiation by restricting the radiation beam using proper collimation. Additionally, placing lead shielding between the gonads and the radiation source is appropriate when the clinical objectives of the examination are not compromised.

Sternum

The position of the sternum with respect to the denser thoracic structures, both bony and soft, makes it one of the more difficult structures to radiograph satisfactorily. Few problems are involved in obtaining a lateral projection, but, because of the location of the sternum directly anterior to the thoracic spine, an AP or PA projection contains little useful diagnostic information. To separate the vertebrae and sternum, it is necessary to rotate the body from the prone body position or to angle the central ray medially. The exact degree of angulation required depends on the depth of the chest; deep chests require less angulation than shallow chests (Figs. 9-9 and 9-10).

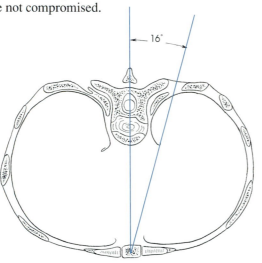

Fig. 9-9. Drawing of 26 cm chest.

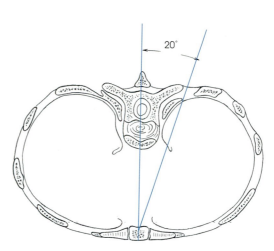

Fig. 9-10. Drawing of 18 cm chest.

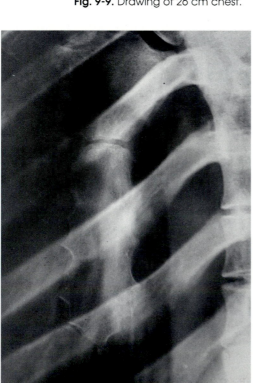

Fig. 9-11. PA oblique sternum. LAO.

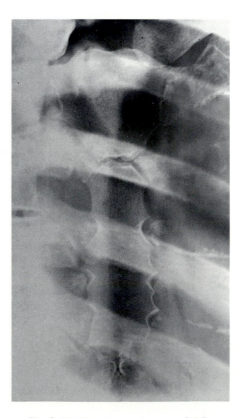

Fig. 9-12. PA oblique sternum. RAO.

(Courtesy Kalma Butler, R.T.)

Although angulation of the body or the central ray to project the sternum to the right of the thoracic vertebrae clears the sternum of the vertebrae, it superimposes the sternum over the posterior ribs and the lung markings (Fig. 9-11). If the sternum is projected to the left of the thoracic vertebrae, it is also projected over the heart and other mediastinal structures (Fig. 9-12). The superimposition of the homogeneous density of the heart can be used to advantage, as seen by comparing the two radiographs.

The pulmonary structures, particularly of elderly persons and of heavy smokers, can cast confusing markings over the sternum, unless the motion of *shallow* breathing is used to eliminate them. If motion is desired, the exposure time should be long enough to cover several phases of shallow respiration (Figs. 9-13 and 9-14). The mA must be relatively low to achieve the desired mAs.

If the female patient has large, pendulous breasts, they should be drawn to the sides and held in position with a wide bandage to prevent them from overlapping the sternum and to obtain closer proximity of the sternum to the cassette. This is particularly important in the lateral projection, in which the breast can obscure the inferior portion of the sternum.

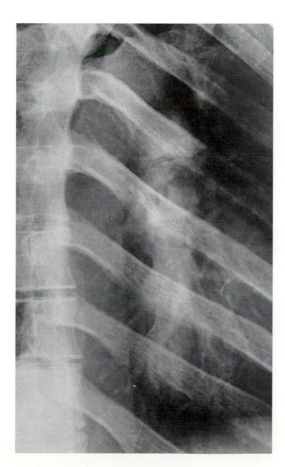

Fig. 9-13. Suspended respiration

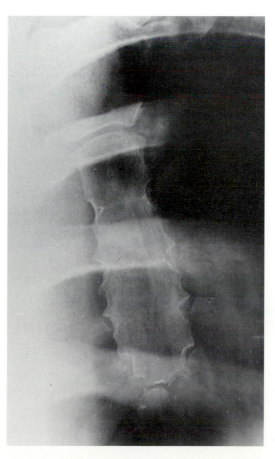

Fig. 9-14. Shallow breathing during exposure.

Sternum

 ### PA OBLIQUE PROJECTION
RAO position

Film: 10 × 12 in (24 × 30 cm) lengthwise.

Position of patient

- With the patient prone, adjust into an RAO position to use the heart as previously described.
- Have the patient support himself or herself on the forearm and flexed knee.

Position of part

- Align the patient's body so the long axis of the sternum is centered to the midline of the grid.
- Adjust the elevation of the left shoulder and hip so that the thorax is rotated just enough to prevent superimposition of the vertebrae and sternum.
- Estimate the average 15 to 20 degrees of rotation with sufficient accuracy by placing one hand on the patient's sternum and the other hand directly above it on his or her thoracic vertebrae to act as guides while adjusting the degree of obliquity (Fig. 9-15).
- Center the cassette midway between the jugular notch and the xiphoid process at the approximate level of the seventh thoracic vertebra.
- *Shield gonads.*
- Respiration: When breathing motion is to be used, instruct the patient to take slow, shallow breaths during the exposure. When a short exposure time is to be used, instruct the patient to hold his or her breath at the end of exhalation to obtain a more uniform density.
- On trauma patients, this projection is obtained with the patient supine utilizing the LPO position and an AP oblique projection.

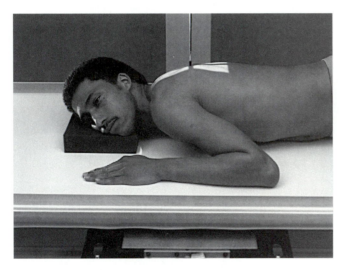

Fig. 9-15. PA oblique sternum. RAO.

Central ray

- Direct the central ray perpendicular to the midsternum. It enters the *elevated side* of the posterior thorax approximately 1 inch lateral to the median sagittal plane.

Structures shown

This image shows a slightly oblique projection of the sternum (Fig. 9-16). The detail demonstrated depends largely on the technical procedure employed. If breathing motion is used, the pulmonary markings will be obliterated.

□ Evaluation criteria

The following should be clearly demonstrated:

- Entire sternum from jugular notch to the tip of the xiphoid process.
- Reasonably good visibility of the sternum through the thorax, including:
  - □ Blurred pulmonary markings if breathing technique was used.
- Minimally obliqued sternum and thorax, as demonstrated by:
  - □ Sternum projected just free of superimposition from vertebral column.
  - □ No rotation of sternum.
  - □ Minimally obliqued vertebrae to prevent excessive rotation of sternum.
  - □ The lateral portion of the manubrium and sternoclavicular joint, free of superimposition by the vertebrae.
- Sternum projected to overlie the cardiac shadow.

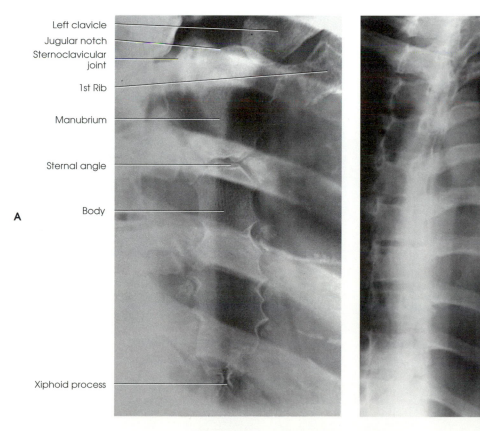

Left clavicle
Jugular notch
Sternoclavicular joint
1st Rib
Manubrium
Sternal angle
Body
Xiphoid process

A

B

Fig. 9-16. A and **B,** PA oblique sternum. RAO.

(**B,** courtesy Carol Corder, R.T.)

Sternum

 LATERAL PROJECTION
R or L position
Upright

Film: 10 × 12 in (24 × 30 cm) lengthwise.

Position of patient

- Place the patient in a lateral position, either seated or standing, before a vertical grid device.
- Use a 72-inch SID to reduce magnification of the sternum.

Position of part

- Have the patient sit or stand straight.
- Adjust the height of the film so that its upper border is 1½ inches above the jugular (manubrial) notch.
- Rotate the shoulders posteriorly.
- Have the patient lock the hands behind the back.
- Center the sternum to the midline of the grid.
- Being careful to keep the median sagittal plane of the body vertical, place the patient close enough to the grid so that he or she can rest the shoulder firmly against it.
- Adjust the patient so that the broad surface of the sternum is perpendicular to the plane of the film (Fig. 9-17).
- Have the breasts of female patients drawn to the sides and held in position with a wide bandage so that their shadows will not obscure the lower portion of the sternum.
- For a direct lateral projection of the sternoclavicular region only, center a vertically placed 8 × 10 in (18 × 24 cm) cassette at the level of the jugular notch.
- *Shield gonads.*
- Ask the patient to suspend respiration at the end of deep inhalation to obtain sharper contrast between the posterior surface of the sternum and the adjacent structures.

Central ray

- Direct the central ray perpendicular through the lateral border of the mid-sternum at the level of the seventh thoracic vertebra.

Structures shown

A lateral image of the entire length of the sternum is demonstrated (Fig. 9-18) showing the superimposed sternoclavicular joints and medial ends of the clavicles. A lateral of the sternoclavicular region only is shown in Fig. 9-19.

□ Evaluation criteria

The following should be clearly demonstrated:

- Sternum in its entirety.
- The manubrium, free of superimposition by the soft tissue of the shoulders.
- The sternum, free of superimposition by the ribs.
- Reduced magnification of the sternum if a 72-inch SID is used.
- The lower portion of the sternum unobscured by the breasts of a female patient. A second radiograph may be needed with increased penetration.

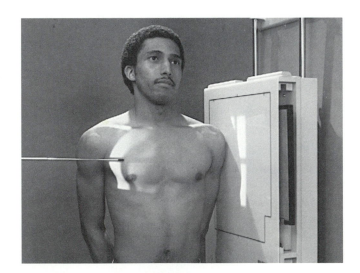

Fig. 9-17. Lateral sternum.

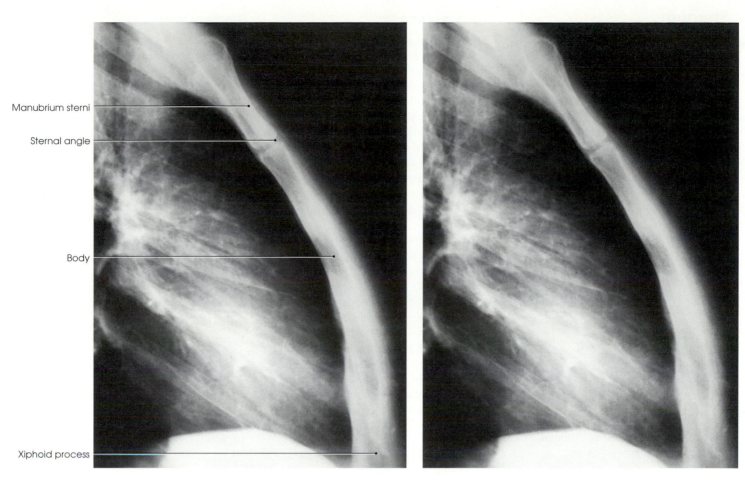

Manubrium sterni

Sternal angle

Body

Xiphoid process

Fig. 9-18. Lateral sternum.

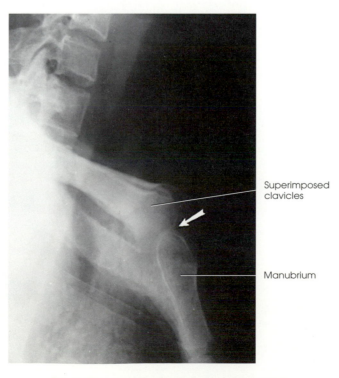

Superimposed
clavicles

Manubrium

Fig. 9-19. Lateral sternoclavicular joint *(arrow)*.

Sternum

 LATERAL PROJECTION
R or L position
Recumbent

Film: 10 × 12 in (24 × 30 cm) length-wise.

Position of patient

- Place the patient in the lateral recumbent position.
- Center the long axis of the sternum to the midline of the grid.
- Flex the patient's hips and knees to a comfortable position.

Position of part

- Extend the arms over the head to prevent them from overlapping of the sternum.
- Rest the patient's head on the dependent arm or a pillow (Fig. 9-20).
- If necessary, place a support under the lower thoracic region to position the long axis of the sternum horizontally.
- Adjust the rotation of the body so that the broad surface of the sternum is perpendicular to the plane of the film.
- Center the sternum to the midline of the grid.
- Apply a compression band across the hips for immobilization, if necessary.
- *Shield gonads.*
- Respiration is suspended at the end of deep inhalation to obtain high contrast between the posterior surface of the sternum and the adjacent structures.
- In cases of severe injury the patient can be examined using the dorsal decubitus position. In this case a grid-front cassette or a stationary grid should be used as shown in Fig. 9-21.

Central ray

- Direct the central ray perpendicular through the sternum to the cassette.

Structures shown

The lateral aspect of the entire length of the sternum is shown (Fig. 9-22).

☐ Evaluation criteria

The following should be clearly demonstrated:

- A lateral image of the sternum in its entirety.
- The sternum, free of superimposition by the soft tissue of the shoulders or arms.
- The sternum, free of superimposition by the ribs.
- Magnification of the sternum, due to the increased OID.
- The inferior portion of the sternum unobscured by the breasts of a female patient. A second radiograph may be needed with increased penetration.

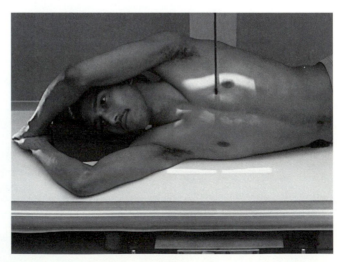

Fig. 9-20. Lateral sternum.

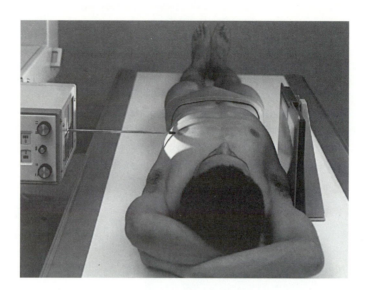

Fig. 9-21. Dorsal decubitus position for lateral sternum.

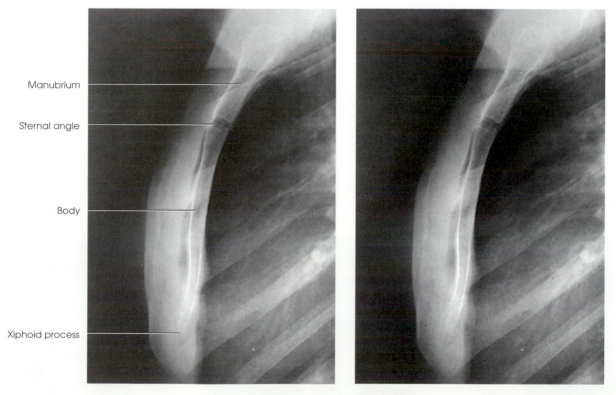

Manubrium

Sternal angle

Body

Xiphoid process

Fig. 9-22. Lateral sternum.

Sternoclavicular Articulations

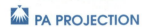
PA PROJECTION

Film: 8 × 10 in (18 × 24 cm) crosswise.

Position of patient

- Place the patient in the prone position.
- Center the median sagittal plane of the body to the midline of the grid.
- Adapt the same procedure for use with the patient who is standing or seated upright.

Position of part

- Center the cassette at the level of the spinous process of the third thoracic vertebra, which lies posterior to the jugular (manubrial) notch.
- Place the arms along the sides of the body with the palms facing upward.
- Adjust the shoulders to lie in the same transverse plane.
- For a bilateral examination, rest the patient's head on the chin and adjust it so that the median sagittal plane is vertical.

- For a unilateral projection, ask the patient to turn the head to face the affected side and then to rest the cheek on the table (Fig. 9-23). The rotation of the head rotates the spine slightly away from the side being examined and thus gives better visualization of the lateral portion of the manubrium.
- *Shield gonads.*
- Ask the patient to suspend respiration at the end of exhalation to obtain a more uniform density.

Central ray

- Direct the central ray perpendicular to the third thoracic vertebra.

Structures shown

A PA projection of the sternoclavicular joints and the medial portions of the clavicles (Figs. 9-24 and 9-25).

☐ Evaluation criteria

The following should be clearly demonstrated:

- ▪ Both sternoclavicular joints and medial ends of the clavicles.
- ▪ Sternoclavicular joints visible through the superimposing vertebral and rib shadows.
- ▪ No rotation present on a bilateral examination; slight rotation present on a unilateral examination.

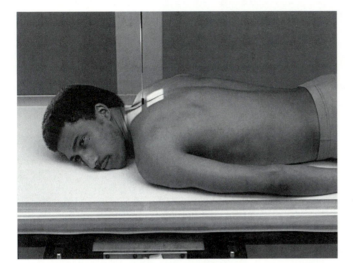

Fig. 9-23. Unilateral examination to demonstrate left sternoclavicular articulation.

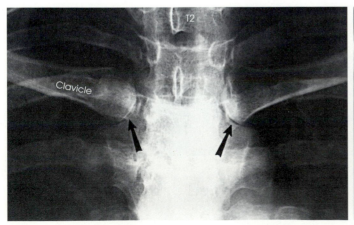

Fig. 9-24. Bilateral sternoclavicular joints *(arrows)*.

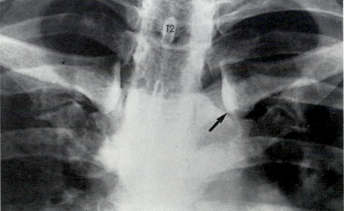

Fig. 9-25. Unilateral sternoclavicular joint *(arrow on right)*.

Sternoclavicular Articulations

 PA OBLIQUE PROJECTION
RAO or LAO position

Film: 8 × 10 in (18 × 24 cm) crosswise.

Body rotation technique

Position of patient

- Place the patient in a prone or seated-upright position.

Position of part

- Keeping the affected side adjacent to the film, oblique the patient enough to project the vertebrae well behind that of the sternoclavicular joint closest to the film. This will usually be about 10° to 15°.
- Then, adjust the patient's position to center the joint to the midline of the grid device.
- Adjust the shoulders to lie in the same transverse plane.
- Center the cassette at the level of the sternoclavicular joint (Fig. 9-26).
- *Shield gonads.*
- Ask the patient to suspend respiration for the exposure.

Central ray

- Direct the central ray perpendicular through the sternoclavicular joint closest to the film.
- See p. 416 for structures shown and evaluation criteria.

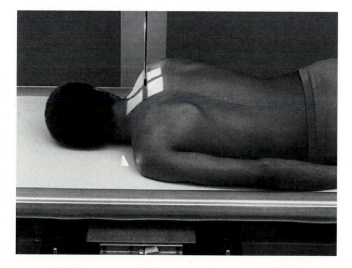

Fig. 9-26. PA oblique sternoclavicular joint. LAO.

Sternoclavicular Articulations

PA OBLIQUE PROJECTION
Central ray angulation technique:
NON-BUCKY TECHNIQUE

Position of patient

- Place the patient in the prone position.
- Adjust a grid cassette directly under the upper chest.
- Center the cassette to the level of the sternoclavicular joints.
- To avoid grid cut-off, place the grid on top of the x-ray table with its long axis running *perpendicular* to the long axis of the table.

Position of part

- Extend the arms along the sides of the body with the palms of the hands facing upward.
- Adjust the shoulders to lie in the same transverse plane.
- Ask the patient to rest the head on the chin or rotate the chin toward the side of the joint being radiographed (Fig. 9-27).

Central ray

- From the side opposite that being examined, direct the central ray to the midpoint of the cassette at an angle of 15 degrees toward the median sagittal plane of the body. A small angle is satisfactory in examinations of the sternoclavicular articulations because there is only a slight anteroposterior overlapping of the vertebrae and these joints.

Structures shown

A slightly oblique image of the sternoclavicular joint is demonstrated by either method. Because the joint is closer to the plane of the film, less distortion is obtained with the central ray angulation method than with the body rotation method (Figs. 9-28 and 9-29).

□ Evaluation criteria

The following should be clearly demonstrated:

- Sternoclavicular joint of interest in center of radiograph. Manubrium and medial end of clavicle included.
- Open sternoclavicular joint space.
- Sternoclavicular joint of interest directly in front of the vertebral column with minimal obliquity.
- Reasonably good visibility of the sternoclavicular joint through the superimposing rib and lung fields.

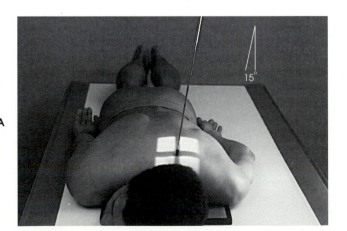
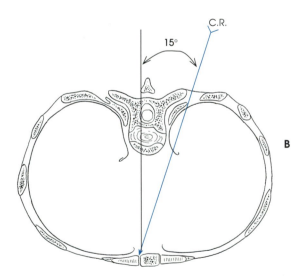

Fig. 9-27. PA oblique sternoclavicular joint. Central ray angulation.

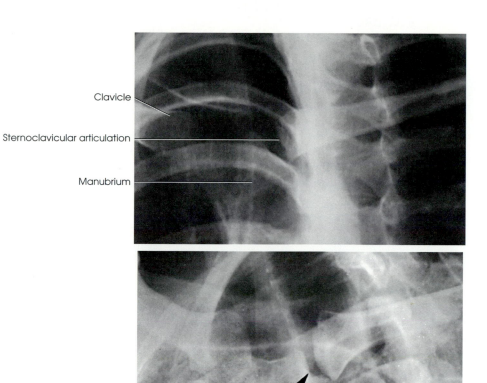

Clavicle

Sternoclavicular articulation

Manubrium

Fig. 9-28. PA oblique projection, sternoclavicular joint. LAO position. Joint closest to film shown *(arrow)*.

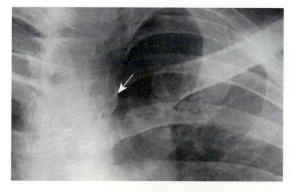

Fig. 9-29. Central ray angulation for sternoclavicular joint farthest from x-ray tube *(arrow)*.

Sternoclavicular Articulations

AXIOLATERAL PROJECTION
KURZBAUER METHOD

Film: 8 × 10 in (18 × 24 cm) lengthwise.

Position of patient

- Have the patient lie in the lateral recumbent position on the affected side, with the sternoclavicular region centered to the midline of the grid.
- Flex the patient's hips and knees in a comfortable position.

[1]Kurzbauer R: The lateral projection in the roentgenography of the sternoclavicular articulation, AJR 56:104-105, 1946.

Position of part

- Have the patient fully extend the arm of the affected side and grasp the end of the table for support.
- Make any necessary adjustment to center the sternoclavicular articulation to the midline of the grid.
- Place the uppermost arm along the side of the body.
- Have the patient grasp the dorsal surface of the hip to hold the shoulder in a depressed position. The extension of the affected shoulder, along with the depression of the uppermost shoulder, prevents superimposition of the two articulations.
- Adjust the thorax to place the anterior surface of the manubrium perpendicular to the plane of the film (Figs. 9-30 and 9-31).
- Adjust the cassette so that its midpoint will be centered to the central ray.
- Although the best result is obtained with the patient in the recumbent position, a comparable image can be made in the upright position if the affected shoulder cannot be laid on.
- *Shield gonads.*
- Ask the patient to suspend respiration at the end of full inhalation.

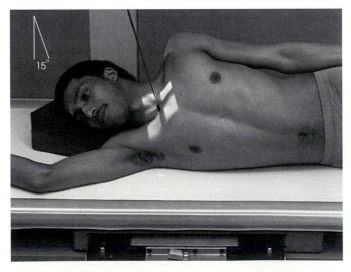

Fig. 9-30. Axiolateral sternoclavicular joint.

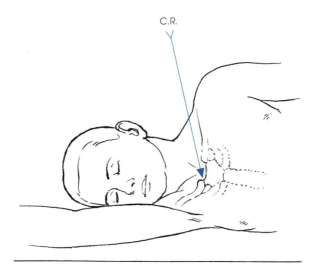

Fig. 9-31. Axiolateral sternoclavicular joint.

Central ray

- Direct the central ray through the sternoclavicular articulation closest to the film at an angle of 15 degrees caudad.

Structures shown

This image shows an unobstructed axiolateral projection of the sternoclavicular articulation closest to the film (Fig. 9-32).

□ Evaluation criteria

The following should be clearly demonstrated:
- Sternoclavicular joint on affected side.
- The sternoclavicular articulations, free of superimposition by the shoulders.

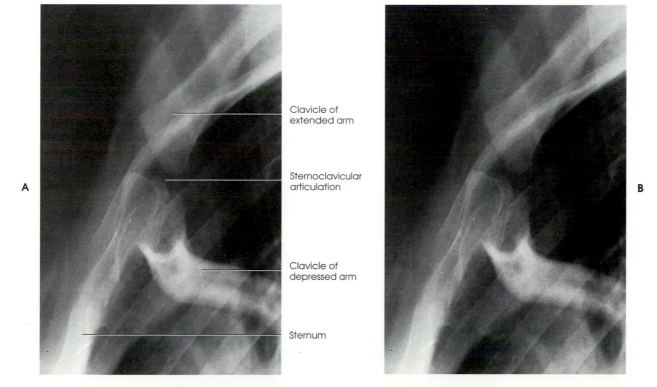

A   Clavicle of extended arm   Sternoclavicular articulation   Clavicle of depressed arm   Sternum   B

Fig. 9-32. Axiolateral sternoclavicular joint.

Ribs

In radiography of the ribs, a 14 × 17 in (35 × 43 cm) cassette should be used to identify the ribs involved and to determine the extent of trauma or pathologic condition. Projections can be made in recumbent and upright positions. If the area in question is localized to the first or last rib, additional images may be required to better demonstrate the affected area (Fig. 9-33).

After localizing the lesion, determine (1) the position required to place the affected rib region parallel with the plane of the film and (2) whether the radiograph should be made to include the ribs above or below the diaphragm.

The anterior portions of the ribs, usually referred to simply as the anterior ribs, are often examined with the patient facing the film for a PA projection (Fig. 9-34). The posterior portion of the ribs, or posterior ribs, are more commonly radiographed with the patient facing the x-ray tube, as for an AP projection (Fig. 9-35). The posterior ribs are well shown in the AP projection if the SID is 36 inches or more.

The axillary portion of the ribs is best shown using an oblique projection. Because the lateral projection results in superimposition of the two sides, it is generally used only in the investigation of fluid and/or air levels.

When the ribs that are superimposed over the heart are involved, the body must be rotated to project the ribs free of the heart shadow, or the radiographic exposure must be increased to compensate for the density of the heart. While the anterior and posterior ends are superimposed, the left ribs are cleared of the heart when using the LAO position (Fig. 9-36) or RPO position (Fig. 9-37). These two body positions place the right-sided ribs parallel with the plane of the film and are reversed to obtain comparable projections of the left-sided ribs. Selection of technical factors that will result in a short scale radiograph are often used.

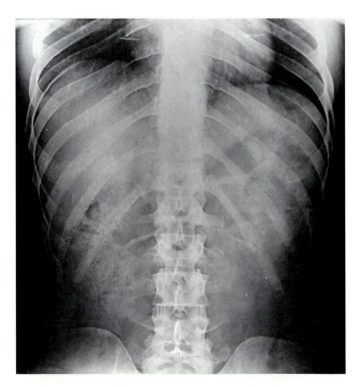

Fig. 9-33. AP projection lower ribs.

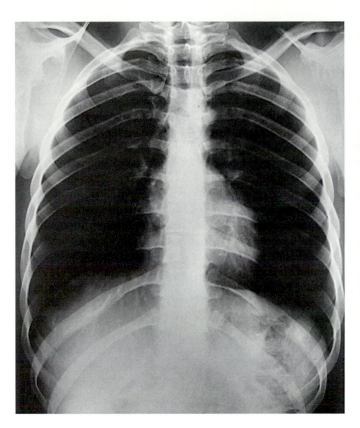

Fig. 9-34. PA ribs.

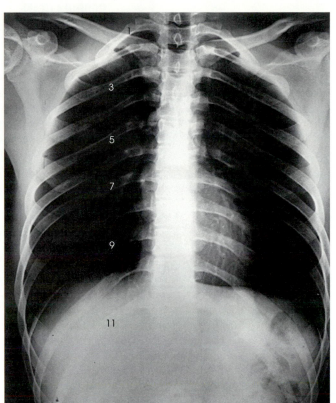

Fig. 9-35. AP ribs.

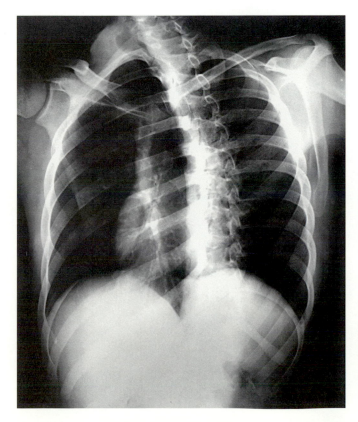

Fig. 9-36. PA oblique ribs. LAO.

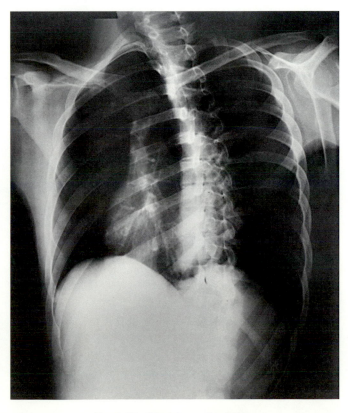

Fig. 9-37. AP oblique ribs. RPO.

RESPIRATION

In radiography of the ribs, the patient is usually examined with respiration suspended in either inspiration or expiration. Occasionally, shallow breathing may be used to obliterate lung markings. If this technique is used, breathing must be shallow enough to ensure that the ribs are not elevated or depressed as described in the anatomy portion of this chapter. Examples of shallow breathing and suspended respiration are compared in Figs. 9-38 and 9-39.

Rib fractures can cause a great deal of pain and hemorrhage due to the closely related neurovascular structures. This commonly makes it difficult for the patient to breathe deeply for the required radiograph. Deeper inspiration will be attained if the patient fully understands the importance of expanding the lungs and if the exposure is made after the patient takes the second deep breath.

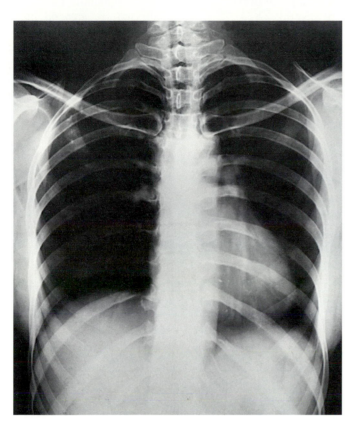

Fig. 9-38. Shallow breathing technique.

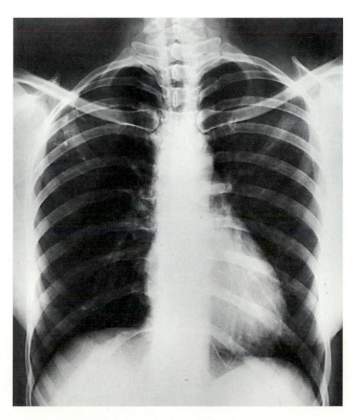

Fig. 9-39. Suspended respiration technique.

Upper Anterior Ribs

PA PROJECTION

Film: 14 × 17 in (35 × 43 cm) length-wise.

Position of patient

- Position the patient for a PA projection, either upright or recumbent.
- Because the diaphragm descends to its lowest level in the upright position, use the standing or seated-upright position for projections of the upper ribs when the patient's condition permits (Fig. 9-40). The upright position is also valuable for demonstrating fluid levels in the chest.

Position of part

- Center the median sagittal plane of the body to the midline of the grid.
- Adjust the cassette position to project approximately 1½ inches above the upper border of the shoulders to include the upper ribs.
- Rest the patient's hands against the hips with the palms turned outward to rotate the scapulae away from the rib cage.
- Adjust the shoulders to lie in the same transverse plane.
- If the patient is prone, rest the head on the chin and adjust the median sagittal plane to be vertical (Fig. 9-41).
- Affected ribs are often imaged unilaterally using 11x14 in (30 x 35 cm) film for contrast improvement.

- For hypersthenic patients with wide rib cages, include the entire lateral surface of the affected rib area on the radiograph. This may require moving the patient laterally to include all of the affected ribs.
- *Shield gonads.*
- Ask the patient to suspend respiration at the end of *full inhalation* to depress the diaphragm as much as possible.

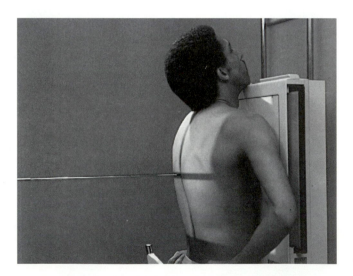

Fig. 9-40. PA upright ribs.

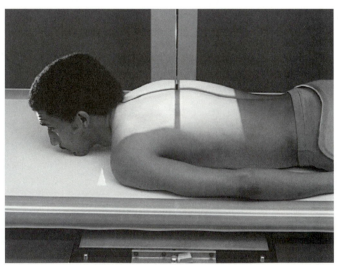

Fig. 9-41. PA recumbent ribs.

Central ray

- Direct the central ray perpendicular to the center of the film at the level of the seventh thoracic vertebra for the upper ribs.
- As a useful option for demonstrating the seventh, eighth, and ninth ribs, move the x-ray tube so that the central ray is approximately 5 inches above the midpoint of the film; then angle the central ray to coincide with the center of the film. In the latter case, high centering aids in projecting the diaphragm below that of the affected rib.

Structures shown

The PA projection best demonstrates the ribs above the diaphragm (Figs. 9-42 and 9-43).

□ Evaluation criteria

The following should be clearly demonstrated:

- First through ninth ribs in their entirety, the posterior portions lying above the diaphragm.
- First through seventh anterior ribs from both sides in their entirety and above the diaphragm.
- In a unilateral examination, ribs from the opposite side may not be entirely included.
- Ribs, visible through the lungs, with sufficient contrast.

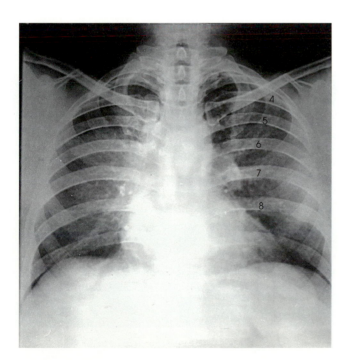

Fig. 9-42. PA ribs, normal centering.

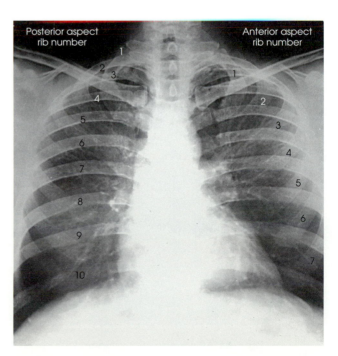

Fig. 9-43. PA ribs, high centering.

Upper anterior ribs

Posterior Ribs

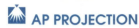 **AP PROJECTION**

Film: 14 × 17 in (35 × 43 cm) length-wise.

Position of patient

- Have the patient face the x-ray tube, either upright or recumbent.
- When the patient's condition permits, use the upright position for ribs above the diaphragm and the supine position for ribs below the diaphragm to permit gravity to assist in moving the patient's diaphragm.

Position of part

- Center the median sagittal plane of the body to the midline of the grid.

  #### Ribs above diaphragm
- Place the cassette lengthwise 1½ inches above the upper border of the shoulders centered at the seventh thoracic vertebra.
- Rest the patient's hands, palms outward, against the hips or extend the arms to the vertical position with the hands under the head. This will move the scapula off the ribs (Fig. 9-44).
- Adjust the shoulders to lie in the same transverse plane, and rotate them forward to draw the scapulae away from the rib cage.
- *Shield gonads.*
- Ask the patient to suspend respiration at the end of *full inhalation* to depress the diaphragm.

Ribs below diaphragm
- Place the crosswise cassette in the Bucky tray with the caudal edge positioned at the level of the crest of the ilium. Such positioning assures inclusion of the lower ribs because of the divergent x-rays.
- Adjust the shoulders to lie in the same transverse plane.
- Place the arms in a comfortable position (Fig. 9-45).
- *Shield gonads.*
- Respiration is suspended at the end of *full exhalation* for the purpose of elevating the diaphragm.

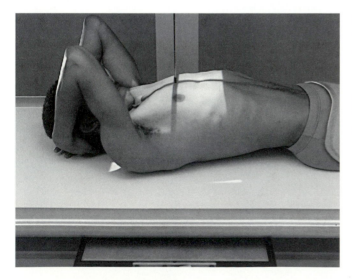

Fig. 9-44. AP ribs above diaphragm.

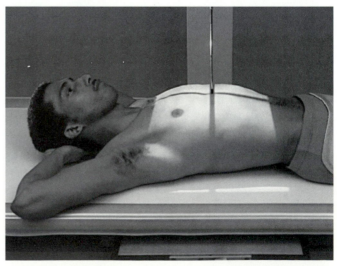

Fig. 9-45. AP ribs below diaphragm.

Central ray

- With the central ray *perpendicular* to the plane of the film, center to the approximate level of:
  - the *seventh thoracic vertebra for the ribs above* the diaphragm or
  - the *twelfth thoracic vertebra for ribs below* the diaphragm when the cassette is crosswise, or at the tenth thoracic vertebra when the cassette is longitudinally placed.

Structures shown

The AP projection shows the posterior ribs above or below the diaphragm, according to the region examined (Figs. 9-46 and 9-47).

□Evaluation criteria

The following should be clearly demonstrated:

- For ribs above the diaphragm, first through tenth posterior ribs from both sides in their entirety.
- For ribs below the diaphragm, eighth through twelfth posterior ribs on both sides in their entirety.
- Ribs, visible through the lungs or abdomen.
- In a unilateral examination, ribs from the opposite side may not be entirely included.

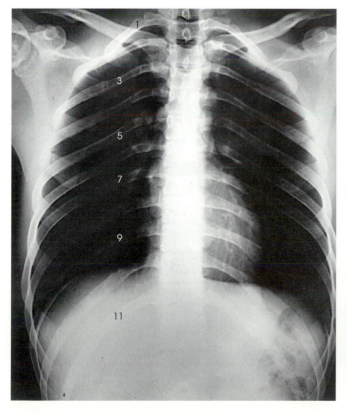

Fig. 9-46. AP ribs above diaphragm.

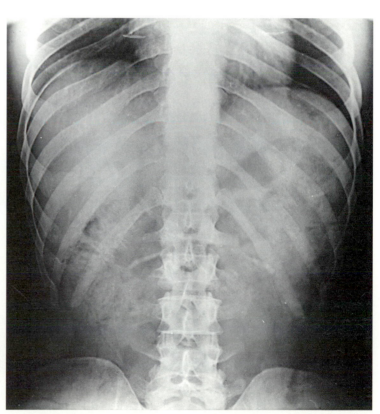

Fig. 9-47. AP lower ribs.

Ribs: Axillary

 AP OBLIQUE PROJECTION

RPO or LPO position

Film: 14 × 17 in (35 × 43 cm) length-wise.

Position of patient

- Examine the patient in the upright or recumbent position.
- Unless contraindicated by the patient's condition, use the upright position for ribs above the diaphragm and the recumbent position for ribs below the diaphragm. Gravity assists by moving the diaphragm.

Position of part

- Position the body for a 45-degree AP oblique projection using the RPO or LPO position. *Place the affected side closest to the film.*
- Center the affected side on a longitudinal plane drawn midway between the median sagittal plane and the lateral surface of the body.
- Position this plane to the midline of the grid.
- If the patient is in the recumbent position, support the elevated hip.
- Abduct the arm of the affected side and elevate it to carry the scapula away from the rib cage.
- Rest the hand on the patient's head if placed in the upright position (Fig. 9-48), or place it under or above the head if in the recumbent position (Fig. 9-49).

- Abduct the opposite limb with the hand on the hip.
- Center the cassette at the seventh thoracic vertebra with the top 1½ inches above the upper border of the shoulder for ribs above the diaphragm; for ribs below the diaphragm, place the bottom of the cassette at the level of the crest of the ilium. The cassette will be centered at the level of the tenth thoracic vertebra.
- Center the cassette midway between these points for an initial projection, if necessary.
- *Shield gonads.*
- Respiration is suspended at the end of deep *exhalation* for ribs *below* the diaphragm and at the end of full *inhalation* for ribs *above* the diaphragm.

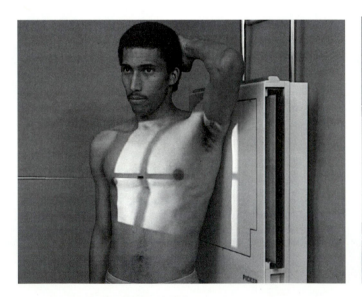

Fig. 9-48. *Upright* AP oblique ribs. LPO.

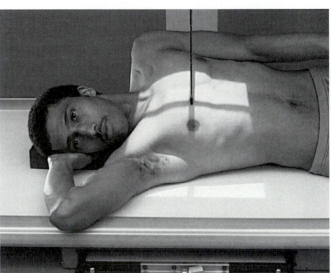

Fig. 9-49. *Recumbent* AP oblique ribs. RPO.

Central ray

- With the central ray directed *perpendicularly* to the plane of the film, center *midway between the median sagittal plane and the lateral border of the affected ribs* at the level of:
  - the *seventh thoracic vertebra* for upper ribs or
  - the *tenth thoracic vertebra* for lower ribs.

Structures shown

In these images the axillary portion of the ribs are projected free of self-superimposition (Fig. 9-50).

Ribs: axillary

□ Evaluation criteria

The following should be clearly demonstrated:

- Approximately twice as much distance between the vertebral column and the lateral border of the ribs on the affected side as there is on the unaffected side.
- Axillary portion of the ribs free of superimposition.
- First through tenth ribs visible above the diaphragm for upper ribs.
- Eighth through twelfth ribs visible below the diaphragm for lower ribs.
- Ribs, visible through the lungs or abdomen according to the region examined.

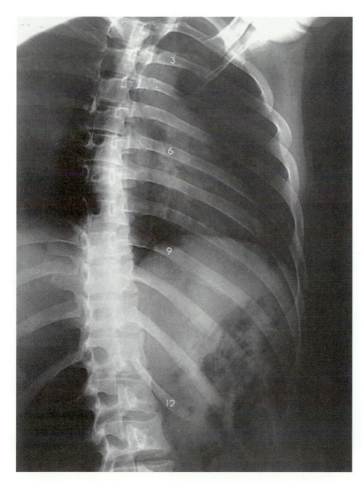

Fig. 9-50. AP oblique lower ribs. LPO.

Ribs: Axillary

▲ PA OBLIQUE PROJECTION
RAO or LAO position

Film: 14 × 17 in (35 × 43 cm) lengthwise.

Position of patient

- Examine the patient in the upright or recumbent position.
- Unless contraindicated by the patient's condition, use the upright position for ribs above the diaphragm and the recumbent position for ribs below the diaphragm. Gravity assists by moving diaphragm.

Position of part

- Position the body for a 45-degree PA oblique projection using the RAO or LAO position. Place the affected side *away* from the film (Fig. 9-51).
- If the patient is in the recumbent position, have him or her rest on the forearm and flexed knee of the elevated side (Fig. 9-52).
- Align the body so that a longitudinal plane drawn midway between the midline and the lateral surface of the body is centered to the midline of the grid.

- Center the cassette at the seventh thoracic vertebra with the top 1½ inches above the upper border of the shoulder for ribs above the diaphragm; for ribs below the diaphragm, place the bottom of the cassette at the level of the crest of the ilium, centered at the level of the tenth thoracic vertebra.
- *Shield gonads.*
- Respiration is suspended at the end of *full exhalation* for ribs below the diaphragm and at the end of *full inhalation* for ribs above the diaphragm.

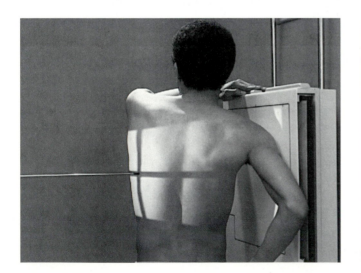

Fig. 9-51. *Upright* PA oblique ribs. RAO.

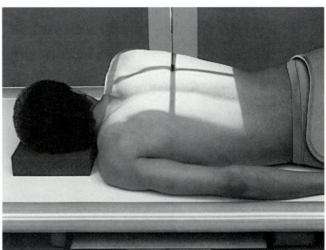

Fig. 9-52. *Recumbent* PA oblique ribs. LAO.

Central ray

- For an image of the upper ribs, with the central ray perpendicular to the plane of the film, center midway between the midline and the lateral border of the body at the level of the seventh thoracic vertebra for upper ribs.
- For an image of the lower ribs, with the central ray perpendicular to the plane of the film, center midway between the midline and the lateral border of the body at the level of the tenth thoracic vertebra.

Structures shown

In these images, the axillary portion of the ribs is projected, free of bony superimposition (Fig. 9-53).

□Evaluation criteria

The following should be clearly demonstrated:

- Approximately twice as much distance between the vertebral column and the lateral border of the ribs on the affected side as there is on the unaffected side.
- Axillary portion of the ribs free of superimposition.
- First through tenth ribs visible above the diaphragm for upper ribs.
- Eighth through twelfth ribs visible below the diaphragm for lower ribs.
- Ribs, visible through the lungs or abdomen according to the region examined.

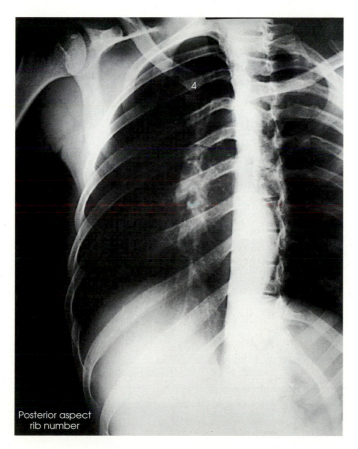

Posterior aspect
rib number

Fig. 9-53. PA oblique ribs. LAO.

Costal Joints

AP AXIAL PROJECTION

This projection is recommended for the demonstration of the costal joints in cases of rheumatoid spondylitis.

Film: 11 × 14 in (30 × 35 cm) lengthwise.

Position of patient

• Place the patient in the supine position.
• The head should rest directly on the table to avoid accentuating the dorsal kyphosis.

Position of part

• Center the median sagittal plane to the midline of the grid.
• If the patient has an accentuated dorsal kyphosis, extend the arms over the head; otherwise the arms may be placed along the sides of the body.
• Adjust the shoulders to lie in the same transverse plane (Fig. 9-54).
• With the cassette in the Bucky tray, adjust its position so that the midpoint of the film will coincide with the central ray. The film will project approximately 4 inches beyond the upper border of the shoulders.
• Apply compression across the thorax, if necessary.
• *Shield gonads.*
• Ask the patient to suspend respiration at the end of full inhalation because the lung markings are less prominent at this phase of breathing.

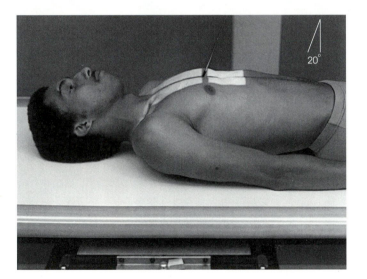

Fig. 9-54. AP axial costal joints.

Central ray

- Direct the central ray to exit the sixth thoracic vertebra at an average angle of 20 degrees cephalad; it enters the midline about 2 inches above the xiphoid process.
- Increase the central ray angulation slightly (5 to 10 degrees) when examining patients who have an accentuated dorsal kyphosis.

Structures shown

The costovertebral and costotransverse joints are demonstrated (Fig. 9-55).

□ **Evaluation criteria**

The following should be clearly demonstrated:

- ■ Open costovertebral and costotransverse joints.

NOTE: On large-boned subjects it may be necessary to examine the two sides separately to demonstrate the costovertebral joints. This is done by alternately rotating the body approximately 10 degrees medially; the elevated side is best demonstrated.

Hohmann and Gasteiger[1] state that in their studies of the costal joints (costovertebral and costotransverse) they have found that the central ray must usually be angled 30 degrees cephalad on the average patient. They increase the central ray angulation to 35 to 40 degrees when accentuated kyphosis is present, and in cases of severe curvature of the spine they also elevate the pelvis on a suitable support. For localized studies the central ray may be centered to T4 for the upper area and to T8 for the lower area.

---

[1]Hohmann D and Gasteiger W: Roentgen diagnosis of the costovertebral joints, Fortschr Roentgenstr 112:783-789, 1970. (In German.) Abstract: Radiology 98:481, 1971.

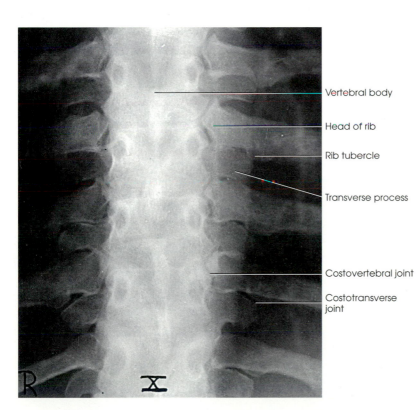
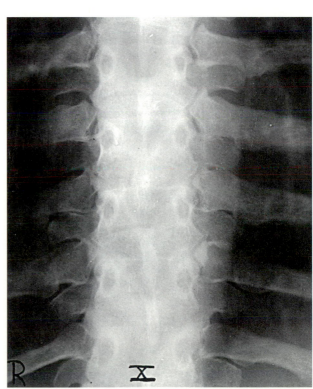

Vertebral body

Head of rib

Rib tubercle

Transverse process

Costovertebral joint

Costotransverse joint

Fig. 9-55. AP axial costal joints.

(Courtesy Dr. A. Justin Williams.)

Chapter 10

THORACIC VISCERA

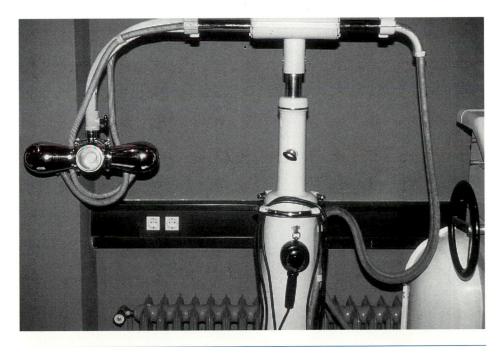

A portable radiographic unit from the early 1940s. Note the exposed bare glass ends of the x-ray tube. A spring-wound mechanical timer is hanging on the vertical support.

Body Habitus

The general form, or *habitus,* of the body determines the size, shape, position, tonus, and movement of the internal organs. For a description of the different body forms and how each appears on radiographs involving the thoracic area, see "Body habitus" in Chapter 3. Chest radiographs are included for the four body types: the hypersthenic, sthenic, asthenic, and hyposthenic (see Figs. 3-7 to 3-10 in Chapter 3).

Respiratory System

The thoracic cavity is bounded by the walls of the thorax, extends from the superior thoracic aperture (thoracic inlet) to the diaphragm, and contains the thoracic viscera. The superior thoracic aperture (thoracic inlet) is bounded laterally by the first pair of ribs. Its plane slants obliquely anteriorly and inferiorly from the level of the superior border of the first thoracic vertebra to the jugular (manubrial or suprasternal) notch.

The *thoracic viscera* (Fig. 10-1) consist of the lungs and the mediastinal structures, the mediastinum containing all thoracic organs except the lungs.

The *mediastinum* is the potential space between the lungs. It extends from the superior aperture of the thorax (thoracic inlet) inferiorly to the diaphragm. It is bounded anteriorly by the sternum and posteriorly by the vertebral column. The portion lying above the heart is called the *superior mediastinum.* The lower portion is subdivided into the *anterior mediastinum,* the shallow space in front of the heart; the *middle mediastinum,* which is the largest part and is occupied by the heart; and the *posterior mediastinum,* which lies behind the heart. The radiographically important mediastinal structures are the heart and the great blood vessels (the anatomy of which is described in Chapter 26), the trachea, the esophagus, and the thymus gland.

The *respiratory system proper* consists of the larynx (Chapter 15), trachea, bronchi, and two lungs. The air passages of these organs communicate with the exterior through the pharynx, mouth, and nose, each of which, in addition to other described functions, is considered a part of the respiratory apparatus.

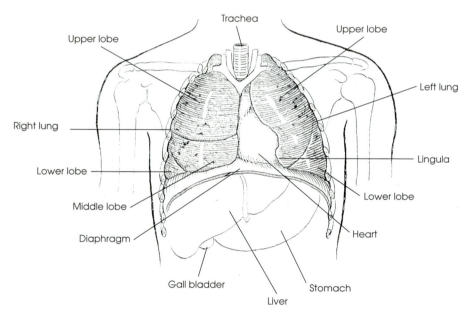

Fig. 10-1. Anterior aspect of lungs in relation to surrounding structures.

The *trachea* is a fibrous, muscular tube with 16 to 20 C-shaped cartilaginous rings embedded in its walls for greater rigidity (Fig. 10-2). Measuring approximately ¾ inch (2 cm) in diameter and 4½ inches (11 cm) in length, the tube is flattened behind. The cartilaginous rings are incomplete posteriorly and extend around the anterior two thirds of the tube. The trachea lies in the midline of the body anterior to the esophagus in the neck. However, in the thorax the trachea is shifted slightly to the right of the midline as a result of the arching of the aorta. The trachea follows the curve of the vertebral column and extends from its junction with the larynx at the level of the sixth cervical vertebra inferiorly through the mediastinum to about the level of the space between the fourth and fifth thoracic vertebrae. The last tracheal cartilage is elongated and has a hook-like process, the *carina,* extending posteriorly on its inferior surface. At the carina, the trachea divides, or bifurcates, into two lesser tubes, the main, or primary, bronchi, one of which enters the right lung and the other the left lung.

The *main* (primary) *bronchi* slant obliquely inferiorly to their entrance into the lungs, where they branch out to form the right and left bronchial branches (Figs. 10-2 and 10-3). The right main (primary) bronchus is shorter, wider, and more vertical than the left main bronchus. Because of the more vertical position and greater diameter of the right main bronchus, foreign bodies entering the trachea are more likely to pass into the right bronchus than into the left bronchus.

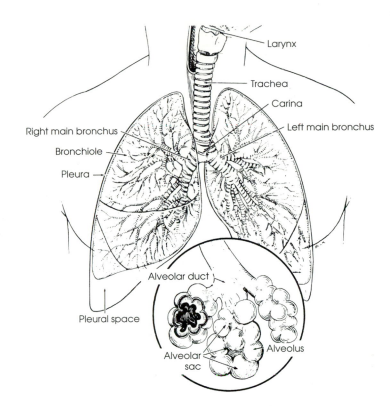

Fig. 10-2. Anterior aspect of respiratory system.

(From Thibodeau GA: Anthony's textbook of anatomy and physiology, ed 13, St Louis, 1990, Mosby.)

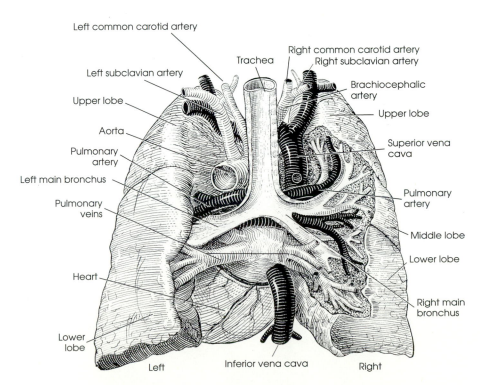

Fig. 10-3. Posterior aspect of heart, great vessels, lungs, trachea, and bronchial trees. (Pulmonary veins are shaded to match the shading of arteries, since both carry oxygenated blood. Similarly, pulmonary arteries are shaded to match the shading of veins.)

After entering the hilum, each main bronchus divides, sending branches to each lobe of the lung (three to the right lung and two to the left lung). These *lobar branches* further divide and decrease in caliber. The bronchi continue dividing and end in minute tubes called the *terminal bronchioles*. The terminal bronchiole communicates with an alveolar duct. Each duct ends in one or more alveolar sacs, the walls of which are lined with many alveoli (Fig. 10-2).

The *lungs* are the organs of respiration (Figs. 10-4 and 10-5). They comprise the mechanism for introducing oxygen into, and removing carbon dioxide from, the blood. The lungs are composed of a light, spongy, highly elastic substance, the *parenchyma,* and are covered by a layer of serous membrane. Situated one on each side in the thoracic cavity, the lungs fill all the costomediastinal recess not occupied by the mediastinal structures. Each lung presents a rounded *apex* that reaches above the level of the clavicles into the root of the neck and a broad *base* that, resting on the obliquely placed diaphragm, reaches lower in back and at the sides than in front. The right lung is about 1 inch shorter than the left lung as a result of the large space occupied by the liver, and it is broader than the left lung because of the position of the heart. The lateral, or costal, surface of each lung conforms with the shape of the chest wall. The inferior surface of the lung is concave, fitting over the diaphragm, and the lateral margins are thin. During inspiration the lateral margins descend into the costodiaphragmatic recess of the parietal pleura. In radiology, this is called the *costophrenic angle*. The mediastinal surface is concave with two depressions: the cardiac impression (fossa) for the accommodation of the heart and the hilum (hilus) for the accommodation of the bronchi, pulmonary blood vessels, lymph vessels, and nerves. The cardiac impression (fossa), which is deeper on the left lung than on the right, lies below and in front of the hilar depression.

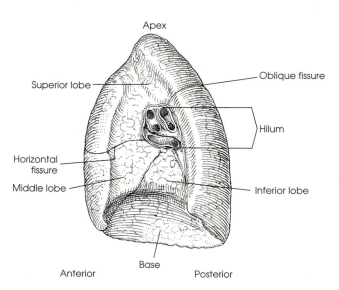

Fig. 10-4. Mediastinal aspect of right lung.

Each lung is enclosed in a double-walled, serous membrane sac called the *pleura*. The inner layer of the pleural sac, called the *pulmonary* or *visceral pleura*, closely adheres to the surface of the lung, extends into the *interlobar fissures*, and is continuous with the outer layer at the hilum. The outer layer, called the *parietal pleura*, lines the wall of the cavity occupied by the lung, being reflected over the adjacent mediastinal structures, and closely adheres to the upper surface of the diaphragm and the inner surface of the chest wall. The two layers are moistened by serum to move easily on each other and thus prevent friction between the lungs and chest walls during respiration. The space between the two pleural walls is called the *pleural cavity.* The narrow space between the costal and diaphragmatic portions of the parietal pleura, where it dips below the lateral margin of the lung, is the *costodiaphragmatic recess* (costophrenic, or phrenicocostal, sinus).

Each lung is divided into *lobes* by deep fissures. The fissures lie in an oblique plane from above inferiorly and anteriorly so that the lobes overlap each other in the AP (anteroposterior) direction. The *oblique fissures* divide the lungs into *superior* (upper) and *inferior* (lower) *lobes.* The superior lobes lie above and are anterior to the inferior lobes. The right superior lobe is further divided by a *horizontal fissure,* creating a right *middle lobe* (Fig. 10-4). The left lung has no horizontal fissure and thus no middle lobe (Fig. 10-5). The portion of the left lobe that corresponds in position to the right middle lobe is called the *lingula.* The lingula is a tongue-shaped process on the anterior-medial border of the left lung. It fills the space between the chest wall and the heart (see Fig. 10-1).

Each of the five lobes comprises closely bound but individual *bronchopulmonary segments.* Each of these segments in turn is composed of several smaller units called *primary lobules.* The primary lobule is the anatomic unit of lung structure and comprises a terminal bronchiole with its expanded alveolar duct and alveolar sac. The walls of the alveoli are thin and delicate; they support the fine network of pulmonary capillaries in which the blood receives its fresh supply of oxygen.

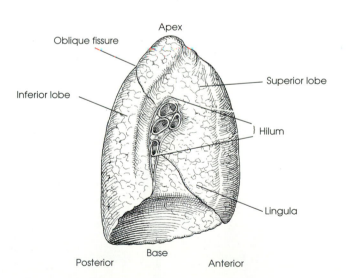

Fig. 10-5. Mediastinal aspect of left lung.

Mediastinal Structures

The *mediastinum* is the area of the thorax bounded by the sternum anteriorly, the spine posteriorly, and the lungs laterally. The structures associated with the mediastinum are the heart and its great vessels, the trachea, the esophagus, and the thymus, as well as the lymphatics and nerves, fibrous tissue, and fat.

The *esophagus* is the part of the digestive canal that connects the pharynx with the stomach. It is a narrow, musculomembranous tube about 9 inches (23 cm) in length. It begins at the level of the sixth cervical vertebra, where it is continuous with the pharynx, and reaches to the level of about the eleventh thoracic vertebra, where it ends at the esophagogastric junction (esophageal orifice) of the stomach. Following the curves of the vertebral column, the esophagus descends through the posterior part of the mediastinum and then runs anteriorly to pass through the esophageal hiatus of the diaphragm. The esophagus normally has two narrowed areas: one at its superior end, where it enters the thorax, and one at its inferior end at the hiatus in the diaphragm. It also has two indentations: one at the aortic arch and one where it is crossed by the left bronchus.

The esophagus lies just in front of the vertebral column with its anterior surface in close relation to the trachea, aortic arch, and heart, which makes it valuable in certain heart examinations. When the esophagus is filled with barium sulfate, the posterior border of the heart and aorta are outlined well in lateral and oblique projections (Figs. 10-6 and 10-7). Frontal, oblique, and lateral images are often used in examinations of the esophagus. Radiography of the esophagus is discussed later in this chapter.

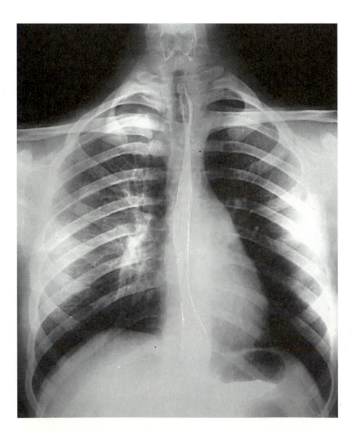

Fig. 10-6. Esophagus with walls coated with barium sulfate.

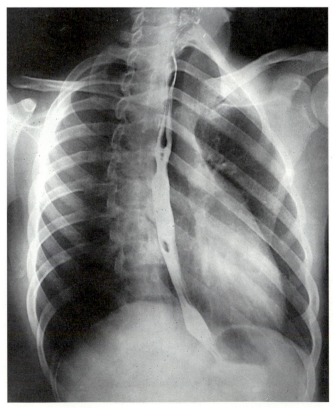

Fig. 10-7. PA oblique projection with barium-filled esophagus. RAO position.

(Courtesy W. William Pollino.)

The *thymus gland* has been identified as the primary control organ of the lymphatic system. It is responsible for producing the hormone *thymosin,* which plays a critical role in the development and maturation of the immune system. It consists of two pyramid-shaped lobes that lie in the lower neck and superior mediastinum, anterior to the trachea and great vessels of the heart and posterior to the manubrium sterni. The thymus reaches its maximum size at puberty, with a weight of 35 to 40 gm, and then gradually undergoes atrophy until it almost disappears (Figs. 10-8 and 10-9).

In older individuals, the lymphatic tissue is replaced by fat. At its maximum development, the thymus rests on the pericardium and reaches as high as the thyroid gland. When the thymus is enlarged in infants and young children, it can press on the retrothymic organs, displacing them posteriorly and causing respiratory disturbances. A radiographic examination may be made in both the AP and lateral projections. Exposures should be made at the end of full inhalation for optimal image contrast.

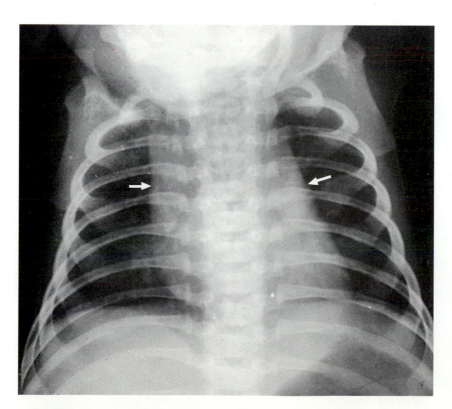

Fig. 10-8. PA chest radiograph showing mediastinal enlargement caused by thymus hypertrophy *(arrows).*

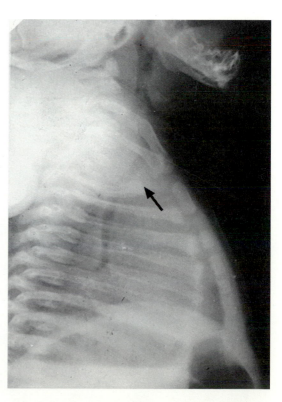

Fig. 10-9. Lateral chest radiograph demonstrating enlarged thymus *(arrow).*

General positioning considerations

For radiography of the heart and lungs, the patient is placed in an *upright position* whenever possible to prevent engorgement of the pulmonary vessels and to allow gravity to depress the diaphragm. In the recumbent position, gravitational force causes the abdominal viscera and diaphragm to move superiorly, compress the thoracic viscera, and prevent full expansion of the lungs. Although the difference is not great in hyposthenic persons, it is marked in hypersthenic individuals. Figs. 10-10 and 10-11 illustrate the effect of body position; both projections were made on the same subject. The left lateral chest position (Fig. 10-12) is most commonly employed because it places the heart closer to the film, resulting in a less magnified heart image. (See Figs. 10-12 and 10-13 for comparison of right and left lateral chest images.)

A *slight amount of rotation* from the PA or lateral projections causes considerable distortion of the heart shadow. To preclude this distortion, the body must be carefully positioned and immobilized using the following procedure:

- **PA Criteria**
  - Instruct the patient to sit or stand upright. If standing, the weight of the body must be equally distributed on the feet.
  - Position the patient's head upright, facing directly forward. Have the patient depress the shoulders and hold them in contact with the grid device to carry the clavicles below the lung apices. Except in the presence of an upper thoracic scoliosis, a faulty body position can be detected by the asymmetrical appearance of the sternoclavicular joints. Compare the clavicular shadows in Figs. 10-14 and 10-15.

- **Lateral Criteria**
  - Place the side of interest against the film holder.
  - Have the patient stand so the weight is equally distributed on the feet. The patient should not lean toward, or away from, the film holder.
  - Raise the patient's arms to prevent the soft tissue of the arms from superimposing the lung fields.
  - Instruct the patient to face straight ahead and raise the chin.
  - To determine rotation, examine the posterior aspects of the ribs. Radiographs without rotation will show superimposed posterior ribs as shown in Figs. 10-12 and 10-13.

- **Oblique Criterion**
  - For oblique projections, have the patient rotate the hips with the thorax and point the feet directly forward. The shoulders should lie in the same transverse plane on all radiographs.

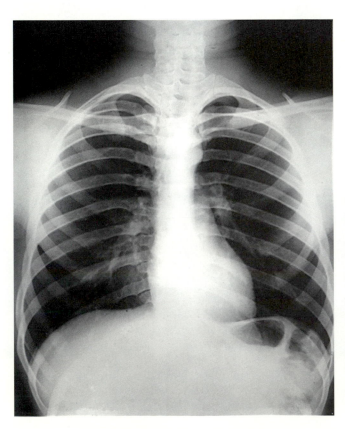

Fig. 10-10. Upright chest radiograph.

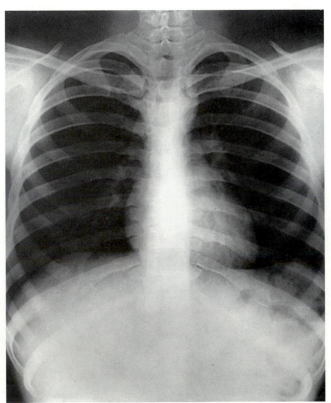

Fig. 10-11. Prone chest radiograph.

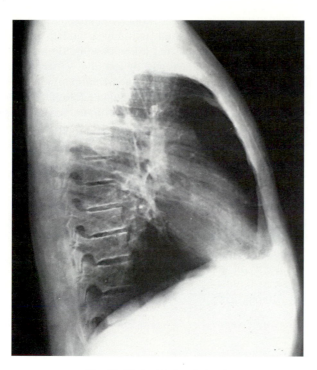

Fig. 10-12. Left lateral chest.

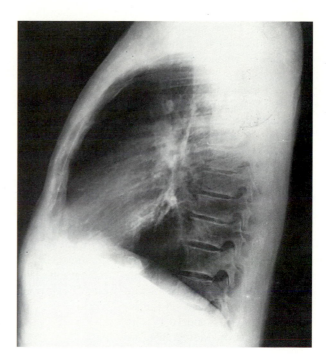

Fig. 10-13. Right lateral chest.

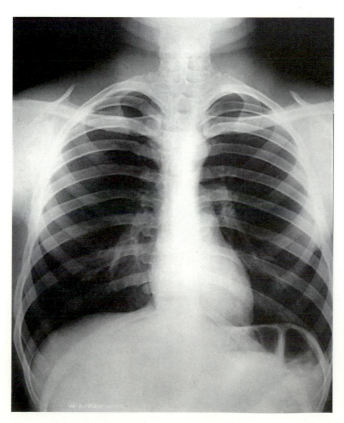

Fig. 10-14. PA chest without rotation.

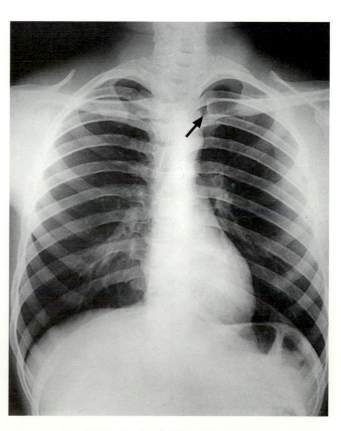

Fig. 10-15. PA chest with rotation *(arrow)*.

Breathing instructions

During *normal inspiration,* the costal muscles pull the anterior ribs superiorly and laterally, the shoulders rise, and the thorax expands from front to back and from side to side. These changes in the height and AP dimension of the thorax must be considered when positioning the patient.

Deep inspiration causes the diaphragm to move inferiorly, resulting in elongation of the heart. Radiographs of the heart should therefore be obtained at the end of normal inhalation to prevent distortion. More air is inhaled during the second breath, and without strain, than during the first breath.

When a pneumothorax (the presence of gas or air in the pleural cavity) is suspected, one exposure is often made at the end of full inhalation and another at the end of full exhalation to demonstrate small amounts of free air in the pleural cavity that might be obscured on the inhalation film (Figs. 10-16 and 10-17). Inhalation and exhalation radiographs are also used to demonstrate the movement of the diaphragm, the occasional presence of a foreign body, and atelectasis.

Technical procedure

The projections required for an adequate demonstration of the thoracic viscera are usually requested by the attending physician, according to the clinical history of the patient. The PA projection of the chest is the most common projection and is used in all lung and heart examinations. Right and left oblique and lateral projections are also employed, as required, as a supplement to the PA projection. It is often necessary to improvise variations of the basic positions to project a localized area free of superimposed structures.

The exposure factors and accessories employed in examining the thoracic viscera depend on the radiographic characteristics of the existent pathologic condition. Normally, chest radiography uses a high kilovoltage (kVp) to penetrate and demonstrate all thoracic anatomy on the radiograph. The kilovoltage can be lowered if exposures are made without using a grid.

However, if the selected kilovoltage is too low, the radiographic contrast may be too high resulting in few shades of gray. On such a radiograph the lung fields may appear properly penetrated, but the mediastinum will appear underexposed. If the selected kilovoltage is too high, the contrast may be too low, which does not allow for demonstration of the finer lung markings. Adequate kilovoltage will penetrate the mediastinum and demonstrate a faint shadow of the spine. Whenever possible, an SID of 72 inches (180 cm) is used to minimize magnification of the heart shadow and to obtain sharper outlines of the delicate lung structures (Fig. 10-18).

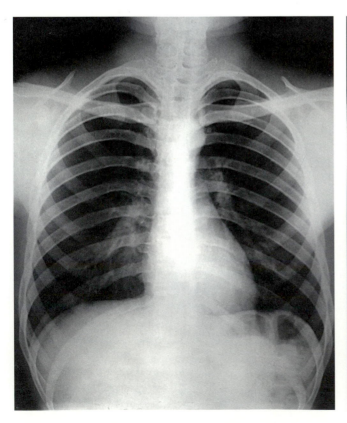

Fig. 10-16. PA chest, inhalation.

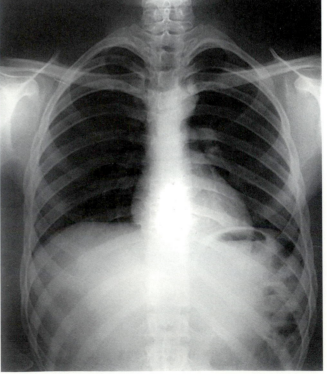

Fig. 10-17. PA chest, exhalation.

A grid technique is recommended for opaque areas within the lung fields and to demonstrate the lung structure through thickened pleural membranes. See Figs. 10-19 and 10-20 for comparison.

Radiation protection

Protection of the patient from unnecessary radiation is a professional responsibility of the radiographer. (See Chapter 1 for specific guidelines.) In this chapter, the *"Shield gonads"* statement indicates that the patient is to be protected from unnecessary radiation by restricting the radiation beam using proper collimation. In addition, placing lead shielding between the gonads and the radiation source is appropriate when the clinical objectives of the examination are not compromised. An example of a properly placed lead shield is demonstrated in Fig. 10-27.

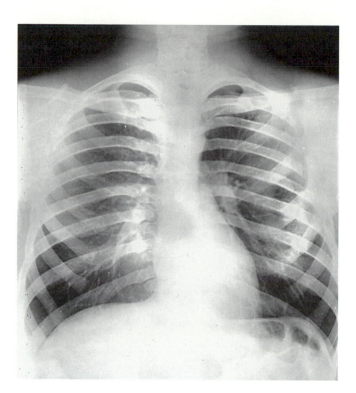

Fig. 10-18. Radiograph taken at SID of 36 inches shows magnified heart shadow.

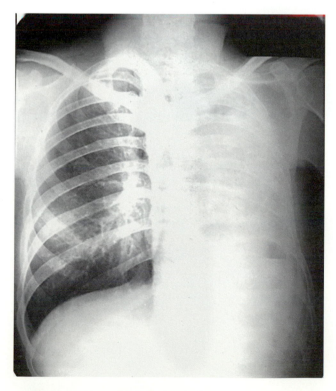

Fig. 10-19. Non-grid radiograph demonstrating pathologic condition on same patient as in Fig. 10-20.

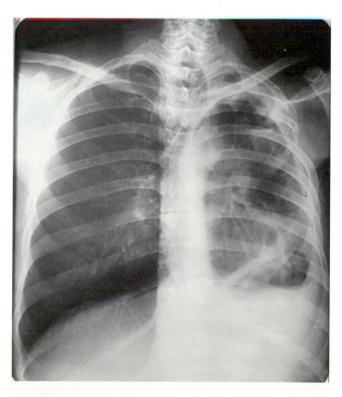

Fig. 10-20. Grid film of same patient as in Fig. 10-19.

Trachea
AP PROJECTION

When preparing to radiograph the trachea for the AP projection, use a grid technique to minimize secondary radiation, because the kilovoltage must be high enough to penetrate both the sternum and the cervical vertebrae.

Film: 10 × 12 in (24 × 30 cm) lengthwise.

Position of patient

- Examine the patient in either the supine or upright position.

Position of part

- Center the median sagittal plane of the body to the midline of the grid.
- Adjust the shoulders to lie in the same transverse plane.
- Extend the neck slightly and adjust it so that the median sagittal plane is perpendicular to the plane of the film (Fig. 10-21).
- Center the cassette at the level of the manubrium.
- *Shield gonads.*
- *Respiration:* Instruct the patient to inhale slowly *during* the exposure to ensure that the trachea is filled with air.

Central ray

- Direct the central ray perpendicular through the manubrium to the center of the cassette.

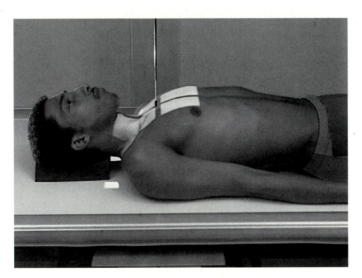

Fig. 10-21. AP trachea.

Structures shown

An AP projection shows the outline of the air-filled trachea, which, under normal conditions, is superimposed on the shadow of the cervical vertebrae (Fig. 10-22).

Evaluation criteria

The following should be clearly demonstrated:

- Area from the mid-cervical to the mid-thoracic region.
- Air-filled trachea.
- No rotation.

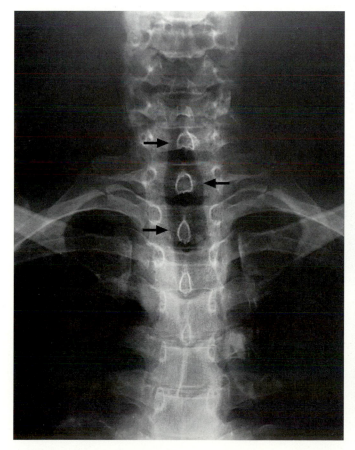 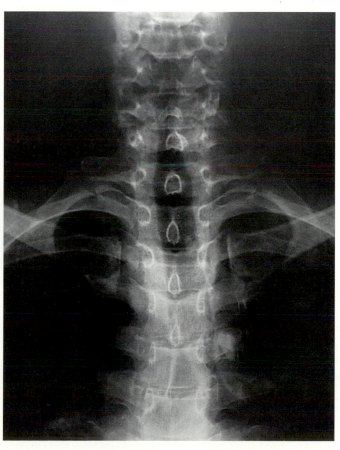

Fig. 10-22. AP trachea during inhalation demonstrating air-filled trachea (*arrows*).

Trachea and Superior Mediastinum

LATERAL PROJECTION
R or L position

Film: 10 × 12 in (24 × 30 cm) or 11 × 14 in (30 × 35 cm) lengthwise.

Position of patient

• Place the patient in a lateral position, either seated or standing, upright before a vertical grid device. If standing, the weight of the body must be equally distributed on the feet.

Position of part

• Instruct the patient to clasp the hands behind the body and then rotate the shoulders posteriorly as far as possible (Fig. 10-23). This will prevent their superimposed shadows from obscuring the structures of the superior mediastinum. If necessary, immobilize the arms in this position with a wide bandage.

• Adjust the patient's position to center the trachea to the midline of the film. The trachea lies in the coronal plane that passes approximately midway between the jugular notch and the median coronal plane.

• Adjust the height of the cassette so that the upper border of the film is at or above the level of the laryngeal prominence.

• Readjust the position of the body, being careful to have the median sagittal plane vertical and parallel with the plane of the film.

• Extend the neck slightly.

• *Shield gonads.*

• *Respiration:* Make the exposure *during slow inhalation* to ensure that the trachea is filled with air.

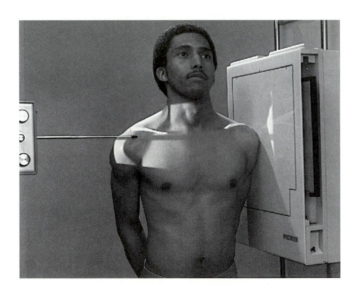

Fig. 10-23. Lateral trachea and superior mediastinum.

Central ray

- Direct the central ray horizontally through a point midway between the jugular notch and the anterior border of the head of the humerus for the superior mediastinal structures (Fig. 10-24, *A*) and from 4 to 5 inches (10 to 13 cm) lower for the demonstration of the entire chest (Fig. 10-24, *B*). A 14 × 7 inch cassette is required for the full chest projection.

Structures shown

A lateral projection demonstrates the air-filled trachea and the regions of the thyroid and thymus glands. This projection first described by Eiselberg and Sgalitzer,[1] is used extensively to demonstrate retrosternal extensions of the thyroid gland, thymic enlargement in infants (in the recumbent position), and the opacified pharynx and upper esophagus, as well as the trachea and bronchi. It is also used for foreign body localization.

[1]Eiselberg A and Sgalitzer DM: X-ray examination of the trachea and the bronchi, Surg Gynecol Obstet 47:53-68, 1928.

□ Evaluation criteria

The following should be clearly demonstrated:

- Area from the mid-cervical to the mid-thoracic region.
- The trachea and superior mediastinum free of superimposition by the shoulders.
- Air-filled trachea.
- No rotation.

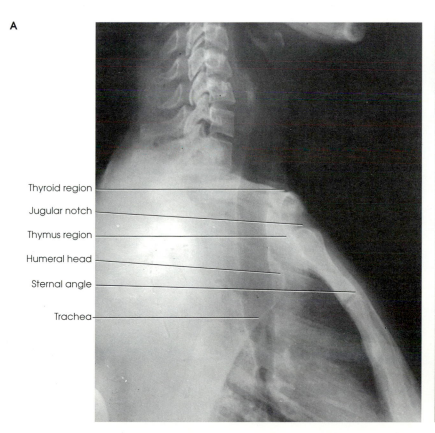

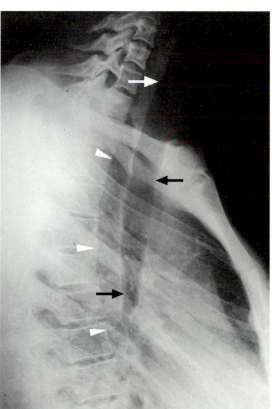

Thyroid region

Jugular notch

Thymus region

Humeral head

Sternal angle

Trachea

Fig. 10-24. A, Lateral superior mediastinum. **B,** Thoracic mediastinum with air-filled trachea *(arrows)* and esophagus *(arrowheads).*

Trachea and superior mediastinum

Trachea and Pulmonary Apex

AXIOLATERAL PROJECTION
R or L position
TWINING METHOD

This projection is used to obtain an axiolateral image of the apex of the lung nearest the film and the trachea and superior mediastinum on patients who cannot rotate their shoulders posteriorly enough for a true lateral projection.

Film: 10 × 12 in (24 × 30 cm) lengthwise.

Position of patient

- Seat or stand the patient before a vertical grid device, with the affected side toward the cassette.

Position of part

- Elevate the arm adjacent to the cassette in extreme abduction, flex the elbow, and place the forearm across or behind the head.
- Center the film to the region of the trachea at the level of the axilla.
- Have the patient rest the shoulder firmly against the grid device for support.
- Depress the opposite shoulder as much as possible.
- Adjust the body in a true lateral position, with the median sagittal plane parallel with the plane of the film (Fig. 10-25).

- *Shield gonads.*
- *Respiration:* For the trachea, instruct the patient to inhale slowly *during* the exposure. For the lung apex, make the exposure at the end of *full inhalation.*

Central ray

- Direct the central ray through the adjacent supraclavicular impression at an angle of 15 degrees caudad. It exits the dependent axilla.

Structures shown

This axiolateral projection demonstrates the air-filled trachea and the apex of the lung closest to the cassette (Fig. 10-26).

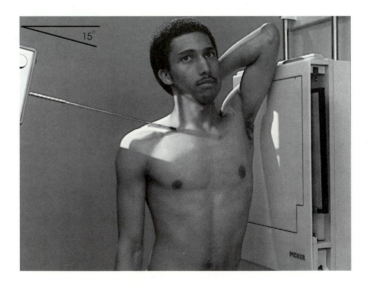

Fig. 10-25. Axiolateral trachea and pulmonary apex.

□ Evaluation criteria

The following should be clearly demonstrated:

- Shoulders well separated from each other.
- Area from the mid-cervical to the mid-thoracic region.
- Air-filled trachea.
- No rotation.

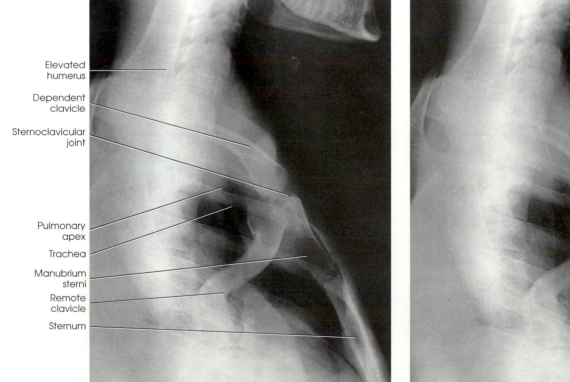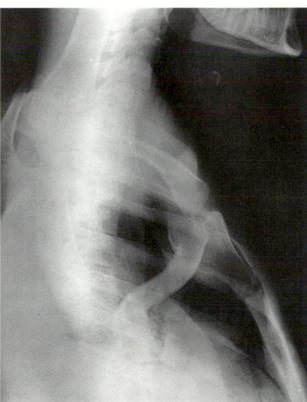

Elevated humerus

Dependent clavicle

Sternoclavicular joint

Pulmonary apex

Trachea

Manubrium sterni

Remote clavicle

Sternum

Fig. 10-26. Axiolateral trachea and pulmonary apex.

Chest: Lungs and Heart

⚜ PA PROJECTION

The recommended SID for this projection is 72 inches (180 cm) to decrease the magnification of the heart.

Film: 14 × 17 in (35 × 43 cm) lengthwise, or crosswise for the hypersthenic patient.

Position of patient

- If possible, examine the patient in the upright position, either standing or seated, so that the diaphragm will be at its lowest position and engorgement of the pulmonary vessels is avoided. The central ray object-to-image receptor relationship is the same for the prone position as for the upright position.

Position of part

- Place the patient, with arms hanging at sides, before a vertical grid device.
- Adjust the height of the cassette so that the upper border of the film is about 1½ to 2 inches (3 to 5 cm) above the relaxed shoulders (or approximately 4 inches [10 cm] above the jugular notch).
- Center the median sagittal plane of the body to the midline of the cassette.
- Have the patient stand straight, with the weight of the body equally distributed on the feet.
- Extend the chin over the top of the grid device and adjust the head so the median sagittal plane is vertical.
- Ask the patient to pronate the arms, resting the backs of the hands low on the hips, below the level of the costophrenic angles. This maneuver rotates the scapulae laterally so that they are not superimposed over the lungs.
- Adjust the shoulders to lie in the same transverse plane, depress them to carry the clavicles below the apices, and then rotate them forward (Figs. 10-27 and 10-28).

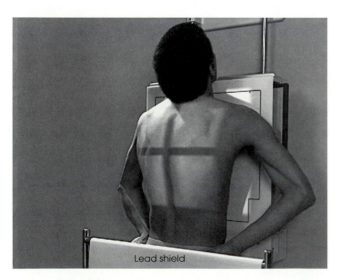

Fig. 10-27. Patient positioned for PA chest.

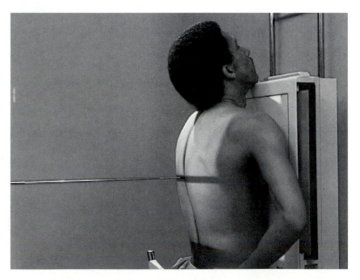

Fig. 10-28. PA chest.

- Instruct the patient to keep the shoulders in contact with the grid device.
- Aid the patient who is unsteady because of age and/or illness in maintaining the position by placing a restraining band around the patient.
- When a restraining band is necessary, exercise care to adjust the arms to rotate the scapulae away from the lung fields as much as possible.
- If an immobilization band is used, exercise care to avoid rotating the body when applying the band. The least amount of rotation will result in considerable distortion of the heart shadow.
- If a woman's breasts are large enough to be superimposed over the lower part of the lung fields, ask the patient to pull them upward and laterally. Have the patient hold them in place by leaning against the film holder (Figs. 10-29 and 10-30).
- *Shield gonads:* Place a lead shield between x-ray tube and patient's pelvis as shown.

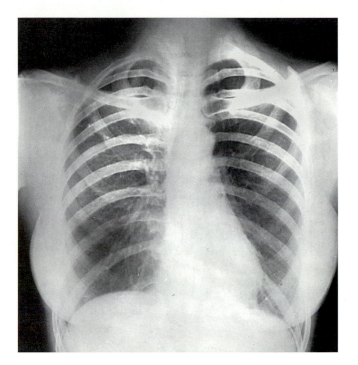

Fig. 10-29. Breasts superimposed over lower lungs.

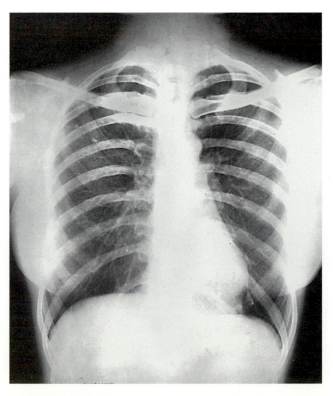

Fig. 10-30. Correct placement of breasts.

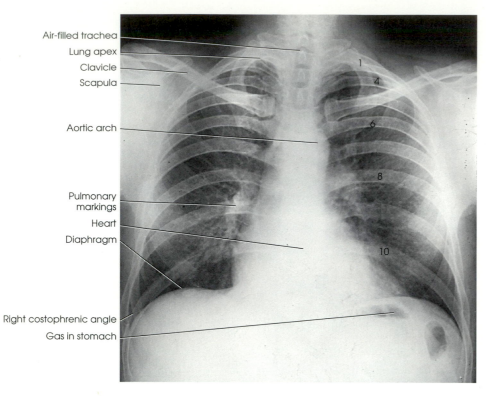

Air-filled trachea
Lung apex
Clavicle
Scapula

Aortic arch

Pulmonary markings
Heart
Diaphragm

Right costophrenic angle
Gas in stomach

Fig. 10-31. Inhalation (posterior rib numbers).

- *Respiration:* Expose general survey films at the end of full inhalation to show the greatest possible area of lung structure. The lungs will expand more on the *second breath* than on the first and without strain to the patient. For certain conditions, such as pneumothorax, the presence of a foreign body, and fixation of the diaphragm, radiographs are sometimes made at the end of both inhalation and exhalation (Figs. 10-31 and 10-32).

Central ray

- Adjust the collimator and direct the central ray perpendicular to the median sagittal plane to the center of the film at the level of the seventh thoracic vertebra.

Structures shown

A PA projection of the thoracic viscera shows the air-filled trachea, the lungs, the diaphragmatic domes, the heart and aortic knob, and, if enlarged laterally, the thyroid or thymus gland (Figs. 10-33 and 10-34). The vascular markings are much more prominent on the projection made at the end of exhalation. The bronchial tree is shown from an oblique angle. The esophagus is well demonstrated when filled with a barium sulfate suspension.

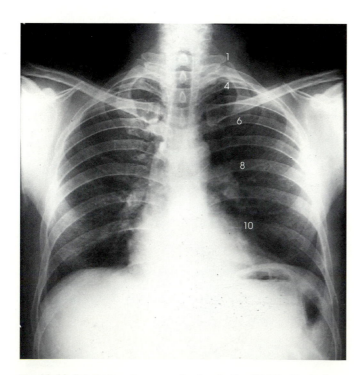

Fig. 10-32. Exhalation (same patient as in Fig. 10-31). (Posterior rib numbers).

□ Evaluation criteria

The following should be clearly demonstrated:

- Sternal ends of the clavicles equidistant from the vertebral column.
- Trachea visible in the midline unless pathologic change is present.
- Scapulae projected outside the lung fields.
- 2 inches (5 cm) of lung apex visible above the clavicles.
- Ten posterior ribs visible above the diaphragm.
- Distance from the vertebral column to the lateral border of the ribs equidistant on each side.
- Small amount of the heart visible on the right side of the vertebral column.
- Lateral aspects of the lung fields including the costophrenic angles.
- Sharp outlines on heart and diaphragm.
- Faint shadow of the ribs and superior thoracic vertebrae visible through the heart shadow.
- The lung fields.
- Lung markings visible from the hilum to the periphery of the lung.
- With inspiration and expiration chest images: the expiration radiograph should demonstrate the diaphragm at a higher level so that at least one fewer rib is seen within the lung field.

NOTE: Inferior lobes of both lungs should be carefully checked for adequate penetration on women with large, pendulous breasts.

Cardiac studies with barium

PA chest radiographs are often obtained with the patient swallowing a bolus of barium sulfate to outline the posterior heart and aorta. The barium used in cardiac examinations should be thicker than that used for the stomach to make it descend more slowly and adhere to the esophageal walls. Have the patient take two or three swallows of barium and hold in the mouth until ready to make the exposure. The exposure is made after the patient takes a deep breath and then swallows the bolus of barium (Fig. 10-6).

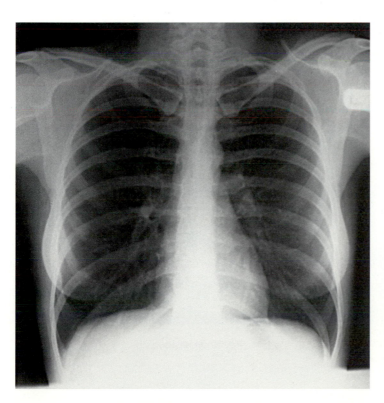

Fig. 10-33. PA chest, female.

(Courtesy Elizabeth Zuffuto, R.T.)

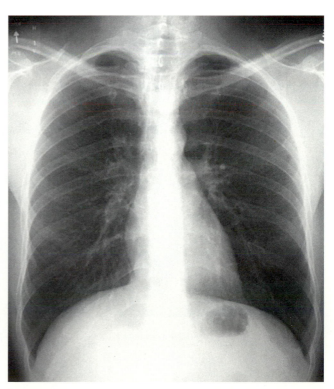

Fig. 10-34. PA chest, male.

(Courtesy Frank J. Brewster, R.T.)

Chest: Lungs and Heart

LATERAL PROJECTION
R or L position

The recommended SID for this projection is 72 inches (180 cm) to compensate for the magnification of the heart caused by the increased OID.

Film: 14 × 17 in (35 × 43 cm) lengthwise.

Position of patient

- If possible, examine the patient in the upright position, either standing or seated, so the diaphragm will be at its lowest position and engorgement of the pulmonary vessels is avoided.
- Turn the patient to a lateral position, arms by the sides.
- Use the left lateral position, with the left side against the film, to show the heart and left lung; use the right lateral position to best demonstrate the right lung.

Position of part

- Adjust the position of the patient so that the median sagittal plane of the body is parallel with the film and the adjacent shoulder is touching the grid device.
- Adjust the height of the cassette so that the upper border of the film is about 1½ to 2 inches (4 to 5 cm) above the shoulders.
- Center the thorax to the grid; the median coronal plane will lie about 2 inches (5 cm) posterior to the midline of the grid.
- Have the patient sit or stand straight, elevate the chin, and look straight ahead.
- Have the patient extend the arms directly upward, flex the elbows, and, with the forearms resting on his or her head, grasp the elbows to hold the arms in position (Figs. 10-35 and 10-36).
- If the patient is unsteady, place an IV stand in front of him or her, and have the patient extend the arms and grasp the standard as high as possible for support.

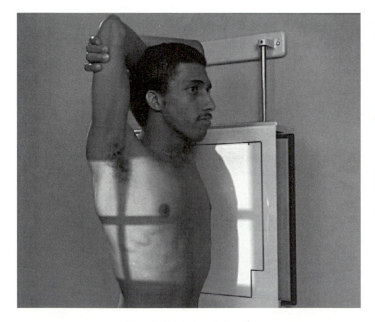

Fig. 10-35. Lateral chest.

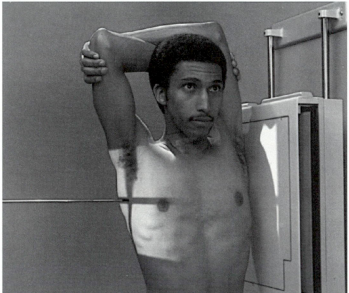

Fig. 10-36. Lateral chest.

- Recheck the position of the body; the median sagittal plane must be vertical. Depending on the width of the shoulders, the lower part of the thorax may be a greater distance from the film, but this position is necessary to obtain true structural outlines. Having the patient *lean* against the grid device (foreshortening) results in distortion of all thoracic structures (Fig. 10-37). *Forward bending* also results in distorted structural outlines (Fig. 10-38).
- *Shield gonads.*

- *Respiration:* Make the exposure at the end of *full inhalation,* preferably at the end of the second breath, to show the greatest possible area of lung structure.

Central ray

- Direct the central ray perpendicular to the midline of the film. It should enter the patient 2 inches (5 cm) anterior to the median coronal plane at the level of the seventh thoracic vertebra.

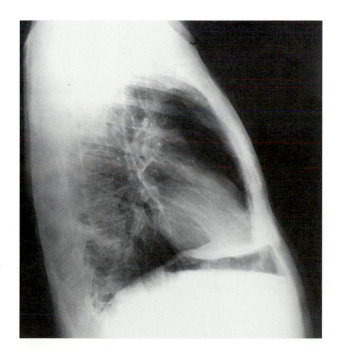

Fig. 10-37. Foreshortening.

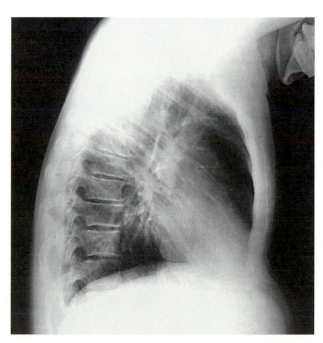

Fig. 10-38. Forward bending.

Structures shown

The preliminary left lateral chest position is used to demonstrate the heart and aorta and left-sided pulmonary lesions (Figs. 10-39 and 10-40); the right lateral chest position is used to demonstrate right-sided pulmonary lesions (Fig. 10-41). These lateral projections are employed extensively to demonstrate the interlobar fissures, to differentiate the lobes, and to localize pulmonary lesions.

□Evaluation criteria

The following should be clearly demonstrated:

- Superimposition of the ribs posterior to the vertebral column.
- The arm or its soft tissues do not overlap the superior lung field.
- Long axis of lung fields demonstrated in vertical position, without forward-backward leaning.
- Lateral sternum with no rotation.
- Costophrenic angles and the apices of the lungs.
- Penetration of the lung fields and heart.
- Open thoracic intervertebral spaces, except in patients with scoliosis.
- Sharp outlines on heart and diaphragm.
- Hilum in the approximate center of the radiograph.

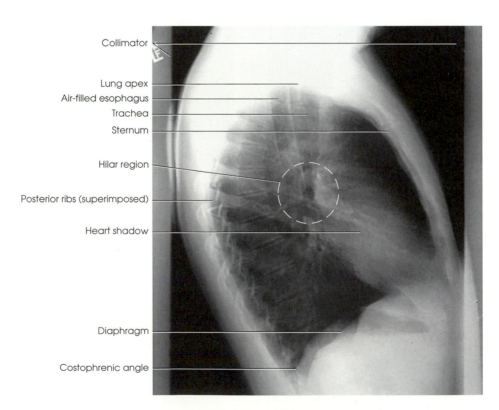

Collimator
Lung apex
Air-filled esophagus
Trachea
Sternum
Hilar region
Posterior ribs (superimposed)
Heart shadow
Diaphragm
Costophrenic angle

Fig. 10-39. Left lateral chest.

(Courtesy Frank J. Brewster, R.T.)

Cardiac studies with barium

The left lateral position is traditionally used during cardiac studies with barium. Follow the same procedure described in the PA chest on p. 455.

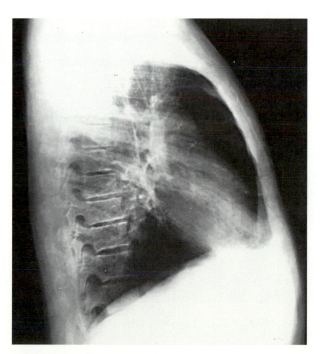

Fig. 10-40. Left lateral chest. (Compare heart shadows with radiograph of same patient in Fig. 10-41.)

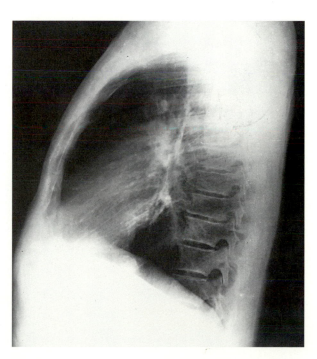

Fig. 10-41. Right lateral chest (same patient as in Fig. 10-40).

Chest: Lungs and Heart

 ### PA OBLIQUE PROJECTION
RAO and LAO positions

The recommended SID is 72 inches (180 cm) to compensate for the magnification of the heart caused by the increased OID.

Film: 14 × 17 in (35 × 43 cm) lengthwise.

Position of patient

- Maintain the patient in the same position, standing or seated upright, that was used for the PA projection.
- Instruct the patient to let the arms hang free, and, unless otherwise specified, have the patient turn approximately 45 degrees toward the left side for an LAO position and approximately 45 degrees toward the right side for an RAO position.

- Ask the patient to stand or sit straight; when standing, the weight of the body must be equally distributed on the feet to prevent unwanted rotation.
- Check the cassette centering used for the PA projection to be certain the cassette projects far enough above the upper border of the shoulders (approximately 2 to 3 inches [5 to 8 cm]) to clear the identification marker.
- For PA oblique projections, the side of interest is generally the side *farthest* from the film. The resulting image demonstrates the greatest area of the elevated lung. However, the lung closest to the film is also imaged, and diagnostic information is often obtained for that side.

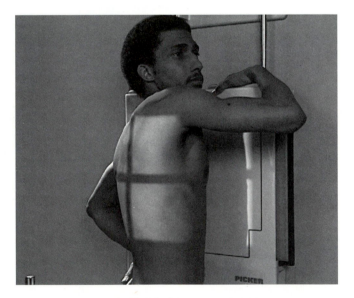

Fig. 10-42. PA oblique chest. LAO.

Position of part

LAO position

- Rotate the patient to place the left shoulder and breast in contact with the grid device, and center the chest to the film. The center of the cassette will coincide with a plane midway between the *lateral margins of the body*.
- Instruct the patient to place the left hand on the hip with the palm down.

- Adjust the rotation of the body to 45 degrees for preliminary examinations of the chest and, for the purpose of separating the shadows of the aorta and the spine, 55 to 60 degrees for studies of the heart and great vessels.
- Ask the patient to raise the right arm to shoulder level and grasp the side of the vertical grid device for support.
- Adjust the shoulders to lie in the same horizontal plane, and instruct the patient to not rotate the head (Fig. 10-42).

RAO position

- Reverse the previously described position, placing the right shoulder in contact with the grid device.
- Adjust the rotation of the body to 45 degrees unless requested otherwise (Figs. 10-43 and 10-44).
- *Shield gonads*.
- *Respiration:* Make the exposure at the end of full inhalation.

Central ray

- Direct the central ray perpendicular to the center of the film at the level of the seventh thoracic vertebra. The central ray enters the body midway between the lateral surface of the elevated side and the spine.

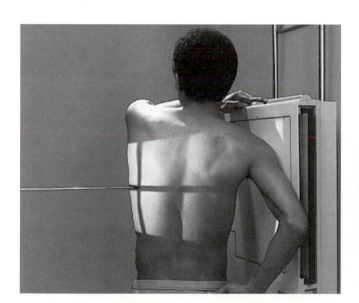

Fig. 10-43. PA oblique chest. RAO.

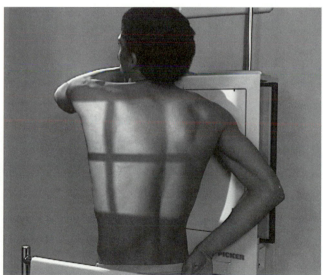

Fig. 10-44. PA oblique chest. RAO.

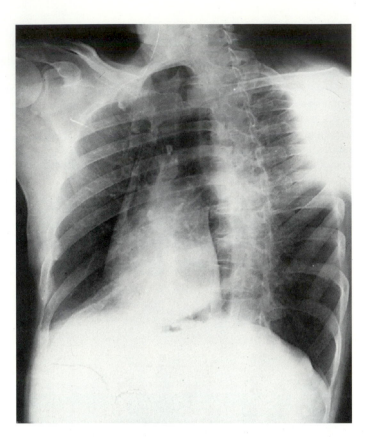

Fig. 10-45. PA oblique chest. LAO.

Structures shown

LAO position

The maximum area of the right lung field (side farthest from the film) is demonstrated with its posterior portion superimposed by mediastinum. The anterior portion of the left lung is superimposed by the shadow of the spine (Figs. 10-45 and 10-46). Also shown are the trachea and its bifurcation (the carina), the entire right branch of the bronchial tree, and a foreshortened image of the left lung. The heart, the descending aorta (lying just in front of the spinal shadow), the arch of the aorta, and the pulmonary artery are also presented.

RAO position

The maximum area of the left lung field (side farthest from the film) is demonstrated with its posterior portion superimposed by the shadow of the mediastinum. The anterior portion of the right lung is superimposed by the spine (Figs. 10-47 and 10-48). Also shown are the trachea and entire left branch of the bronchial tree, as well as a foreshortened image of the right lung. This position gives the best image of the left atrium, the left main branch of the pulmonary artery, the anterior portion of the apex of the left ventricle, and the right retrocardiac space. When filled with barium, the esophagus is shown clearly in the RAO and LAO positions (Fig. 10-48).

NOTE: The radiographs on this page, like all radiographs in this text, are printed as if the reader is looking at the patient's anterior body surface. (See Displaying Radiographs, in Chapter 1.)

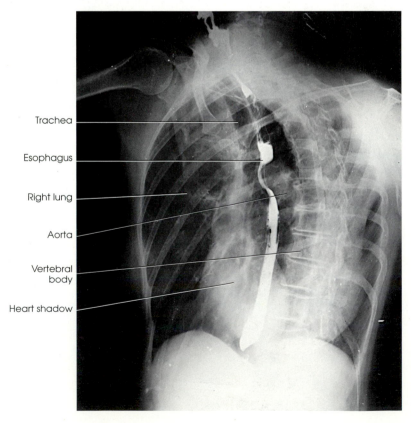

Trachea

Esophagus

Right lung

Aorta

Vertebral body

Heart shadow

Fig. 10-46. PA oblique chest. LAO with barium-filled esophagus.

□ Evaluation criteria

The following should be clearly demonstrated:

- Approximately twice as much distance between the vertebral column and the outer margin of the ribs on the remote side of the film compared with the dependent side.
- Both lungs in their entirety.
- Visible identification markers.
- The lung fields.
- The heart and mediastinal structures within the lung field of the elevated side in oblique images of 45 degrees.

Barium studies

The RAO and LAO positions are routinely used during cardiac studies with barium. Follow the same procedure described in the PA chest section on p. 455.

NOTE: A lesser-degree oblique position has been found to be of particular value in the study of pulmonary diseases. The patient is turned only slightly (10 to 20 degrees) from the RAO or LAO body positions. This slight degree of obliquity rotates the superior segment of the respective lower lobe from behind the hilum and displays the medial part of the right middle lobe or the lingula of the left upper lobe free from the hilum. These areas are not clearly shown in the standard "cardiac oblique" of 45- to 60- degree rotation, largely because of superimposition of the spine.

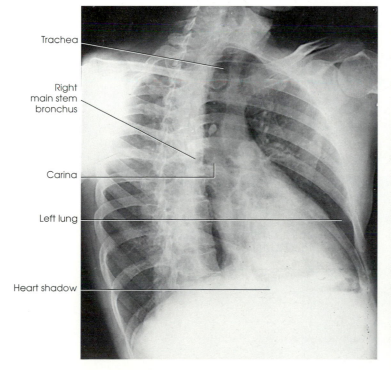

Trachea
Right main stem bronchus
Carina
Left lung
Heart shadow

Fig. 10-47. PA oblique chest. RAO.

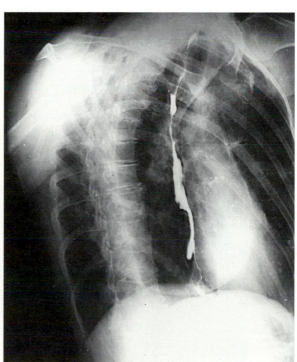

Fig. 10-48. PA oblique chest. RAO.

Chest: Lungs and Heart

 ### AP OBLIQUE PROJECTION
RPO and LPO positions

RPO and LPO positions are used when the patient is too ill to be turned in to the prone position and sometimes as supplementary positions in the investigation of specific lesions. They are also used with the recumbent patient in contrast studies of the heart and great vessels.

One point the radiographer must bear in mind is that the *RPO corresponds to the LAO* and that the *LPO corresponds to the RAO* position. For AP oblique projections, the side of interest is generally the side *closest* to the film. The resulting image demonstrates the greatest area of the lung closest to the film. However, the lung farthest from the film is also imaged, and diagnostic information is often obtained for that side. The recommended SID is 72 inches (180 cm) to compensate for the magnification of the heart caused by the increased OID.

Film: 14 × 17 in (35 × 43 cm) lengthwise.

Position of patient

- With the patient supine or facing the x-ray tube, either upright or recumbent, adjust the cassette so that the upper border of the film is about 2 to 3 inches (5 to 8 cm) above the shoulders.

Position of part

- Rotate the patient toward the correct side, adjust the thorax at a 45-degree angle, and center the chest to the grid.
- If the patient is recumbent, support the elevated hip and arm. A plane midway between the margins of the body surface will coincide with the center of the cassette.
- Flex the elbows and place the hands on the hips with the palms facing outward, or pronate the hands beside the hips. The arm closest to the film may be raised as long as the shoulder is rotated anteriorly.
- Adjust the shoulders to lie in the same transverse plane in a position of forward rotation (Figs. 10-49 and 10-50).
- *Shield gonads.*
- *Respiration:* Make the exposure at the end of *full inhalation.*

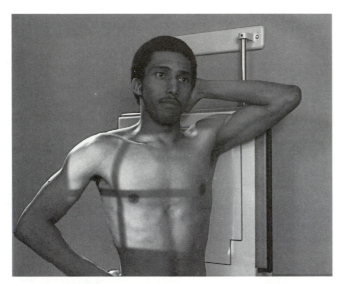

Fig. 10-49. *Upright* AP oblique chest. LPO.

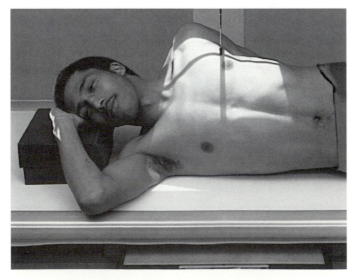

Fig. 10-50. *Recumbent* AP oblique chest. RPO.

Thoracic viscera

Central ray

- Direct the central ray perpendicular to the center of the film at the level of the seventh thoracic vertebra.

Structures shown

This radiograph presents an AP oblique projection of the thoracic viscera similar to the corresponding PA oblique projection (Fig. 10-51). An RPO position is comparable to an LAO position. However, the lung field of the elevated side usually appears shorter because of magnification of the shadow of the diaphragm. The heart and great vessels also cast magnified shadows as a result of being farther from the film.

□ Evaluation criteria

The following should be clearly demonstrated:
- Approximately twice as much distance between the vertebral column and the outer margin of the ribs on the dependent side compared with the remote side.
- Both lungs in their entirety.
- Visible identification markers.
- The lung fields and mediastinal structures.

Chest: lungs and heart

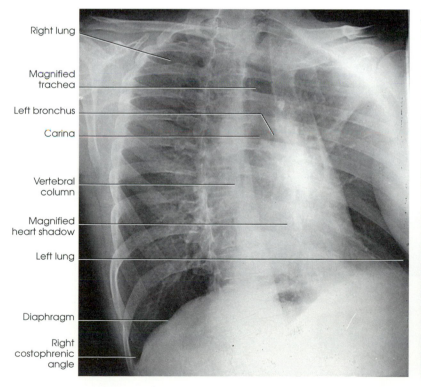
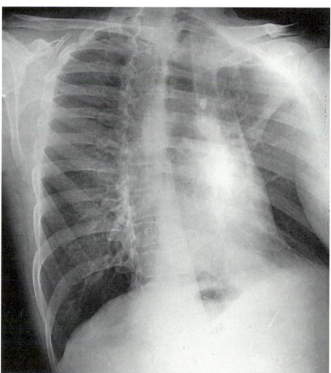

Right lung
Magnified trachea
Left bronchus
Carina
Vertebral column
Magnified heart shadow
Left lung
Diaphragm
Right costophrenic angle

Fig. 10-51. AP oblique chest. LPO.

Chest

 ### AP PROJECTION

The supine position is used when the patient is too ill to be turned to the prone position; it is sometimes used as a supplementary projection in the investigation of certain pulmonary lesions. Use of a 72-inch (180 cm) or a 60-inch (150 cm) SID is recommended if it can be attained using the equipment available.

Film: 14 × 17 in (35 × 43 cm) lengthwise.

Position of patient

- Place the patient in the supine, or upright, position with the back against the grid.

Position of part

- Center the median sagittal plane of the chest to the cassette.
- Adjust it so that the upper border of the film is approximately 2 to 3 inches (5 to 8 cm) above the shoulders.
- If possible, flex the elbows, pronate the hands, and place the hands on the hips to draw the scapulae laterally. This maneuver is often impossible because of the condition of the patient.
- Adjust the shoulders to lie in the same transverse plane (Fig. 10-52).
- *Shield gonads.*
- *Respiration:* Make the exposure at the end of *full inhalation.*

Central ray

- Direct the central ray perpendicular to the center of the film at the level of the seventh thoracic vertebra.

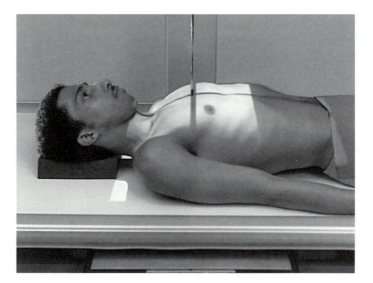

Fig. 10-52. AP chest.

Structures shown

An AP projection of the thoracic viscera (Fig. 10-53) demonstrates an image somewhat similar to that of the PA projection (Fig. 10-54). Being farther from the film, the heart and great vessels are magnified, as well as engorged, and the lung fields appear shorter because abdominal compression moves the diaphragm to a higher level. The clavicles are projected higher, and the ribs assume a more horizontal appearance.

□Evaluation criteria

The following should be clearly demonstrated:

- Medial portion of the clavicles equidistant from the vertebral column.
- Trachea visible in the midline.
- Clavicles lying more horizontal and obscuring more of the apices than in the PA projection.
- Distance from the vertebral column to the lateral border of the ribs equidistant on each side.
- Small amount of the right atrium visible on the right side of the vertebral column.
- Lateral aspects of the lung fields including the costophrenic angles.
- Faint image of the ribs and thoracic vertebrae visible through the heart shadow.
- The lung fields.
- Pleural markings visible from the hilar regions to the periphery of the lungs.

NOTE: Resnick[1] recommends an angled AP projection to free the basal portions of the lung fields from superimposition by the anterior diaphragmatic, abdominal, and cardiac structures. He reports that this projection also differentiates middle lobe and lingular processes from lower lobe disease. For this projection the patient may be either upright or supine, and the central ray is directed to the midsternal region at an angle of 30 degrees caudad. Resnick states that a more suitable angulation may be chosen by studying the preliminary films.

[1]Resnick D: The angulated basal view: a new method for evaluation of lower lobe pulmonary disease, Radiology 96:204-205, 1970.

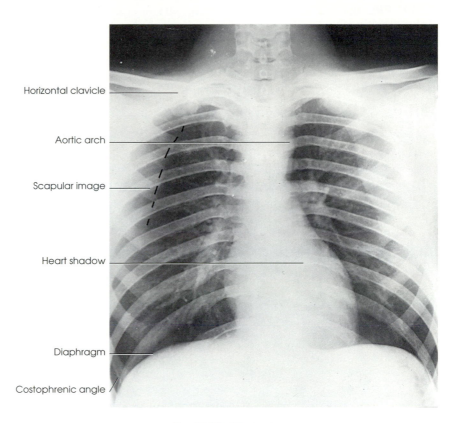

Horizontal clavicle

Aortic arch

Scapular image

Heart shadow

Diaphragm

Costophrenic angle

Fig. 10-53. AP chest.

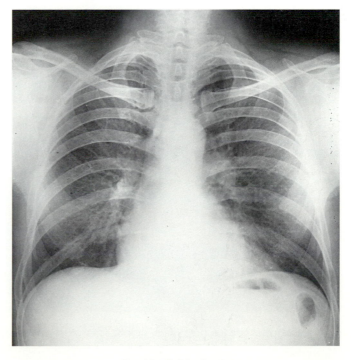

Fig. 10-54. PA chest.

Thoracic viscera

Pulmonary Apices

AP AXIAL PROJECTION
Lordotic position
LINDBLOM METHOD

Film: 14 × 17 in (35 × 43 cm) length-wise.

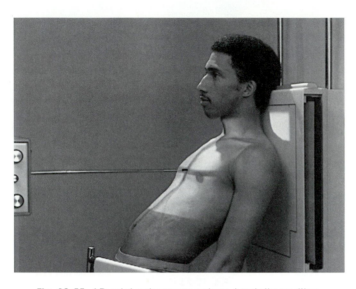

Fig. 10-55. AP axial pulmonary apices. Lordotic position.

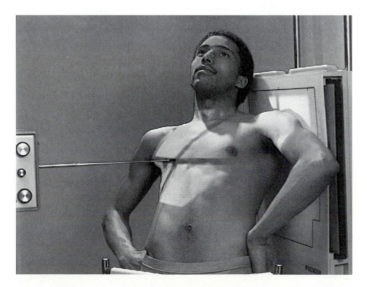

Fig. 10-56. AP axial oblique pulmonary apices. LPO lordotic position.

Position of patient

• Using a recommended 72-inch (180 cm) SID, place the patient in the upright position, facing the x-ray tube standing approximately 1 foot in front of the vertical grid device.

Position of part

• Adjust the height of the cassette so that the upper margin of the film will be about 3 inches (7.5 cm) above the upper border of the shoulders when the patient is adjusted in the lordotic position.

Lordotic position

• Adjust the patient for the AP axial projection, with the median sagittal plane centered to the midline of the grid (Fig. 10-55).

Oblique lordotic positions—LPO or RPO

• Rotate the body approximately 30 degrees away from the position used for the AP projection, with the affected side toward and centered to the grid (Fig. 10-56).

• With the patient in either of the preceding positions, have the patient flex the elbows and place the hands, palms out, on the hips.

• Have the patient lean backward in a position of extreme lordosis and rest the shoulders against the vertical grid device.

• *Shield gonads.*

• *Respiration:* Make the exposure at the end of *full inhalation.*

Central ray

• With the central ray directed perpendicular at the level of the midsternum, center to the center of the film.

Structures shown

The AP axial (Fig. 10-57) and AP axial oblique (Fig. 10-58) images of the lungs demonstrate the apices and conditions such as interlobar effusions.

☐Evaluation criteria

The following should be clearly demonstrated:

Lordotic position

- Clavicles lying superior to the apices.
- Sternal ends of the clavicles equidistant from the vertebral column.
- Apices and lungs in their entirety.
- Clavicles lying horizontally with their medial ends overlapping only the first or second ribs.
- Ribs distorted with their anterior and posterior portions somewhat superimposed.

Oblique lordotic position

- Dependent apex and lung of the affected side in its entirety.

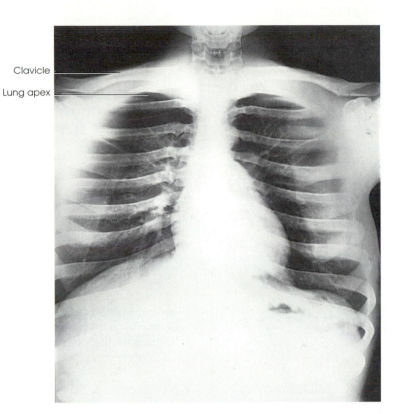

Clavicle

Lung apex

Fig. 10-57. AP axial pulmonary apices. Lordortic position.

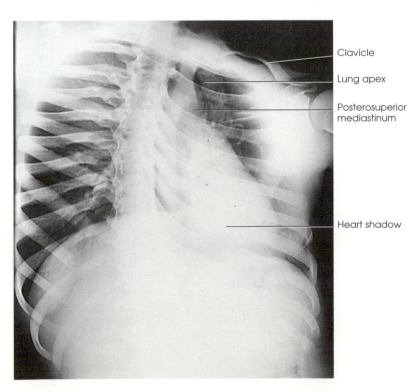

Clavicle

Lung apex

Posterosuperior mediastinum

Heart shadow

Fig. 10-58. AP axial oblique pulmonary apices. LPO lordotic position.

Pulmonary Apices
PA AXIAL PROJECTION

The recommended SID is 72 inches (180 cm) to compensate for the magnification caused by the increased OID.

Film: 10 × 12 in (24 × 30 cm) or 11 × 14 in (30 × 35 cm) crosswise.

Position of patient

- Position the patient, either seated or standing, before a vertical grid device. If the patient is standing, the weight of the body must be equally distributed on the feet.

Position of part

- Adjust the height of the cassette so that the film is centered at the level of the jugular notch.
- Center the median sagittal plane of the body to the midline of the cassette and rest the chin against the grid device.
- Adjust the head so that the median sagittal plane is vertical. Flex the elbows and place the hands, palms out, on the hips.
- Depress the shoulders, rotate them forward, and adjust them to lie in the same transverse plane.
- Instruct the patient to keep the shoulders in contact with the grid device to move the scapulae from the lung fields (Fig. 10-59).
- *Shield gonads.*
- *Respiration:* Make the exposure at the end of *full inhalation* or optionally at *full exhalation.* The clavicles are elevated by inhalation and depressed by exhalation; the apices move little, if at all, during either phase of respiration.

Central ray

Inhalation
- Direct the central ray 10 to 15 degrees cephalad through the third thoracic vertebra to the center of the film.

Exhalation (optional)
- Direct the central ray perpendicular to the plane of the film, and center at the level of the third thoracic vertebra.

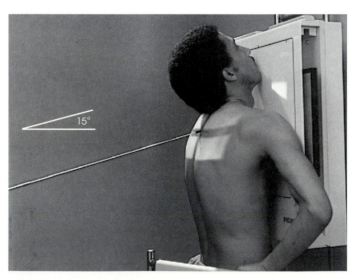

Fig. 10-59. PA axial pulmonary apices.

Structures shown

The apices will be projected above the shadows of the clavicles in the PA axial and PA projections (Figs. 10-60 and 10-61).

☐ Evaluation criteria

The following should be clearly demonstrated:

- Apices in their entirety.
- Along with the apices, only the adjacent superior lung region.
- Clavicles lying below the apices.
- Medial portion of the clavicles equidistant from the vertebral column.

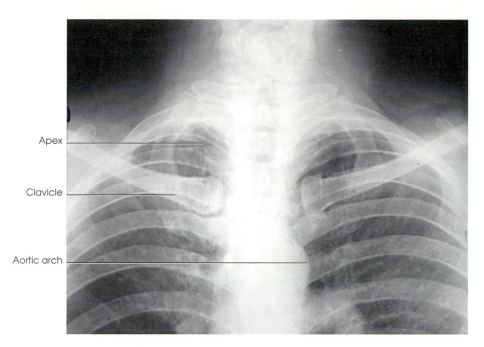

Apex

Clavicle

Aortic arch

Fig. 10-60. AP axial pulmonary apices. *Inhalation* with central ray angled.

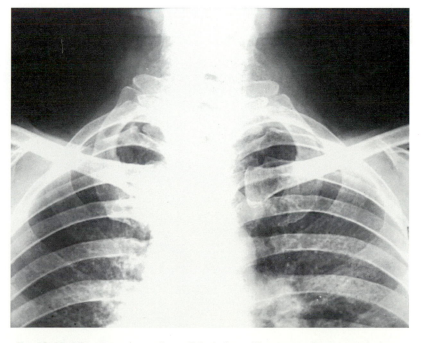

Fig. 10-61. AP pulmonary apices. *Exhalation* with perpendicular central ray.

Pulmonary Apices

AP AXIAL PROJECTION

The recommended SID is 72 inches (180 cm) to compensate for the magnification caused by the increased OID.

Film: 10 × 12 in (24 × 30 cm) or 11 × 14 in (30 × 35 cm) crosswise.

Position of patient

- Examine the patient in the upright or supine position.

Position of part

- Center the film to the median sagittal plane at the level of the second thoracic vertebra, and adjust the body so it is not rotated.
- Flex the elbows and place the hands on the hips with the palms out, or pronate the hands beside the hips.
- Place the shoulders back against the grid and adjust them to lie in the same transverse plane (Fig. 10-62).
- *Shield gonads.*
- *Respiration:* Expose at the end of *full inhalation.*

Central ray

- With the patient in the upright or supine position, direct the central ray to enter the manubrium at an angle of 15 or 20 degrees cephalad to the center of the film.

Structures shown

An AP axial projection demonstrates the apices lying below the clavicles (Fig. 10-63).

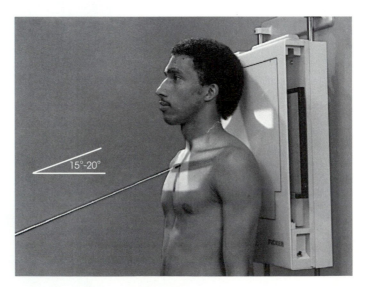

Fig. 10-62. AP axial pulmonary apices.

□ Evaluation criteria

The following should be clearly demonstrated:

- Clavicles lying superior to the apices.
- Sternal ends of the clavicles equidistant from the vertebral column.
- Apices included in their entirety.
- Only the apices and adjacent superior lung region.
- Clavicles lying horizontally with their medial ends overlapping only the first or second ribs.
- Ribs distorted with their anterior and posterior portions somewhat superimposed.

NOTE: The AP axial projection is used in preference to the PA axial projection for patients whose clavicles occupy a high position, as well as for hypersthenic persons, to separate the apical and clavicular shadows without undue distortion of the apices.

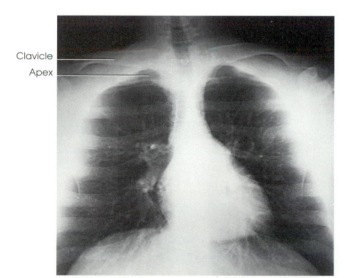 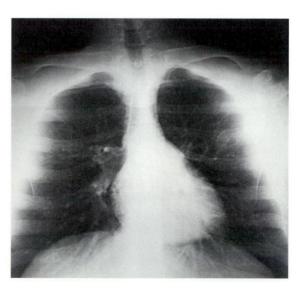

Clavicle

Apex

Fig. 10-63. AP axial pulmonary apices.

PULMONARY APICES

PA AXIAL PROJECTION
Lordotic position
FLEISCHNER METHOD

The recommended SID is 72 inches (180 cm) to compensate for the magnification caused by the increased OID.

Film: 14 × 17 in (35 × 43 cm) lengthwise.

Position of patient

- Position the patient upright, facing the vertical grid device.

Position of part

- Adjust the height of the cassette so that the upper margin of the film is about 1 inch below the upper border of the shoulders *when the patient is standing upright.* With the patient in the lordotic position, the lungs will be correctly projected on the film.
- Center the median sagittal plane of the body to the midline of the grid.
- Have the patient grasp the grid device, brace the abdomen against it, and then lean backward in a position of extreme lordosis. The thorax should be inclined posteriorly approximately 45 degrees (Figs. 10-64 and 10-65).
- *Shield gonads.*
- *Respiration:* Make the exposure at the end of *full inhalation.*

Central ray

- Direct the central ray perpendicular to the fourth thoracic vertebra.

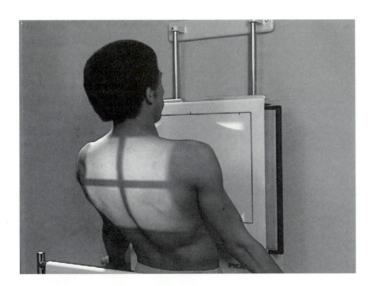

Fig. 10-64. PA axial pulmonary apices. Lordotic position.

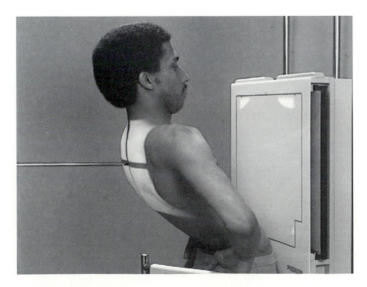

Fig. 10-65. PA axial pulmonary apices. Lordotic position.

Structures shown

The PA axial projection demonstrates interlobar effusion and collapse of the right middle lobe. This positioning places the horizontal fissure parallel with the x-ray beam (Fig. 10-66).

A similar radiograph can be obtained by adjusting the patient in the prone position and directing the central ray 45 degrees caudad (Fig. 10-67).

Kjellberg[1] recommends a prone position with a 30-degree caudal angulation of the central ray for the demonstration of minimal mitral disease.

☐ **Evaluation criteria**

The following should be clearly demonstrated:

- Clavicles lying superior to the apices.
- Sternal ends of the clavicles equidistant from the vertebral column.
- Apices and lungs in their entirety.
- Clavicles lying horizontally with their medial ends overlapping only the first or second ribs.
- Ribs distorted with their anterior and posterior portions somewhat superimposed.

[1]Kjellberg SR: Importance of prone position in the roentgenologic diagnosis of slight mitral disease, Acta Radiol 31:178-181, 1949.

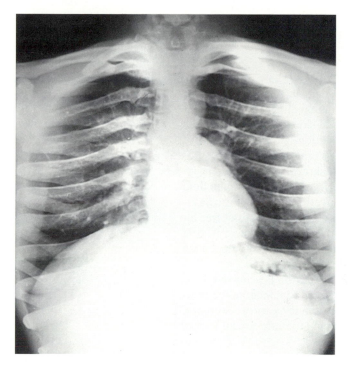

Fig. 10-66. Upright PA axial pulmonary apices. Lordotic position.

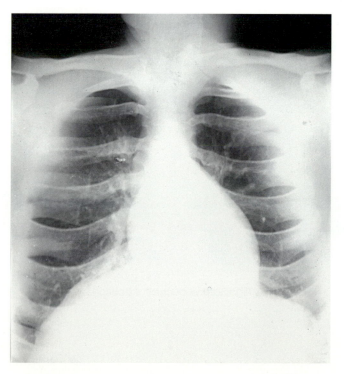

Fig. 10-67. Prone axial pulmonary apices with 45-degree caudal central ray.

Thoracic viscera

Lungs and Pleurae

AP PROJECTION
R or L lateral decubitus positions

Film: 14 × 17 in (35 × 43 cm) lengthwise.

Position of patient

- Place the patient in a lateral decubitus position, lying on either the affected or the unaffected side, as indicated by the existing condition. A small amount of fluid in the pleural cavity is, in most instances, best shown with the patient lying on the affected side, where the fluid will not be overlapped by the mediastinal shadows. A small amount of free air in the pleural cavity is generally best demonstrated by the patient lying on the unaffected side.
- The best visualization is achieved if the patient is allowed to remain in the position for five minutes prior to exposure. This allows fluid to settle and air to rise.

Position of part

- If the patient is lying on the affected side, elevate the body 2 to 3 inches (5 to 8 cm) on a suitable platform or a firm pad.
- Extend the arms well above the head, and adjust the thorax in a true lateral position (Fig. 10-68).
- Place the anterior or the posterior surface of the chest against a vertical grid device.
- Adjust the cassette so that it extends approximately 2 inches (5 cm) beyond the shoulders.
- *Shield gonads.*
- *Respiration:* Expose at the end of *full inhalation.*

Central ray

- Direct the central ray *horizontal* and perpendicular to the seventh thoracic vertebra.

Structures shown

An AP projection demonstrates the change in fluid position and reveals any previously obscured pulmonary areas or, in the case of a suspected pneumothorax, the presence of any free air (Figs. 10-69 to 10-71). The lateral decubitus positions can also be performed using a PA projection. The patient faces the vertical grid device with arms above the head.

This application of the lateral decubitus position was first recommended by Rigler[1] and later by Abo.[2]

---

[1]Rigler LG: Roentgen diagnosis of small pleural effusions, JAMA 96:104-108, 1931.
[2]Abo S: Roentgenographic detection of minimal pneumothorax in the lateral decubitus position, AJR 77:1066-1070, 1957.

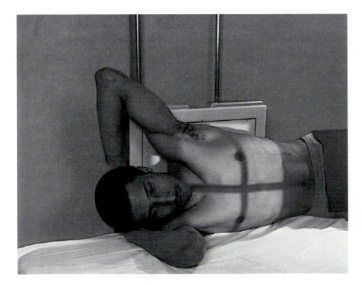

Fig. 10-68. AP projection. Right lateral decubitus position.

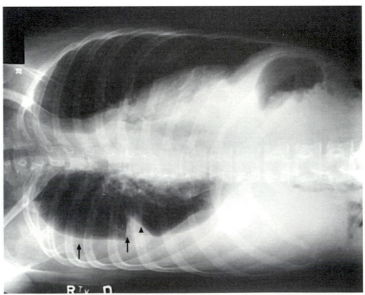

Fig. 10-69. AP projection. Right lateral decubitus position showing fluid level *(arrows)* on side down. Note fluid in lung fissure *(arrowhead)*.

(Courtesy Terry Doherty, R.T.)

□ Evaluation criteria

The following should be clearly demonstrated:

- No rotation of the patient from a true frontal position, as evidenced by the clavicles being equidistant from the spine.
- Affected side in its entirety.
- Apices.
- Proper identification visible to indicate that decubitus was performed.
- Patient's arms not visible in the field of interest.

NOTE: An exposure made with the patient leaning directly laterally from the upright PA position is sometimes an advantage in the demonstration of fluid levels in pulmonary cavities. Ekimsky[3] recommends this position, with the patient leaning laterally 45 degrees, for the demonstration of small pleural effusions. Ekimsky reports that the inclined position is simpler to perform than the decubitus position and states that it is equally satisfactory.

[3]Ekimsky B: Comparative study of lateral decubitus views and those with lateral body inclination in small pleural effusions, Vestn Rentgenol Radiol 41:43-49, 1966. (In Russian.) Abstract: Radiology 87:1135, 1966.

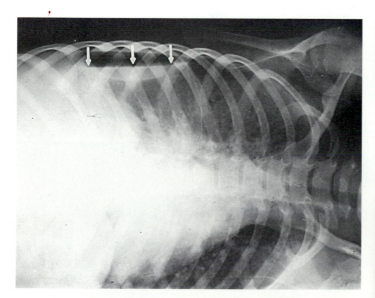

Fig. 10-70. AP projection. Left lateral decubitus position on same patient as in Fig. 10-71. *Arrows* indicate air-fluid level (air on side up).

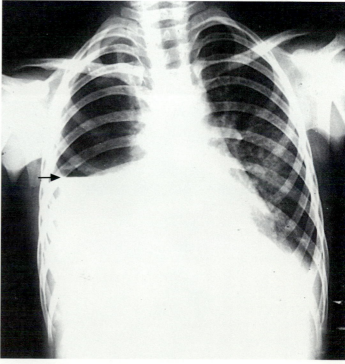

Fig. 10-71. Upright PA chest. *Arrow* indicates air-fluid level.

Lungs and Plurae

✦ LATERAL PROJECTION
Ventral or dorsal decubitus positions

Film: 14 × 17 in (35 × 43 cm) lengthwise.

Position of patient

- With the patient in a prone or supine position, elevate the thorax 2 to 3 inches (5 to 8 cm) on folded sheets or a firm pad, centering the thorax to the grid.
- The best visualization is achieved if the patient is allowed to remain in the position for five minutes prior to exposure. This allows fluid to settle and air to rise.

Position of part

- Adjust the body in a true prone or supine body position, and extend the arms well above the head.
- Place the affected side against a vertical grid device, and adjust it so that the top of the film extends to the level of the laryngeal prominence (Fig. 10-72).
- *Shield gonads.*
- *Respiration:* Make the exposure at the end of *full inhalation.*

Central ray

- With the central ray directed *horizontal* and perpendicular to the film, center to the median coronal plane and the center of the film.

Structures shown

A lateral projection in the decubitus position shows a change in position of fluid and reveals pulmonary areas that are obscured by the fluid in standard projections (Figs. 10-73 and 10-74).

☐ Evaluation criteria

The following should be clearly demonstrated:
- Entire lung fields, including the anterior and posterior surfaces.
- No rotation of the thorax from a true lateral position.
- Upper lung field not obscured by the arms.
- Proper identification visible to indicate the decubitus was performed.
- The sixth thoracic vertebra in the center of the film.

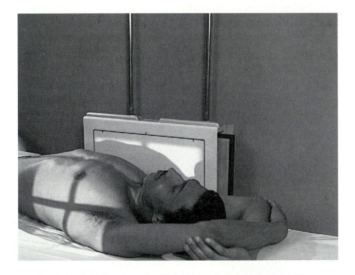

Fig. 10-72. Lateral projection. Dorsal decubitus position.

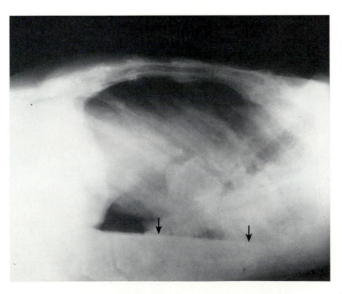

Fig. 10-73. Lateral projection. Dorsal decubitus position. *Arrows* indicate air-fluid level.

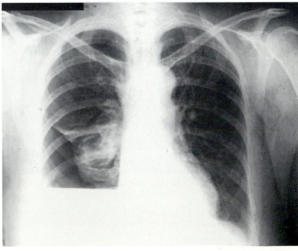

Fig. 10-74. Upright PA chest on same patient as in Fig. 10-73.

Bronchography

NOTE: This description of bronchography has been reduced from that in earlier editions. For those interested in an expanded description, please see volume 3 of the fourth or fifth edition of this text.

Bronchography is the term applied to the specialized radiologic examination of the lungs and bronchial tree by means of introducing an opaque contrast medium into the bronchi (Figs. 10-75 and 10-76). This mode of examination has been employed in the investigation of conditions such as hemoptysis, bronchiectasis, chronic pneumonia, bronchial obstruction, pulmonary tumors, cysts and cavities, and bronchopleural-cutaneous fistulae.

In years past, bronchography was routinely performed in radiology departments; but today it is performed only as a very specialized procedure, partly because of computed tomography, improved diagnostic techniques available in nuclear medicine, and the development of the fiberoptic bronchoscope. The fiberoptic bronchoscope has had a profound effect. In bronchography, the lung can be imaged down to the level of the fifth bronchial division. In fiberoptic bronchoscopy, the bronchoscope can be placed in the trachea and advanced directly into the lung to the second division level. The greatest advantage of the bronchoscope, however, is that a biopsy of lung tissue can be obtained during bronchoscopy; a biopsy is not obtained during routine bronchography. Additionally, some pulmonary masses that years ago would have required surgical removal are now successfully managed with antibiotics.

Numerous iodinated media, both aqueous and oily, are available for bronchography. However, the oily media are more generally used.

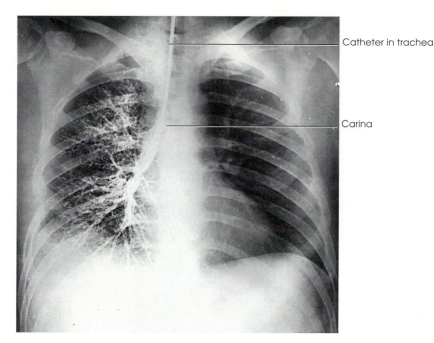

Catheter in trachea

Carina

Fig. 10-75. PA for right lung.

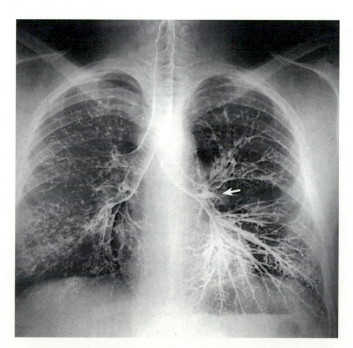

Fig. 10-76. PA showing obstruction of main lingular branch bronchus, left superior lobe *(arrow).*

Contrast Medium Instillation

There are several ways of introducing the contrast medium into the bronchial tree. Following administration of a local anesthetic to the throat and larynx, a catheter, or cannula, may be used to drop the contrast medium on the base of the anesthesized tongue, causing the contrast medium to flow into the bronchial tree without penetrating any patient surface. The technique used most often is to advance a catheter across the larynx. The contrast medium may be injected into the superior trachea for a bilateral examination, or the catheter may be further advanced into the right or left main bronchus to examine the side of interest. In a seldom-used approach, the trachea is directly punctured, with the contrast medium being injected through a catheter, or cannula, which results in the distribution of contrast medium into one or both lungs.

Once the contrast medium has been introduced, the distribution through the bronchial branches depends on gravity; therefore, the direction of flow must be guided by body position. Guidance of the contrast medium generally occurs during fluoroscopy.

Resulting radiographic images may include (1) a supine AP projection; (2) an upright PA projection (Figs. 10-75 and 10-76); (3) supine, or upright, oblique positions; (4) a lateral position (Fig. 10-77); and (5) images of small portions of interest (Figs. 10-78 and 10-79). Exposure factors must be increased from normal chest technique to penetrate the contrast medium.

At the conclusion of the examination, the patient coughs and expectorates as much of the contrast agent as possible. Any contrast medium remaining in the lungs is eventually excreted via the urinary system.

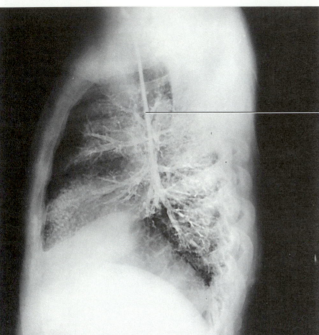

Intratracheal catheter

Fig. 10-77. Right lateral.

(Courtesy Dr. Hugh M. Wilson.)

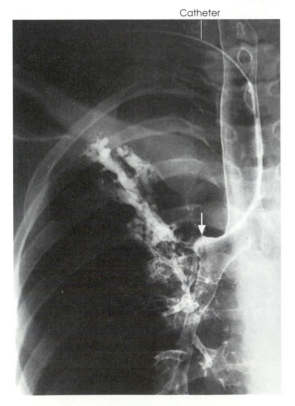

Catheter

Fig. 10-78. PA of right superior lobe showing partial occlusion of right superior lobe bronchus (*arrow*). Post obstructive bronchiectasis was found.

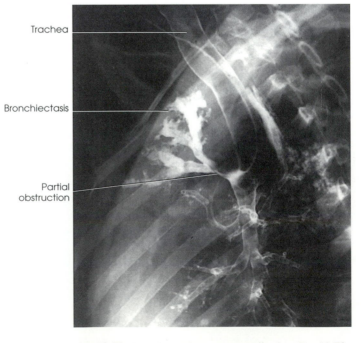

Trachea

Bronchiectasis

Partial obstruction

Fig. 10-79. Right lateral on same patient as Fig. 10-78.

(Courtesy Dr. Constantine Cope.)

Chapter 11

LONG BONE MEASUREMENT

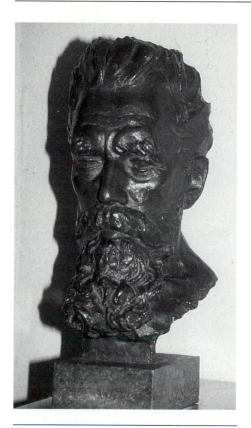

A bust of Dr. Roentgen on display in the Roentgen Museum.

ORTHOROENTGENOGRAPHY

Radiation protection
Position of patient
Position of part
Localization of joints
Computed tomography technique

Radiography provides the most reliable means of obtaining accurate measurements of the length of long bones, specifically of length differences between the two sides. Studies are occasionally made of the upper limbs, but the procedure is most frequently applied to the lower limbs. Various radiographic methods have been devised for long bone measurement, only a few of which are considered here. For a detailed description of the different procedures and their modifications, see the bibliography for a listing of original papers.

Radiation Protection

Limb length differences, which are not uncommon in children, result from any one of a variety of disorders. Patients may require yearly examinations for evaluation of any inequality in growth. More frequent examinations may follow surgical intervention to equalize limb length. One treatment method is to control the growth of the normal side. This is usually done by means of a metaphysial-epiphysial fusion at the distal femoral or proximal tibial level. Another treatment technique is to increase the growth of the shorter limb. This is done by surgically cutting the femur and/or tibia-fibula. A frame is then placed around the cut ends extending to the outside of the body. Gradual pressure on the frame separates the bone, extends the leg, and promotes healing at the same time. Patients have interval checkups extending over a period of years. It is therefore necessary to guard their well-being by gonad shielding and by avoiding unnecessary repeat exposures through careful positioning, secure immobilization, and accurate centering of a closely collimated beam of radiation.

Position of Patient

Three exposures are made of each limb, and the accuracy of the examination depends on the patient not moving the limb or limbs being examined even slightly. Small children must be carefully immobilized to prevent motion. If movement of the limb occurs before the examination is completed, all radiographs may need to be repeated.
- Place the patient in the supine position for all techniques, and examine both sides for comparison.
- When a soft tissue abnormality (swelling or atrophy) is causing rotation of the pelvis, elevate the low side on a radiolucent support to overcome the rotation, if necessary.

Position of Part

- Adjust the limb to be examined, immobilizing it, for an AP projection.
- If the two lower limbs are examined simultaneously, separate the ankles 5 or 6 inches (13 to 15 cm) and place the specialized ruler under the pelvis and extending down between the legs. If they are examined separately, the patient is usually positioned with a special ruler beneath each limb.
- When the knee of the abnormal side cannot be fully extended, flex the normal knee to the same degree and support each knee on one of a pair of *identical-sized* supports to ensure that the joints are flexed to the same degree and are equidistant from the film.

Localization of Joints

- For the methods that require centering over the joints, localize each joint accurately and mark to indicate the centering point.
- Both sides are examined for comparison, and, because there is usually a bone-length discrepancy, mark the joints of each side. Do this with a skin-marking pencil after the patient is placed in the supine position.
- For the upper limb, place the mark for the shoulder joint over the superior margin of the head of the humerus; for the elbow joint, ½ to ¾ inch (1 to 1.5 cm) below the plane of the epicondyles of the humerus (depending on the size of the patient); and for the wrist, midway between the styloid processes of the radius and ulna.
- For the lower limb, locate the *hip joint* by placing a mark 1 to 1¼ inches (2 to 3 cm), according to the size of the patient, laterodistally at a right angle to the midpoint of an imaginary line extending from the anterior superior iliac spine to the symphysis pubis.
- Locate the *knee joint* just below the apex of the patella at the level of the depression between the femoral and tibial condyles.
- Locate the *ankle joint* directly below the depression midway between the malleoli.

In all radiographs made by a single x-ray exposure, the radiographic image is larger than the part of the body examined. This occurs because the x-ray photons start at a very small area on the target of the x-ray tube and diverge as they travel in straight lines through the body to the film. This is diagrammed in Fig. 11-1. This magnification can be decreased by putting the part of the body examined as close to the film as possible and making the distance between the x-ray tube and image receptor as long as possible (a procedure sometimes referred to as teleoroentgenography). However, it is possible to learn the exact length of a child's limb bones by using a radiographic technique called orthoroentgenology.

Using a single x-ray cassette, with the metal measurement ruler placed between the patient's lower limbs, three exposures are made on the same film.

The following steps are observed:
- Position the x-ray tube directly over the hip, and make the first exposure (Fig. 11-2, *A*).
- Then, move the x-ray tube to directly over the knee joint, and make a second exposure (Fig. 11-2, *B*).
- Finally, move the x-ray tube to directly over the tibiotalar joint, and make a third exposure (Fig. 11-2, *C*).
- Three exposures can be made on one film by narrow collimation and careful centering to the upper, middle, and lower thirds of the cassette.

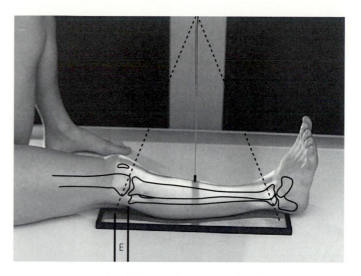

Fig. 11-1. Conventional radiographs are magnified (elongated) images. Proximal elongation in above example is equal to the distance E. Similar elongation occurs distally.

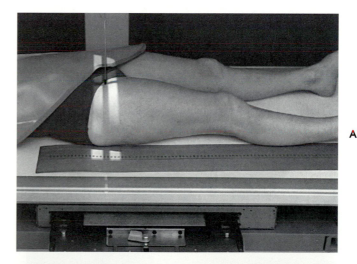

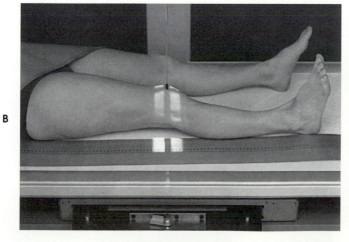

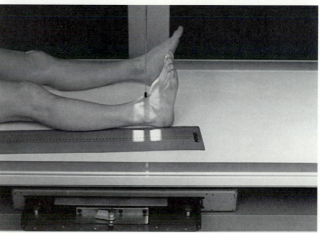

Fig. 11-2. Patient positioned for orthoroentgenographic measurement of lower limb. Central ray is centered over the **A,** hip joint; **B,** knee joint; and **C,** ankle joint. (Metal ruler placed near lateral aspect of leg for photographic purposes. Ruler normally placed between the limbs as shown in Fig. 11-4.)

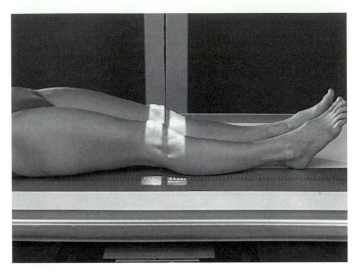

Fig. 11-3. Bilateral leg length measurement. (Metal ruler placed beside leg for photographic purposes. See Fig. 11-4 for proper placement of ruler.)

- For all three exposures, place the central ray perpendicular to, and passing directly through, the specified joint—hence the term orthoroentgenology, from the Greek *orthos*, meaning straight.
- Do not move the limb between exposures. Because the film is in the Bucky tray for all exposures, including that of the ankle, exposure factors must be modified accordingly.

If the child holds the leg perfectly still while the three exposures are made, the true distance from the proximal end of the femur to the distal end of the tibia can be directly measured on the film.

Place a special metal ruler (engraved with radiopaque centimeter or one-half inch marks that show when a radiograph is made) under the leg and on top of the table (Fig. 11-2).

- If the film is placed in the Bucky tray and then moved between the exposures, as described in Fig. 11-2, the length of the femur and tibia can be calculated by subtracting the numerical values projected over the two joints obtained by simultaneously exposing the patient and the metal ruler.

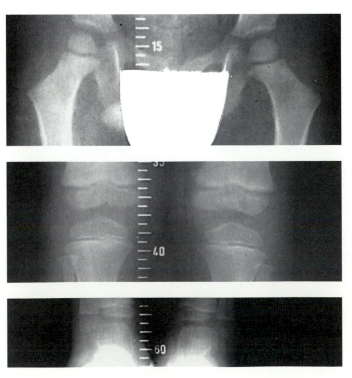

Fig. 11-4. Orthoroentgenogram for leg measurement.

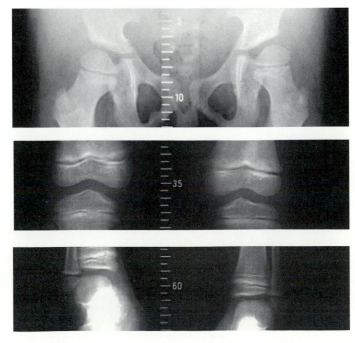

Fig. 11-5. Leg measurement showing right leg shorter than left.

Another method of measuring the lengths of the femurs and tibias is to examine both limbs simultaneously (Figs. 11-3 and 11-4):

- Adjust the lower limbs in the anatomical position; slight medial rotation.
- Tape the special metal ruler to the top of the table so that part of it is included in each of the exposure fields. This records the position of each joint.
- Place a cassette in the Bucky tray and shift it for centering at the three joint levels without moving the patient.
- Make three exposures on one 14×17 in (35×43 cm) or 11×14 in (30×35 cm) film. Limb length can then be quickly determined.
- To perform the above procedure, center the median sagittal plane of the patient's body to the midline of the grid.
- Center the cassette and the tube successively at the previously marked level of the hip joints, the knee joints, and the ankle joints for simultaneous bilateral projections, as seen in Figs. 11-3 and 11-4.

- When there is a difference in level between the contralateral joints, center the film and the tube midway between the two levels.

The orthoroentgenographic method is reasonably accurate if the limbs are of almost the same length. When there is more than a slight discrepancy, as seen in Fig. 11-5, the principles of orthoroentgenography are violated, because it is not possible to place the center of the x-ray tube exactly over both knee joints and make a single exposure or exactly over both ankle joints and make a single exposure. A compromise is made by centering midway between the two joints. But now there is bilateral distortion as a result of the diverging x-ray beam. In Fig. 11-5, the measurement obtained of the right femur is somewhat shorter than it really is, whereas the measurement of the left femur is somewhat longer.

- To correct this problem, examine each limb separately (Fig. 11-6).

- Center the limb being examined on the grid and place the special ruler beneath the limb.
- Make a closely collimated exposure over each joint. This restriction of the exposure field not only increases the accuracy of the procedure but also considerably reduces radiation exposure—and most important is a reduction of radiation exposure to the gonads.
- After the joint localization marks are made, position the patient and apply local gonad shielding.
- Adjust the collimator to limit the exposure field as much as possible.
- With successive centering to the localization marks, make exposures of the hip, knee, and ankle.
- Repeat the procedure for the opposite limb.
- Use the same approach to measure the lengths of the long bones in the upper limbs (Fig. 11-7).

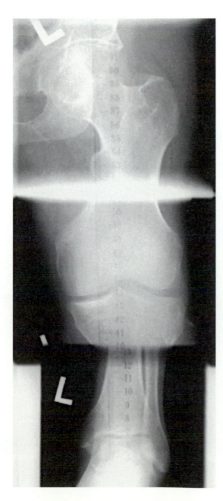

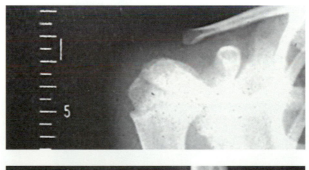

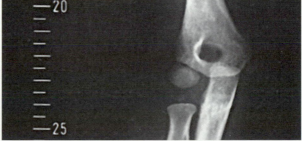

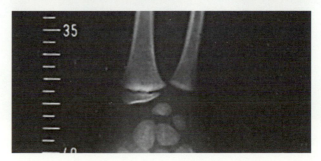

Fig. 11-6. Unilateral leg measurement.

(Courtesy Charles McCartly, R.T.)

Fig. 11-7. Measurement of upper limb.

Computed Tomography Technique

Helms and McCarthy[1] report a method for measuring discrepancies in leg length using computed tomography. Temme, Chu, and Anderson[2] compared conventional orthoroentgenograms with computed tomography in long bone measurements. They concluded that the CT scanogram is more consistently reproduced and that it causes less radiation exposure to the patient than the conventional radiographic approach. In this approach the following steps are observed:

- Take CT localizer, or scout, images of the femurs and tibias.
- Then place cursors over the respective hip, knee, and ankle joints as described earlier in this chapter. To similarly study the upper limb, obtain a scout image of the humerus, radius, and ulna.
- Then, place CT cursors over the shoulder, elbow, and wrist joints, and obtain the measurements. The measurements are displayed on the CRT, as seen in Figs. 11-8 to 11-10.

The accuracy of the examination depends on proper placement of the cursor. To improve accuracy, Helms and McCarthy place the cursors three times and average the values.

The authors report radiation dose reductions from 50 to 200 times when this method is compared with conventional radiography. The time required to perform the examination is approximately the same as for conventional radiography.

[1]Helms CA and McCarthy S: CT scanograms for measuring leg length discrepancy, Radiology 252:802, 1984.
[2]Temme JB, Chu W, and Anderson JC: CT scanograms compared with conventional orthoroentgenograms in long bone measurement, Radiol Technol 59:65-68, 1987.

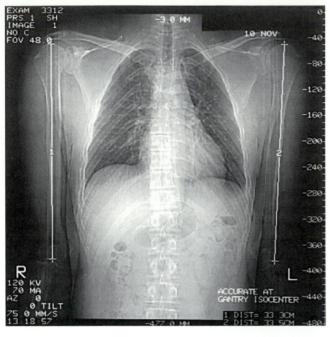

Fig. 11-8. CT measurement of arms. Note arm labels and measurements in right lower corner.

(Courtesy James B. Temme, R.T.)

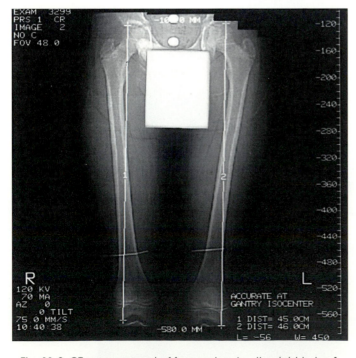

Fig. 11-9. CT measurement of femurs showing the right to be 1 cm shorter than the left.

(Courtesy James B. Temme, R.T.)

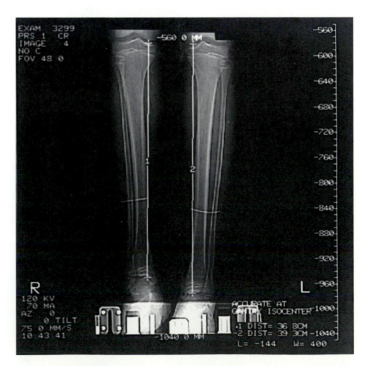

Fig. 11-10. CT measurement of legs on same patient as in Figs. 11-8 and 11-9.

(Courtesy James B. Temme, R.T.)

Long bone measurement

Chapter 12

CONTRAST ARTHROGRAPHY

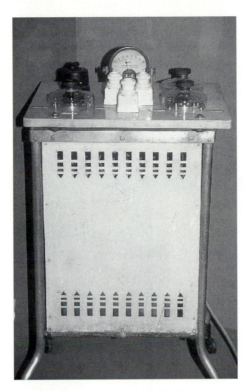

A radiographic unit from 1920 with a marble top. Note the glass insulating covers surrounding the electrical controls and protecting the operator from electrical shock. Compare this unit to the non-insulated unit shown at the beginning of Chapter 3.

The introduction and development of magnetic resonance imaging (MRI) have significantly reduced the number of arthrograms performed in radiology departments. Because MRI is a noninvasive imaging technique, the knee, wrist, hip, shoulder, temporomandibular joint, and other joints previously evaluated by contrast arthrography are now studied using MRI, as seen in Fig. 12-1. As a result, radiographic contrast arthrography has increasingly specialized functions.

Arthrography (Gr. *arthron,* joint) is radiography of a joint or joints. *Pneumoarthrography, opaque arthrography,* and *double-contrast arthrography* are terms used to denote radiologic examinations of the soft tissue structures of joints (menisci, ligaments, articular cartilage, bursae) following the injection of one or two contrast agents into the capsular space. A gaseous medium is employed in pneumoarthrography, a water-soluble iodinated medium in opaque arthrography (Fig. 12-2), and a combination of both in double-contrast arthrography. Although contrast studies may be made on any encapsuled joint, the knee has been the most frequent site of investigation. Other joints examined by contrast arthrography include the shoulder, hip, wrist, and temporomandibular joints.

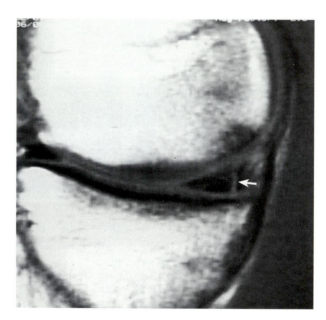

Fig. 12-1. Noninvasive MRI of knee showing torn medial meniscus (*arrow*).

Arthrogram examinations are usually performed with a local anesthetic. The injection is made under careful aseptic conditions, usually in a combination fluoroscopic-radiographic examining room, which should be carefully prepared in advance. The sterile items required, particularly the length and gauge of the needles, vary according to the part being examined. The sterile tray and the nonsterile items should be set up on a conveniently placed instrument cart or a small two-shelf table.

After aspirating any effusion, the radiologist injects the contrast agent or agents and manipulates the joint to ensure proper distribution of the contrast material. The examination is usually performed by fluoroscopy and spot films. Conventional radiographs may then be taken when special images, such as an axial projection of the shoulder or an intercondyloid fossa position of the knee, are desired.

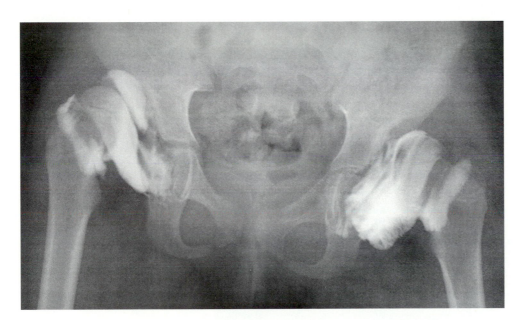

Fig. 12-2. Bilateral opaque arthrogram of hip joints in patient with bilateral congenital dislocations.

(Courtesy Dr. William B. Seaman.)

Contrast Arthrography of Knee

VERTICAL RAY METHOD

Contrast arthrography of the knee by the vertical ray method requires the use of a stress device. The following steps are observed:

- Place the limb in the frame to widen or "open up" the side of the joint space under investigation. This widening, or spreading, of the intrastructural spaces permits better distribution of the contrast material around the meniscus.
- After the contrast material is injected, place the limb in the stress device (Fig. 12-3). For the delineation of the medial side of the joint, for example, place the stress device just above the knee, and the lower leg is laterally stressed.

- When contrast arthrograms are to be made by conventional radiography, turn the patient to the prone position, and fluoroscopically localize the centering point for each side of the joint. The mark ensures accurate centering for closely collimated studies of each side of the joint and permits multiple exposures to be made on one cassette. The images obtained of each side of the joint usually consist of an AP projection and a 20-degree right and left AP oblique projection.
- Obtain the oblique position by leg rotation or central ray angulation (Figs. 12-4 to 12-6).

Following completion of these studies the frame is removed for a lateral and an intercondyloid fossa projection.

NOTE: Anderson and Maslin[1] recommended that tomography be used in knee arthrography, a technique that can frequently be used to advantage in other contrast-filled joint capsules.

---

[1]Anderson PW and Maslin P: Tomography applied to knee arthrography, Radiology 110:271-275, 1974.

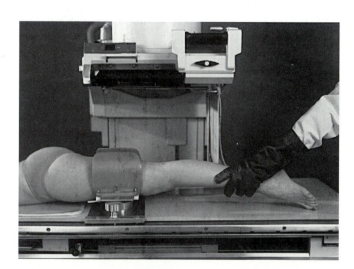

Fig. 12-3. Patient lying on lead rubber for gonad shielding and positioned in stress device on fluoroscopic table.

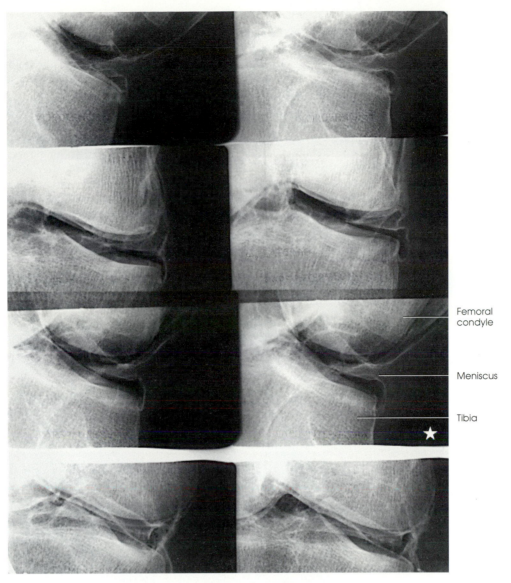

Femoral condyle

Meniscus

Tibia

Fig. 12-4. Vertical ray double-contrast knee arthrogram.

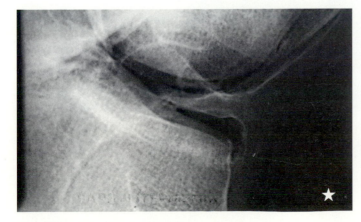

Fig. 12-5. Enlarged image of frame with star seen in Fig. 12-4.

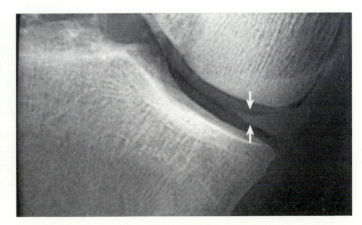

Fig. 12-6. Knee pneumoarthrogram showing normal lateral meniscus *(arrows)* surrounded above and below with air.

Double-Contrast Arthrography of Knee
HORIZONTAL RAY METHOD

The horizontal central ray method of performing double-contrast arthrography of the knee was first described by Andrén and Wehlin,[1] and later by Freiberger, Killoran, and Cardona.[2] It was found that by using a horizontal x-ray beam position and a comparatively small amount of each of the two contrast agents, improved double-contrast delineation of the knee joint structures could be obtained. This is because the excess of the heavy iodinated solutions drains into the dependent part of the joint, leaving only the desired thin opaque coating on the gas-enveloped uppermost part, the part then under investigation.

[1]Andrén L and Wehlin L: Double-contrast arthrography of knee with horizontal roentgen ray beam, Acta Orthop Scand 29:307-314, 1960.
[2]Freiberger RH, Killoran PJ, and Cardona G: Arthrography of the knee by double contrast method, AJR 97:736-747, 1966.

Medial meniscus

- Adjust the patient in the semiprone position that places the posterior aspect of the medial meniscus uppermost (Figs. 12-7 and 12-8).
- To widen the joint space, manually stress the knee.
- Direct the central ray along the line that is drawn on the medial side of the knee and center to the meniscus.
- With rotation toward the supine position, turn the leg 30 degrees for each of the succeeding five exposures.
- Direct the central ray along the localization line.

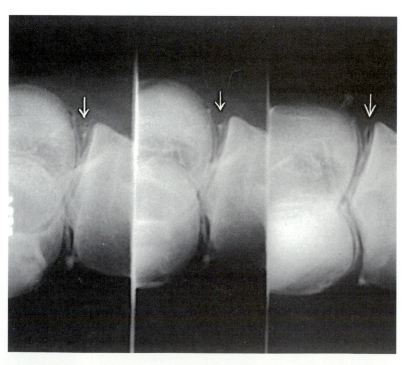

Fig. 12-7. Medial meniscus. Tear in posterior half. Note irregular streaks of positive contrast material within meniscal wedge (arrows).

Lateral meniscus

- Adjust the patient in the semiprone position that places the posterior aspect of the lateral meniscus uppermost (Fig. 12-9).
- To widen the joint space, manually stress the knee.
- As with the medial meniscus, make six images on one cassette.
- With movement toward the supine position, rotate the leg 30 degrees for each of the consecutive exposures, from the initial prone oblique position to the supine oblique position.
- Adjust the central ray angulation as required to direct it along the localization line and center to the meniscus.

NOTE: For the demonstration of the cruciate ligaments after filming of the menisci,[1] the patient is asked to stand and then to sit with the knee flexed 90 degrees over the side of the radiographic table. A firm cotton pillow is then adjusted under the knee so that some forward pressure is applied to the leg. With the patient holding a grid cassette in position, a closely collimated and slightly overexposed lateral position is taken.

---

[1]Mittler S, Freiberger RH, and Harrison-Stubbs M: A method of improving cruciate ligament visualization in double-contrast arthrography, Radiology 102:441-442, 1972.

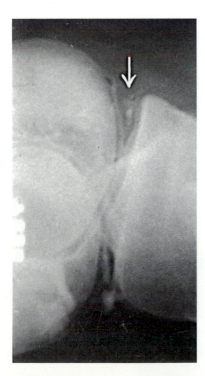

Fig. 12-8. Enlarged image showing tear in medial meniscus on same patient as in Fig. 12-7.

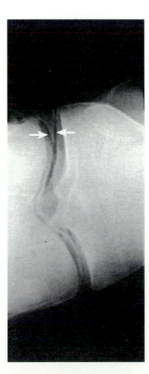

Fig. 12-9. Normal lateral meniscus (*arrows*) on same patient as in Figs. 12-7 and 12-8.

Wrist Arthrography

The primary indications for wrist arthrography are trauma, persistent pain, or limitation of motion. Following injection of the contrast material (approximately 1.5 to 4 ml) through the dorsal wrist at the articulation of the radius, scaphoid, and lunate, the wrist is gently manipulated to disperse the contrast medium. The projections most commonly used are the PA, lateral, and both obliques (Figs. 12-10 and 12-11). Fluoroscopy or tape recording of the wrist during rotation is recommended for exact detection of contrast medium leaks.

Hip Arthrography

Hip arthrography is performed most often on children to evaluate congenital hip dislocation before treatment (Fig. 12-2) and following treatment (Figs. 12-12 and 12-13). In adults, the primary use of hip arthrography is to detect a loose hip prosthesis or to confirm the presence of infection. The cement used to fasten hip prosthesis components has barium sulfate added to make the determination of the cement and the cement-bone interface radiographically visible (Fig. 12-14). Although the addition of barium sulfate to the cement is an advantage in confirming proper seating of the prosthesis, it makes evaluation of the same joint by arthrography difficult. Because both the cement and the contrast material produce the same approximate radiographic density, a subtraction technique is recommended, either photographic subtraction as seen in Figs. 12-15 and 12-16 (see Volume 2, Chapter 26) or digital subtraction as seen in Figs. 12-17 and 12-18 (see Volume 3, Chapter 33). A common puncture site for hip arthrography is ¾ in (2 cm) distal to the inguinal crease and ¾ in (2 cm) lateral to the palpated femoral pulse. To reach the joint capsule, it is helpful to use a spinal needle.

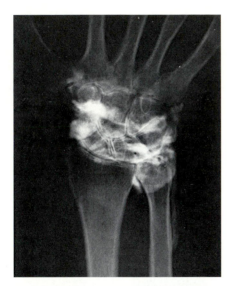

Fig. 12-10. Opaque arthrogram of wrist. Rheumatoid arthritis.

(Courtesy Dr. Robert H. Freiberger.)

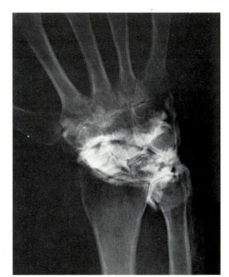

Fig. 12-11. PA arthrogram with wrist in radial flexion.

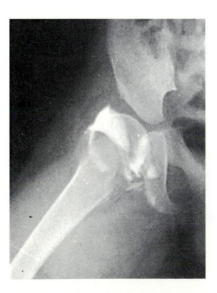

Fig. 12-12. AP opaque arthrogram showing treated congenital right hip dislocation on same patient as in Fig. 12-2.

(Courtesy Dr. William B. Segman.)

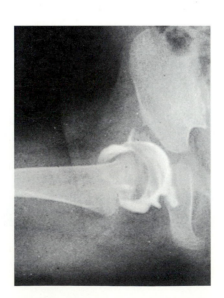

Fig. 12-13. Axiolateral "frog" right hip of patient treated for congenital dislocation of hip.

(Courtesy Dr. Robert H. Freiberger.)

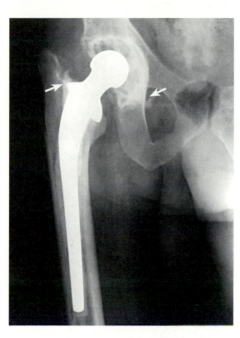

Fig. 12-14. AP hip radiograph showing radiopaque cement *(arrows)* used to secure hip prosthesis.

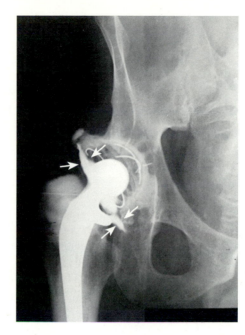

Fig. 12-15. AP hip arthrogram showing hip prosthesis in proper position. Cement with radiopaque additive difficult to distinguish from contrast medium used to perform arthrogram *(arrows)*.

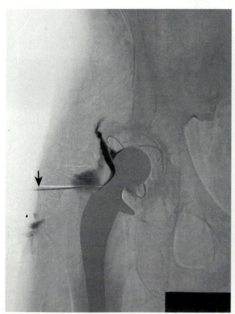

Fig. 12-16. Normal photographic subtraction AP hip arthrogram on same patient as in Fig. 12-14. Contrast medium (black image) readily distinguished from hip prosthesis by subtraction technique. Contrast medium does not extend inferiorly below the level of the injection needle *(arrow)*.

(Courtesy Dr. Javier Beltran.)

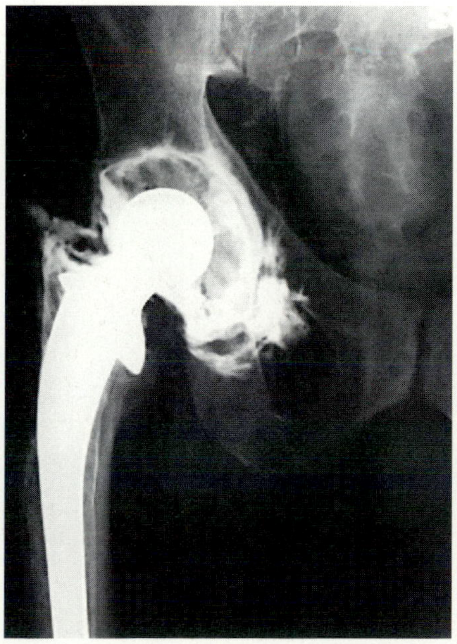

Fig. 12-17. AP hip radiograph following injection of contrast medium.

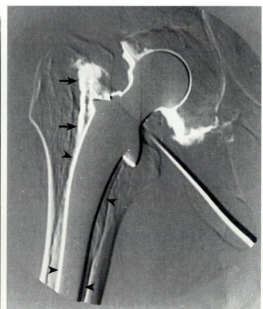

Fig. 12-18. Digital subtraction hip arthrogram on same patient as in Fig. 12-17. Contrast medium around the prosthesis in proximal lateral femoral shaft *(arrows)* indicates a loose prosthesis. Lines on the medial and lateral aspect of the femur *(arrowheads)* are a subtraction registration artifact caused by slight patient movement during the injection of contrast medium.

(Courtesy Dr. Javier Beltran.)

Shoulder Arthrography

Arthrography of the shoulder is performed primarily for the evaluation of either partial or complete tears in the rotator cuff or the glenoidal labrum, persistent pain or weakness, or frozen shoulder. A single-contrast technique (Fig. 12-19) or a double-contrast technique (Fig. 12-20) may be used.

The usual injection site is approximately ½ in (1 cm) inferior and lateral to the coracoid process. The joint capsule is usually deep, so a spinal needle is recommended.

For the single-contrast shoulder arthrogram (Fig. 12-21), the physician injects approximately 10 to 12 ml of positive contrast medium.

For double-contrast examinations, inject approximately 3 to 4 ml of positive contrast medium and 10 to 12 ml of air.

The projections most often used are the AP (both internal and external rotation), 30-degree AP oblique, axillary (Figs. 12-22 and 12-23), and tangential (see Volume 1, Chapter 5 for positioning description).

Following the performance of the double-contrast shoulder arthrogram, some patients may be examined using computed tomography (CT). CT images may be taken at each approximate 5 mm through the shoulder joint. In shoulder arthrography, CT has been found to be very sensitive and reliable in diagnosis; compare radiographic and CT images of the same patient (Figs. 12-20 and 12-24).

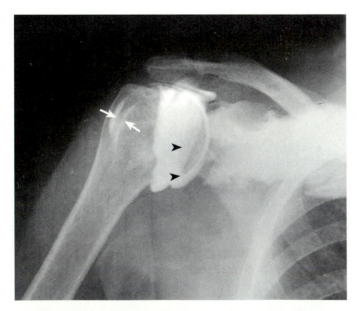

Fig. 12-19. Normal AP single-contrast shoulder arthrogram with contrast medium surrounding the biceps tendon sleeve lying in the intertubercular (bicipital) groove *(arrows)*. The axillary recess is filled but has a normal medial filling defect *(arrowheads)* created by the glenoid labrum.

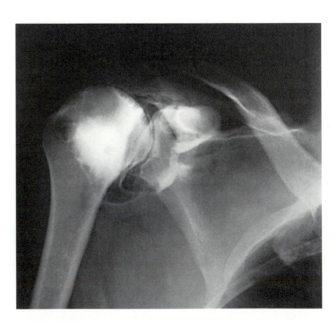

Fig. 12-20. Normal AP double-contrast shoulder arthrogram.

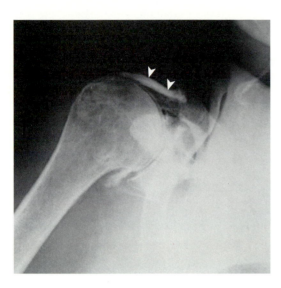

Fig. 12-21. Single-contrast arthrogram showing rotator cuff tear *(arrows).*

(Courtesy Dr. Javier Beltran.)

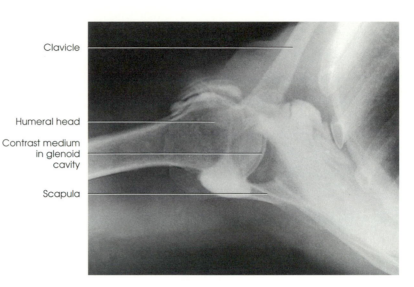

Clavicle

Humeral head

Contrast medium
in glenoid
cavity

Scapula

Fig. 12-22. Normal axillary single-contrast shoulder arthrogram.

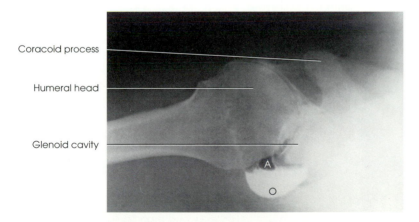

Coracoid process

Humeral head

Glenoid cavity

Fig. 12-23. Normal axillary double-contrast shoulder arthrogram projection of a patient in the supine position showing opaque medium *(O)* and air- *(A)* created density anteriorly.

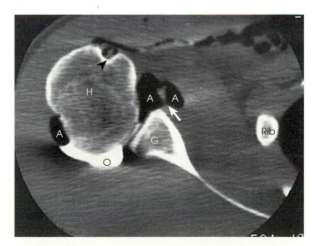

Fig. 12-24. CT shoulder arthrogram. Radiographic arthrogram on this patient was normal as seen in Fig. 12-20. CT shoulder arthrogram demonstrates small chip fracture *(arrow)* on the anterior surface of the glenoid cavity. Head of humerus *(H)*, air surrounding biceps tendon *(arrowhead)*, air contrast medium *(A)*, opaque contrast medium *(O)*, and glenoid portion of scapula *(G)*.

(Courtesy Dr. Javier Beltran.)

Temporomandibular Joint (TMJ) Arthrography

CT evaluation of the temporomandibular joint replaced many temporomandibular joint arthrograms because CT is a noninvasive method of investigation. In many institutions, MRI has replaced CT, because MRI is also a noninvasive procedure and the diagnostic value of MRI has been well established (Fig 12-25).

Contrast arthrography of the temporomandibular joint is useful in diagnosing abnormalities of the articular disk *(discus articularis),* the small oval plate located between the condyle of the mandible and mandibular fossa. Abnormalities can be the result of trauma or a stretched or loose posterior ligament that allows the disk to be anteriorly displaced, causing pain.

Single-contrast opaque arthrography of the temporomandibular joint, although relatively uncomfortable for the patient, is easy to perform; it requires 0.5 to 1 ml of contrast medium. The puncture site is approximately ½ in (1 cm) anterior to the tragus of the ear. The following steps are observed:

- Generally, before the arthrogram is performed, take preliminary tomographic images with the patient's mouth in both the closed and open positions.
- After injection of the contrast medium, fluoroscopically observe the joint and take spot films to evaluate mandibular motion.

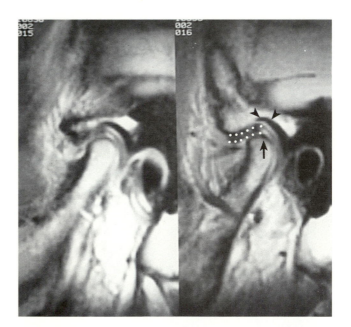

Fig. 12-25. Open-mouth lateral MRI of the temporomandibular joint, showing mandibular condyle *(arrow),* mandibular fossa of temporal bone *(arrowheads),* and the articular disk *(dots).*

Tomograms and/or radiographs (Fig. 12-26 and 12-27) are generally taken of the patient with the mouth in the closed, partially open, and fully open positions.

Other Joints

Although essentially any joint can be evaluated by arthrography, the preceding joints are the ones most often investigated. For additional references on arthrography, see the bibliography at the end of this volume.

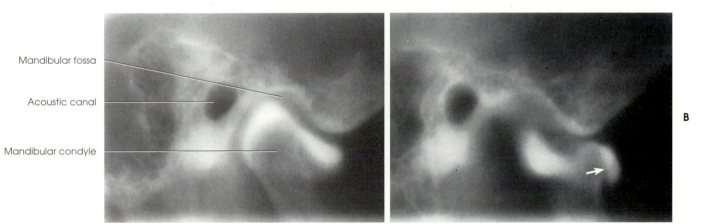

Mandibular fossa

Acoustic canal

Mandibular condyle

A

B

Fig. 12-26. Postinjection tomographic arthrogram of temporomandibular joint taken with patient's mouth closed *(A)* and fully open *(B)*. Positive contrast medium anterior to condyle *(arrow)* demonstrates anterior dislocation of the meniscus.

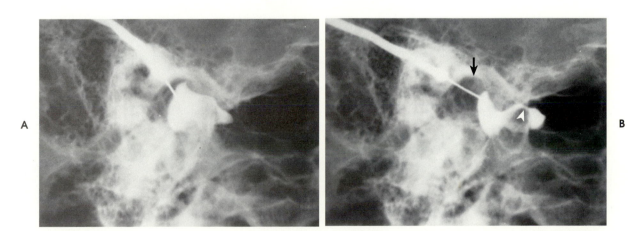

A

B

Fig. 12-27. Postinjection radiographs on same patient as in Fig. 12-26. Dislocated meniscus is shown with the mouth half open **(A)** and completely open **(B)**. Mandibular fossa *(arrow)* and condyle *(arrowhead)* are shown.

Chapter 13

FOREIGN BODY LOCALIZATION AND TRAUMA RADIOGRAPHY GUIDELINES

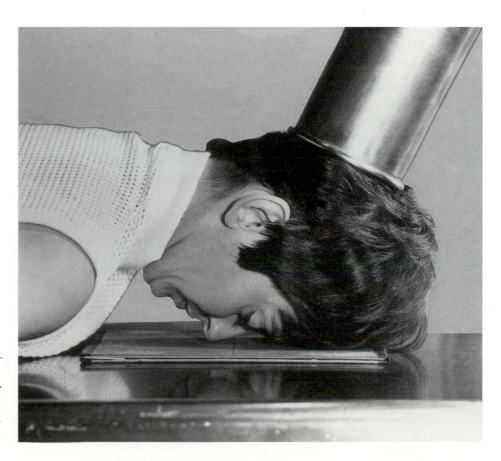

To reduce the possibility of screen artifacts, localization of foreign bodies was often accomplished using a cardboard holder (without intensifying screens).

FOREIGN BODY LOCALIZATION

Any alien object that has entered the body by any route is called a *foreign body*. A wide variety of foreign materials enter the body under many different circumstances—some by way of a puncture wound, others by way of a natural orifice (Figs. 13-1 to 13-3). A majority of these objects must be removed by a surgical procedure. The referring physician depends on the radiology department to verify the presence of, and to determine the nature and exact site of, any such objects so that the physician can determine the best procedure for its removal.

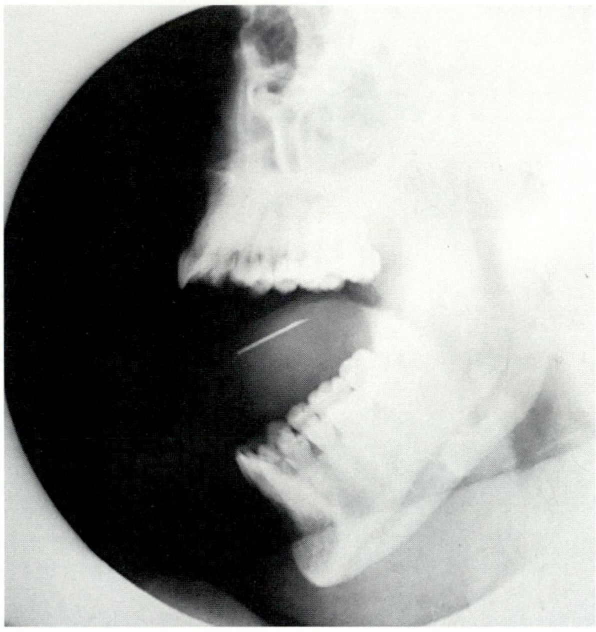

The objective of this section is to describe the most commonly employed radiologic examinations for the detection and localization of foreign bodies in regions other than the eye (for which see Volume 2, Chapter 20). The bibliography contains a listing of papers detailing other techniques for foreign body localization.

In civilian practice the most frequently encountered foreign bodies are those which have been aspirated or swallowed and tissue-penetrating materials such as needles, broken glass, and wood and metal splinters. Children sometimes insert a foreign object into the nose, ear, or genital orifice. An object lodged in one of these areas can usually be removed without referring the patient to the radiology department. When referral is necessary, the examination consists of obtaining radiographs made in at least two planes. Industrial areas and high crime areas frequently give rise to foreign body traumas comparable to those sustained on battlefields. These injuries often cause extensive bone and/or soft tissue damage by the impact of high-velocity objects.

Aspirated and swallowed foreign bodies are discussed under this heading because the examinations employed for the detection and localization of objects entering by way of the mouth are limited to the two systems involved (Figs. 13-4 to 13-6).

Fig. 13-1. Lateral open-mouth facial bones showing a pin in the tongue.

(Courtesy Valerie Sasson, R.T.)

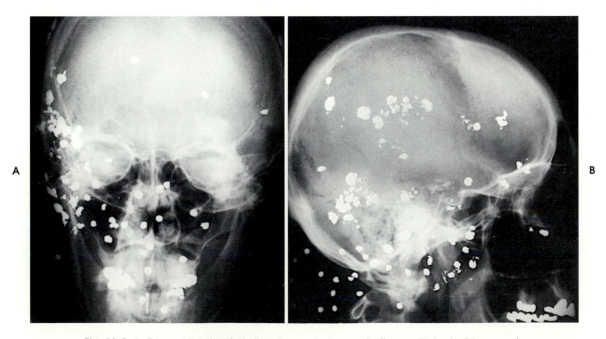

Fig. 13-2. A, PA and **B,** lateral, skull radiograph demonstrating multiple shell fragments lodged in the superficial tissues of the cranium, face, and neck.

(Courtesy D. Peter Kuum.)

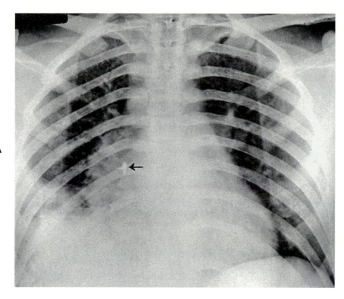

A

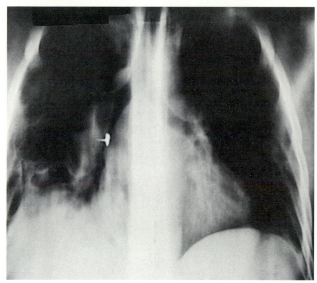

B

Fig. 13-3. Patient treated for chronic pneumonia with symptoms of cough, foul-smelling sputum, and intermittent fever. The frontal radiograph, **A,** reveals pneumonia in the right lower lung and the presence of a foreign body *(arrow).* Tomography, **B,** profiled a thumb-tack lodged in the right lower lobe bronchus adjacent to the hilum. The thumbtack was removed bronchoscopically.

(Courtesy Dr. Bernard S. Epstein.)

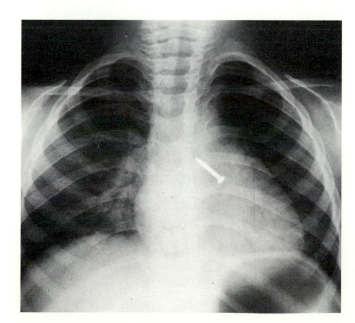

Fig. 13-4. Nail aspirated into left bronchus.

(Courtesy Dr. Milton Elkin.)

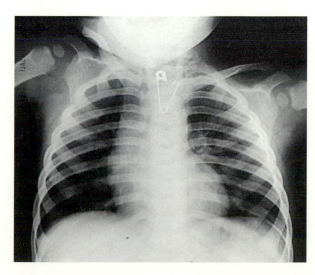

Fig. 13-5. Open safety pin lodged in esophagus of 13-month-old boy.

(Courtesy Dr. Milton Elkin.)

Penetrating foreign bodies are localized by both radiographic and fluoroscopic techniques. The radiographic techniques are generally preferred because they afford a permanent record, and, after preliminary screening by the radiologist, they can be carried out by the radiographer (Fig. 13-7). During fluoroscopic screening, the radiologist may place a mark on the skin surface, anteriorly or posteriorly, immediately over the center of the image of the foreign body. Then, by turning the patient or by the parallax method, a mark may be placed on the body at the exact site of the object to indicate its depth. These marks can be used by the radiographer as centering points in positioning the patient and by the surgeon as reference points for surgery.

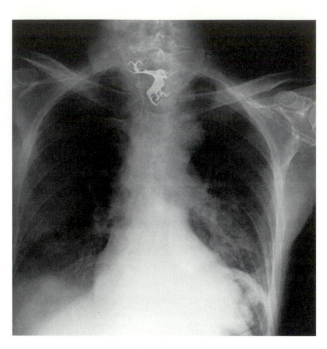

Fig. 13-6. Portable chest radiograph located the patient's missing dental partial.

(Courtesy Dianna Childs, R.T.)

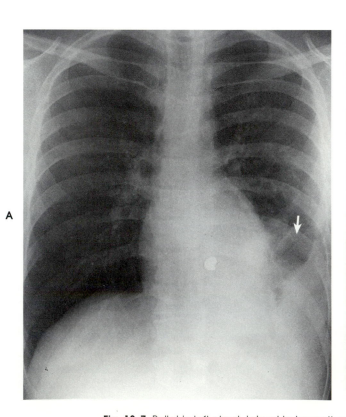

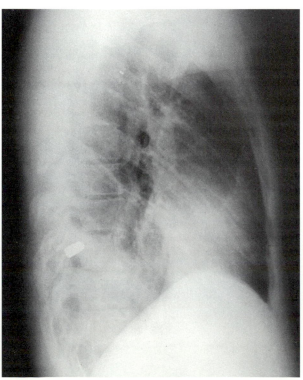

Fig. 13-7. Bullet in left chest, lateral to lower thoracic spine. No bone injury. Left pleural effusion seen on PA *(arrow)*, **A,** and left lateral image, **B.** Fluid mostly lateral and posterior.

(Courtesy Dr. William H. Shehadi.)

Preliminary Considerations

Careful attention to each of the factors affecting recorded radiographic detail is important in every examination, but it is nowhere more crucial than for the detection of low-density foreign bodies. The factors discussed here are of particular importance.

FOCAL SPOT

A small focal spot is a prerequisite for maximum recorded detail. Pitting, cracking, and rippling the anode result from overloading and overheating. These irregularities on the face of the target produce radiation emitted in all directions, causing serious loss of recorded detail. Using the tube within the limits shown on its rating chart, which should be prominently displayed in every control booth, will prevent target damage.

SCREENS

Dust and other extraneous particles, nicks, scratches, and stains produce shadows that can simulate small foreign bodies. Imperfect intensifying screen contact produces blurring similar to that produced by motion. These imperfections can result from careless handling of cassettes and improper care of the contained screens.

EXPOSURE FACTORS

The exposure factors must be adjusted according to the tissue density of the part examined, and involuntary motion must be compensated for by the appropriate technique. For the demonstration of both bony and soft tissue structures in thick parts, a long scale of gray tones is generally desirable.

Fragments of low-density materials such as plastic, wood, and glass are most frequently found in the superficial tissues. The detection of these materials generally requires a short-scale contrast. It is important that thick surgical dressings be removed for the x-ray exposures, leaving only a thin layer of sterile gauze. However, remove the dressings only if so permitted.

The detection of glass fragments presents the greatest problem. There are more than 70,000 types of glass, each of which has a particular chemical composition. Many of the glasses contain a high enough percentage of lime and/or metallic oxide (iron, gold, lead, copper, etc., added to obtain specific colors) to render them sufficiently opaque to cast a shadow through the surrounding tissues. Others are composed of a high percentage of silicon (silica glass) with a low lime and metallic content. Failure to detect this type of glass does not preclude its presence.

POSITIONING OF PATIENT

Positioning of the patient is of prime importance in foreign body localization where even slight rotation of the patient or part can result in erroneous depth measurements. Positioning the patient for AP or PA, and lateral projections must be exact. Optimum oblique and tangential projections are usually determined under fluoroscopic control to enable the radiologist to place the skin mark tangent to the film.

MOTION

Motion of the part, voluntary or involuntary, causes blurring and loss of recorded detail. This can obscure the presence of objects of low density and/or small size. For maximum recorded detail, every effort must be made to control motion of body parts before an exposure is made. This must be done by means other than compression. Compression reduces tissue thickness, which results in erroneous depth measurements. Length of exposure is the only means of overcoming the problem of involuntary motion.

EQUIPMENT

Precision depth-measurement techniques require exact centering of the tube within its housing and the exact measurement of target-film and target-shift distances.

The distance markings on the x-ray tube stand must be checked for accuracy so that exact compensation can be made for any discrepancy. The source-to-image receptor distance (SID) used for precision depth localization must be exact.

Penetrating Foreign Bodies
INITIAL EXAMINATION

The purpose of the initial examination is to verify the presence of suspected single or multiple foreign bodies and to determine their nature, size, shape, and location and the extent of bony and/or soft tissue trauma. In the presence of severe injury, one or more initial radiographs may be all that can be obtained.

The smaller parts of the limbs do not usually require a preliminary radiograph. The foreign body is most often near the site of entry, and the following steps are observed:

- Direct the central ray exactly through the foreign body.
- Obtain right-angle AP, or PA, and lateral projections as shown in Fig. 13-8.
- Indicate the site of the puncture wound on these studies by placing a lead marker on the film exactly opposite the wound.
- Obtain additional projections as indicated.

The initial examination of thick parts may be carried out by a preliminary radiograph or fluoroscopy when the skull, chest, or abdominopelvic regions are involved (Figs. 13-9 to 13-11). Scout radiographs must be large enough to include the entire region under investigation. The angle of entrance of high-velocity objects such as bullets and fragments of metal must also be taken into account. High-velocity objects entering at an angle usually lodge some distance from the puncture wound.

Preliminary screening expedites the examination because it enables the physician (1) to quickly locate radiopaque foreign bodies, whether near or far from the site of entry, (2) to determine whether the object is located within deep structures or in the periphery of a rounded area where it is best shown by tangential projections, (3) to determine the localization technique best suited to the circumstances, and (4) to mark the skin overlying the shadow of the foreign body in two or more planes. When the foreign body is distant from natural reference points (joints or other bony parts), a metal marker may be attached to the skin for the surgeon's use as a reference point. Emergency radiology departments keep a supply of sterile wire rings and crosses for this purpose.

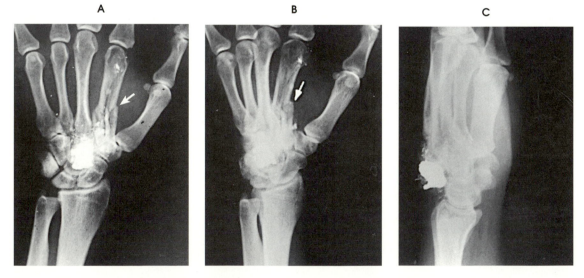

Fig. 13-8. Metallic foreign body (bullet) in dorsal aspect of wrist with comminuted fracture of second metacarpal *(arrow).*

(Courtesy Dr. Albert A. Dunn.)

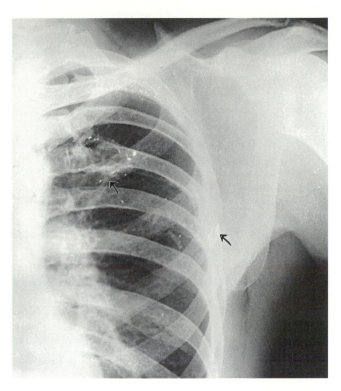

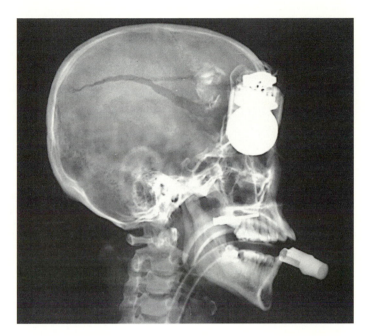

Fig. 13-9. Old, healed bullet wound fractures involving fifth rib laterally and posteriorly. Note track of lead deposits extending through soft tissues along path traveled by bullet *(arrows)*.

Fig. 13-10. Battlefield injury resulting in extensive bone and brain damage caused by hand grenade embedded in forehead.

(Courtesy Dr. Harold G. Jacobson.)

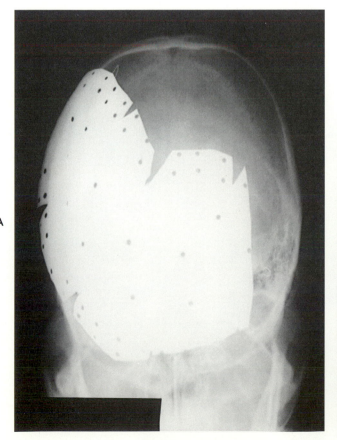

A

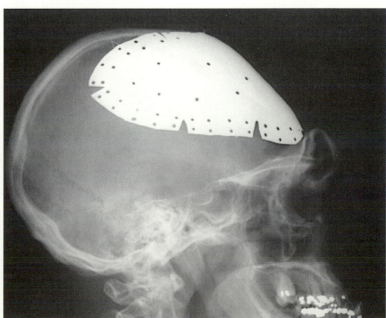

B

Fig. 13-11. A, Occipital (Towne method), and **B,** lateral radiographs of battlefield injury victim with cranial plate covering brain.

(Courtesy Dr. Peter Kuum.)

RADIOGRAPHIC LOCALIZATION TECHNIQUES

Radiographic localization techniques are the following:

1. Right-angle projections
2. Oblique projections
3. Tangential projections
4. Single-film triangulation

Radiographic foreign body localization is performed after the surgeon has determined the route and body placement to be used for the removal of the foreign body. The localization images are then made with the patient adjusted in the body position to be used for surgery. The images must always be large enough to include natural reference points, unless wire or other suitable markers have been attached to the skin or over a wound to serve this purpose.

Computed tomography is often used to localize foreign bodies. Magnetic resonance is cautiously used *only* after the composition of the foreign body is known to be non-ferrous.

Right-angle projections

The right-angle technique of localization consists of taking exact right-angle AP, PA, and lateral projections, with the central ray directed through the foreign body (Fig. 13-12).

Thick parts, particularly the chest and abdominopelvic regions, require the following procedure:

- Adjust the patient in the body position to be used in the operating room for the surgical removal of the foreign body.
- Mark the skin overlying the site of the foreign body in both frontal and lateral planes.
- Direct the central ray through the center of the foreign body for accurate localization of the object. If the centering is not accurate, the shadow of the foreign body will be cast by divergent radiation emitted from the periphery of the tube target. The distance of the image displacement and the resultant error in localization will depend on the distance between the foreign body and the film and on the source-to-image receptor distance SID as well as the distance of off-centering.

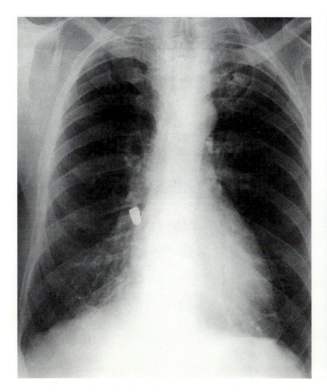
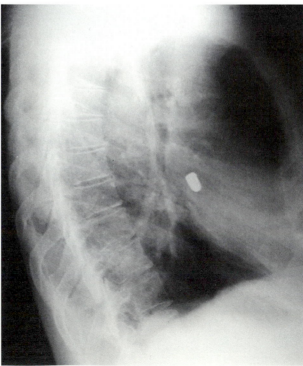

Fig. 13-12. AP and lateral projections. Bullet in right chest of patient who has been asymptomatic for 15 years following shooting.

- Except for the hands and feet, whenever possible, obtain biplane projections. This is particularly important in the presence of pointed and sharp-edged objects, where movement of the patient could result in deeper penetration of the object with further soft tissue trauma. Biplane projections are also important when a foreign body is located where there is a possibility of a shift in its position, as in the mediastinum and abdominopelvic areas.
- When there is a possibility of movement of a foreign body, resulting from its unstable location or from movement of the patient during transfer from radiology to surgery, verify the location of the object with right-angle images in the operating room immediately before the operation.

• • •

Not only are the foregoing techniques the simplest and most universally used procedures for the localization of penetrating foreign bodies—they are usually the only ones required.

Oblique projections

Oblique projections are used to separate overlapping structures in any region. They are particularly useful in determining the relationship of superimposed bone and foreign body images to demonstrate whether the object is embedded in the bone or is lodged in the adjacent soft tissues.

Tangential projections

Tangential projections are useful in foreign body detection when the physical configuration of the body part allows the central ray to "skim" between the foreign body and the primary body part. It is most useful for the evaluation of superficial foreign bodies in limbs.

Single-film triangulation

The single-film triangulation technique is a precise way of depth localization, requiring the following steps:
- Measure accurately and record the *exact* source-to-image receptor distance (SID) and tube-shift distance (TSD) used.
- Keep the patient and the film stationary for two exposures on one film.
- Measure accurately and record the uppermost skin surface-to-film distance. The latter measurement is used in the final step of the depth calculation.

Any practical SID may be used—30, 36, or 40 inches (75 to 100 cm). The TSD may be 4, 6, 8, or 10 inches (10 to 15 cm). The greater the object-to-image receptor distance (OID), the greater the image shift distance (ISD). For this reason a shorter TSD can be used for objects near the surface but a longer TSD is more satisfactory for deep-seated objects, because it ensures adequate separation of the images. The tube is shifted at right angles to the long axis of elongated objects. This prevents possible difficulty in measuring the exact image-shift on partially superimposed shadows of slender or tapered objects.

Application of procedure

- Adjust the patient in an exact supine or prone body position as required to place him or her in the position to be used for the surgical removal of the foreign body.
- Center the central ray to the skin mark overlying the site of the foreign body.
- With the film in a Bucky tray, center it to the skin mark.
- Carefully measure the uppermost skin-to-image receptor distance in the plane of the foreign body, and record this measurement with the SID and TSD.
- Make the first exposure using one-half of the exposure time required for a conventional radiograph of the part.
- Shift the tube an *exact distance,* transversely or longitudinally as required, and, without disturbing the patient or film, make the second exposure using the same factors as for the first exposure. These two "half exposures" produce a radiographic density comparable to that obtained with a single full exposure of the region (Fig. 13-13). When a wide tube shift is used, adjust the collimator for the second (off-center) exposure to avoid a cutoff, as shown by the transverse line seen in Fig. 13-14. The upper right-hand corner cutoff was made by the gonad shield.
- Process the film in the usual manner.

Depth calculation

- From the same point on each image, measure the exact distance between the two images cast on the radiograph by the foreign body.
- With the three known factors, SID, TSD, and ISD, calculate the foreign body-image receptor distance using the following formula:

$$\frac{SID \times ISD}{TSD + ISD} =$$

Foreign body-image receptor distance

Example: Assuming an SID of 40 inches, a TSD of 6 inches, and an ISD of 1 ½ inches, calculate the foreign body-film distance as follows:

$$(40 \times 1.5) \div (6 + 1.5) = 8 \text{ inches}$$

- Then, calculate the depth of the foreign body below the skin surface by subtracting the foreign body-image receptor distance from the skin-image receptor distance. Assume the latter measurement to be 10 inches (25 cm). Using the result of the above example, 10 minus 8 equals 2, which places the foreign body 2 inches (5 cm) below the skin surface.

- The measurements can be graphically reproduced on a sheet of paper, using a scale of ¼ to 1 inch, by drawing a set of triangles (Fig. 13-15) as follows:
  - Draw a line representing the SID, line AB.
  - Draw a line representing the TSD, line AC.
  - Draw a line representing the ISD, line BD.
  - Draw a line from C to D.
  - Draw a line representing the skin surface, line SS.

The location of the foreign body (FB) is where line CD intersects line AB.

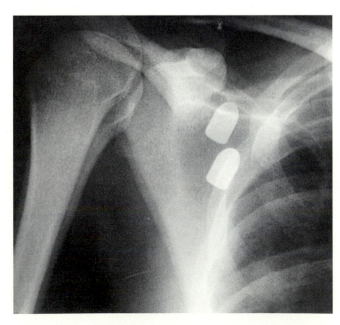

Fig. 13-13. Triangulation technique for locating single bullet.

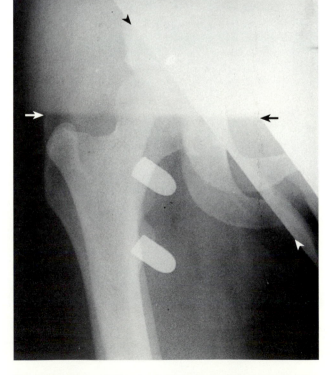

Fig. 13-14. Triangulation technique radiograph showing the line caused by intentionally off-centered collimated x-ray beam for second exposure *(arrows)* and diagonal lines *(arrowheads)* caused by gonad shield.

FLUOROSCOPIC LOCALIZATION TECHNIQUES

Fluoroscopic localization techniques are the following:

1. Parallax method
2. Right-angle method
3. Profunda method

The fluoroscopic methods of foreign body localization can be performed quickly and therefore are used when circumstances indicate that speed is of greater importance than the permanent record afforded by the somewhat more time-consuming radiographic techniques.

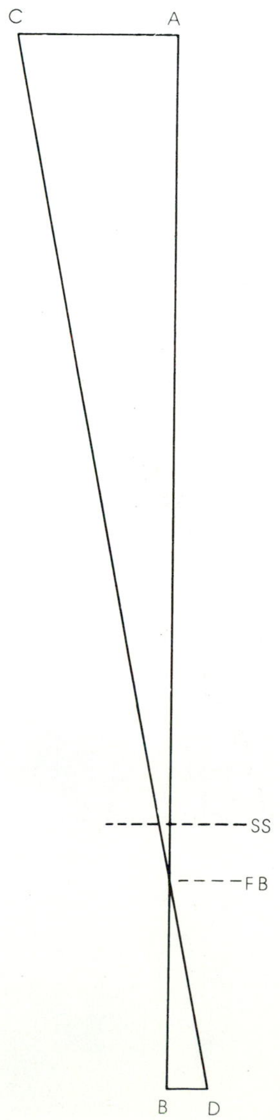

Parallax method

The parallax method is based on the principle that the images cast by two objects equidistant from the fluoroscopic screen will move together at the same amplitude when the fluoroscope and tube are simultaneously moved back and forth across them. A metal indicator (a round-headed screw in the end of a wooden rod or stick serves the purpose well) is used for parallax localization of the depth of foreign bodies.

The following steps are observed by the fluoroscopist:

- After locating the foreign body, close the diaphragm shutters down to the size of the object to direct the central ray through its center.
- Mark the skin, or tape with a suitable metallic marker in position to indicate the exact site of the foreign body in the frontal plane.
- Place the metal indicator against the side of the body, and, holding it in an exactly horizontal position, move the screen back and forth while raising or lowering the indicator until the images of the foreign body and the indicator move at the same amplitude.
- Make a mark on the side of the body to indicate the depth of the foreign body.

The parallax method is the technique of choice when the patient cannot be turned for right-angle projections. It may also be used for depth localization in such regions as the shoulder, buttocks, and upper thigh.

Right-angle method

The right-angle method is applicable when turning the patient is not contraindicated by his or her condition or by the nature or location of the foreign body. The following procedure is used:

- Locate and suitably mark the exact site of the foreign body in the frontal plane.
- Then, repeat the procedure with the patient in the lateral position.

Profunda method

The profunda method consists of removing a foreign body under fluoroscopic guidance. The procedure can be time consuming, and because of the radiation dose to both patient and surgeon, the use of this method is generally discouraged.

Fig. 13-15. Graphic representation of location of foreign body *(FB). SS,* skin surface.

Aspirated and Swallowed Objects

Infants and young children instinctively investigate things by taste as well as by sight and touch. The result is that anything they can grasp they put into their mouths; therefore foreign bodies are frequently aspirated or swallowed (Figs. 13-16 and 13-17). In adults the most frequent foreign body traumas under this heading may be fragments of bone (commonly fish or chicken bones), a bolus of solid food, and dental appliances (see also Fig. 13-6). Adults are also prone to hold between their teeth such items as rings and open safety pins (Figs. 13-18 and 13-19). Some craftsmen, most notably carpenters and those in the sewing trades, find it expedient to fill their mouths with such items as tacks, small nails, and pins, to be fed out for rapid use in their work. Many mentally disturbed patients have a compulsion to swallow objects and manage to swallow some of a surprisingly large size (Fig. 13-20).

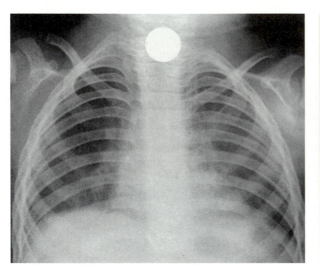

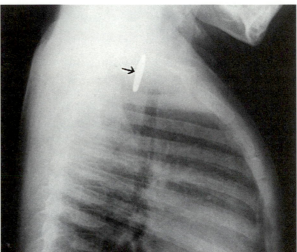

Fig. 13-16. Coin in lower cervical esophagus.

(Courtesy Dr. William H. Shehadi.)

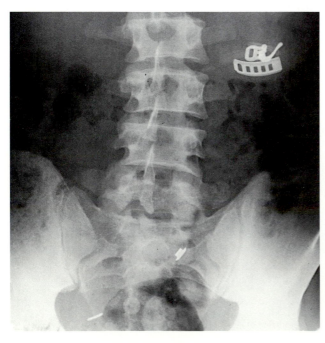

Fig. 13-17. Swallowed rubber boot clip and fastener.

(Courtesy Dr. Peter Kuum.)

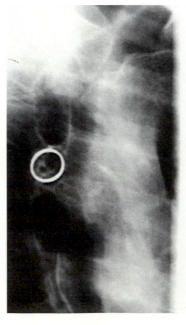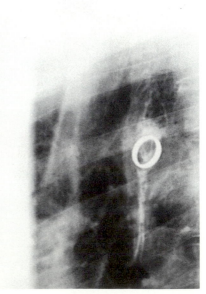

Fig. 13-18. Wedding ring in upper esophagus.

A foreign body that enters the mouth may start a gag reflex and be expelled immediately. When this occurs, a search should be made to recover and identify the object, thus obviating the need for futile and unnecessary radiologic examination of the patient.

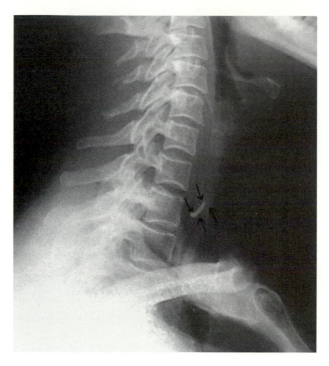

Fig. 13-19. Chicken bone in lower cervical esophagus.

(Courtesy Dr. William H. Shehadi.)

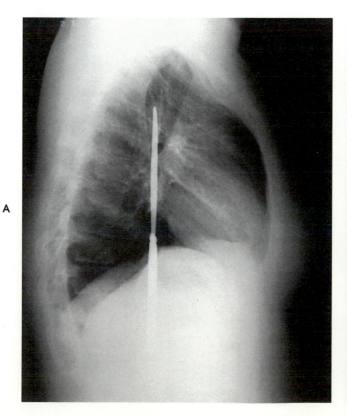 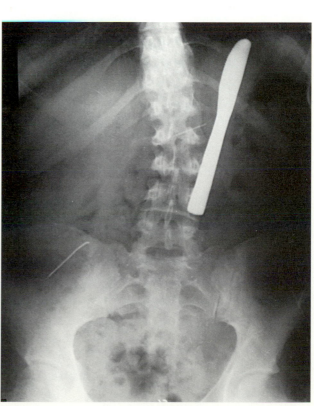

A B

Fig. 13-20. A, Lateral chest showing table knife in esophagus. **B,** AP abdomen showing different table knife and other small straight foreign bodies. Same patient as in **A** at a later date.

More frequently the foreign body is retained and will be aspirated or swallowed (Fig. 13-21). Rarely, it will be dislodged superiorly from the oral pharynx into the nasopharynx. If aspirated into air passages, the foreign body will be above the diaphragm in the neck or chest. If swallowed, the foreign body will pass beyond the oropharynx and may lodge or become impacted in the cervical or thoracic portion of the esophagus, or it may travel on into the stomach and intestines (Figs. 13-22 and 13-23).

The patient's symptoms will usually, but not always, indicate whether a foreign body has been aspirated or swallowed. When there is any doubt, particularly in the case of infants and young children, the preliminary radiographic survey should include the body of the patient from the level of the external acoustic meatuses to the level of the anal canal—the neck, chest, abdomen, and pelvis—that is, from the level of the highest external orifice to the level of the lowermost orifice. Once the location of the foreign body has been determined, accurate localization and follow-up radiographs to determine its progress will depend on its size and shape and on the degree of impaction, if any.

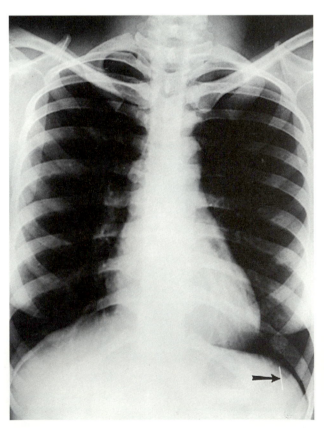 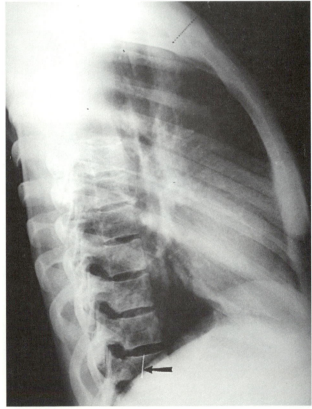

Fig. 13-21. Straight pin aspirated into posterior basal bronchus *(arrows).*

(Courtesy Dr. Harold G. Jacobson.)

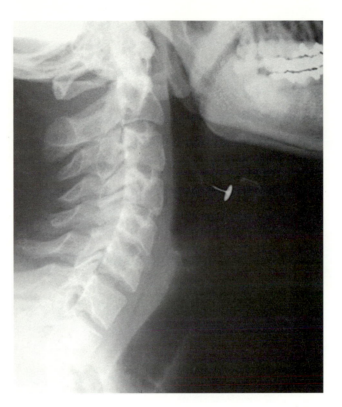

Fig. 13-22. Thumbtack (aspirated) lodged on epiglottis. The tack was spontaneously expelled when the patient coughed.

(Courtesy Dr. William H. Shehadi.)

A   B   C

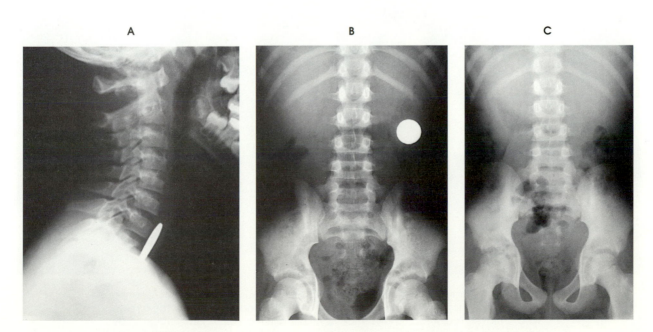

Fig. 13-23. A, Twenty-five cent piece in the lower cervical esophagus. **B,** Interval radiograph shows the coin in the stomach, and **C,** to have been expelled.

(Courtesy Dr. William H. Shehadi.)

Usually the only problem encountered in the detection of radiopaque foreign materials in the respiratory and alimentary tracts is the control of involuntary motion. This must be achieved by patient cooperation and/or rapid exposure times.

Radiolucent foreign bodies require the use of a contrast medium to coat the object or localize the site of foreign body obstruction and to demonstrate the condition of the soft tissues at the site where the foreign body is lodged (Fig. 13-24).

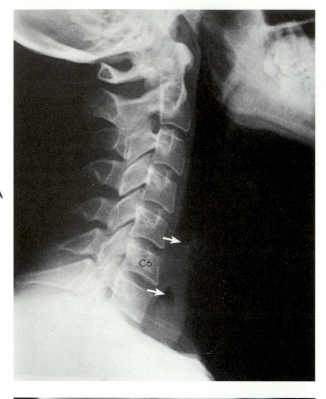

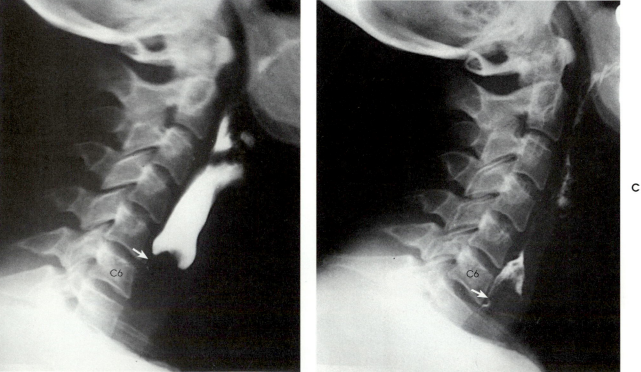

Fig. 13-24. A, Impacted, nonopaque meat bolus *(arrow)* causing widening of esophagus. **B,** Complete obstruction by meat bolus causes barium to stop at the site of the foreign body. **C,** Delayed radiograph shows small trickle of barium bypassing the foreign body posteriorly.

Aspirated Foreign Bodies

INFANTS AND YOUNG CHILDREN

Because an aspirated object can be quickly drawn into a distal branch of the airways, the initial radiographs of infants and young children should be large enough to include the entire respiratory system. The following steps are observed:

- Obtain an AP projection of the head and neck and a lateral image of the neck.
- When placing the films, align the top border of the film at the level of the external acoustic meatuses to include the entire nasopharynx. This is necessary for the detection of an object that rarely is, but may possibly have been, explosively dislodged from a lower level only to become lodged in the nasopharynx.
- Ensure that the lower edge of the film used for the AP projection of the neck and chest extends well below the level of the diaphragm.
- Place infants in an upright immobilizing device or in a supine and immobilized position.
- If the infant is supine, obtain the lateral projection by the cross-table technique.
- Employ the recommended infant technique, which is always based on the shortest possible exposure time. On viewing the initial image, the physician will determine if further projections are indicated.

OLDER CHILDREN AND ADULTS

Aspirated foreign bodies may lodge in the larynx or trachea or in a main bronchus, most frequently in the right bronchus because of its larger diameter and more vertical direction. Small objects sometimes pass on to occlude one of the smaller bronchial branches where exact localization of the site of obstruction may require bronchoscopy.

Larynx and upper trachea

Radiopaque foreign bodies lodged in the larynx and upper trachea are clearly shown on AP and lateral projections. The lateral projection of the trachea and mediastinum (Volume 1, Chapter 10) is sometimes useful, particularly with short-necked, high-shouldered subjects, and employs the following procedure:

- Center the films and the central ray to the laryngeal prominence.
- Decrease the exposure technique to better visualize the soft tissue structures.

Radiolucent foreign bodies require the use of a contrast medium. This procedure, laryngography, is carried out under fluoroscopic visualization, with spot films, conventional radiographs, and tomography being used as indicated.

Trachea and bronchial tree

Radiography of the intrathoracic respiratory system usually consists of two PA projections; the following steps are observed:

- Place a marker indicating the correct phase of respiration on each film.
- Take the first radiograph on deep inspiration and the second radiograph on maximum expiration.[1] Interference with air flow caused by bronchial obstruction will result in interference of air flow in the affected segment of the lung.
- Compare the two images; this interference of air flow will be demonstrated by no change in the radiolucency of the lung in the affected area.
- When the affected side is determined, make a corresponding lateral image. Depending on the nature of the foreign body and its site, further studies and/or bronchoscopy may be indicated.

---

[1]Griffiths DM, and Freeman NV: Expiratory chest x-ray examination in the diagnosis of inhaled foreign bodies, Br Med J 288:1074-1075, 1984.

Swallowed Foreign Bodies
INFANTS AND YOUNG CHILDREN

Preliminary images of infants and young children should include the entire alimentary canal, irrespective of the time lapse between the accident and the radiography; the following steps are observed:

- As with aspirated foreign bodies, make a mandatory lateral projection of the neck and nasopharynx.
- To best obtain this projection, use the cross-table technique for ease of positioning and immobilization of small and/or uncooperative children.
- Use a 14 × 17 in (35 × 43 cm) film, which is large enough for the AP projection of the neck and body of small infants. A smaller film is used for the lateral.
- Make two exposures, one for the neck and chest areas and one for the abdominopelvic areas, for larger children.
- Employ the routine rapid-exposure infant technique for these studies.

The radiologist determines the nature and site of nonopaque objects under fluoroscopic visualization with the use of a contrast medium to coat the object or localize the site of obstruction.

Smooth-surfaced foreign bodies such as coins and marbles are usually followed with 24-hour interval radiographs to verify their clearance of the pylorus and the ileocecal valve, until a final radiograph confirms that the foreign object is no longer in the body. An object presenting the possibility of perforation, such as an open safety pin, is followed at more frequent intervals.

OLDER CHILDREN AND ADULTS
Pharynx and upper esophagus

Radiopaque foreign bodies lodged in the pharynx and upper esophagus can usually be clearly shown with one or two lateral soft tissue radiographs of the neck.

- In the preliminary exam, make one exposure on deep expiration to depress the shoulders and one at the height of deglutition to elevate the superior end of the esophagus (Volume 2, Chapter 15, see coverage of the lateral soft palate, pharynx, and larynx).
- Make a lateral retrosternal projection to obtain delineation of the upper end of the esophagus on short-necked, high-shouldered subjects. (See the discussion pertaining to the transshoulder lateral, Twining method, for trachea and pulmonary apex in Volume 1, Chapter 10.)
- As with infants and young children, identify and localize nonopaque foreign bodies in this region with the use of a contrast medium administered under fluoroscopic control, followed by radiographs as necessary.

Esophagus, stomach, and intestines

When a foreign body is not found in the pharynx, it is customary to take a PA oblique projection in the RAO position of the esophagus and an AP projection of the abdomen before fluoroscopy with the administration of a contrast medium. This precludes the possibility of obscuring a foreign object with the opaque medium.

One of the water-soluble iodinated media for the investigation of esophageal foreign bodies may be used. The water-soluble medium localizes a nonopaque foreign body by giving an opaque coating, localizes the site of obstruction, and permits better evaluation of any possible soft tissue trauma. The water-soluble medium does not adhere to the foreign body and therefore will not interfere with its endoscopic removal. Barium suspensions adhere to a foreign body, rendering it slippery and difficult for the physician to grasp and remove with an esophagoscope.

Foreign bodies that have reached the stomach but present no danger of perforation are followed with interval images to verify their passage through the pylorus and ileocecal valve. A final radiograph confirms that the object has been discharged from the body.

Patients who have experienced trauma are often referred to the radiology department for examination. The patient is often unable to move and assume the position used for routine radiographic examinations. Whether the examination is relatively simple or complex, professional judgment, ingenuity, and creativity are required on the part of the radiographer.

After the patient has been evaluated by a physician, it is the responsibility of the radiographer performing the examination to move the radiographic and accessory equipment around the patient to avoid causing additional injury or discomfort. The radiographer must exercise sound judgment and discretion and not move the patient in any manner that will cause additional injury.

It is not possible within the space of this text to describe all approaches and modifications needed to obtain radiographs of the critically injured patient. Each patient requires special attention and a slightly different approach, simply because each injured patient is unique. Therefore the following general trauma positioning guidelines must be considered:

- Do not move the patient unless absolutely necessary. If necessary, obtain the assistance of qualified personnel. Move the patient only after determining that it is safe to do so as judged by competent medical personnel.
- Obtain a minimum of two radiographs for each body part. In general, try to obtain them at 90-degree angles to each other.

- If the patient is conscious and coherent, explain exactly what you are going to do *before* moving the patient. If a choice exists regarding more than one approach, ask the patient which would be more comfortable.
- Maintain the routine central ray entrance and exit points as close together as possible for the body part being radiographed.
- Place the cassette (with or without a grid assembly) adjacent to the part being radiographed to center the part of interest to the film.
- When radiographing long bones, include both joints if possible. If this is not possible, include the joint closest to the injury, and obtain a separate radiograph of the other joint of the long bone.
- Do not remove splints or bandages unless instructed to do so. Removal of splints could lead to vascular or nerve injury by bone fragments.

Trauma radiography guidelines

Reversing/Modifying a Projection

The fourth guideline on the previous page stresses the need to maintain the central ray's entrance and exit points as close as possible. Let's apply this guideline by assuming that a patient is brought to the trauma center having sustained injury to the facial area. The patient is conscious, and an image of the facial bones is but one of the radiographic examinations to be performed. Depending on the clinical condition, and cooperation offered by the patient, several radiographic approaches appear possible for completing the examination.

It must be realized that the majority of critically injured patients arrive in the trauma center in the *supine body position*. Therefore the patient is most often radiographed in the supine position. To show progression and development of reversing a position to obtain the diagnostic radiograph, the following sequence is presented:

- The usual way of obtaining a Water's method, parietoacanthial projection (described in Volume 2, Chapter 21), is to align the median sagittal plane perpendicular to the plane of the film and have the orbitomeatal line form an angle of 37 degrees with the plane of the film as depicted in Figs. 13-25 and 13-26.
- If the patient is unable to assume the above *upright* position precisely, modify the approach as follows:
- The first step in modifying a position is to mentally remove the film but maintain the central ray entrance and exit points as diagrammed in Fig. 13-27.
- If the patient is able to safely assume the upright body position represented in Fig. 13-28, the line representing the central ray will remain unchanged. Instead of angling the patient's head, angle the central ray to coincide with the entrance and exit points normally used.
- If the patient is brought to the radiographic room for the parietoacanthial projection in the *prone* position or if the patient is able to assume this position most comfortably, perform the radiograph normally as illustrated in Fig. 13-29.
- Should the patient be unable to assume this prone position with the chin extended, mentally remove the cassette as before (Fig. 13-30). A *similar* radiographic image will be obtained if the entrance and exit points of the central ray and film alignment are maintained as seen in Fig. 13-31.

As stated earlier, in the majority of trauma cases, the patient is brought into the radiographic room in the *supine* position. The facial bones can be radiographically demonstrated (slightly magnified as a result of the increased object-image receptor distance) if the same central ray and image receptor relationship is maintained as previously described. The technique for obtaining a facial bone radiograph on the supine trauma patient is illustrated in Figs. 13-32 and 13-33. The following points should be kept in mind:

- Remember that most patients who have sustained trauma to the facial bones have the possibility of having received trauma to the cervical spine or other body areas.
- Do not flex or extend the patient's neck to obtain the orientation of the central ray and the film as depicted in the above illustrations. Instead, increase or decrease the central ray angulation to keep the same geometric arrangement.

It must be emphasized that in the above examples the resulting radiograph for the different approach will not be identical, but it will be *similar*. The preliminary radiograph is the basis for making the initial patient diagnosis. Following the initial diagnosis, the patient may be further evaluated if movement of the patient is not contraindicated.

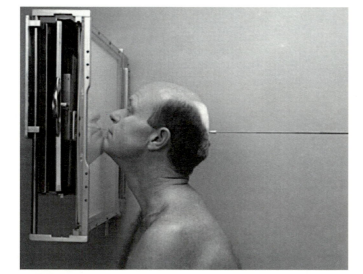

Fig. 13-25. Routine positioning to obtain a Water's method, parietoacanthial projection.

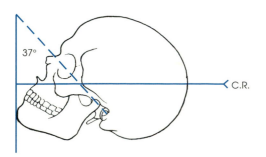

Fig. 13-26. Routine upright radiography.

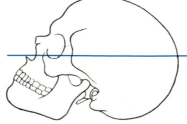

Fig. 13-27. Upright radiography with film line removed.

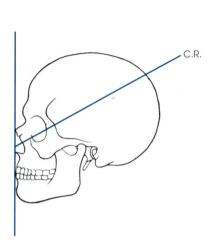

Fig. 13-28. Upright position with angled central ray.

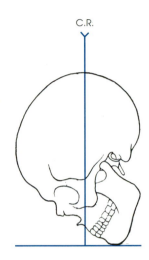

Fig. 13-29. Normal table radiography.

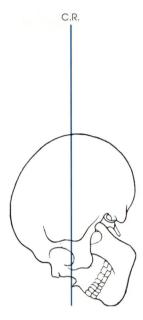

Fig. 13-30. Table radiography with film line removed.

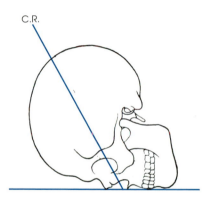

Fig. 13-31. Prone position requiring caudal central ray angulation.

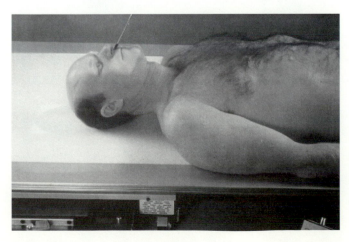

Fig. 13-32. Supine position requiring cephalic central ray angulation.

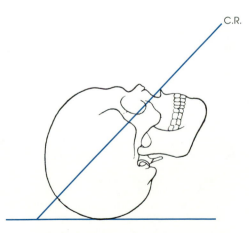

Fig. 13-33. Patient positioned for AP axial projection of facial bones.

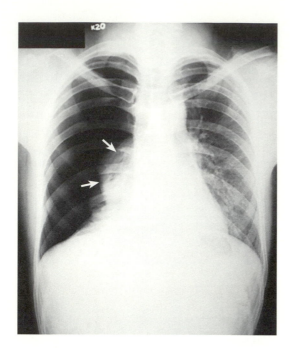

Fig. 13-34. Expiration PA chest radiograph taken of patient having received blunt trauma to the right chest. Pneumothorax seen on right side (*arrows* show the collapsed lung around the hilum with free air in the thoracic cavity).

(Courtesy Sharon A. Coffey, R.T.)

Trauma Radiographs

Representative trauma cases are shown in Figs. 13-34 to 13-61 to illustrate the wide range of patient conditions that result from trauma. In all cases, the patient must be individually evaluated and handled with extreme care, with radiographs often taken through the rescue-squad backboard. In working with the trauma patient, the radiographer must make professional judgments and routinely modify the approach used to obtain the radiographs needed to make the patient diagnosis.

The general positioning guidelines presented here are intended to introduce the reader to the concept of adapting to radiograph the patient in the body position in which he or she arrives in the radiology department. Additional trauma radiography information is presented in other chapters. For specific information on radiography of a trauma patient involving the cervical spine, see Chapter 8.

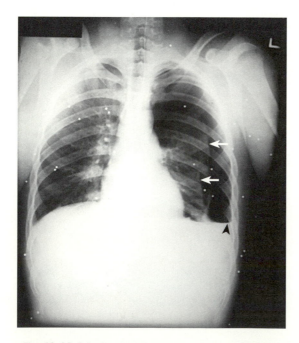

Fig. 13-35. PA chest radiograph of innocent bystander. Multiple buckshot caused hydropneumothorax (*arrows* show margin of collapsed lung with free air laterally, and *arrowhead* shows fluid level at costophrenic angle of left lung).

(Courtesy Sharon A. Coffey, R.T.)

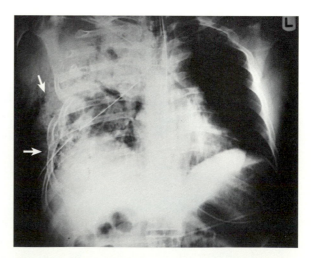

Fig. 13-36. AP chest radiograph of patient who received a crushing injury. Chest tube and multiple rib fractures are seen on the right side. Free air is also seen in soft tissue *(arrows)* lateral to the multiple rib fractures.

(Courtesy Sharon A. Coffey, R.T.)

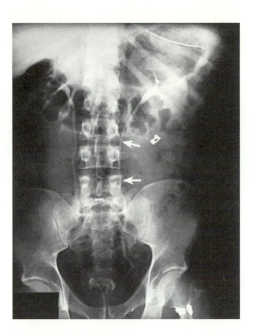

Fig. 13-37. Intravenous urogram of gunshot wound victim. Bullet entered point marked by surgical clip in upper left quadrant and stopped in the left hip area. Note medial displacement of left, contrast-filled ureter *(arrows)* caused by retroperitoneal hemorrhage.

(Courtesy Sharon A. Coffey, R.T.)

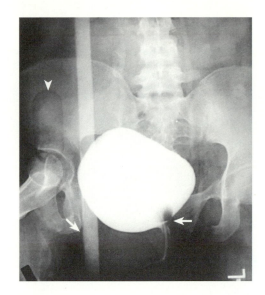

Fig. 13-38. AP projection with cystography of pelvis of auto accident victim. Note diastasis of pelvis (separation of pubic symphysis) *(arrows)*. Vertical line and ovoid artifact *(arrowhead)* are the result of properly performing the examination on a rescue squad backboard.

(Courtesy Sharon A. Coffey, R.T.)

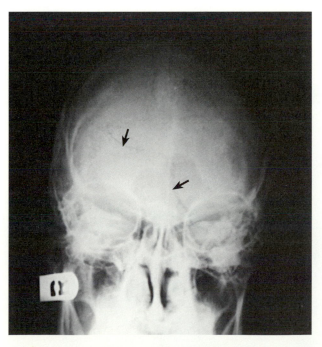

Fig. 13-39. AP projection of skull showing fracture extending from posterior to anterior surface *(arrows)*.

(Courtesy Sharon A. Coffey, R.T.)

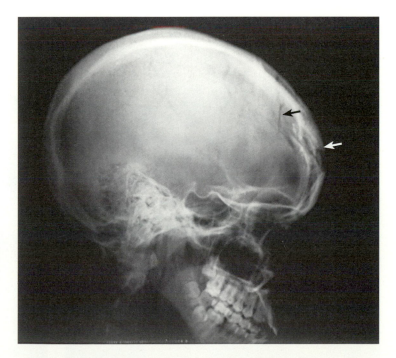

Fig. 13-40. Cross-table lateral skull of auto accident victim showing frontal skull fracture caused by contact with dashboard.

(Courtesy Sharon A. Coffey, R.T.)

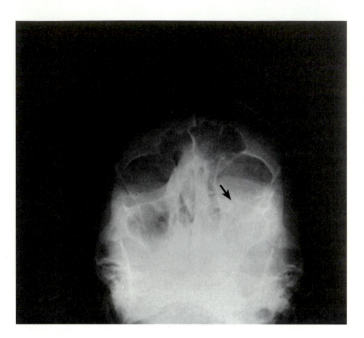

Fig. 13-41. Water's method, acantoparietal projection, of supine patient. Patient was struck with a baseball bat in the left maxillary area. (This radiograph was obtained as demonstrated in Fig. 13-32.) Fracture of floor of left orbit is seen *(arrow)* with related cloudiness of the maxillary sinus caused by fluid accumulation.

(Courtesy Sharon A. Coffey, R.T.)

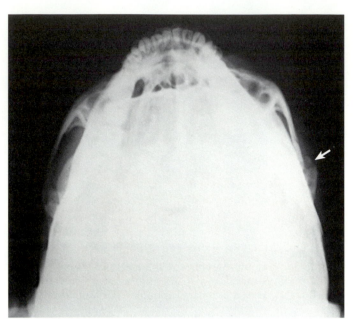

Fig. 13-42. Submentovertical projection demonstrating normal zygomatic arch *(right)* and depressed fracture *(arrow)* of left zygomatic arch caused by patient being struck during a fistfight.

(Courtesy Sharon A. Coffey, R.T.)

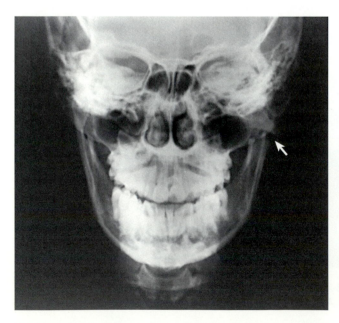

Fig. 13-43. PA projection of mandible showing fracture of left mandibular neck *(arrow)*. Fracture resulted from patient's chin striking the steering wheel during an auto accident.

(Courtesy Sharon A. Coffey, R.T.)

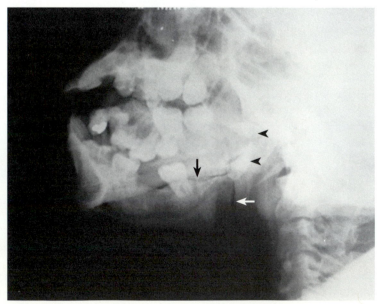

Fig. 13-44. Oblique mandible of fistfight victim showing fracture *(arrows)* extending from mandibular angle superiorly and anteriorly into mandibular body. Tooth also fractured *(arrowheads)*.

(Courtesy Sharon A. Coffey, R.T.)

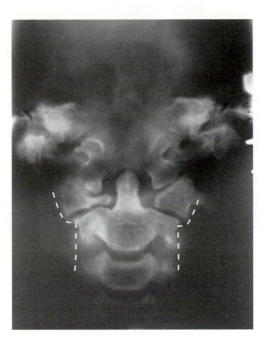

Fig. 13-45. AP tomogram of cervical vertebrae of patient who fell and landed on his head. Bursting-type Jefferson fracture caused lateral displacement of both halves of C1.

(Courtesy Sharon A. Coffey, R.T.)

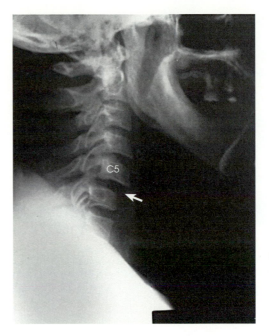

Fig. 13-46. Cross-table lateral cervical spine showing anterior subluxation *(arrow)* of C5 and C6 as a result of the patient diving into a shallow swimming pool.

(Courtesy Sharon A. Coffey, R.T.)

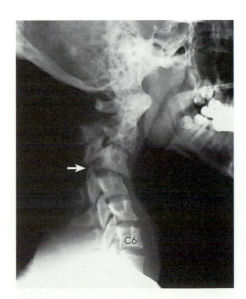

Fig. 13-47. Cross-table lateral cervical spine showing facet dislocation *(arrow)* of C3 and C4 of patient who fell down a flight of stairs. The patient walked away from the hospital 6 weeks later.

(Courtesy Sharon A. Coffey, R.T.)

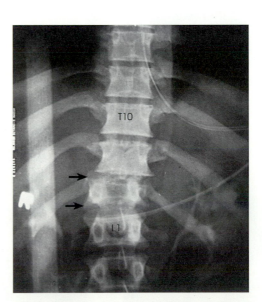

Fig. 13-48. AP thoracic spine of a patient thrown from a horse. Compression fracture of T12 *(arrows)* and loss of alignment of spine at level of T11 to T12 are demonstrated. Contrast-filled kidneys are seen as well as vertical artifact caused by correctly taking radiographs of patient while on rescue-squad backboard support.

(Courtesy Sharon A. Coffey, R.T.)

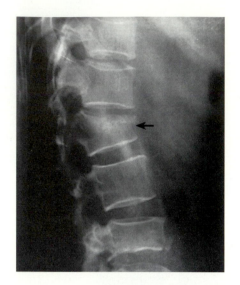

Fig. 13-49. Cross-table lateral lumbar spine showing compression fracture of body of L2 *(arrow)* caused by patient slipping and landing on back side.

(Courtesy Sharon A. Coffey, R.T.)

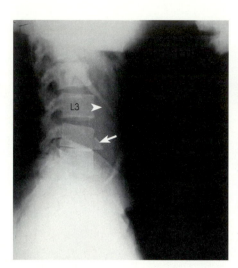

Fig. 13-50. Cross-table lateral lumbar spine of patient whose car was hit by a train, resulting in a compression fracture of L4 and L5 with an anteriorly displaced bone chip *(arrow)*. Bone chip caused localized swelling anteriorly, displacing the contrast-filled ureter *(arrowhead)*.

(Courtesy Sharon A. Coffey, R.T.)

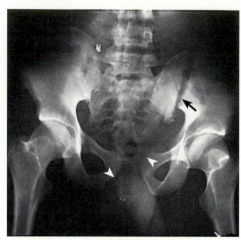

Fig. 13-51. AP projection of pelvis of teacher run over by a school bus. Projection demonstrates separation of the pubic bones *(arrowheads)* anteriorly and the associated fracture of the ilium on the left *(arrow)*. Patient died as a result of hypovolemic shock, a common body response to such trauma.

(Courtesy Sharon A. Coffey, R.T.)

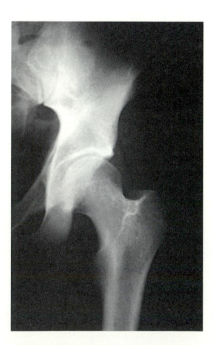

Fig. 13-52. AP projection of hip taken to rule out a hip fracture on a patient who fell inside her house. No fracture is seen on this initial radiograph. A second radiograph taken to complete the diagnosis showed a fracture (see Fig. 13-53).

(Courtesy Sharon A. Coffey, R.T.)

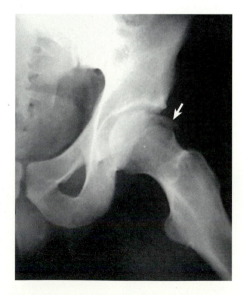

Fig. 13-53. Frog leg lateral hip of same patient as in Fig. 13-52 taken after no fracture was seen on initial radiograph. Note chip fracture of femoral head *(arrow)*. The need for a minimum of two images for each body part is demonstrated by this case.

(Courtesy Sharon A. Coffey, R.T.)

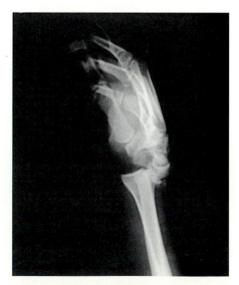

Fig. 13-54. Lateral wrist of patient thrown from a motorcycle resulting in posterior carpal dislocation.

(Courtesy Sharon A. Coffey, R.T.)

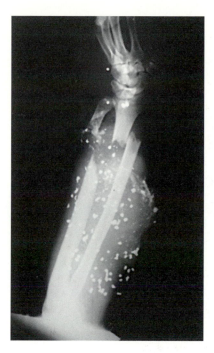

Fig. 13-55. Gunshot wound fracture of radius and ulna with extensive soft tissue damage.

(Courtesy Sharon A. Coffey, R.T.)

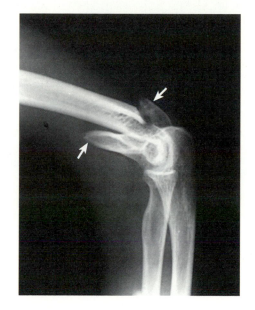

Fig. 13-56. Lateral elbow of patient who fell from a tree, fracturing the distal humerus and splitting the distal articular surface of the humerus *(arrows)*.

(Courtesy Sharon A. Coffey, R.T.)

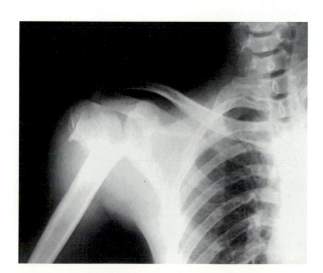

Fig. 13-57. AP shoulder of patient who fractured the surgical neck of the humerus in a fall.

(Courtesy Sharon A. Coffey, R.T.)

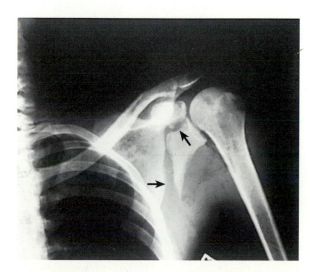

Fig. 13-58. AP projection of shoulder of auto accident victim. Patient had the arm out the window of the car at the time of the accident. Note fracture of scapula through glenoid cavity and extending inferiorly *(arrows)*.

(Courtesy Sharon A. Coffey, R.T.)

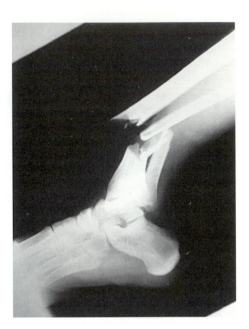

Fig. 13-59. Skiing accident showing compound fracture of the tibia and fibula on this lateral image.

(Courtesy Sharon A. Coffey, R.T.)

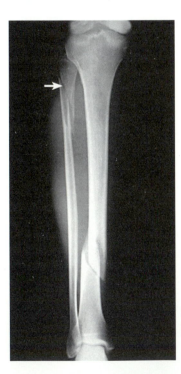

Fig. 13-60. AP lower leg showing fracture of distal tibia with accompanying spiral fracture of the proximal fibula. This radiograph demonstrates the importance of including the entire length of any long bone in the limb.

(Courtesy Sharon A. Coffey, R.T.)

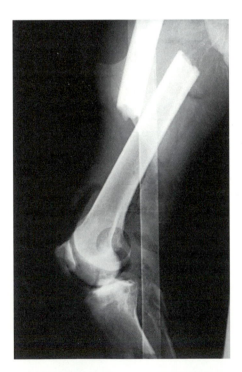

Fig. 13-61. An industrial accident resulted in this fracture of the femur. Patient was radiographed on rescue-squad backboard with the proximal femur seen in the AP projection. The fractured distal femur was rotated, resulting in the lateral image of the distal femur.

(Courtesy Sharon A. Coffey, R.T.)

GLOSSARY

Selected Medical Terms Used In This Text

A

a-, an- (before a vowel). Prefixes signifying without, lack of; as *atypical*, not characteristic of type, and *anemia*, lack of blood or of blood quality.

ab-, abs- Prefix signifying away from, departure; as *abduct*, to draw away from median plane or axis, and *abnormal*, deviation from usual structure or condition.

abdomen (ab-dō'men). Part of body lying between thorax and pelvis; cavity extending from diaphragm to pelvic floor.

abduct (ab-dukt'). To draw away from midsagittal plane, as in moving an arm or leg laterally.

abnormal (ab-nor'-mal). Irregular; deviation from usual form or condition.

abrade (ab-rād'). To rub or scrape off outer layer of a surface.

abrasion (ab-rā'zhun). Act of abrading; an area where skin or mucous membrane has been abraded.

abscess (ab'ses). Localized pus collection in a cavity, resulting from tissue disintegration.

absorb (ab-sorb'). To suck in, as a sponge; to assimilate fluids or other substances from skin, mucous surfaces, or absorbing vessels; energy transferred to tissue, e.g., from radiation.

absorption (ab-sorp'shun). Sucking up or assimilation of fluids, gases, or other substances by absorbing tissues and vessels of body.

acanthomeatal line (a-kan"thō-me-ā'tal). Imaginary line extending from external auditory meatus to acanthion.

acanthion (a-kan'thē-on). Point at center of base of anterior nasal spine.

accessory (ak-ses'or-e). Additional, supplementary; as an *accessory* organ that contributes subordinately to function of a similar but more important organ.

acinus (as'i-nus). Any one of smallest lobules of a racemose gland; one of saclike terminations of a passage, as air sacs, or alveoli, of lungs.

acoustic (a-koos'tik). Pertaining to sound or to organs of hearing.

acromegaly (ak"ro-meg'al-ē). Chronic metabolic disease characterized by permanent enlargement of bones and soft tissues of face as well as of hands and feet.

acute (a-kūt'). Having a sudden onset and running a short but relatively severe course, as an *acute* disease; opposed to chronic.

ad- Prefix signifying toward; as *adduct*, movement toward central axis of body.

Addison's planes (ad'i-sonz). Imaginary planes used to divide abdomen into nine regions for descriptive purposes.

adduct (a-dukt'). To draw toward median plane or axis, as drawing an extremity medially.

adeno- (ad'en-ō-), **aden-** A gland; of or pertaining to a gland; as *adenitis*, inflammation of a gland.

adenoma (ad"e-nō'mah). Benign tumor of glandular origin.

adenopathy (ad"e-nop'ath-ē). Any disease of glands.

adherent (ad-hēr'ent). Clinging or sticking to or together; that which adheres, as a covering membrane.

adhesion (ad-hē'zhun). Union or sticking together of two surfaces as result of inflammatory process, as pleural *adhesions*.

adipose (ad'i-pōs). Fat; of a fatty nature; fat in cells of adipose tissue.

adnexa (ad-nek'sah). Appendages or conjoined parts; as *adnexa* uteri, the ovaries and oviducts.

adrenal (ad-rē'nal). Situated adjacent to kidneys, pertaining to adrenal glands or bodies, also called suprarenal glands.

aer- (ā'er-), **aer-i, aer-o.** Air; combining forms denoting relation to air or gas.

aerated (ā'er-āt-ed). Filled with air, as lungs; charged with air or gas.

afferent (af'er-ent). Conveying inward from periphery to center; applied to nerves and to blood and lymphatic vessels; opposed to efferent.

aggregate (ag're-gāt). Grouped or clustered together; as an *aggregate* gland.

ala (ā'lah). Wing; winglike process or part.

alar (ā'lar). Pertaining to an ala or alae; as *alar* processes of sacrum.

algia (-al'ji-ah). Suffix denoting pain; as *arthralgia*, pain in a joint.

aliment (āl'i-ment). That which nourishes; food or alima (a-li'mah); any nutritive substance.

alimentary (al"i-men'ta-rē). Of or pertaining to nutrition or aliment; as *alimentary* canal, the gastrointestinal tract.

alveolar (al-vē'ō-lar). Pertaining to an alveolus or alveoli of mandible or lungs.

alveolus (al-vē'ō-lus). Small cavity or pit; socket for tooth, acinus, or compound gland; terminal air sac of a bronchiole.

ambi- (am'bē-). Prefix meaning both; as *ambilateral*, pertaining to or affecting both sides; bilateral.

amnion (am'nē-on). Thin, inner membrane of closed sac; bag of waters surrounding fetus in utero.

amphiarthrosis (am-fe-ar-thrō'sis). Articulation admitting but little motion, as between vertebral bodies.

amplitude. Length of travel described by tube during a tomographic motion; 45-degree circular tomographic motion will have greater amplitude than linear motion of same degree.

ampulla (am-pul'ah). Any flasklike or saccular dilatation of a canal; as rectal *ampulla*.

anal (ā'nal). Pertaining to anus.

analgesia (an"al-jē'zē-ah). Diminished sensibility to pain.

analogous (a-nal'o-gus). Having analogy; corresponding in function in certain particulars to an organ or part of different structures; cf. homologous.

anatomic (an"a-tom'ik). Of, pertaining to, or dealing with body structure.

anatomy (a-nat'o-mē). Science dealing with structure of body and relation of different parts.

anesthesia (an"es-thē'zē-ah). Local or general loss of feeling or sensation; anesthesia may be produced by administration of anesthetic agent or by disease.

anesthetic (an"es-thet'ik). Agent capable of producing anesthesia.

aneurysm (an'ū-rizm). Abnormal, saccular dilation of wall of blood vessel, containing blood and usually forming pulsating tumor.

angiocardiography (an"jē-ō-kar"dē-og'–rah-fē). Radiographic demonstration of the heart and great vessels during injection of contrast medium.

angiography (an"jē-og'ra-fē). Study of blood and lymphatic vessels; radiographic depiction of blood vessels after injection of radiopaque contrast substance.

angioma (an"jē-ō'mah). Tumor composed largely of blood or lymph vessels.

ankylosis (ang"ki-lō'sis). Abnormal union of two or more normally separate bones; immobility of a joint.

anomaly (a-nom'al-ē). Marked irregularity or deviation from normal standard of structural formation.

ante- (an'te-). Prefix denoting before (in time or place); as *anteversion*, forward displacement of an organ, and *antenatal*, occurring before birth.

antegrade (an'te-grād). Moving in the direction considered normal.

anterior (an-ter'i-er). Pertaining to, designating, or situated in forward part of body or of an organ.

anteroposterior (AP) (an"ter-ō-pos-ter'i-er). Directed or extending from front to back.

anthropologic base line. As established at Munich Congress in 1877, anthropologic base line of skull passes from lowest point of inferior margin of orbit to center of superior margin of external auditory meatus; line is also known as Frankfurt horizontal plane, German horizontal plane, Reid's base line, and eye-ear plane; infraorbitomeatal line, or Virchow's plane *(which see),* is more widely used in radiographic positioning, because it is more easily localized and it parallels anthropologic base line closely enough for radiographic purposes.

anti- (an'ti-). Prefix signifying against, counter, opposite; as *antitoxin,* against poison.

antiseptic (an"ti-sep'tik). Opposing decay or putrefaction; any substance that will prevent or arrest growth of microorganisms without necessarily destroying them; cf. disinfectant.

antrum (an'trum). Cavern or cavity within a bone, especially maxillary air sinus.

anus (ā'nus). Terminal opening of alimentary canal; orifice through which fecal material is expelled.

aperture (ap'er-chūr). Opening, orifice, or mouth.

apex (ā'peks). Tip or pointed extremity of any conical structure.

apnea (ap-nē'ah). Suspended respiration; transient cessation of breathing following forced respiration; as deglutition *apnea,* temporary cessation of respiration activity during swallowing.

apophyseal (ap-of-iz'e-al). Of or pertaining to an apophysis; apophysial.

apophysis (a-pof'i-sis). Any outgrowth or offshoot; process of bone, especially articular processes of vertebral arches.

appose (a-pōz'). To bring two surfaces in juxtaposition or proximity, as in reduction of a fracture.

apposition (ap"o-zish'un). Contact of adjacent parts; act of apposing or state of being apposed.

aqua (ak'wah). Latin for water; used in pharmacy in sense of liquid or solution.

aqueduct (ak'wē-dukt). Canal for transmission of a liquid; as *aqueduct* of Sylvius, passage connecting third and fourth ventricles of brain.

aqueous (a'kwe-us). Of or of the nature of water; watery.

areola (a-re-ō'-lah). Minute space or interstice in a tissue; colored ring around mammary nipple.

areolar (a-re'o-lar). Of or pertaining to areola; containing interstitial areolae.

arteriography (ar-ter"e-og'ra-fe). Radiographic examination of arteries during injection of contrast medium.

artery (ar'ter-e). Any one of vessels conveying blood from heart to various parts of body.

arthritis (ar-thri'tis). Inflammation of joints.

arthrosis (ar-thro'sis). Any joint or juncture uniting two bones.

articulation (ar-tik"u-la'shun). Joint between bones.

ascites (a-sī'tēz). Collection of serous fluid in peritoneal cavity; abdominal dropsy.

asepsis (a-sep'sis). Methods of preventing and of maintaining freedom from infection; state of being free from septic or putrefactive matter.

aseptic (a-sep'tik). Free from septic material; substances capable of destroying pathogenic germs; cf. antiseptic.

asis (-ā-sis). Combining form from -sis, used after nouns ending in *a* to denote action; as *metastasis,* transfer of a disease from a primary site of infection to another part or parts of body.

aspirate (as'pi-rāt). To remove or draw off by suction; to tap; to treat by aspiration.

aspiration (as"pi-rā'shun). A drawing out by suction; removal of fluids from a cavity by means of an aspirator; commonly called tapping.

assimilation (a-sim"i-lā'shun). Conversion or absorption of nutritive material into living tissue; anabolism or constructive metabolism.

asthenia (as-thē'ne-ah). Loss of strength; general debility.

asthenic (as-then'ik). Pertaining to asthenia or weakness; a bodily habitus characterized by slender build and poor muscular development.

asthma (az'mah). Disease characterized by recurrent attacks of paroxysmal breathing, with sense of suffocation.

ataxia (a-tak'si-ah). Condition characterized by inability to coordinate voluntary muscular movements.

atelectasis (at"e-lek'ta-sis). Defective aeration of pulmonary alveoli at birth; collapse or partial collapse of one or more of pulmonary lobes after birth.

atony (at'o-ne). Lack of normal tone or vitality; weakness; especially, deficient tonicity of contractile muscles.

atresia (ah-trē'zhe-ah). Absence or closure of a natural passage.

atrophic (a-trof'ik). Wasted; pertaining to or characterized by atrophy.

atrophy (at'ro-fe). Wasting away, or emaciation, of body or of any part; diminution in size of an organ or part.

atypical (a-tip'i-kal). Unusual; not characteristic of the type.

auditory (aw'di-tō"re). Of or pertaining to sense or organs of hearing.

auricle (aw'rik'l). Protruding portion of external ear; pinna or flap of ear; small, pouched portion of each of two atria of heart.

auricular line (aw-rik'u-lar). Line passing through external auditory meatuses and perpendicular to Frankfurt horizontal plane.

auricular point. Center of external auditory meatus.

auto- (aw'tō). Prefix signifying self; as *autointoxicant,* a virus generated within body.

axial (ak'se-al). Pertaining to axis of a body, part, or thing; directed along axis, or center line.

axilla (ak-sil'ah). Armpit or fossa beneath junction of arm and shoulder.

axillary (ak'si-ler"e). Of or pertaining to armpit, or axilla.

axis (ak'sis). Straight line, real or imaginary, passing through center of a body or thing and around which body or part revolves or is supposed to revolve; second cervical vertebra.

azygos (az'i-gos). An unpaired part, especially an azygous vein or an azygous lobe of lung.

B

barium (bar'e-um). Chemical element belonging to alkaline earth metals; symbol, Ba; atomic weight 137.36. The soluble compounds or salts of barium are poisonous. Chemically pure (USP) barium sulfate ($BaSO_4$) is a heavy, white, insoluble compound of barium and sulfuric acid and is used as a contrast medium in radiography because of its high radiopacity.

basion (bā'se-on). Center of anterior margin of foramen magnum.

benign (be-nīn'). Of mild character; as *benign* tumor, not malignant.

bi- (bī) **(bis-, twice; di-, twice).** Prefix signifying two or twice; as *bilateral,* having or pertaining to two symmetric sides, and *biarcuate,* twice curved.

bifurcate (bī'fur-kāt). To fork or divide into two branches.

bifurcation (bī"fur-kā'shun). Division into two branches; point of division.

bilateral (bīlat'er-al). Two-sided; pertaining to two sides.

bio- (bī'o-) **(Gr.** *bios,* life]. prefix signifying relation to life; as *biology,* science dealing with living organisms.

bismuth (biz'muth). Metallic element, the salts of which are used chiefly in medicine, by mouth in treatment of certain gastrointestinal conditions and by intramuscular injection in treatment of syphilis. Bismuth salts are radiopaque.

BNA. Abbreviation for Basle Nomina Anatomica or for anatomic terminology adopted by Anatomical Society at Basel, Switzerland, in 1895.

body-section radiography. Technical procedure in which any selected plane of body is depicted distinctly by moving film and x-ray tube in opposite directions to blur superjacent and subjacent structures; also called planigraphy, laminagraphy, stratigraphy, and tomography.

bolus (bō'lus). Round mass of anything, especially a soft mass of masticated food ready for swallowing; a dose of IV medication injected all at once.

bougi (bōō-zhē'). Tapering instrument used to dilate tubular passages.

brachial (brāke-al). Pertaining to arm; as *brachialgia,* pain in arm.

brachiocubital (brā"ke-o-kū'bit-al). Pertaining to arm and forearm.

brachy- (brak'e-). Prefix meaning short; as *brachyfacial,* a short, broad face.

brachycephalic (brak"e-se-fal'ik). A head of short, broad type.

brady- (brad'e-). Prefix meaning slow; as *bradycardia* (also called brachycardia), abnormal slowness of heart action.

bregma (breg'mah). Point on surface of cranium at junction of coronal and sagittal sutures.

bronchiectasis (brong"ke-ek'ta-sis). Dilation of a bronchus or bronchi, which may be saccular or cylindrical.

bronchiogenic (brong"ke-o-jen'ik). Of bronchial origin.

bronchitis (brong-kī'tis). Inflammation, acute or chronic, of bronchial passages.

bronchography (brong-kog'ra-fe). Radiographic examination of lungs and bronchial trees after bronchi have been filled with radiopaque contrast substance.

buccal (buk'al). Of or pertaining to a bucca, or cheek; as *buccal* cavity, space between teeth and cheeks.

bursa (bur'sah). Small, fluid-containing sac interposed between surfaces that glide on each other and that would otherwise cause friction.

bursitis (bur-sī'tis). Inflammation of a bursa, sometimes attended with formation of concretions or calculi.

c

c. Symbol for Latin *cum,* with.

calcareous (kal-kar'e-us). Consisting of or containing lime or calcium.

calcific (kal-sif'ik). Having or forming lime or calcium salts.

calcification (kal"si-fi-kā'shun). Deposition of calcium salts in a tissue; preliminary process in formation of bone; a calcified part or calcific deposit.

calculus (kal'ku-lus). Abnormal concretion formed in any part of body, usually in various reservoirs of body and in their passages; as biliary *calculi,* or gallstones, located mainly in gallbladder and biliary ducts, urinary *calculi,* located in any part of urinary tracts, and renal *calculi,* occurring in kidneys. (See *concretion.*)

callous (kal'us). Hard, horny; as thickened area of skin; a callosity.

callus (kal'us). Substance deposited around the healing fragments of fractured bone and ultimately converted into bone as it repairs.

Camper line (Pieter Camper, Dutch physician, 1722-1789). Line extends from lower posterior border of wing of nose to center of tragus.

cancer (kan'ser). Malignant growth or tumor; cf. carcinoma; tends to invade and metastasize.

cannula (kan'u-lah). Small, tubular instrument used for insertion, usually with a trocar, into a body cavity, as in a paracentesis.

cannulation (kan"u-la'shun). Insertion of a cannula into a body orifice or cavity.

canthus (kan'thus). Angle on each side of eye where upper and lower eyelids meet.

capillary (kap'i-ler-e). Any one of minute, thin-walled vessels that connect arterioles with venules to form networks in practically all parts of body.

carcinoma (kar"si-nō'mah). Malignant tumor originating in epithelial tissue and tending to spread, or metastasize, to other parts of body; a cancer.

cardia (kar'de-ah). Upper, or esophageal, orifice of stomach; pertaining to or in relation to heart.

cardio- (kar'de-ō-), **cardi-** (kar'de-). Prefix indicating relation to heart.

cardioangiography (kar"de-o-an"je-og'ra-fe). Radiographic demonstration of heart and great vessels during injection of opaque contrast medium; also called angiocardiography.

cardiospasm (kar'de-o-spazm). Spasmodic contraction of cardiac sphincter of stomach.

caries (kā'ri-ēz). Molecular decay and subsequent suppuration of bone; gradual disintegration, as distinguished from mass destruction from necrosis; tooth decay.

cata- (kat'ah-). Prefix signifying down, lower, against, in accordance with; as *catabasis,* stage of decline of a disease, and *catastaltic,* restraining, as an agent that tends to check a process.

cathartic (ka-thar'tik). Medicine producing evacuations by stool or catharsis; mild purgative.

catheter (kath'e-ter). Tubular instrument for passage through a canal to withdraw or instill fluid or to distend canal.

cauda (kaw'dah). Tail or tail-shaped appendage; as *cauda equina,* tail-like termination of spinal cord, which consists of sacral nerves.

caudad (kaw'dad). In a caudal direction; toward tail; opposed to cephalad.

cele (-sēl). Suffix signifying tumor or hernia; as *cystocele,* hernial protrusion of urinary bladder.

celiac, coeliac (sē'le-ak). Pertaining to abdomen; as *celiotomy,* surgical incision into abdominal cavity.

celiocentesis (sē"le-o-sen-tē'sis). Surgical puncture of abdomen; tapping.

cellulitis (sel"u-lī'tis). Inflammation of connective cellular tissue, especially of subcutaneous areas.

centesis (sen-tē'sis). Surgical puncture of a cavity; tapping.

centi- (sen'ti-). Prefix denoting a hundred or a hundredth part; used chiefly in metric system, as in *centimeter.*

centigrade (sen'ti-grād). Temperature scale graduated into 100 equal divisions called degrees; centigrade thermometer (also called Celsius thermometer), a thermometer having 0° as freezing point of water and 100° as boiling point of water. For conversion to degrees Fahrenheit, multiply degrees centigrade by ⅘ and add 32.

cephalad (sef'al-ad). In a cranial direction, toward head; opposed to caudad.

cephalic (se-fal'ik). Of or pertaining to cranium; directed toward head end of body.

cephalo- (sef'al-o-), **cephal-** Prefix indicating relation to cranium; as *cephalotrypesis* (sef"al-o-tri-pē'sis), trephination of cranium.

cerebellum (ser-e-bel'um). The little brain; part of brain lying in inferior occipital fossa below cerebrum and behind fourth ventricle, pons, and upper part of medulla. Responsible for muscle coordination.

cerebral (ser'e-bral). Of or pertaining to brain, specifically to cerebrum.

cerebro- (ser'e-bro-). Prefix indicating relation to brain; as *cerebrospinal,* pertaining to or affecting brain and spinal cord.

cerebrum (ser'e-brum). Largest and main part of brain, its two hemispheres filling upper and greatest portion of cranial cavity.

cervical (ser'vik-al). Of or pertaining to neck or any necklike part.

cervico- (ser'vi-ko-), **cervic-** Prefix indicating relation to neck or to cervix of any organ; as *cervicooccipital,* pertaining to neck and occiput, and *cervicitis,* inflammation of neck of uterus.

cervix (ser'viks). Neck or necklike portion of any organ; as *cervix uteri,* narrow lower portion of uterus.

cholangeitis, cholangitis (kol"an-jī'tis). Inflammation of bile ducts.

cholangiography (ko-lan″je-og′ra-fe). Radiographic demonstration of bile ducts after they have been filled with radiopaque medium; cholangiography may be performed in operation room while biliary tract is exposed or in radiology department.

chole- (kol′e-), **cholo-** Prefix signifying relation to bile or to biliary tract; as *cholecyst*, gallbladder, and *cholecystectomy*, surgical removal of gallbladder.

cholecystitis (kol″e-sis-tī′tis). Inflammation of gallbladder.

cholecystography (kol″e-sis-tog′ra-fe). Radiographic demonstration of gallbladder following administration of substance that will render organ radiopaque.

choledochogram (ko-led-o′ko-gram). Radiograph of common bile duct while it is filled with contrast medium.

choledochography (ko-led-o-kog′ra-fe). Radiographic demonstration of common bile duct while it is filled with opaque medium administered by ingestion or injection.

choledochus (ko-led′o-kus). Common bile duct.

cholegraphy (ko-leg′ra-fi). Radiologic examination of biliary tract by means of contrast medium.

cholelithiasis (kol″e-li-thī′a-sis). Condition favoring formation of or of being affected with biliary concretions or calculi.

cholesteatoma (ko″les-te-a-tō′mah). Tumor containing cholesterol and fatty tissue, occurring in the middle ear.

chondro- (kon′dro-), **chondr-** Prefix signifying relation to cartilage; as, *chondroma*, benign tumor composed of cartilage, and *chondrocostal*, pertaining to ribs and rib cartilages.

chorea (ko-rē′ah). A nervous disease characterized by spasmodic twitching of muscles; most common in children. Types include St. Vitus' dance and Huntington's chorea.

chorion (ko′re-on). Outer membrane of protective covering that envelops fetus.

chronic (kron′ik). Continuing for a long time; as a *chronic* disease, one which is characterized by a protracted course; opposed to acute.

cicatricial (sik″a-trish′al). Pertaining to or having character of a scar or cicatrix.

cicatrix (sik′a-triks). Scar or scarlike mark; contracted fibrous tissue that forms at site of a wound during process of healing.

cirrhosis (sir-ō′sis). Disease associated with increase in fibrous tissue followed by contraction; specifically, chronic disease of liver in which organ may diminish in size (atrophic cirrhosis) or may increase in size (hypertrophic cirrhosis).

cleido- (klī′do-), **cleid-** Prefix indicating relation to clavicle; as *cleidocostal*, pertaining to clavicle and ribs, and *cleidarthritis*, gouty pain in clavicular region.

clysis (klī′sis). Washing out of a body cavity, as by lavage; an irrigation.

coagulation (ko-ag″u-lā′shun). Act or state of changing from liquid to gelatinous or solid mass; as clotting or *coagulation* of freshly drawn blood.

coalescence (ko″a-les′ens). Growing together or fusion of parts, as in a wound.

cohesion (ko-he′zhun). Molecular attraction or force that causes particles of a substance to cohere or cling together as in a mass.

colitis (ko-lī′tis). Inflammation of colon.

collateral (ko-lat′er-al). Having indirect relation to; secondary or accessory in function.

colo- (ko′lo-; kol′o-). Prefix denoting relation to colon; as *colocentesis*, surgical puncture of colon.

columella (kol″u-mel′ah). A little column; any part likened to a column; as *columella nasi*, nasal septum.

coma (ko′mah). State of profound unconsciousness caused by disease or injury and from which patient cannot be aroused.

comatose (kōm′a-tōs). Resembling or affected with coma; lethargic.

comminuted (kom″i-nūt′ed). Broken into small pieces; splintered, as in a *comminuted fracture*.

compound (kom′pound). Distinct, homogeneous substance composed of two or more chemically combined elements that have lost their original identity and cannot be separated by other than chemical means; cf. mixture, solution.

compound fracture. Fracture having an open wound extending into site of fracture.

concentric (kon-sen′trik). Having a common center, as graduated circles, one within the other; directed toward or converging at a common center; opposed to eccentric.

concretion (kon-kre′shun). A solid, stony mass formed by succeeding layers of mineral salts surrounding a foreign body, such as a grain of sand.

condyle (kon′dīl). Rounded, knucklelike articular process on a bone; applied mainly to rounded articular eminences that occur in pairs, as those of occipital bone, mandible, and femur.

confluent (kon′flu-ent). Coming together; meeting or merging.

congenital (kon-jen′i-tal). Existing at birth; acquired or developed in utero.

congestion (kon-jes′chun). Abnormal accumulation of fluid in any body organ or area, commonly blood; hyperemia.

coniosis (ko″ne-ō′sis). Pulmonary disease caused by inhalation of dust.

consolidation (kon-sol″i-dā′shun). Process of solidification in porous tissue as result of disease, as of lung in pneumonia and tuberculosis.

constriction (kon-strik′shun). Narrowing of lumen or orifice of a passage; a stricture.

contagion (kon-tā′jun). Communication of disease by direct or indirect contact; contagious disease, one that is readily transmissible from one to another without immediate contact.

contagious (kon-tā′jus). Transmissible by mediate or immediate contact; generating disease; conveying contagion.

contra- (kon′trah-). Prefix signifying against, in opposition; as *contraindication*, a symptom that opposes a treatment otherwise advisable.

contralateral (kon″tra-lat′er-al). Occurring on or associated in function with a similar part on opposite side.

contusion (kon-tū′zhun). Bruise; injury to subcutaneous tissue, with effusion of blood throughout area, but without breaking the skin.

coracoid (kor′a-koid). Process of bone projecting upward and forward from upper part of neck of scapula, called coracoid process because of its resemblance to a crow's beak.

corium (ko′re-um). Layer of skin below the epidermis.

coronal plane (ko-rō′nal). Plane or section passing from side to side parallel with coronal suture, at right angles to median sagittal plane of body.

coronoid (kor′o-noid). Shaped like beak of a crow; process on anterior surface of upper extremity of ulna; process on anterior surface of mandibular ramus.

corpus (kor′pus). Latin for body; main part of any organ; mass of specialized tissue.

costal (kos′tal). Of or pertaining to a rib or ribs.

costo- (kos′to-). Prefix signifying relation to ribs; as *costogenic*, originating in a rib.

costophrenic (kos″to-fren′ik). Pertaining to ribs and diaphragm; as *costophrenic* angle, angle formed by ribs and diaphragm and occupied by phrenicostal sinus of pleural cavity.

cox- (koks), **coxo-** Prefixes denoting relation to hip or hip joint; as *coxalgia*, pain in hip, and *coxofemoral*, pertaining to hip and thigh.

coxa (kok′sah). Hip or hip joint.

cranial (kra′ne-al). Of or pertaining to cranium.

cranio- (kra′ne-o-). Prefix denoting relation to cranium; as *craniofacial*, pertaining to cranium and face.

crater (kra′ter). A pit; a bowl-shaped depression.

crepitation (krep″i-tā′shun). Crackling or grating sound, such as that produced by rubbing together two ends of a fractured bone; crepitant rales, crackling sound heard on auscultation in certain lung diseases.

crepitus (krep′i-tus). Crackling noise; crepitation; noise produced by rubbing fragments of fractured bones or rales in lung.

crisis (kri′sis). Turning point in a disease; change that indicates whether symptoms will begin to subside or to increase in severity.

cum (kum). Latin for with; symbol is c̄.

cumulative (kū′mu-lā″tiv). Composed of added parts; increasing in intensity of action after successive additions; cumulative force or action.

cutaneous (kū-tā′ne-us). Of or pertaining to skin or cutis.

cutis (kū′tis). Corium or dermis; true skin as distinguished from epidermis.

cyanosis (sī″a-nō′sis). Bluish or purplish coloration of skin and mucous membrane resulting from deficient oxygenation of blood.

cyst (sist). Any normal fluid-containing sac or pouch, such as gallbladder and urinary bladder; any encapsulated or encysted collection of fluid or semifluid material formed as a result of disease.

cystitis (sis-tī′tis). Inflammation of urinary bladder.

cystography (sis-tog′ra-fe). Radiographic examination of urinary bladder after it has been filled with contrast medium.

cystoscopy (sis-tos′ko-pe). Visual inspection of interior of urinary bladder by means of cystoscope.

D

dacryo- (dak′ri-o-), **dacry-** (dak′ri-). Combining form denoting relation to tears or to lacrimal apparatus; as *dacryocyst,* lacrimal sac, and *dacryocystography,* radiography of lacrimal drainage system.

debility (de-bil′i-te). Weakness; lack or loss of strength.

deciduous (de-sid′u-us). Temporary; that which falls off or is shed, as *deciduous* teeth.

decubitus (de-kū′bi-tus). Lying down; as dorsal *decubitus,* lying on back.

defecation (def″e-kā′shun). Act or process of expelling fecal material from bowel.

deglutition (de″glū-tish′un; deg″lu-tish′un). Swallowing; act or process of swallowing.

demarcation (dē″mar-kāshun). Act or process of marking off boundaries; line of separation, as between healthy and diseased tissue.

dens (denz). Odontoid process of second cervical vertebra; a tooth.

dentition (den-tish′un). Eruption, or cutting, of teeth; form and general arrangement of teeth.

denture (den′tūr). Full set of teeth; artificial teeth.

depression (de-presh′un). Hollow area; concavity; decrease of functional activity or mental vitality.

dermato- (der′ma-to-). Prefix denoting relation to skin; as *dermatoma,* a skin tumor.

dermis (der′mis). Skin; specifically, corium, or true skin.

detergent (de-ter′jent). Any cleansing agent; a medicine used to cleanse wounds.

dextral (deks′tral). Of or pertaining to right side; opposed to sinistral.

dextro- (deks′tro-). Prefix denoting relation to right side; as *dextrocardia,* transposition of heart to right side of chest.

dextrosinistral (deks″tro-sin′is-tral). Extending from right to left; as a *dextrosinistral* plane.

diagnosis (dī″ag-nō′sis). Art or act of determining character of a disease from existing symptoms; also, conclusion reached.

diaphysis (dī-af′i-sis). Shaft, or main part, of a long bone.

diarrhea (dī″a-rē′ah). Frequent discharge of loose or fluid fecal material from bowels.

diarthrosis (dī″ar-thrō′sis). Joint that permits free movement, such as hip or shoulder joint (also called synovial joint).

diastole (dī-as′to-lē). Phase of rhythmic dilation or relaxation of heart and arteries; correlative to dystole.

digestion (di-jes′chun). Process of converting food into chyme and chyle so that it can be absorbed and assimilated.

diploë (dip′lo-ē). Cancellous osseous tissue occupying space between two tables of cranial bones.

dis- (dis-). Prefix denoting absence, reversal, or separation.

disarticulation (dis″ar-tik″u-la′shun). Amputation at a joint with separation of joint.

disinfectant (dis″in-fek′tant). Any agent (heat or chemical) that destroys disease microbes but does not ordinarily injure spores; cf. germicide.

dispersion (dis-per′shun). Act of separating or state of being separated, as finely divided particles of a substance dispersed through a suspension medium.

distal (dis′tal). Remote from origin or head of a part; as *distal* end of a long bone; opposed to proximal.

diverticulitis (di″ver-tik″u-lī′tis). Inflammation of a diverticulum or diverticula.

diverticulosis (di″ver-tik″u-lo′sis). Multiple diverticula of any cavity or passage, most commonly of colon.

diverticulum (di″ver-tik′u-lum). A blind sac or pocket branching off from a main cavity or canal.

dolicho- (dol′i-ko-). Prefix meaning long and narrow; as *dolichofacial,* a long, narrow face.

dolichocephalic (dol″i-ko-se-fal′ik). Having a long, narrow head.

dorsal (dor′sal). Pertaining to or situated near back of body or an organ; opposed to ventral.

dose (dōs). Proper quantity of a medicine to be taken at one time or within a specified time; quantity of x-radiation administered therapeutically at one time or over a period of time.

dropsy (drop′se). Abnormal accumulation of fluid in cellular tissue or in a cavity of body (also called hydrops).

drug (drug). Any chemical substance used, internally or externally, in treatment of disease.

dys- (dis-). Prefix denoting (1) difficulty or pain, as *dyspnea,* labored or painful breathing, or (2) abnormality or impairment, as *dysarthrosis,* malformation of a joint, and *dystrophia,* defective nutrition.

dyspnea (disp-nē′ah). Labored or painful breathing.

dysuria (dis-u′ri-ah). Difficult or painful urination.

E

ec- (ek-). Prefix meaning out or out of; as *eccyesis,* extra-uterine pregnancy, and *ecchymosis,* extravasation of blood; also, resulting discoloration of skin.

eccentric (ek-sen′trik). Situated off center; not having same center; opposed to concentric.

ecto- (ek′to-), **ect-** Prefix denoting without, on the outer side, external; as *ectopic,* out of normal position, and *ectocondyle,* external condyle of a bone.

ectomy (ek′to-me). Suffix denoting surgical removal of; as *cholecystectomy,* removal of gallbladder.

edema (e-dē′mah). Abnormal accumulation of fluid in tissues or cavities of body, resulting in puffy swelling when present in subcutaneous tissues or in distention when in abdominal cavity; dropsy is the old term.

edentulous (e-den′tu-lus). Without teeth; edentate.

efferent (ef′er-ent). Conveying outward from center toward periphery; applied to nerves and to blood and lymphatic vessels; opposed to afferent.

effusion (ef-ū′zhun). Escape of fluid from vessels into tissues or cavities of body.

egest (e-jest′). To expel or excrete waste material from body; opposed to ingest.

elephantiasis (el"e-fan-ti'a-sis). Chronic disease in which affected part undergoes extensive enlargement and skin becomes thick, rough, and fissured, so that it resembles an elephant's hide.

em-, en- Prefixes meaning in; as *empyema*, pus in a cavity, and *encysted*, enclosed in a sac.

emaciation (e-ma"si-a'shun). Wasted; condition of becoming lean or emaciated.

embolism (em'bo-lizm). Obstruction of a blood vessel by an embolus or plug carried in from a larger vessel, usually a blood clot.

embolus (em'bo-lus). Clot of blood, air bubble, or other obstructive plug conveyed by bloodstream and lodging in smaller vessel; cf. thrombus.

emesis (em'e-sis). Act of vomiting.

emetic (e-met'ik). Any means employed to produce vomiting; a medicine that causes vomiting.

emphysema (em"fi-se'mah). Swelling produced by an accumulation of gas or air in interstices of connective tissues; dilation of pulmonary alveoli.

empyema (em"pi-e'mah). Accumulation of pus in a body cavity; most frequently in pleural cavity.

emulsion (e-mul'shun). Oily or resinous substance suspended in an aqueous liquid by mucilaginous or other emulsifying agent.

en-, em- Prefixes meaning in; as *empyema*, pus in a cavity, and *encysted*, enclosed in a sac.

encephalo- (en-sef'a-lo-). Prefix signifying relation to brain.

encephalography (en-sef"a-log'ra-fe), Radiographic examination of brain after ventricles have been filled with contrast medium; pneumoencephalography.

encysted (en-sist'ed). Enclosed in a sac or cyst.

endo- (en'do-). Prefix meaning within; occupying an inward position; as *endocarditis*, inflammation of lining membrane of heart, and *endoscope*, instrument that permits visual examination of interior of a hollow viscus, such as urinary bladder.

endocrine (en'do-krin). Secreting internally, as ductless glands; pertaining to endocrine glands such as pituitary, thyroid, pineal body, and lymphatic system.

endoscopic retrograde cholangiopancreatography (ERCP). Radiographic examination of pancreatic and biliary duct performed by injection of contrast media into these ducts; contrast media is injected through a catheter positioned with use of fiberoptic scope.

endoscopy (en-dos'ko-pe). Visual inspection of gastrointestinal tract with fiberoptic scope.

endosteal (en-dos'te-al). Of or pertaining to endosteum, vascular tissue lining medullary cavity of bones.

enema (en'e-mah). Fluid injected into rectum to clean the bowel or to administer food or a drug.

enteric (en-ter'ik). Of or pertaining to intestines.

enteritis (en-ter-i'tis). Inflammation of intestine, specifically of small intestine.

entero- (en'ter-o-), **enter-** Prefix denoting relation to intestine; as *enteroptosis*, a dropping or downward displacement of intestines.

enterostomy (en"ter-os'to-me). Surgical formation of an opening into intestine through abdominal wall; as gun-barrel *enterostomy*, operation in which each segment of divided intestine is brought to a separate opening on surface of abdominal wall.

enuresis (en"u-re'sis). Involuntary discharge of urine; incontinence of urine, especially at night.

epi- (ep'i), **ep-** Prefix meaning on, above, on the outside, over; as *epicostal*, situated on a rib, *epigastric*, situated above stomach, and *epidermis*, outermost layer of skin.

epiphysis (e-pif'i-sis). Center of ossification separated during growth from main body of a bone by cartilage that subsequently ossifies to unite two parts of bone, epiphysis and diaphysis.

epiphysitis (e-pif"i-si'tis). Inflammation of an epiphysis or of cartilage separating it from diaphysis.

ERCP. See endoscopic retrograde cholangiopancreatography.

erosion (e-ro'zhun). Irregular or uneven wearing or eating away, beginning at surface of a part, as an ulcerative or necrotic process.

eructation (e"ruk-ta'shun). Act of discharging or belching gas from stomach; a belch.

erythema (er"i-the'mah). Morbid redness of skin caused by capillary congestion resulting from irritation or any form of inflammatory process.

etiology (e"ti-ol'o-je). Science or doctrine of causation; investigation or assignment of cause of a disease.

eu- (u-). Prefix signifying well; as *eupnea*, normal breathing; opposed to dys-.

evagination (e-vaj"i-na'shun). Turned inside out; protrusion of a part or organ.

eventration (e"ven-tra'shun). Protrusion of intestines from abdomen.

eversion (e-ver'shun). Act of turning or state of being turned outward or inside out.

evert (e-vert'). To turn outward or inside out.

ex- (eks-). Prefix denoting out, out of, or away from; as *excavation*, a hollowing out, and *excrete*, throwing off of waste material.

excreta (eks-kre'tah). Waste materials excreted or separated out by an organ; waste products cast out from body.

excretion (eks-kre'shun). Throwing off of waste matter.

excretory (eks'kre-to"re). Of or pertaining to excretion.

exo- (sk'so-), **ex-** Prefix meaning outward or outside; as *exogenous*, growing from or on the outside of a part of body; originating outside body.

exostosis (eks"os-to'sis). Spur, or osseous outgrowth, from a bone or tooth.

extension (eks-ten'shun). Movement of a joint or joints that brings parts of an extremity or of body into or toward a straight line.

extra- (eks'tra-). Prefix meaning on outside, beyond, in addition; as *extragastric*, situated or occurring outside stomach.

extravasation (eks-trav"a-sa'shun). Escape of fluid from a vessel into surrounding tissues; said of blood, lymph, and serum.

extrinsic (eks-trin'sik). Originating outside of part involved.

exudate (eks'u-dat). Adventitious material exuded or discharged on injured or diseased tissues.

F

facet (fas'et). Any plane, circumscribed surface; as an articular facet on a bone.

Fahrenheit (fah'ren-hit). Pertaining to thermometric scale invented by Gabriel Daniel Fahrenheit. On Fahrenheit thermometer, freezing point of water is 32° above zero point, and boiling point of water at 212°. Cf. centigrade.

febrile (fe'bril). Pertaining to fever; feverish.

fecal (fe'kal). Relating to or of nature of feces.

feces (fe'sez). Excrement, or waste products, of food digestion discharged from bowels.

fenestra (fe-nes'trah). Small aperture, or opening, as in certain bones.

fetid (fet'id). Having offensive smell.

fetography (fe-tog'ra-fe). Radiographic examination of fetus in utero.

fibroma (fi-bro'mah). Benign tumor composed mainly of fibrous tissue.

fibrosis (fi-bro'sis). Formation of fibrous tissue in any organ or region; replacement of normal tissue with fibrous tissue.

fissure (fish'ur). Any narrow furrow, cleft, or slit, normal or otherwise.

fistula (fis'tu-lah). Abnormal passage leading from an abscess cavity or from a hollow organ to surface of body or from one hollow organ to another.

flaccid (flak'sid). Without firmness or tone; flabby, as a *flaccid muscle*.

flatulence (flat'u-lens). Gaseous distention of stomach or intestines.

flatus (fla'tus). Gas generated in stomach or intestines and passed through the rectum.

flexion (flek'shun). Bending of a joint in which angle between parts is decreased; forward bending; opposite of extension.

flocculent (flok'u-lent). Containing soft flakes or shreds, as in a *flocculent* precipitate.

flux (fluks). Flow of either energy or a liquid; an excessive discharge, as from the bowels.

focal plane. Plane of tissue that is maximumly in focus on a tomogram.

focal plane level. Height from level of focal plane to tabletop.

fontanel (fon'ta-nel). Any one of intervals or soft spots between angles of parietal bones and adjacent bones of cranium in an infant.

formula (for'mu-lah). Prescribed ingredients, with proportions, for preparation of a medicine; prescription; combination of symbols to express chemical constituents of a body.

fossa (fos'ah). A pit, cavity, or depression; as acetabular *fossa*, supraclavicular *fossa*, and nasal *fossae*.

fovea (fo've-ah). Pit or cup-shaped depression.

Fowler's position (fow'lerz). Position in which head end of body is elevated, usually about 30 degrees.

Frankfurt plane or line. See anthropologic base line.

fremitus (frem'i-tus). Palpable vibration or thrill; as tussive *fremitus*, vibration felt through head on humming with mouth closed.

frenulum (fren'u-lum). Small fold of mucous membrane serving to support or restrain movements of a part.

fulcrum. Pivot point or axis about which tube and film rotate during a tomographic motion.

fundus (fun'dus). Base or deepest part of a hollow organ; part farthest from opening, as cardiac end of stomach.

furuncle (fu'rung-k'l). A boil; a localized, pus-filled skin infection.

G

gall (gawl). Bitter, brownish or greenish yellow fluid secreted by liver; bile.

ganglion (gang'gle-un). Any aggregation of nerve cells forming a nerve center; small cystic tumor occurring on a tendon, usually about wrist or ankle.

gangrene (gang'gren). Necrosis of tissue caused by interference with blood supply to part, usually accompanied with putrefaction.

gas gangrene. Gangrene occurring chiefly in lacerated wounds and in which tissues become impregnated with gas produced by a mixed infection of bacteria, including gas bacillus.

gastr- (gas'tr-), **gastro-** Prefix signifying relation to stomach; as *gastritis, gastroenterostomy.*

gastric (gas'trik). Of or pertaining to stomach.

gastroentero- (gas"tro-en'ter-o-), **gastroenter-** Prefix denoting relation to stomach and intestine; as *gastroenteroptosis*, prolapse or downward displacement of stomach and intestines.

gavage (gah"vahzh'). Feeding by stomach tube.

genic (-jen'ik). Combining form meaning causing, giving origin to, or arising from; as *osteogenic*, originating in bone.

German horizontal plane. Base line of cranium; anthropologic base line.

germicide (jer'mi-sid). Any agent that destroys germs; cf. antiseptic and disinfectant.

gingivae (jin-ji've); **sing. gingiva** (jin-ji'vah). Gums.

gingival (jin'ji-val). Of or pertaining to gums.

glabella (glah-bel'ah). Smooth space on forehead between superciliary arches, which corresponds in position with eyebrows.

glabelloalveolar line (glah-bel'o-al-v-'o-lar). Imaginary line extending from glabella to upper alveolus; localization plane of face.

glabellomeatal line (glah-bel"o-al-v-'o-lar). Imaginary line extending from glabella to external auditory meatus; localization line used in skull radiography.

glenoid (gle'noid). Smooth, shallow depression; specifically, glenoid fossa of scapula.

glioma (gli-o'mah). Malignant tumor originating in supportive or connective tissue of central nervous system.

glossa (glos'ah). Greek for tongue.

glossal (glos'al). Of or pertaining to tongue; lingual.

gonion (go'ne-on). Tip of angle of mandible.

granulation (gran-u-la'shun). Formation of small grains or particles; any small, granule-like mass of abnormal tissue projecting from surface of an organ; formation in a wound of small, rounded granules of new tissue during healing process.

gravel (grav'el). Deposit of small, stonelike concretions in kidneys and urinary bladder; calculi.

gravid (grav'id). Pregnant. A condition containing a developing young.

groin (groin). Depression between lower part of abdomen and thigh, or region around depression; inguen, or inguinal region.

groove (groov). Shallow, linear depression, or furrow in a part, especially in bone.

Grossman principle. Tomographic principle in which fulcrum or axis of rotation remains at a fixed height. The focal plane level is changed by raising or lowering the tabletop through this fixed point to the desired height.

gumma (gum'ah). Soft, gummy, granulomatous tumor of syphilitic origin, occurring in third stage of disease.

gynecology (gin"e-kol'o-je). Branch of medicine that treats women's diseases occurring in genital, urinary, and rectal regions.

H

habitus (hab'it-us) **(Latin for habit).** Fixed practice established by frequent usage; bodily appearance; general form or architecture of body.

haustrum (haws'trum); **pl. haustra** (-trah). Any one of recesses formed by sacculations of colon.

hem-, haem-, hemo- Prefix denoting blood or relation to blood; as *hematuria*, presence of blood in urine.

hemangioma (he-man"je-o'mah). Tumor consisting of newly formed blood vessels.

hematoma (he"mah-to'mah). Tumor or swelling containing effused blood.

hemi- (hem'i-). Prefix signifying one half; pertaining to or affecting one side of body; as *hemiplegia*, paralysis of one side of body.

hemoptysis (he-mop'ti-sis). Presence of blood in sputum; expectoration of blood.

hemorrhage (hem'o-rij). Discharge of blood from vessels in any region; bleeding.

hemorrhoid (hem'o-roid). Vascular tumor situated at orifice of or within anal canal.

hepatic (he-pat'ik). Of or pertaining to liver.

hepato- (hep'a-to-), **hepat-** Prefix signifying relation to liver; as *hepatomegalia*, enlargement of liver.

hernia (her'ne-ah). Protrusion of a part of an organ through normal or abnormal opening in wall of its natural cavity; a rupture.

herniation (her-ne-a'shun). Hernial protrusion; formation of a hernia.

herpes (her'pez). Acute inflammation of skin or mucous membrane, in which clusters of small vesicles form and tend to spread.

hetero- (het'er-o-). Prefix signifying other, or other than usual; difference or dissimilarity between constituents; to or from a different source; opposite of homo-.

heterogeneous (het"er-o-je'ne-us). Differing in kind or nature; composed of unlike elements or ingredients or having dissimilar characteristics; opposed to homogeneous.

heterogenous (het"er-oj'e-nus). Arising or originating outside body; opposed to autogenous.

hiatus (hi-ā'tus). An opening; a space, gap, or fissure for transmission of a nerve, vessel, or tubular passage.

hilum (hi'lum). Depression on a gland or organ that marks site of entrance and exit of nerves, vessels, and ducts; as *hilum* of kidney or of lung.

hilus (hi'lus). Same as hilum.

homeo-, homoeo- (ho'me-o-). Prefix meaning like, similar; as *homeomorphous*, of similar structure and form.

homo- (ho'mo-). Prefix meaning one and same, common, similar; as *homodox, homocentric, homologue;* opposed to hetero-.

homogeneous (ho"mo-jē'ne-us). Of same kind or nature; composed of similar elements or ingredients or having similar uniform characteristics; opposed to heterogeneous.

homologous (ho-mol'o-gus). Corresponding in position or structure but not necessarily resembling in function; cf. analogous.

hydro- (hi'dro-). Prefix meaning water or denoting some relation to water or to hydrogen.

hydrocele (hi'dro-sēl). An accumulation of fluid, usually in a sacculated cavity such as scrotum.

hydrocephalus (hi'dro-sef'a-lus). Condition characterized by excessive amount of cerebrospinal fluid in cerebral ventricles, accompanied by dilatation of ventricles, and causing atrophy of brain substance and enlargement of head.

hydronephrosis (hi'dro-nef-rō'sis). Accumulation of urine in pelvis of kidney, caused by obstruction of ureter, with resultant dilatation of renal pelvis and atrophy of organ itself.

hydrops (hi'drops). Excessive accumulation of fluid in a cavity of body; dropsy.

hyper- (hi'per). Prefix meaning over; above in position; beyond usual or normal extent or degree; excessive; opposite of hypo-.

hypermotility (hi"per-mo-til'i-te). Excessive movement or motility of involuntary muscles, especially those of gastrointestinal tract.

hyperplasia (hi"per-pla'ze-ah). Increase in number of cells in a body part (opposite of hypertrophy).

hyperpnea (hi"perp-nē'ah). Abnormally rapid respiratory movements.

hypersthenic (hi"per-sthen'ik). Excessive strength or tonicity of body or of any part; type of bodily habitus characterized by massive proportions.

hyperthyroid (hi"per-thī'roid). Excessive functional activity of thyroid gland, pertaining to hyperthyroidism.

hypertrophic (hi"per-trof'ik). Pertaining to or affected with hypertrophy.

hypertrophy (hi-per'tro-fe). Morbid increase in size of an organ or part caused by increase in size of cells.

hypo- (hi'po-). Prefix meaning under; below or beneath in position; less than usual or normal extent or degree; deficient; opposite of hyper-.

hyposthenic (hi"pos-then"ik). Lack of strength or tonicity; type of bodily habitus characterized by slender build, a modification of more extreme asthenic type.

hypothyroid (hi"po-thī'roid). Deficient functional activity of thyroid gland, pertaining to hypothyroidism.

hysteresis (his"ter-ē'sis). Lagging or retardation of one of two associated phenomena; failure to act in unison.

hystero- (his'ter-o-), **hyster-** Prefix denoting relation to uterus; as *hysterectomy*, surgical removal of uterus.

hysterography (his"ter-og'ra-fe). Radiographic examination of uterus after injection of contrast medium; uterography.

hysterosalpingography (his"ter-o-sal-ping-gog'ra-fe). Radiographic examination of uterus and oviducts after injection of contrast medium; uterosalpingography.

I

-iasis (-ī'a-sis). Suffix denoting morbid or diseased condition; as *elephantiasis, nephrolithiasis, dracontiasis.*

idio- (id'i-o-). Combining form denoting self-produced; as *idiopathic*, self-originated, of unknown cause.

ileac (il-e-ak). Pertaining to ileum or to ileus; cf. iliac.

ileo- (il'e-o-). Prefix denoting some relation to ileum; as *ileocolic, ileocecal, ileotomy.*

ileum (il'e-um). Terminal three fifths of small intestine, part extending from jejunum to cecum; cf. ilium.

ileus (il'e-us). Condition caused by intestinal obstruction, marked by severe pain in and distention of abdomen.

iliac (il'e-ak). Of or pertaining to ilium; cf. ileac.

ilium (il'e-um). Wide upper one of three bones composing each os coxa, or hip bone (half of pelvic girdle; cf. ileum).

im-, in- Prefixes meaning in, within, or into, as in *immersion, injection;* also, not, non-, un-, as in *imbalance, inactive, incurable.*

impacted (im-pak'ted). Firmly wedged or lodged in position; forcibly driven together, as two ends of a bone in an *impacted* fracture.

incipient (in-sip'e-ent). Beginning to exist; commencing; as the *incipient* or initial stage of a disease.

incisura (in"si-sū'rah). Notch or cleft; deep indentation.

incisure (in-sizh'ūr). Notch; cut or gash.

incontinence (in-kon'ti-nens). Inability of any of organs to restrain a natural evacuation; involuntary discharges; as *incontinence* of urine or feces.

induration (in"du-rā'shun). Hardening or hardened tissue resulting from inflammation or congestion.

infarct (in'farkt). Circumscribed area of necrosis of tissue, resulting from obstruction of local blood supply by an embolus or a thrombus.

infection (in-fek'shun). Communication of disease germs to body tissues by any means.

infectious (infek'shus). Contaminated or charged with disease germs; readily communicable by infection but not necessarily contagious; cf. contagious.

inferior (in-fer'ier). Situated lower or nearer to bottom or base; below.

inferosuperior (in'fer-o-su-per'i-er), Directed or extending from below upward; caudocranial.

infiltration (in"fil-tra'shun). Filtering into or penetration of tissues by a substance not normal to them.

inflammation (in"fla-mā'shun). Morbid condition produced in tissues by an irritant; natural reaction to irritation wherein plasma and blood cells are excluded at site of infection or injury in attempt to heal damage; it is manifested by redness, swelling, and pain.

infra- (in'frah-). Prefix meaning below; as *infraorbital*, situated below orbit.

infraorbitomeatal line (in"frah-or"bit-o-me-a'tal). Also known as Virchow's plane (vē'kōz). A line that extends from center of inferior orbital margin to center of tragus and that is used in radiography for adjustment of base of cranium. Because this line closely parallels anthropologic base line, it is frequently denoted by this and other terms applied to anthropologic base line.

infundibulum (in"fun-dib'u-lum). Any conical or funnel-shaped structure or passage.

infusion (in-fū'zhun). Process of introducing a solution into a vessel or a hollow viscus by gravity pressure; cf. injection, instillation, insufflation.

ingest (in-jest'). To take in for digestion; to eat; to take anything by mouth.

inguinal (ing'gui-nal). Of or pertaining to region of inguen or groin, region between abdomen and thigh.

inion (in'i-on). External occipital protuberence.

injection (in-jek'shun). Forcible introduction, usually by syringe, of a liquid, gas, or other material into a part of body, a vessel, a cavity, an organ, or subcutaneous tissue; cf. infusion, instillation, insufflation.

inorganic (in″or-gan′ik). Not organic in origin; pertaining to or composed of substances other than animal or vegetable; inanimate matter; as *inorganic* elements.

inspissated (in-spis′a-ted). Thickened by evaporation or by absorption of fluid content; as *inspissated* pus.

instillation (in″stil-lā′shun). To drop in; process of introducing a liquid into a cavity drop by drop; cf. infusion, injection, insufflation.

insufflation (in″su-flā′shun). Act of blowing air or gas (or a powder or vapor) into a cavity of body, as into colon for double-contrast enema; cf. infusion, injection, instillation.

inter- (in′ter-). Prefix signifying between; as *interlobar*, situated between two lobes; cf. intra-.

intercostal (in″ter-kos′tal). Pertaining to or situated in spaces between ribs.

interpediculate (in″ter-pe-dik′u-lāt). Of or pertaining to space between pedicles of neural arch.

interpupillary line (in″ter-pu′pi-ler″e). Imaginary line passing through pupils of eyes; used in radiography in adjustment of head in an exact lateral position.

interstice (in-ter′stis). Small gap or space in a tissue; an interval.

interstitial (in″ter-stish′al). Of or pertaining to spaces, or interstices, of a tissue.

intra- (in′trah-). Prefix meaning within or into; as *intralobar*, within a lobe, and *intravenous*, injected into a vein; cf. inter-.

intrinsic (in-trin′sik). Situated or originating entirely within an organ or part; opposite of extrinsic.

invaginated (in-vaj′i-nāt″ed). Condition of being drawn inward to become ensheathed, as a covering membrane turning backward to form a double-walled cavity.

invert (in′vert). To turn inward; as to *invert* foot.

involuntary (in-vol′un-ter″e). Movement not under control of the will, as that of cardiac, gastrointestinal, and other involuntary muscles.

ipsilateral (ip″si-lat′er-al)**(L. ipse, self).** Located on or pertaining to same side.

itis (-ī′tis). Suffix signifying inflammation of specified part; as *arthritis, appendicitis, bronchitis.*

J

jaundice (jawn′dis). Morbid condition caused by obstruction of biliary passages; it is characterized by a yellowish discoloration of skin, eyes, and secretions of body resulting from absorption of accumulation of bile pigments from blood.

jejuno- (je-ju′no), **Jejun-** Prefix signifying some relation to jejunum; as *jejunoduodenal, jejunitis, jejunectomy, jejunostomy.*

jejunum (je-ju-num). Middle division of small intestine, extending from duodenum to ileum.

joint mouse (joint mous). Small, movable calcific body in or near a joint, most commonly knee joint.

jugular (jug′u-lar). Of or pertaining to region of throat or neck, specifically to jugular vein.

juxta- (juks′tah-). Prefix meaning by side of, near; as *juxtaspinal, juxtopyloric, justa-articular*, situated or occurring near part specified.

juxtaposition (juks″tah-po-zish′un). A placing or being placed end to end or side by side; apposition.

K

keloid (kē′loid). New growth or tumor of skin consisting of dense, fibrous tissue, usually resulting from hypertrophy of cicatrix, or scar.

KUB. Abbreviation for kidney, ureter, and bladder.

kymography (kī-mo′-gra-fe). Radiographic recording of involuntary movements of such viscera as heart, stomach, and diaphragm, and motion, as in blood vessels.

kyphoscoliosis (kī″fo-sko″li-ō′sis). Backward and lateral curvature of spine.

kyphosis (kī-fō-sis). Acute curvature of spine, usually of thoracic region, with convexity backward; humpback.

kyphotic (kī-fot′ik). Relating to or affected with kyphosis.

L

labial (lā′be-al). Of or pertaining to lips, or labia.

labium (lā′bi-um). A lip; any lip-shaped part.

lacerated (las′er-āt″ed). Torn or mangled; not clean-cut; a wound inflicted by tearing.

lacrimal (lak′ri-mal). Pertaining to or situated near lacrimal, or tear, gland; as *lacrimal* duct, *lacrimal* bone.

lacuna (la-kū′nah). A small pit or depression; a minute cavity.

lambda (lam′dah). Eleventh Greek letter (Λ, λ); point of junction of lambdoidal and sagittal sutures of cranium, site of posterior fontanel.

lamina (lam′i-nah). Thin, flat plate or layer; flattened posterior portion of neural arch, which extends from pedicle to midsagittal plane, where it unites with contralateral lamina or neurapophysis.

laminagraphy (lam″i-nag′ra-fe). See tomography.

laminated (lam′i-nāt″ed). Separated into or made up of thin, flat plates or layers; arranged in layers.

laminectomy (lam″i-nek′to-me). Excision of posterior part of neural arch.

laminography. See tomography.

laparo- (lap′a-ro-), **lapar-** Prefix signifying relation to flank, side of body extending between ribs and ilium or, more loosely, to abdominal wall; as *laparotomy*, surgical incision into abdominal wall.

laryngo- (lăr-in′go), **laryng-** Prefix denoting relation to larynx; as *laryngotracheal, laryngitis.*

laryngogram (la-rin′go-gram). Radiograph of larynx.

larynogography (lăr″in-gog-ra-fe). Radiographic examination of larynx with aid of contrast medium.

larynx (lăr′ingks). Modified upper extremity of trachea; organ of voice.

latent (lā′tent). Not apparent or manifest; dormant.

laterad (lat′er-ad). Directed toward side.

lateral (lat′er-al). Pertaining to side.

lavage (lah″vahzh′). Washing out of an organ, especially irrigation of stomach.

laxative (laks′a-tiv). Mild cathartic.

lesion (lē′zhun). Injury or local pathologic change in structure of an organ or part.

lien (lī′en). Latin for spleen.

lienal (lī-ē′nal). Of or pertaining to spleen.

lienitis (lī″e-ne′tis). Inflammation of spleen.

lieno- (lī-ē′no-), **lien-** Prefix signifying relation to spleen; as *lienorenal*, pertaining to spleen and kidney.

lienography (lī″en-og′ra-fe). Radiographic examination of spleen after injection of contrast medium.

linea (lin′e-ah). Latin for line; any normal strip, mark, or narrow ridge.

lingua (ling′gwah). Latin for tongue.

lingual (ling-gwal). Of or pertaining to tongue; glossal.

lipo- (lip′o-), **lip-** Prefix meaning fat, fatty; as *lipomyoma*, a tumor composed of muscular and fatty elements.

lipoma (li-pō′mah). Tumor composed of fatty tissue.

lith (-lith). Suffix meaning a concretion or calculus; as *phlebolith*, a concretion or calculus in a vein.

lithiasis (li-thī′a-sis). Formation of concretions or calculi in body, especially in urinary passages and gallbladder.

litho- (lith′o-), **lith-** Prefix meaning calculus or concretion; as *lithonephritis*, inflammation of kidney caused by presence of calculi.

lithotomy position (lith-ot′o-me). Position in which body is supine, legs flexed on thighs, and thighs flexed on abdomen and abducted; also called dorsosacral position.

localize (lō′kal-īz). To restrict or limit to one area or part.

localized (lō′kal-īzd). Restricted to a limited area; not general.

locular (lok'u-lar). Divided into small compartments or loculi; pertaining to a loculus or loculi.

loculus (lok'u-lus). Small cavity, compartment, or chamber; a recess or cell, as cells of ethmoidal sinuses.

loin (loin). The portion of the body located between the ribs and crests of ilia and lateral to spine.

longitudinal (lon"ji-tū'di-nal). Extending lengthwise, as distinguished from traverse; axial, as *longitudinal* plane of posterior teeth extends anteroposteriorly with long axis of mandible.

lordosis (lor-dō'sis). Curvature of spine with forward convexity.

lumbar (lum'bar). Of or pertaining to loin; vertebrae situated in region of loin.

lumen (lū'men). Cavity or clear space of a tubular passage such as an artery, a bronchus, or intestine.

luxation (luks-ā'shun). Act or condition of being dislocated or luxated; dislocation.

lymph (limf). Transparent, nearly colorless fluid contained in lymphatics.

lymphatics (lim-fat'iks). Lymphatic system; lymphatic glands and lymphatic vessels, which pervade body and which collect and convey lymph.

M

macerate (mas'er-āt). To soften and separate parts of by soaking or steeping, with or without heat.

maceration (mas"er-ā'shun). Process of becoming macerated.

macro- (mak'ro-), **macr-** Prefix signifying excessive development, especially elongation; as *macrocephalic*, an unusually large head; also, morbid enlargement; as *macrencephaly*, hypertrophy or enlargement of the brain; opposed to micro-.

mal- (mahl-). Prefix meaning ill, bad, badly; as *malalignment, malfunction, maldevelopment.*

mal (mahl). Disease; usually qualified, as *mal de mer, petit mal.*

malacia (mă-lā'shi-ah). Morbid softening of any tissue; as *osteomalacia,* softening of bone.

malignant (ma-lig'nant). Virulent; having a tendency to cause death; as a *malignant* tumor.

mammary (măm'ah-re) **(L. *mamma*, breast).** Of or pertaining to breast, or mamma (măm'ah).

mammilla (mă-mil'ah). Mammary nipple; any nipple-shaped part.

mammillary line (măm'i-ler"e). Imaginary line passing vertically through one mammilla or passing horizontally through mammillae.

mammography (măm-og'ra-fe). Radiologic examination of breasts; also called mastography.

masto- (mas'to-), **mast-** (Gr. mastos, breast). Prefix denoting relation to breast, as in *mastocarcinoma, mastitis.*

mastography (mas-tog'ra-fe). Same as mammography.

maximum (mak'si-mum). Greatest appreciable or allowable; opposite of minimum.

meatus (me-ā'tus); **pl. meatuses** (-iz). Natural passage or canal, especially external orifice of such a passage.

mediad (mē'di-ad). Directed toward midsagittal plane.

medial (mē-di-al). Situated in or occurring near middle in relation to another part; nearer center, or median sagittal plane, mesial.

median (mē'di-an). Having a central position; in middle; mesial.

mediastinum (mē"di-as-ti'num). Space between pleural sacs of lungs, sternum, and thoracic spine; it contains heart and all thoracic viscera except lungs.

mediate (mē'di-it). Indirect; effected by a secondary or intervening cause or medium; not immediate.

mediate (mē'di-āt). To effect by mediation; to intervene.

medulla (me-dul'ah). Marrow of bones; inner substance of an organ, such as that of kidney; tapering terminal portion of brain, medulla oblongata.

medullary (med'ū-ler"e). Pertaining to any medulla; consisting of or resembling marrow.

mega- (meg'ah-), **meg-** Prefix meaning large, as in *megacephalic;* also, a million times, as in *megohm.*

megacolon (meg"ah-kō'lon). Abnormally large colon.

megalo- (meg'a-lo-), **megal-** Prefix meaning large, great, abnormal enlargement; as *megalo-esophagus, megalakria, acromegaly.*

meninges (me-nin'jēz). Three membranes (dura mater, arachnoid, and pia mater) that form protective covering of brain and spinal cord.

meniscus (me-nis'kus). Interarticular, crescent-shaped fibrocartilage, especially of knee.

mental (men'tal) **(L. *mentum*, chin; *mens*, mind).** Of or pertaining to chin or mind.

mesati- (mes'ah-ti-). Prefix meaning medium, as *mesatipelvic,* having a medium-sized pelvis.

mesaticephalic (mes"ah-ti-se-fal'ik). Having a head of medium or average proportions; midway between brachycephalic and dolichocephalic; same as mesocephalic.

mesentery (mes'en-ter"e). Fold of peritoneum that invests intestines and attaches them to posterior wall of abdominal cavity.

mesial (mē'zi-al). Situated near or toward midsagittal plane; medial.

mesiodistal (mē"zi-o-dis'tal). Directed laterally or posteriorly from center or median line of dental arch.

mesion (mē'zi-on). Plane that divides body into right and left halves; midsagittal plane.

meso- (mes'o-). Prefix meaning medium, moderate, or middle; as *mesosoma,* having medium stature, *mesosyphilis,* secondary stage of syphilis, and *mesotropic,* located in center of a cavity.

mesocephalic (mes"o-se-fal'ik). Head of medium or average size; same as mesaticephalic.

meta- (met'ah), **met-** Prefix signifying change or transfer, as in *metabolism, metabasis;* along with, after, or next, as in *metatarsus.*

metaphysis (me-taf'i-sis). Zone of spongy bone between cartilaginous epiphyseal plate and diaphysis of a long bone.

metastasis (me-tas'tah-sis). Transfer of a disease from one organ or region to another, as a malignant tumor spreading from initial location to secondary locations in body; secondary growth so produced.

metastasize (me-tas'tah-sīz). To form new or secondary sites of infection in other parts of body by metastasis, as a tumor.

metra (mē'trah). Uterus.

metro- (mē-tro-), **metr-** Prefix denoting relation to uterus, as in *metrocarcinoma, metritis.*

micro- (mī-kro-), **micr-** Prefix meaning small, minute, as in *microbe, microcephaly;* one millionth part of, as in *microfarad.*

microcephalic (mī"kro-se-fal'ik). Having an unusually small head.

micturition (mik"tū-rish'un). Act of urinating.

miscible (mis'i-b'l). Susceptible to being readily mixed; mixable.

mixture (miks'chur). Heterogeneous substance made up of two or more ingredients that retain their own properties and can be separated by mechanical means; cf. compound, solution.

mobility (mo-bil'i-te). Capacity or facility of movement of an organ, such as stomach, gallbladder, or kidney; cf. motility.

mono- (mon'o), **mon-** Prefix meaning one, single, alone; as *monoplegia,* paralysis affecting but one part of body.

morbid (mor'bid). Disease; of or pertaining to an abnormal or diseased condition.

moribund (mor'i-bund). Near death; a dying state.

mortification (mor"ti-fi-kā-shun). Death of a part or localized area of tissue; old term for gangrene.

motility (mo-til'i-te). Capacity to move or contract spontaneously; contractility; cf. mobility.

mucoid (mū'koid). Resembling mucus.

mucosa (mū-kō'sah). Mucous membrane.

mucosal (mū-kō'sal). Of or pertaining to mucous membrane.

mucous (mū'kus). Of or pertaining to mucus.

mucus (mū'kus). Viscid, watery fluid secreted by mucous glands.

Müller maneuver (Johannes Peter Müller, German physiologist, 1801-1858). Forced inspiration against a closed glottis; maneuver is performed by closing mouth, holding nose, and attempting to breathe in.

multi- (mul'ti-). Prefix meaning many, much; as *multilobular*, composed of many lobes.

multipara (mul-tip'a-rah). Woman who has borne two or more children.

mummify (mum'mi-fī). Term that, as used in nursing and radiographic procedures, means to wrap body in a mummy fashion with a sheet, binding arms to sides, to restrain movement during examination or treatment.

myel (mī'el). Spinal cord; myelon.

myelitis (mī"e-lī'tis). Inflammation of spinal cord or of bone marrow.

myelo- (mī'e-lo-), **myel-** Prefix denoting relation to bone marrow or to spinal cord; as *myeloma, myelomeningitis*.

myelography (mī"e-log'ra-fe). Radiographic examination of spinal cord following injection of contrast medium into spinal canal.

myo- (mī'o-), **my-** Prefix signifying relation to a muscle or muscles; as *myocarditis, myositis*.

myoma (mī-ō'mah). Tumor consisting of muscular elements.

N

nares (na'rēz); **sing, naris** (na'ris). Openings of nasal passages; anterior nares are commonly called nostrils.

nasion (na'zi-on). Midpoint of frontonasal suture.

naso- (na'zo-). Prefix denoting relation to nose; as *nasofrontal, nasopharyngeal*.

nates (na-tēz). Buttocks.

nausea (naw'she-ah). Feeling of sickness at stomach, associated with desire to vomit.

navel (na'vel). Cicatrix, or scar, in center of abdomen, marking point of attachment of umbilical cord; umbilicus.

necrosis (ne-kro'sis). Death or mortification of a part of a circumscribed area of tissue.

necrotic (ne-krot'ik). Affected with or pertaining to necrosis, or death of tissue.

neo- (ne'o). Prefix meaning new or recent; as *neonatus*, a newborn infant.

neoplasm (ne'o-plasm). Any new or morbid growth, such as a tumor.

nephro- (nef'ro-), **nephr-** Prefix denoting relation to kidney; as *nephrolith, nephritis, nephrectomy*.

nephrolithiasis (nef"ro-li-thi'a-sis). Condition caused by accumulation of calculi in kidney.

nephroptosis (nef"rop-to'sis). Abnormal dropping or downward movement of kidney.

neural (nū'ral). Pertaining to a nerve of nervous system.

neuro- (nū-ro-), **neur-** Prefix denoting relation to nerves, as in *neurofibroma, neuralgia, neuritis*.

niche (nich). Small recess or hollow space in a wall; abnormal saccular prominence on wall of stomach resulting from an ulcer crater.

nodular (nod'u-lar). Pertaining to or having form of a node or nodule.

nodule (nod-ūl). Small, rounded prominence; a little bump.

norm (norm). Fixed or authoritive standard; a rule; a pattern or model; a type.

normal (nor'mal). Conforming to an established norm or principle; regular; natural; functioning properly.

normal salt solution. A normal or, more correctly, a physiologic salt solution that is approximately isotonic with body fluids. It is a 0.9% solution of sodium chloride.

nullipara (nu-lip'ar-ah). Woman who has never borne a child.

O

obstetrics (ob-stet'riks). Science dealing with pregnancy and parturition; management of childbirth.

occiput (ok'si-put). Back part of cranium.

occlusal (o-klu'sal). Of or pertaining to biting surface of a tooth or teeth.

occlusal line. Imaginary line passing through head at and parallel with biting surface of teeth.

occlusion (o-klu'zhun). Act of closing or occluding, or state of being closed or occluded, as in a stricture of a normal passage; bringing into contact of opposing surfaces of upper and lower teeth.

oedema (e-dē'mah). *See* edema.

ology (-ol'o-je). Suffix meaning a science or branch of knowledge; as *radiology*, science dealing with diagnostic and therapeutic application of x-radiation.

oma (-o'mah); **pl. -omata** (o'mah-tah) or **-omas** (-o'maz). Suffix denoting morbid condition of some type, usually a tumor, such as *carcinoma, fibroma, myoma, sarcoma*.

omentum (o-men'tum). Free folds of peritoneum that connect stomach with adjacent organs; apronlike great *omentum* hanging downward in front of small intestines.

optimum (op'ti-mum). Best; most conducive to success; condition that is best or most favorable; most suitable degree, quantity, or factor for attainment of a given end.

oral (o'ral). Of or pertaining to mouth or to speech sound.

orbitomeatal line (or"bi-to-me-ā'tal). Imaginary line extending from outer canthus to center of tragus; it is used in radiography for localization purposes.

orchio-, orchi-, orchido- Prefix denoting testes.

organic (or-gan'ik). Of or pertaining to an organ or organs; consisting of or affecting organic structure; also (in chemistry) pertaining to carbon compounds, those of artificial origin as well as those derived from living organisms.

orifice (or'i-fis). Opening, or aperture, of any body cavity.

ortho- (or'tho-), **orth-** Prefix meaning straight or normal; correct or true; as *orthodontic, orthographic, orthuria*, and *orthostatic*, standing upright, caused by or pertaining to standing erect.

orthopedics (or"tho-pe'diks). Branch of surgery dealing with correction or prevention of deformities and with treatment of diseases of bones.

os (os); **pl ora** (o'rah) **(L. oris, mouth).** A mouth; any mouthlike orifice; as *os uteri*.

os (os); **pl. ossa** (os'ah) **(L. ossis, bone).** A bone; as *os calcis, os coxae, os magnum*.

os innominatum (os in-nom"i-nā'tum). Innominate bone; old term for os coxa.

osis (-o'sis); **pl. -oses** (-o'sez). Suffix denoting state or condition; as *psychosis, stenosis, sclerosis*.

ossification (os"i-fi-kā'shun). Formation of bone; process of changing into bone.

osteo- (os'te-o-), **oste-** Prefix denoting relation to bone; as *osteoma*, a benign bony tumor.

osteomalacia (os"te-o-mal-a'shi-ah). Chronic disease characterized by gradual softening of bones, with resultant deformities.

osteomyelitis (os"te-o-mi-el-i'tis). Inflammation of marrow and medullary portion of a bone.

oteoporosis (os"te-o-po-ro'sis). Condition characterized by absorption or rarefaction of bone so that tissue becomes thin and porous.

ostium (os'ti-um). Small mouthlike orifice, especially opening into a tubular passage such as an oviduct.

(o)-stomy (Gr. *stomos*, mouth). Suffix signifying surgical formation of an artificial mouth or opening into some part or between two parts; as *enterostomy,* formation of an opening into intestines through abdominal wall, and *gastroenterostomy,* formation of an artificial opening between stomach and small intestine.

otic (o′tik). Of or pertaining to ear; auditory.

otitis (o-ti′tis). Inflammation of ear; as *otitis media,* inflammation of middle ear.

(o)-tomy (Gr. *-tomia*, cutting). Suffix signifying surgical incision of, usually for the purpose of draining; as *cholecystotomy, nephrotomy, osteotomy.*

oviduct (o′vi-dukt). Duct, or passage, extending, one on each side, from uterus to ovary; fallopian tubes.

oxycephalic (ok″si-se-fal′ik). Having an unusually high vertex; a steeple-shaped head.

P

pachy- (pak′e-). Prefix meaning thick, dense; as *pachypleuritis,* inflammation of pleura attended with thickening of membranes.

pachycephalic (pak″e-se-fal′ik). Having unusually thick, dense cranial walls.

Paget's disease (paj′ets). Osteitis deformans; chronic disease of bones, characterized by irregular rarefaction and thickening, enlargement, and deformity.

palsy (pawl′ze). Loss of power of voluntary movement or sensation, partial or complete, of any part of body; paralysis.

para- (par′ah), **par-** Prefix denoting the following: irregular or abnormal, as in *paranoia, parachroia, parachroma;* resembling in form (said of diseases), as in *paraparesis, parapneumonia, paratyphoid;* near, beside, alongside of, as in *paracystic, parathyroid;* accessory to, as in *paranasal sinuses.* Cf. peri-.

paracentesis (par″ah-sen-te′sis). Surgical puncture of a cavity of body for withdrawal of fluid; tapping.

paralysis (pah-ral′i-sis). Loss of function or sensation, partial or complete, in any part of body through injury or disease of nerve supply; palsy.

paralysis agitans (aj′i-tanz). Chronic, progressive disease of old age, characterized by muscular tremor, weakness, and peculiar gait; shaking palsy or Parkinson's disease.

parenchyma (pah-reng′ki-mah). Essential, functional tissue of an organ as distinguished from its stroma or framework.

paries (pā′ri-ēz); **pl. parietes** (pah-rī-e-tēz). A wall, especially wall of a hollow organ or cavity.

parietal (pah-rī′e-tal). Of or pertaining to parietes, or walls of a cavity.

parotid (pah-rot′id). Situated near ear; specifically, *parotid* gland, largest of salivary group, which is located on side of face in front of and below ear.

parotitis (par″ot-i′tis). Inflammation of parotid glands; mumps.

parturition (par″tū-rish′un). Process of bringing forth young; labor; childbirth.

patent (pā′tent). Open, patulous, unoccluded; as lumen of a vessel.

patho- (path′o-), **path-** Prefix denoting disease; as *pathogenic,* causing or giving origin to disease.

pathology (pah-thol′o-je). Scientific study of essential nature of diseases, structural and functional alterations caused by them; condition or changes produced by disease.

p.c. Abbreviation for Latin *post cibum,* after food.

pediatrics (pe″de-at′riks). Science that treats diseases of children.

pedicle (ped′i-k'l) **(L. *pediculus*, little foot).** Short stem or stalklike part; a pedicle or peduncle; specifically, anterolateral part of each side of neural arch, connecting laminae with body of vertebra.

pedicular (pe-dik′u-lar) **(L. *pedicularis*, louse).** Pertaining to lice; lousy.

pediculate (pe-dik′u-lāt) **(L. *pediculatus*).** Of or pertaining to a pedicle or pedicles.

peduncular (pe-dung′ku-lar). Of or pertaining to a peduncle or pedicle.

pelvimetry (pel-vim′e-tre). Measurement of size and capacity of pelvis.

peri- (per′i-). Prefix meaning around, about, all around, near; as *periapical,* around the apex of a tooth.

periosteum (per″i-os′te-um). Fibrous membrane that closely invests all parts of surface of a bone, except articular surfaces.

periphery (pe-rif′er-e). External part of an organ; circumference.

peristalsis (per″i-stal′sis). Rhythmic contractions by which tubular passages such as alimentary canal, force their contents onward.

petrous (pet′rus; pē′trus). Resembling a stone or rock; specifically, pertaining to petrosa or *petrous* portion of temporal bone.

pH. Symbol used to denote negative logarithm of hydrogen ion concentration in gram atoms per liter.

phleb- (fleb-), **phlebo-** Suffix denoting relation to a vein; as *phlebitis, phlebolith.*

phlebogram (fleb′o-gram). Radiograph of veins following injection of radiopaque substance; also called a venogram.

phonate (fō′nāt). To utter throaty or laryngeal, usually prolonged, vowel sounds with minimum aid from lips.

phrenic (fren′ik) **(Gr. *phren, phrenos*, diaphragm, mind).** Of or pertaining to diaphragm or to mind; phrenic nerve.

phrenico- (fren′i-ko). Prefix signifying some relation to phrenic nerve; as *phrenicotomy.*

phreno- (fren′o), **phren-** Prefix denoting relation to diaphragm, as in *phrenogastric, phrenohepatic,* or to mind, as in *phrenopathy, phrenoplegia.*

physiology (fiz″i-ol′o-je). Scientific study of functions of tissues and organs, as distinguished from anatomy, the study of their structure.

placenta (plah-sen′tah). Flat, cakelike mass; specifically, vascular organ through which fetus communicates with mother by means of umbilical cord.

placentography (plas″en-tog′ra-fē). Radiographic examination of gravid uterus for localization of placenta.

plane (plān). Any flat surface, real or imaginary.

planigraphic principle. Tomographic principle in which fulcrum or axis of rotation is raised or lowered to alter level of focal plane; the tabletop height remains constant.

planigraphy (plah-nig′ra-fe). See tomography.

plantar (plan′tar). Pertaining to the sole of the foot.

platy- (plat′i-), **plat-** Prefix meaning broad, flat; as *platycephalic,* having a broad, flat head.

pleural (ploor′al). Of or pertaining to pleura or pleurae.

pleurisy (ploor′i-se). Inflammation of pleura, usually attended with exudation into pleural cavity.

plica (pli′kah). A fold; as *plica sublingualis,* fold of mucous membrane on each side of floor of mouth overlying sublingual gland.

-pnea (-p′ne′ah). Suffix meaning breath; as in eupnea, dyspnea.

pneumo- (nū′mo-) **(Gr. *pneumon*, lung; *pneuma*, air).** Prefix denoting relation to lungs or to air or other gas; as *pneumonia, pneumonic, pneumothorax, pneumocystography, pneumoperitoneum.*

pneumoconiosis (nu″mo-ko″ne-o′sis). Condition characterized by permanent deposition of particulate matter of substantial amounts in the lungs. Deposition is usually of environmental or occupational nature.

pneumothorax (nū″mo-tho′raks). Accumulation of air or other gas in pleural cavity, usually induced for therapeutic purposes but, occasionally spontaneously as a result of injury or disease.

poly- (pŏl′e-). Prefix meaning many, much, often; as *polycystic, polygraph, polymorphous.*

polyp (pol′ip). Projection of hypertrophied mucous membrane in a body cavity such as nose, paranasal sinuses, and urinary bladder; a polypus.

popliteal (pop-lit′e-al). Of or pertaining to part of knee behind joint.

porus (pō′rus). Latin for pore or opening; meatus; as *porus acusticus internus*, internal auditory meatus.

post- Prefix meaning behind, after, later; as *postnasal, postpartum, postdiastolic*.

post cibum (post sī′bum). Latin for after food; abbreviation, p.c.

posterior (pos-ter′i-er). Pertaining to, designating, or situated in back part of body or of an organ.

posteroanterior (pos″ter-ō-an-ter′i-er). Directed or extending from back to front.

pre- (prē-). Prefix signifying before in time or place; as *prenatal, prevertebral*.

primigravida (pri″mi-grav′i-dah). Woman pregnant for first time.

primipara (pri-mip′ah-rah). Woman who is bearing or has borne her first child.

pro- (prō-). Prefix signifying forward, to front, according to; as *project, progress, prolapse, proportion*.

procto- (prok-to-), **proct-** Prefix denoting relation to anus and rectum; as *proctopolypus, proctoscope, proctitis*.

prognosis (prog-nō′sis). Forecast of course and probable outcome of a disease.

pronation (prō-nā′shun). Medial rotation of hand so that it faces downward or backward; act of lying face down; opposite of supination.

prone (prōn). Lying face down; having palm of hand facing downward or backward.

prophylaxis (prō″fi-lak′sis). Protection from or prevention of disease; protective or preventive treatment.

prostato- (pros′tah-to-) **prostat-** Prefix denoting relation to prostate gland; as *prostatocystitis, prostatitis*.

prostatography (pros″tah-tog′ra-fē). Radiographic examination of prostate gland.

protuberance (pro-tū′ber-ans). Any projecting part; a swelling; general term for a process or projection.

proximal (prok′si-mal). Toward beginning or source of a part; toward head end of body; opposed to distal.

pseudo- (sū′do-), **pseud-** Prefix meaning false; illusory; having a deceptive resemblance to; as *pseudoankylosis, pseudoparalysis, pseudoarthrosis*.

P.S.P. Abbreviation commonly used for a kidney function test with use of either phenolsulfonphthalein or indigo carmine.

psychiatry (sī′kī′ah-trē). Science that treats mental disorders, psychoses, and neuroses.

psycho- (sī′kō-), **psych-** Prefix denoting relation to mind or mental processes, as in *psychogenic, psychoneurosis, psychosis*.

psychology (sī-kol′o-jē). Science that deals with mind in all its aspects; study of mental activity and behavior.

ptosis (tō-sis). Prolapse, or dropping, of an organ from its normal position; usually used as a suffix, as in *enteroptosis, gastroptosis, visceroptosis*.

puerile (pū′er-il). Of or pertaining to a child or children or to childhood; immature; juvenile.

puerperal (pū-er′per-al). Of or pertaining to childbirth; as *puerperal* sepsis, *puerperal* fever.

pulmonary, pulmonic (pul′mo-ner-ē; pul-mon′ik) **(L. *pulmo*, lung).** Of or pertaining to lungs.

purgative (pur′gah-tiv). Purging or strong cathartic medicine, causing extensive evacuations. These agents are more drastic in action than laxative or cathartic groups, which stimulate peristaltic activity and increase tendency to evacuate bowels with a minimum of irritation.

purulent (pū′rōō-lent). Consisting of or of nature of pus or matter; associated with suppuration; as a *purulent* lesion or wound.

pus (pūs). Yellowish, greenish, or brownish exudate generated by suppuration as a result of bacterial infection.

putrefaction (pū″tre-fak′shun). Decomposition of organic (animal or vegetable) matter, with formation of various foul-smelling products; decay.

putrescent (pū-tres′ent). Undergoing decomposition or decay; pertaining to putrefaction; as an offensive or *putrescent* odor.

pyelo- (pī′e-lo), **pyel-** Prefix denoting relation to pelvis of kidney, as in *pyelogram, pyelitis*.

pyo- (pī′o), **py-** Prefix signifying presence of pus; as *pyogenesis, pyonephrosis, pyonephrosis, pyuria*.

Q

quadrant (qwod′rant). A fourth; a quarter; any one of four equal parts of divisions, as of orbit or of abdomen.

quadrate (kwod′rāt). Square or almost square in form; cubical; quadrate lobe of liver.

quickening (kwik′en-ing). First movement of fetus in utero felt by mother, usually occurring about midterm.

R

racemose (ras′e-mōs) **(L. *racemosus*, having clusters like a bunch or grapes).** Compound saccular gland (such as pancreas) having numerous branching ducts ending in acini arranged like grapes on a stalk.

rachio- (rā′ki-o), **rachi-** **(Gr. *rachis*, spine).** Prefix denoting relation to spine, as in *rachiocentesis, rachioplegia, rachitis*.

radio- (rā′di-o) **(L. *radius*, ray).** Prefix denoting (1) radial or radially, as lines *radiating* from a center, (2) radial, as in *radiomuscular*, (3) relation to lateral and larger of bones of forearm, as in *radioulnar, radiohumeral*, and (4) relation to radiant energy, especially to roentgen and radium radiation, as in *radioactive, radiosensitive, radionecrosis*.

radiodontia (rā″di-o-don′shi-ah). Radiographic examination of teeth and their supporting structures.

radiolucent (rā″di-ō-lū′sent). Materials offering little resistance to passage of x-radiation; those that have insufficient physical density to cast an appreciable image on film when exposed to kilovoltages used in radiography of body; cf. radioparent.

radiopaque (rā″di-ō-pāk′). Materials that are impenetrable to x-radiation generated by kilovoltages usually employed in medical radiography.

radioparent (rā″di-ō-pār′ent). Materials wholly transparent to x-radiation; cf. radiolucent.

radius (rā′di-us). Line extending from center to periphery of a circle; semidiameter; lateral and larger bone of forearm.

ramus (rā′mus). Branch or branchlike process, as one of primary divisions of a nerve or blood vessel, or a projecting part of an irregularly shaped bone.

rarefaction (rar″e-fak′shun). State of being or process of becoming thin and porous or less dense without a diminution in size or volume; loss of substance; opposed to condensation and destruction.

recumbent (rē-kum′bent). Reclining; lying down.

reflux (rē′fluks). A flowing back, as return or *reflux* of a fluid.

regurgitation (rē-gur″ji-tā′-shun). To flow or be cast backward, as blood from a heart chamber in insufficiency of a valve; egestion, or casting up, of incompletely digested food.

Reid's base line (rēdz) **(Robert William Reid, Scottish anatomist, 1851-1938).** See anthropologic base line.

renal (rē′nal) **(L. *ren*, kidney).** Of or pertaining to kidney or kidneys.

resorption (rē-sorp′shun). Process of absorbing again; removal by absorption of an exudate or of bone.

respiratory (re-spīr′ah-tō″re; res′pi-rah-to″re). Of or pertaining to respiration or respiratory organs.

retro- (rē′tro; ret′ro-). Prefix signifying backward, as in *retroflexion;* behind, as in *retrosternal;* reversed, or against natural course, as in *retrostalsis*.

retrograde (rē'tro-grad). Directed against natural course; specifically, *retrograde* pyelography, in which contrast solution is injected in a direction contrary to natural flow of urinary secretions (opposite of antegrade).

rhinal (rī'nal). Of or pertaining to nose; nasal.

ruga (rōō'gah); **pl. rugae** (rōō'jē). Wrinkle or fold of mucous membrane; specifically, rugae or folds of gastric mucosa in empty or nearly empty stomach.

S

š. Symbol for Latin *sine,* without.

sac (săk). Soft-walled bag or pouch; any bladderlike organ.

sacculated (săk'u-lāt"ed). Having form of a sac or sacs; characterized by a series of pouched expansions or saccules.

sacralization (sa"kral-i-za'shun). Overdevelopment of one or both of transverse processes of last lumbar segment, with encroachment on or fusion with first sacral segment.

sagittal (saj'i-tal). Of or pertaining to sagittal suture of cranium; pertaining to any plane parallel with median sagittal plane.

sal (sal). Latin for salt.

saline (sā'līn). Consisting of or containing a salt or salts; salty; *saline* solution, especially a physiologic, or so-called normal, salt solution.

salpingo- (sal-ping'go-), **salping-** Prefix denoting some relation to an oviduct or, less commonly, to a eustachian tube.

salpinx (sal'pingks); **pl salpinges** (sal-pin'jēz) **(Gr. *salpinx,* tube).** Oviduct; less commonly, a eustachian tube.

sarcoma (sar-ko'mah). Malignant tumor derived from tissue developed from mesoderm (connective and lymphoid tissue, bone, cartilage, muscle, and part of urogenital organs) and characterized by a fleshy consistency.

sclero- (skler'o-), **scler-** Prefix meaning hard, indurated, fibrous; also denotes relation to sclera of eye.

sclerosis (skle-ro'sis). Hardening, or induration, of tissue, especially of interstitial connective tissue.

scoliosis (skō"li-ō'sis) **(Gr. *skolios,* crooked).** Abnormal lateral curvature of spinal column.

secreta (se-krē-tah). Any product of secretion; the secretions.

secrete (se-krēt'). To separate substances from blood and emit as a secretion.

secretion (se-krē-shun). Process of secreting; also, material secreted.

section thickness. Width of plane of tissue that is maximumly in focus on a tomogram. The section thickness decreases as tomographic angle increases.

sedative (sed'ah-tiv). Medication that has a calming effect.

semi- (sem'i-). Prefix meaning partly; half or approximately half; as *semiflexion, semiprone, semicoma.*

sepsis (sep'sis). Poisoning caused by absorption of pathogenic bacteria and their products from a putrefactive process.

septic (sep'tik). Putrefactive; produced by or caused by pathogenic bacteria.

septum (sep'tum). Any dividing wall or partition.

sequestrum (se-kwes'trum); **pl. sequestra** (se-kwes'-trah). Piece of dead bone that has become detached as a result of trauma or necrosis.

shadowgram, shadowgraph (shad'ō-gram, shad'ō-graf). Radiograph; a roentgenogram.

sialaden (sī-al'ad-en) **(Gr. *sialon,* saliva + *aden,* gland).** Salivary gland.

sialography (sī"al-og'ra-fe). Radiographic examination of a salivary gland or duct after injection of radiopaque contrast medium.

silicosis (sil'i-ko'sis). Condition of lungs caused by prolonged inhalation of dust particles of stone or silica; a type of pneumonoconiosis.

Sim's position (simz). Position in which body is semiprone, lying on left side, with right knee drawn up.

sinciput (sin'si-put). Forehead; anterior part of cranium.

sine (sī'ne). Latin for without; symbol š.

sinistrad (sin'is-trad). Directed toward left; opposite of dextrad.

sinistro- (sin'is-tro-), **sinistr-** Prefix meaning left, as in *sinistrocardia, sinistrocerebral.*

sinus (sī'nus). Cavity of hollow space in bone or other tissue; a dilated channel for passage of venous blood; a suppurating tract.

skiagraph, skiagram (ski'ah-graf, ski'ah-gram). Old term for radiograph or roentgenogram.

solution (so-lū'shun). Homogeneous body (typically liquid but may be gaseous or solid) consisting of two parts: (1) *solvent,* or dissolving substance, and (2) *solute,* or dissolved substance. The molecules of the solute, or dissolved substance, are dispersed among those of the solvent and cannot be filtered out; nor will they settle out on standing. The composition or concentration of a solution can be varied within certain limits. A solution is similar to a compound in that it is homogeneous and similar to a mixture in that its composition is variable.

spasm (spaz'm). Involuntary, convulsive contraction of a muscle or muscles.

specific gravity (spe-sif'ik grav'i-te). Abbreviation, sp. gr.; relative density or weight of any volume of a substance compared with that of an equal volume of water at same temperature and pressure.

sphincter (sfingk'ter). Circular muscle structure that serves to close one of orifices of body; as *sphincter ani, sphincter of Oddi,* pyloric *sphincter.*

spicule (spik'ūl). Minute, needlelike fragment, especially of bone.

spina bifida (spi'nah bif'i-dah). Congenital malformation of vertebral arch in which there is a cleft in a lamina, with or without hernial protrusion of spinal cord and meninges.

spina bifida occulta (ō-kul'tah). Cleft in vertebral arch without herniation of spinal cord and meninges.

spin density. A measure of the concentration of nuclei (number of the nuclei per given volume) contributing to the MR signal by release of energy following *resonance.* One of the major determinants of MR signal strength.

spondylitis (spon"di-lī'tis). Inflammation of a vertebra or vertebrae.

spondylolisthesis (spon"di-lō-lis-thē'sis). Forward displacement of a lumbar vertebra, most frequently of last lumbar segment on sacrum.

stasis (stā'sis). Defective circulation of blood; a slacking or stoppage of normal flow of contents of vessels or of any organ of body.

stellate (stel'āt). Shaped or radiated like a star; as a *stellate* fracture of cranium.

stenosis (ste-nō'sis). Stricture, or narrowing, of lumen or orifice of a passage.

sternal angle (ster'nal ang'l). Angle formed by junction of manubrium and gladiolus, or body, of sternum.

sthenic (sthen'ik). Strength; vigor; opposed to asthenia.

sthenic habitus. Bodily type characterized by strong build; a modification of more massive hypersthenic type.

stoma (stō'mah). Minute, mouthlike aperture; surgically established opening into intestine through abdominal wall; opening established between two anastomosed portions of intestine.

strangulated (strang'gū-lāt"ed). Compressed or constricted to arrest or congest circulation in a part; as a *strangulated* hernia, one in which protruding viscus is so constricted as to stop circulation.

stria (strī'ah); **pl. striae** (strī'ē). A strip or line; a streak, distinguished by color, elevation, or texture.

stricture (strik'tur). Circumscribed narrowing of a canal; a constriction.

stroma (strō'mah). Tissue that forms supporting framework of an organ, as distinguished from its parenchyma, or essential functional elements.

sub- (sub-). Prefix meaning below, under, beneath; as *subnormal, sublingual, subdiaphragmatic.*

subacute (sub'ah-kūt). Between acute and chronic; having some acute symptoms.

subcutaneous (sub"kū-tā'nē-us). Situated beneath skin.

submentovertex (sub"men-tō-ver'teks). Directed from below chin to vertex; pertaining to region beneath chin and vertex; submentovertical.

subphrenic (sub-fren'ik). Situated or occurring below diaphragm.

sulcus (sul'kus). A furrow; a groove; a fissure; especially one of sulci on surface of brain.

super- (sū'per-). Prefix meaning over, above, in excess; as *superimpose, supernumerary, supersaturate.*

supero- (sū'per-o). Prefix meaning above; situated or directed from above.

superoinferior (sū"per-ō-in-fēr'i-er). Directed from above downward; craniocaudal.

supination (sū"pi-nā'shun). Rotation of hand and arm so that palm faces forward; act or state of lying face upward; opposed to pronation.

supine (sū-pīn'). Lying on back; opposite of prone.

suppuration (sup"u-ra'shun). Process of generating and discharging pus.

supra- (sū'prah-). Prefix meaning above, higher in position; as *supraclavicular, suprarenal, supraorbital.*

symphysis (sim'fi-sis). Joint, or line of fusion, between paired bones; as *symphysis pubis, symphysis menti.*

synarthrosis (sin"ar-thrō'sis). Immovable joint (such as a cranial suture) in which only fibrous connective tissue intervenes between bones.

syncope (sing'kō-pē). Temporary suspension of respiration and circulation with loss of consciousness; fainting.

systole (sis'tō-lē). Contraction phase of heartbeat; also contraction itself, by which blood is kept in circulation; correlative to diastole.

T

tachy- (tak'ē-). Prefix meaning fast, swift; as *tachycardia,* rapidity of heart action.

tangent (tan'jent). Touching at a point; meeting a curve or surface at a point and then extending beyond without intersection; as a line or plane *tangent* to a curve, or a curve *tangent* to a line or a surface.

tangential (tan-jen'shal). Directed along or arranged in a tangent, as in adjustment of a structure or a mass so that one or more points of its surface will be tangent to central ray.

tele- (tel'e-; te'le-), **teleo-** Prefix meaning far, at a distance; as *telecardiography.*

teleoroentgenogram (tel"e-o-rent'gen-o-gram"). Radiograph made at a distance of 6 feet.

theca (thē'kah). Protective case or sheath; as *theca vertebralis,* dura mater of spinal cord.

thoracentesis (thō"rah-sen-tē'sis). Surgical puncturing of chest wall for removal of fluid in pleural effusion; tapping; also called pleuracentesis.

thoracic (thō-ras'ik). Pertaining to, or situated in region of chest.

thoracoplasty (thō'rah-kō-plas"tē). Plastic surgery of thorax; especially, resection of a part of several ribs to collapse lung in advanced unilateral tuberculosis.

thrombus (throm'bus). Plug or clot formed in heart or in a blood or lymphatic vessel and remaining at site of formation; cf. embolus.

tomographic angle/arc. Angle described by tube and film during a tomographic motion.

tomography (tō-mog'ra-fē). Special radiographic technique in which all planes of tissue above and below a predetermined plane of tissue are blurred from view by means of synchronously moving the x-ray source and film in opposite directions during exposure.

tone (tōn). Healthy function; resiliency; normal vigor and elasticity; especially, tension of involuntary muscles; tonus.

tonic (ton'ik). Pertaining to or characterized by normal tone or tension, particularly muscular tension; an agent that tends to produce or restore a healthy condition.

topical (top-i-kal). Of or pertaining to a specific spot; local, or for local application; as a *topical* anesthetic.

torsion (tor'shun). Act of turning or twisting or state of being full of turns and twists.

torticollis (tor"ti-kol'is). Irregular contraction of cervical muscles, with twisting of neck and an unnatural position of head; commonly called wryneck.

tortuous (tor'tū-us). Winding; circuitous; full of curves or bends; twisted.

trabecula (trah-bek'ū'lah); pl. **trabeculae** (tra-bec'u-lē). Little beam or crossbar; one of septal membranes in framework of various organs; one of intersecting osseous plates, or cancelli, composing spongy, or cancellous, portion of a bone.

tragus (trā'gus). Cartilaginous projection in front of external auditory meatus.

trans- (trans; also tranz-). Prefix meaning across, through, over; to pass across or through; as *transabdominal,* passing through or across the abdomen, and *transoral,* passing through or across mouth.

transverse (trans-verse'). Crosswise, from side to side; horizontal; opposed to lengthwise and longitudinal.

transverse plane. Plane that divides body or any one of its parts horizontally at any level.

trauma (traw'mah). Injury; condition resulting from injury.

traumatic (traw-mat'ik). Of, pertaining to, or caused by a trauma.

tremor (trem'er; tre'mor). Involuntary trembling or shaking as result of undue strain, weakness, injury, or disease.

Trendelenburg position (tren-del'en-berg). Position in which body is recumbent with feet higher than head for treatment of shock or to displace pelvic organs (on a plane inclined 45 degrees cranially).

trephine (tre-fīn'). Circular saw or trepan for removing a disk of bone, used chiefly in brain surgery for perforating cranium; also, to operate with a trephine or trepan.

trocar (trō'kar). Sharp-pointed, rodlike instrument that is fitted into and used for insertion of a cannula or catheter.

trochanter (trō-kan'ter). One of two protuberances on the proximal end of the femur.

trochanteric (trō"kan-ter'ik). Pertaining to a protuberance at the end of the femur.

tubercle (tū'ber-k'l). Small nodule or prominence; small rounded process on a bone, serving for attachment of muscles or ligaments.

tuberculosis (tū-ber"kū-lō'sis). Infectious disease caused by tubercle bacillus and marked by production of tubercles, fever, night sweats, and progressive emaciation. The lungs are the most common site of infection, but such organs as the intestines, lymph nodes, larynx, kidneys, and bones are frequently involved.

tuberosity (tū"ber-os'i-tē). Broad, roughened process on a bone, serving for attachment of muscles or ligaments.

tumor (tū'mor). Circumscribed swelling; any morbid growth, innocent or malignant; neoplasm.

U

ulcer (ul'ser). Open, suppurating sore occurring on surface of skin or a mucous membrane, as distinguished from an abscess, which is a lesion of deep-seated origin.

umbilical (um-bil'i-kal). Of or pertaining to navel, or umbilicus.

umbilicus (um-bil'i-kus; um"bi-lī'kus). Scar on center of abdomen marking site of attachment of umbilical cord; navel.

uni- (ū′ni-). Prefix meaning one, single, first; as in *unilocular, unidirectional, unigravida.*

unilateral (ū″ni-lat′er-al). Affecting or situated on only one side.

uresis (ū-rē′sis). Discharge of urine; urination.

ureteral (ū-rē′ter-al). Pertaining to ureter.

ureterography (ū-rē″ter-og′ra-fē). Radiographic examination of ureter after injection of radiopaque solution.

urethral (ū-rē′thral). Pertaining to urethra.

urethrogram (ū-rē′thrō-gram). Radiograph of contrast-filled urethra.

urethrography (ū-rē-throg′ra-fē). Radiographic examination of urethra during injection of contrast medium or during voiding.

-uria (ū′rē-ah). Suffix denoting some relation to urine; as *hematuria, dysuria, pyuria.*

uro- (ū′rō-), **ur-** Prefix denoting some relation to urine or to urinary tract, as in *urinalysis, urodynia, urolithiasis.*

urography (ū-rog′ra-fē). Radiographic examination of urinary tract or of any of its parts with contrast medium.

urticaria (ur″ti-kā′rē-ah). Inflammatory skin disease characterized by transient, whitish wheals on a reddish base, causing intense stinging and itching; uredo; nettle rash; hives.

uterine (ū′ter-in). Of or pertaining to uterus.

utero- (ū′ter-ō-), **uter-** Prefix denoting some relation to uterus; as *uterocele, uteroscope, uteritis.*

uterography (ū″ter-og′ra-fē). Radiographic examination of uterus after injection of contrast medium.

uterosalpingography (ū″ter-ō-sal″pin-gog′ra-fē). Radiographic examination of uterus and oviducts after injection of contrast medium; hysterosalpingography.

V

Valsalva maneuver (val-sal′va) **(Antonio Mario Valsalva, Italian anatomist, 1666-1723).** Act of forcing a deep breath against closed glottis. This is achieved by a straining action, as if trying to move the bowels, without blowing out the cheeks or filling the pharynx.

varices (var′i-sēz); **sing. varix** (var′iks). Permanently dilated and tortuous veins; varicosities.

varicose (var′i-kōs). Irregularly dilated; enlarged and tortuous; pertaining to a venous varix or varices.

vas (vas); **pl. vasa** (vā′sah). Vessel or duct; specifically, a blood, spermatic, or lymph vessel.

vascular (vas′kū-lar). Pertaining to or composed of vessels; specifically, pertaining to blood or lymph vessels.

vena (vē′nah); **pl. venae** (vē′nē). Vein.

venogram (vēn′o-gram). Radiograph of veins filled with contrast medium; a phlebogram.

venography (vē-nog′ra-fē). Radiologic examination of veins during injection of radiopaque solution.

ventrad (ven′trad) **(L. venter, belly).** Situated or directed toward abdomen or anterior aspect of body; ventrally.

ventral (ven′tral). Pertaining to abdomen or to anterior aspect of body or a part; designating or situated near anterior aspect.

ventricle (ven′tri-k′l). Cavity of an organ, such as ventricles of brain or of heart.

ventriculography (ven-trik″u-log′ra-fē). Radiographic examination of brain following injection of radioparent medium into ventricles; pneumoventriculography.

vermiform (ver′mi-form). Resembling a worm; as *vermiform* appendix or cecum.

vertex (ver′teks). Top or highest part of head.

verticomental (ver″ti-kō-men′tal). Pertaining to vertex and chin; as a *verticomental* projection of facial bones.

verticosubmental (ver″ti-kō-sub-men′tal). Pertaining to vertex and region of throat below chin; as a *verticosubmental* projection of petrosae.

vesicle (ves′i-k′l). Fluid-containing cavity or sac; blister.

villi (vil′ī); **sing. villus** (vil′us). Minute, threadlike processes that project from specialized mucous membrane, as from mucosa of small intestine.

Virchow's plane (ver′kōz) **(Rudolf Virchow, German pathologist, 1821-1902).** See infraorbitomeatal line.

virulent (vir′u-lent). Extremely poisonous or noxious; violent; malignant.

visceral (vis′er-al). Pertaining to a viscus or viscera.

visceroptosis (vis″er-op-tō′sis). Falling or downward displacement of abdominal organs.

viscid (vis′id). Having a gelatinous or sticky consistency; adherent; viscous.

viscosity (vis-kos′i-tē). State or quality of being thick and sticky; viscid; gluey, glutinous.

viscus (vis′kus). Internal organ, such as heart, kidney, or stomach.

vitiate (vish′i-āt). To render faulty or defective; to impair quality of; to contaminate; to make impure, as air by electrical corona or by products of respiration.

voluntary (vol′un-ter″e). Proceeding in obedience to will; acting according to choice.

vomit (vom′it). Spontaneous expulsion of contents of stomach by mouth; also, the vomited matter.

vomitus (vom′i-tus). Matter ejected from stomach through mouth.

Z

zonography. Tomographic technique that depicts thick sections or zones of tissue by utilizing tomographic angles of 10 degrees or less.

zoster (zos′ter). Acute inflammatory skin disease of nervous origin, causing tenderness, itching, and neuralgic pains; it is characterized by clusters of small vesicles on a reddish base following along course of a peripheral nerve; herpes zoster; zona; shingles.

zygapophyseal (zīg″ap-of-iz′e-al). Of or pertaining to a zygapophysis or to zygapophyses.

zygapophysis (zīg″ah-pof′i-sis) **(Gr. zygon, yoke + apophysis, process).** Yokelike articular process; specifically, one of articular processes of neural arch of a vertebra.

zygion (zig′i-on, zij′i-on). Point at either end of bregmatic diameter of skull.

zygoma (zī-gō′mah). Arch formed by union of malar bone of face and zygomatic process of temporal bone of cranium; also, malar bone.

zygomatic (zī″gō-mat′ik). Of or pertaining to zygomatic arch or to malar bone.

BIBLIOGRAPHY

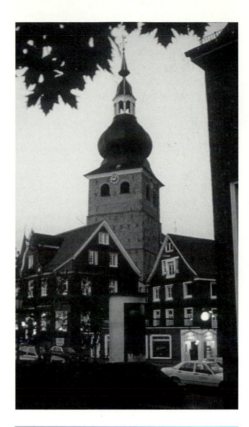

The town square in Lennep, Germany at dusk, with the onion-domed church steeple in the background.

HISTORY

1895 Röntgen WC: Ueber eine neue Art von Strahlen. Part I, Sitzungsber, phys.-med. Gesellsch. Würzburg, pp. 132-141, 1895, English translation in Science 3:Feb 14, 1896.

1896 Röntgen WC: Ueber eine neue Art von Strahlen. Part II, Sitzungsber, phys.-med. Gesellsch. Würzburg, pp. 11-19, 1896, English translation in Science 3:May 15, 1896.

1897 Röntgen WC: Weitere Beobachtungen über X-strahlen, Mitt. Sitzungsberichte Preuss Akad Wess, Physik Math K1, p. 392, 1897.

1905 Albers-Schönberg HE: The development and present state of radiology, Arch Roentgen Ray 10:105, 1905.

1909 Pfahler GE: Notes from some of the roentgen laboratories in Europe, Am Q Roentgenol 2:15-22, 1909-1910.

1923 Grashey R: Wilhelm Conrad Röntgen, Fortschr Roentgenstr 30:409, 1923.

1929 Memenov MI: Das Staatsinstitut für Röntgenologie, Radiologie und Krebsforschung in Leningrad, Fortschr Roentgenstr 40:1069-1087, 1929.

1931 Brown P: Early American roentgenology: manners and men, Radiogr Clin Photogr 7:2-6, 1931.

Glasser O: Dr. W.C. Roentgen and the discovery of the roentgen ray, AJR 25:437-450, 1931.

Hickey PM: The Caldwell lecture, 1928, AJR 25:177-195, 1931.

1932 Glasser O: Reception of Roentgen's discovery in America, Radiogr Clin Photogr 8:2-6, 1932.

O'Hara FS: Looking backward, Radiogr Clin Photogr 8:3-9, 1932.

1934 Crane AW: The research trail of the x-ray, Radiology 23:131-148, 1934.

Curie MS: An editorial by EW Hall, AJR 32:395, 1934.

Donaghey JP: Reminiscences of Röntgen, Radiogr Clin Photogr 10:2-7, 1934.

Forssell G: Marie Curie—in memoriam, Acta Radiol 15:685-688, 1934.

Glasser O: Wilhelm Conrad Röntgen and the early history of roentgen rays, Springfield, Ill, 1934, Charles C Thomas Publisher.

Schinz HR: Röntgen und Zürich, Acta Radiol 15:562-575, 1934.

1936 Brown P: American martyrs to science through the roentgen ray, Springfield, Ill, 1936, Charles C Thomas Publisher.

1937 Glasser O: The life of Röntgen as revealed in his letters, Sci Monthly 45:193-206, 1937.

1938 Pancoast HK: Reminiscences of a radiologist, AJR 39:169-186, 1938.

1939 Casey FS: Early scientists in the field of radiology, Xray Techn 11:88-92, 1939.

1944 Glasser O, et al: Physical foundations of radiology, New York, 1944, Paul B Hoeber Inc.

1945 Case JT: Fifty years of roentgen rays in gastroenterology, AJR 54:607-625, 1945.

Davidoff LM: The development of modern neuroroentgenology, AJR 54:640-642, 1945.

Glasser O: Chronology of Röntgen's life, AJR 54:541-544, 1945.

Glasser O: Fifty years of roentgen rays, Radiogr Clin Photogr 21:58-66, 1945.

Glasser O: Scientific forefathers of Röntgen, AJR 54:545-546, 1945.

Glasser O: WC Röntgen, Springfield, Ill, 1945, Charles C Thomas Publisher.

Hodges PC: Development of diagnostic x-ray apparatus during the first fifty years, Radiology 45:438-448, 1945.

Kirklin BR: Background and beginning of cholecystography, AJR 54:637-639, 1945.

Lough TW: Commemorating a great discovery and half century of its development, Xray Techn 17:325-330, 1945.

Reynolds L: The history of the use of the roentgen ray in warfare, AJR 54:649-672, 1945.

Rigler LG: The development of roentgen diagnosis, Radiology 45:467-502, 1945.

Roesler H: History of the roentgen ray in the study of the heart, AJR 54:647-648, 1945.

Röntgen WC: On a new kind of rays, Reprint from Röntgen's original papers, Radiology 45:428-435, 1945.

Shields DG: Fashion parade of x-ray apparatus 1895-1945, Xray Techn 17:348-360, 1945.

Spillman R: Early history of roentgenology of the sinuses, AJR 54:643-646, 1945.

Wolcott RE: X-ray horizons, Xray Techn 17:337-347, 1945.

1946 Chevalier J: Vie et travaux de Roentgen, J Radiol Electrol 27:107-110, 1946.

Dariaux A: Hommage aux victimes des rayons X, J Radiol Electrol 27:101-104, 1946.

Delherm L: Première communication en France, sur les applications mèdicales de la découverte de Roentgen, J Radiol Electrol 27:105-106, 1946.

Lacharite H: The healing and lethal rays, Xray Techn 18:111-115, 138, 1946.

Ledoux-Lebard R: Les rayons X dans le diagnostic médical, J Radiol Electrol 27:116-125, 1946.

Pilon H: Cinquante ans de construction radiologique, J Radiol Electrol 27:111-115, 1946.

Stolz Sr MF: Contributions of some of Röntgen's predecessors, Xray Techn 18:1-4, 1946.

1947 Fuchs AW: Edison and roentgenology, AJR 57:145-156, 1947.

1951 Scott WG: The development of angiocardiography and aortography, Radiology 56:485-518, 1951.

1952 Leucutia T: Pneumoperitoneum and pneumoretroperitoneum (editorial), AJR 68:655-658, 1952.

1954 Diehl KL: Bronchography: study of its techniques and presentations of improved modification, Arch Otolaryngol 60:277-290, 1954.

Stevenson CA: Development of colon examination, AJR 71:385-397, 1954.

1955 Olson LG: Roentgen's scientific forefathers, Xray Techn 27:184-189, 1955.

1956 Caffey J: The first sixty years of pediatric roentgenology in the United States, AJR 76:437-454, 1956.

Maluf NSR: Role of roentgenology in the development of urology, AJR 75:847-854, 1956.

1958 Glasser O: WC Röntgen, ed 2, Springfield, Ill, 1958, Charles C Thomas Publisher.

Kincaid OW and Davis GD: Abdominal aortography, N Engl J Med 259:1017-1024, 1958.

1960 Scott J: Ancient and modern, Radiography 26:97-107, 1960.

1961 Bull JWD: History of neuroradiology, Br J Radiol 34:69-84, 1961.

Cole WH: Historical features of cholecystography, Radiology 76:354-375, 1961.

Gershon-Cohen J: Breast roentgenology: a historical review. AJR 86:879-883, 1961.

Watson W: 1895 and all that, Radiography 27:305-315, 1961.

1964 Bruwer AJ, editor: Classic descriptions in diagnostic roentgenology, Springfield, Ill, 1964, Charles C Thomas Publisher.

Strain WH et al.: Radiologic diagnostic agents: a compilation, Med Radiogr Photogr 40(suppl):1-110, 1964.

1965 Grigg ERN: The new history of radiology, Radiol Technol 36:229-257, 1965.

Grigg ERN: The trail of the invisible light, Springfield, Ill, 1965, Charles C Thomas Publisher.

Schatzki R: Esophagus: progress and problems: the Caldwell lecture, AJR 94:523-540, 1965.

1974 Kraft E and Finby N: Wilhelm Conrad Roentgen (1845-1923): discoverer of x-ray, NY State J Med 74:2066-2070, 1974.

1976 Morgan KZ: Rolf M Sievert: the pioneer in the field of radiation protection, Health Phys 31:263-264, 1976.

Ramsey LJ: Luminescence and intensifying screens in the early days of radiography, Radiography 42:245-253, 1976.

1978 Eastman TR: History of radiographic technique, Appl Radiol 7:97-100, 1978.

Lang EF: From earlier pages . . . development of a name for radiology. AJR 130:586-587, 1978.

1979 Fischmann E: Retracing Rontgen's discovery, Diagn Imaging 48:294-303, 1979.

1980 Kraft E and Finby N: Rontgen's discovery of x-ray and Lenard's priority claim, NY State J Med 80:1623-1625, 1980.

Ramsey LJ: Some notable early contributors to radiography—Thompson, Jackson, and Campbell Swinton, Radiography 46:289-297, 1980.

Shampo MA and Kyle RA: Thomas A Edison, JAMA 243:1719, 1980.

1981 Bendinger E: The Curies: pioneers and victims of the Atomic Era, Hosp Pract 16:80, 82-84, 1981.

O'Rahilly R: Plain words on planes and sections, Radiol Technol 52:615-617, 1981.

1984 Boag JW: Silvanus Phillips Thompson—some studies in the "prehistory" of X-rays, Br J Radiol 57:1-15, 1984.

Carter P: Recollections of a veteran, Radiography 49:235-238, 1983.

Kischner SG, Kossoff J and Pickens DR: Women in radiology in the United States: 1982 survey of their professional practices, AJR 141:1055-1059, 1984.

Ochsner SF: Perspectives in radiology—1922 to 1982, South Med J 76:1549-1553, 1983.

1987 Lauer OG: Radiography in the united states army during world war II. Part II. Radiol Technol 58:215-224, 1987.

1988 Bassett LW and Gold RH: The evolution of mammography, AJR 150:493-498, 1988.

Healy JW: H.M. Parker lecture. Radiation protection standards: a historical perspective, Health Phys 55:125-130, 1988.

1989 Brodsky A and Kathren RL: Historical development of radiation safety practices in radiology, Radiographics 9:1267-1275, 1989.

1991 Edwards M: Development of radiation protection standards, Radiographics 11:699-712, 1991.

Eisenberg R: Radiology: an illustrated history of radiology, St Louis, 1991, Mosby.

1992 Doby T: Leonardo da Vinci's anatomy revisited, Caduceus 8:23-38, 1992.

Nedd A II: When the solution is the problem: a brief history of the shoe fluoroscope, AJR 158:1270, 1992.

Scatliff JH and Clark JK: How the brain got its names and numbers, AJNR 13:241-248, 1992.

Tauber WB: Clinical consequences of Thorotrast in a long-term survivor, Health Phys 63:13-19, 1992.

JOURNALS ON RADIOGRAPHY

Acta Radiologica, Stockholm, 1921-1962, and continued as both

Acta Radiologica: Diagnosis, Stockholm, 1962- and

Acta Radiologica: Therapy, Stockholm, 1962-1977, and continued as

Acta Radiologica: Oncology, Radiation, Physics, and Biology, 1978-

American Atlas of Stereo-roentgenology, Troy, 1916-1920.

American Journal of Anatomy, New York, 1901-

American Journal of Roentgenology, Pittsburgh, 1913-1923, and continued as

American Journal of Roentgenology and Radium Therapy, Pittsburgh, 1923-1952, and continued as

American Journal of Roentgenology, Radium Therapy, and Nuclear Medicine, Springfield, Ill, 1952-1975, and continued as

AJR Baltimore, 1976-

American Journal of Neuroradiology, Baltimore, MD, 1980.

American Journal of Surgery, New York, 1980-

American Quarterly of Roentgenology, Pittsburgh, 1906-1913.

American X-ray Journal, St Louis, 1897-1904.

Anales del Instituto Municipal de Radiologia y Fisioterapia, Buenos Aires, 1934-1941, and continued as

Archivos del Instituto Municipal de Radiologia y Fisioterapía, Buenos Aires, 1941-

Annales de Radiologie, Paris, 1958.

Annales de Roentgenologie et Radiologie: Journal de l'Institut d'état de Radiologie à Pétersbourg, Pétersbourg, 1922-1928, the international edition of Vestnik Rentgenologii i Radiologii, 1920-

Annali di Radiologia e Fisica Medica, Bologna, 1934-

Annals of Otology, Rhinology and Laryngology, St Louis, 1897-

Annals of Surgery, Philadelphia, 1885-

Applied Radiology, Los Angeles, 1976-

Archives of Radiology and Electrotherapy, London, 1915-1923.

Archivio di Radiologia, Naples, 1925-1956.

Archivos Uruguayos de Medicina, Cirugía y Especialidades, Montevideo, Uruguay, 1932-

Atti del Congresso Italiano di Radiologia Medica, Pavia, Italy, 1914-1959, and continued as

Atti del Congresso Nazionale di Radiologia Medicana Nucleare, 1959-

Australasian Radiology, Sydney, 1957-

British Journal of Radiology, London, 1928-

Bulletins et Mémoirs de la Société d'Electroradiologie Médicale de France, Paris, 1938-1939, and continued as

Journal de Radiologie, d'Electrologie et de Médicine Nucléaire, 1957-

Cardiovascular and Interventional Radiology, 1978.

CRC Critical Reviews in Diagnostic Imaging, Cleveland, 1970-

CT The Journal of Computed Tomography, Baltimore, 1976-

Canadian Journal of Radiography, Radiotherapy, and Nuclear Medicine, Ottawa, 1943-

Canadian Association of Radiologists Journal, Montreal, 1973-

Clinical Imaging, New York, 1977-

Clinical Nuclear Medicine, Philadelphia, 1976-

Computerized Tomography, Elmsford, NY, 1977-

Current Opinions in Radiology, Philadelphia, 1989-1992.

Current Problems in Diagnostic Radiology, Chicago, 1971-

Diagnostic Imaging, Basel, 1974-

Fortschritte auf dem Gebiete der Röntgenstrahlen, Hamburg, 1897-1900, and continued as

Fortschritte auf dem Gebiete der Roentgenstrahlen und der Nuklearnmedizin, Stuttgart, 1956-

Gastrointestinal Radiology, New York, 1976-

Health Physics, Elmsford, NY, 1958-

Investigative Radiology, Philadelphia, 1966-

Journal of the American Medical Association, Chicago, 1883-

Journal of Anatomy, Cambridge, England, 1866-

Journal Belge de Radiologie, Brussels, 1907-

Journal of Bone and Joint Surgery, Boston, 1922-

Journal of Computer Assisted Tomography, New York, 1977-

Journal of Digital Imaging, Philadelphia, 1988-

Journal of the Faculty of Radiologists, 1949-1959, and continued as

Clinical Radiology, Edinburgh, 1950-

Journal of Magnetic Resonance Imaging, Oak Brook, IL, 1991-

Journal of Neuroradiology, Paris, 1978-

Journal de Radiologie, Paris, 1914-

Journal of the Röntgen Society, London, 1904-1923.

Journal of Thoracic Surgery, St Louis, 1931-1959, and continued as

Journal of Thoracic and Cardiovascular Surgery, St Louis, 1959-

Journal of Urology, Baltimore, 1917-

Journal of Vascular and Interventional Radiology, Oak Brook, IL, 1990-

Klinische Wochenschrift, Berlin, 1922-

Laryngoscope, St Louis, 1896-

Medical Imaging, Los Angeles, 1976-

Medical Journal of Australia, Sydney, 1914-

Medical Radiography and Photography, Rochester, NY, 1925-

Neuroradiology, New York, 1970-

Pediatric Radiology, New York, 1973-

Physics in Medicine and Biology, New York, 1956-

Presse Médicale, Paris, 1893-1971, and continued as

Nouvelle Presse Médicale, Paris, 1972-

Quaderni di Radiologia, Belluno, Italy, 1937-

Quarterly Bulletin of Sea View Hospital, New York, 1935-

Radiography . . . Society of Radiographers, London, 1935-1987, and continued as

Radiography and Clinical Photography: Eastman Kodak Co., Rochester, NY, 1930-

Radiography Today, London, 1988-

Radiographics, Easton, PA, 1981-

Radiologe (Der), Berlin, 1961-

Radiología . . . órgano oficial de la Sociedad argentina de radiología, Buenos Aires, 1942-

Radiologia Diagnostica, Berlin, 1960-

Radiologia Medica . . . organo della Societá italiana di radiologia medica, Pavia and Milano, 1914-

Radiologic Clinics of North America, Philadelphia, 1963-

Radiologic Technology, Baltimore, 1963-(formerly X-ray Technician, see below)

Radiologica, Berlin and Leipzig, 1937-1939, and continued as

Fundamenta radiologica, Berlin, 1939-

Radiology Management, American Healthcare Radiology Administrations, Sudbury, Mass, 1978.

Radiology: Radiological Society of North America, Easton, Pa, 1923-

Radiology, section 14 of Excerpta Medica, L Paul, MD, subeditor, Amsterdam, C, The Netherlands, International, 1948.

Röntgenpraxis, Leipzig, 1929-

Scritti Italiani di Radiobiologia Medica, Feltre, Italy, 1934-

Seminars in Roentgenology, New York, 1966-

Skeletal Radiology, New York, 1976-

Southern Medical Journal, Birmingham, Ala, 1908-

Surgery, St Louis, 1935-

Surgery, Gynecology and Obstetrics, Chicago, 1905-

Surgical and Radiologic Anatomy, Paris, 1979-

Topics in Magnetic Resonance Imaging, Frederick, Md, 1988-

Urologic Radiology, Philadelphia, 1979-

Vestnik Rentgenologii Radiologii, Moskva, 1921-

X-ray Technician: American Association of Radiological Technicians, St Paul, Minn, 1929-1963, and continued as

Radiologic Technology, Baltimore, 1963-

X-ray Bulletin: Eastman Kodak Co, Rochester, NY, 1925-1930.

Bibliography

Year Book of Radiology: Year Book Medical Publishers, Inc, Chicago, 1932-1974, and continued as
Year Book of Diagnostic Radiology, Chicago, 1975-

TEXTBOOKS ON RADIOGRAPHY

1901 Williams FH: The roentgen in medicine and surgery, New York, 1901, The Macmillan Co.

1903 Albers-Schönberg HE: Die Röntgentechnik, Hamburg, 1903, Gräfe & Sillem.

1917 Christie AC: A manual of x-ray technic, ed 2, Philadelphia, 1917, JB Lippincott.

1919 Albers-Schönberg HE: Die Röntgentechnik, ed 5, Hamburg, 1919, Gräfe & Sillem.

1920 Hirsch IS: The principles and practice of roentgenological technique, New York, 1920, American X-ray Publishing Co.

1924 Robertson JK: X-rays and x-ray apparatus: an elementary course, New York, 1924, The Macmillan Co.

1926 Grashey R: Allegemeine Aufnahmetechnik und Deutung der Röntgenbilder, Berlin, 1926, Urban & Schwarzenberg.

1927 Fürstenau R, Immelman M, and Schutze J: Leitfaden des Röntgenverfahrens, ed 5, Stuttgart, 1927, Ferdinand Enke.
Lilienfeld L: In Mayer EG and Pardes F, editors: Anordnung der normalisierten Röntgenaufnahmen des menschlichen Körpers, ed 4, Berlin, 1927, Urban & Schwarzenberg.

1928 Jerman EC: Modern x-ray technic, St Paul, Minn, 1928, The Bruce Publishing Co.

1931 Jerman EC et al: X-ray studies in advanced radiographic technic, no 1, Chicago, 1931, General Electric X-ray Corp.

1932 Pillsbury HC, editor: United States Army x-ray manual, ed 2, New York, 1932, Paul B Hoeber.

1934 Palazzi S: Roentgenografia, Milano, 1934, Ulrico Hoepli.

1936 Files GW et al: X-ray studies in advanced radiographic technic, no 2, Chicago, 1936, General Electric X-ray Corp.

1938 Procher P and de Juguelier A: Précis de technique radiographique, Paris, 1938, Gauthier-Villars.

1939 Delherm L and Kahn HLM: Les principales positions utilisées en radiographie, ed 2, Paris, 1939, Norbert Maloine.

1940 Bauer K: A B C der Röntgentechnik, Leipzig, 1940, Georg Thieme.
Davies N and Isenburg U: Standard radiographic positions, London, 1940, Bailliere Tindall & Cox.

1941 McNeill C: Roentgen technique, ed 2, Springfield, Ill, 1941, Charles C Thomas Publisher.
Russell JJ: Outline of modern x-ray technic, ed 3, New York, 1941, Picker X-ray Corp.

1942 Letterman General Hospital, San Francisco, Special Service School: Instructions in the use of roentgen rays and roentgen ray apparatus, San Francisco, 1942.

1943 Files GW et al: Medical radiographic technic, Springfield, Ill, 1943, Charles C Thomas Publisher.

Rhinehardt DA: Roentgenographic technique, ed 3, Philadelphia, 1943, Lea & Febiger.
Sante LR: Manual of roentgenological technique, ed 10, Ann Arbor, Mich, 1943, Edwards Brothers, Inc.

1944 Castillo E: Técnica de la exploración roentgenoscópica roentgenográfica, vol 1, Barcelona, Madrid, 1944, Editorial Labora, SA, p 745.
Military roentgenology: war department technical manual, TM 8-280, Washington, DC, 1944.
Naval medical school: fundamentals of x-ray physics and technique. National Naval Medical Center, Bethesda, Md, 1944.

1945 Janker R: Röntgenaufnahmetechnik, II., vol 1, Leipzig, 1945, Johann Ambrosius Barth.

1947 Hardman GL: Guide to positioning, Radiography 13:42-43, 1947.

1948 Davies N and Isenburg V: Standard radiographic positions, ed 2, Baltimore, 1948, Williams & Wilkins.

1950 Porcher P: Précis de technique radiographique, ed. 3, Paris, 1950, Gauthier-Villars.

1955 Castillo E: Técnica de la exploración roentgenoscópica y roentgenográfica, ed 2, Madrid, 1955, Instituto Radiologico Del Dr. Castillo.

1956 LeDoux-LeBard R and Garcia-Calderon J: Technique du radiodiagnostique, ed 2, Paris, 1956, Masson & Cie.
Sante LR: Manual of roentgenological technique, ed 18, Ann Arbor, Mich, 1956, Edwards Brothers Inc.
Schlosshauer B: Röntgenaufnahmetechnik in der Hals-Nasen-Ohren-Heilkunde, Stuttgart, 1956, Georg Thieme.
Schoen H: Medizinische Röntgentechnik, ed 2, Stuttgart, 1956, Georg Thieme.

1962 Schurleff FE: Children's radiographic technic, ed 2, Philadelphia, 1962, Lea & Febiger.

1964 Bloom WL Jr et al: Medical radiographic technic, ed 3, Springfield, Ill, 1964, Charles C Thomas Publisher.
Clark KC: Positioning in radiography, ed 8, New York and London, 1964, Grune & Stratton.
Jacobi CA and Paris DQ: X-ray technology, ed 3, St Louis, 1964, Mosby.
Vennes CH and Watson JC: Patient care and special procedures in x-ray technology, ed 2, St Louis, 1964, Mosby.

1965 Bauer D deF: A textbook of elementary radiography for students and technicians, Springfield, Ill, 1965, Charles C Thomas Publisher.

1968 Meschan I and Farrer-Meschan RMF: Radiographic positioning and related anatomy, Philadelphia, 1968, WB Saunders.

1969 Schmidt JE: Paramedical dictionary: a practical dictionary for the semimedical and ancillary medical professions, Springfield, Ill, 1969, Charles C Thomas Publisher.

1972 Cullinan JE: Illustrated guide to x-ray technics, Philadelphia, 1972, JB Lippincott.

1973 Clark KC: Positioning in radiography, ed 9 (edited and revised by J McInnes), St Louis, 1973, Mosby.

1974 Watson JC: Patient care and special procedures in radiologic technology, St Louis, 1974, Mosby.

1975 Bushong SC: Radiologic science for technologists: physics, biology, and protection, St Louis, 1975, Mosby.
Snopek AM: Fundamentals of special radiographic procedures, New York, 1975, McGraw-Hill Book Co.

1976 Schertel L, et al: Atlas of xeroradiography, Philadelphia, 1976, WB Saunders.
Snell RS and Wyman AC: An atlas of normal radiographic anatomy, Boston, 1976, Little, Brown & Co.
Warrick CK: Anatomy and physiology for radiographers and radiologic technicians, ed 5, 1976.

1977 Jacobi CA: Textbook of radiologic technology, St Louis, 1977, Mosby.
Norman D, Korobkin M and Newton TH, editors: Computed tomography, St Louis, 1977, Mosby.

1978 Abbott MK: Invasive radiologic diagnostic procedures, Philadelphia, 1978, FA Davis.
Birzle H: Radiology of trauma: textbook and atlas, 1978.
Chesney DN and Chesney MO: Care of the patient in diagnostic radiography, Oxford, 1978, Blackwell Scientific Publications.
Hiss SS: Understanding radiography, Springfield, Ill, 1978, Charles C Thomas Publisher.

1979 Bryan GJ: Diagnostic radiography, New York, 1979, Churchill Livingstone Inc.
Thompson TT: Cahoon's formulating x-ray techniques, Durham, NC, 1979, Duke University Press.
Torres LS and Moore CM: Basic medical techniques and patient care for radiologic technologists, Philadelphia, 1979, JB Lippincott.

1980 Ball JL and Moore AD: Essential physics for radiographers, Boston, 1980, Blackwell Scientific Publications.

1981 Chesney DN and Chesney MO: Radiographic imaging, London, England, 1981, Blackwell Scientific Publications.
Ehrlich RA and Givens EM: Patient care in radiography, St Louis, 1981, Mosby.

1982 Bloomfield JA: Pathology for radiographers and allied health professionals, St Louis, 1982, Mosby.

1984 Bushong SC: Radiologic science for radiologic technologists, ed 3, St Louis, 1984, Mosby.
Curry TS, Dowdy JE and Murry RC: Christensen's introduction to the physics of diagnostic radiology, Philadelphia, 1984, Lea & Febiger.

1985 Selman J: The fundamentals of x-ray and radium physics, ed 7, 1985.
Thompson TT: A practical approach to modern imaging equipment, ed 2, 1985.

1986 Ball JL: Essential physics for radiographers, ed 2, Boston, 1986, Blackwell Scientific Publications.

1988   Bushong SC: Radiologic science for technologists: physics, biology, and protection, ed 4, St Louis, 1988, Mosby.

1989   Ball J and Price T, editors: Chesney' radiographic imaging, ed 5, London, England, 1989, Blackwell Scientific Publications.

1991   Rosen RJ and Nosher J: Angiography and interventional radiology, St Louis, 1991, Mosby.

1992   Bushong SC: Radiologic science for technologists: physics, biology, and protection, ed 5, St Louis, 1992, Mosby.

Carlton RR and Adler AM: Principles of radiographic imaging: an art and a science, Albany, NY, 1992, Delmar Publishers.

Finney WF, Carlton RR, and Adler AM: Principles of radiographic imaging-an art and a science-Laboratory Manual/Workbook, Albany, NY, 1992, Delmar Publishers.

Firooznia H et al: MRI and CT of the musculoskeletal system, St Louis, 1992, Mosby.

Hendee WR and Ritenour ER: Medical imaging physics, ed 3, St Louis, 1992, Mosby.

Russ JC: The image processing handbook, Boca Raton, 1992, CRC Press.

1993   Blickman JG: Pediatric radiology-the requisites, St Louis, 1993, Mosby.

Kath K: Pocket reference to radiographic exposure, St Louis, 1993, Mosby.

Malott JC and Fodor J: The art and science of medical radiography, ed 7, St Louis, 1993, Mosby.

TEXTBOOKS ON POSITIONING

1905   Brühl G: Grundriss und Atlas der Ohrenheikunde, ed 2, Munich, 1905, JF Lehmann.

Grashey R: Atlas typischer Röntgenbilder vom normalen Menschen, Munich, 1905, JF Lehmann.

Schüller A: Die Schädelbasis im Röntgenbilde, Hamburg, 1905, Gräfe & Sillem.

1910   Köhler A: Grenzen des Normalen und Anfänge des Pathologischen im Röntgenbilde, Hamburg, 1910, Gräfe & Sillem.

1912   Denker and Brünings: Die Krankheiten des Ohres und der Luftwege, Jena, 1912, Gustav Fischer.

Grashey R: Atlas typischer Röntgenbilder vom normalen Menschen, ed 2, Munich, 1912, JF Lehmann.

1914   Sonnenkalb V: Die Röntgendiagnostik des Hals-, Nasen-, Ohrenärztes, Jena, 1914, Gustav Fischer.

1918   Holzknecht G: Röntgenologie, ed 2, Berlin, 1918, Urban & Schwarzenberg.

Rhese H: Die Kriegsverletzungen und Kriegserkrankungen von Ohr, Nase und Hals, Wiesbaden, 1918, JF Bergmann.

1920   Law FM: Mastoids roentgenologically considered, Ann Roentgenol 1:1920.

Schaeffer JP: The nose, paranasal sinuses, nasolacrimal passages, and olfactory organ in man, Philadelphia, 1920, P Blakiston's Son & Co.

1923   Sonnenkalb V and Beyer E: Die Röntgendiagnostik von Ohr, Nase und Nebenhöhlen, Rachen, Kehlkopf, Mund und Zähne, Leipzig, 1923, Dr. Werner Klinkhardt, Handbuch Röntgendiagnostik, III, no 3.

1924   Schüller A: Röntgen Diagnostik der Erkrankungen des Köpfes, Berlin, 1924, Urban & Schwarzenberg.

1928   Grashey R: Typische Röntgenbilder vom normalen Menshen. In Lehmann's medizinische Atlanten, ed 5, vol 5, 1928.

1929   Assmann H: Clinical roentgendiagnosis of internal diseases (Die klinische Röntgendiagnostik der inneren Erkrankungen), translated by New York Academy of Medicine Library, Bibliographic Department, March 1929.

Köhler A: Roentgenology, New York, 1929, William Wood & Co.

1930   Mayer EG and Eisinger K: Otologische Röntgendiagnostik, Wien, 1930, Julius Springer, pp 283-304.

1933   Busi A: Tecnica e diagnostica radiologica nelle malattie chirurgiche, C1 TET, 1933.

Davis L: Intracranial tumors, Ann Roentgenol, 1933.

Engel S and Schall L: Handbuch der Röntgendiagnostik und Therapie im Kindesalter, Leipzig, 1933, Georg Thieme.

1934   Codman AE: The shoulder, Boston, 1934, Little, Brown & Co.

1936   Harrison BJM: A textbook of roentgenology, Baltimore, 1936, William Wood & Co.

Hartman E: La radiographie en ophthalmologie, Paris, 1936, Masson & Cie.

1939   Ferguson AB: Roentgen diagnosis of the extremities and spine, Ann Roentgenol, 1939.

1940   Pancoast HK, Pendergrass EP and Schaeffer JP: The head and neck in roentgen diagnosis. Springfield, Ill, 1940, Charles C Thomas Publisher.

1941   Golden R, editor: Diagnostic roentgenology, ed 2, New York, 1941, Thomas Nelson & Sons.

1945   Archer VW: The osseous system, St Louis, 1945, Mosby.

Ferguson AB: Roentgen diagnosis of the extremities and spine, New York, 1945, Paul B Hoeber.

1946   Pillmore GU, editor: Clinical radiology, Philadelphia, 1946, FA Davis.

1947   Ross G, editor: Diagnostic roentgenology, ed 3, New York, 1947, Thomas Nelson & Sons.

1948   Young BR: The skull, sinuses, and mastoids: a handbook of roentgen diagnosis, St Louis, 1948, Mosby.

1949   Merrill V: Atlas of roentgenographic positions, St Louis, 1949, Mosby.

1950   Chaumet G: Traité de radiodiagnostic, ed 2, Paris, 1950, Vigot Frères.

Chaussé C: Premiers elements de radiootologie, Paris, 1950, Masson & Cie.

1955   Bateman JE: The shoulder and environs, St Louis, 1955, Mosby.

1956   Pendergrass EP, Schaeffer JP and Hodes PJ: The head and neck in roentgen diagnosis, ed 2, Springfield, Ill, 1956, Charles C Thomas Publisher.

1957   Gamble FO: Applied foot roentgenology, Baltimore, 1957, Williams & Wilkins.

1959   Merrill V: Atlas of roentgenographic positions, ed 2, St Louis, 1959, Mosby.

1961   Abrams H, editor: Angiography, Boston, 1961, Little Brown & Co.

1962   Bull JW et al: Atlas of myelography, New York, 1962, Grune & Stratton.

Darling DB: Radiography of infants and children, Springfield, Ill, 1962, Charles C Thomas Publisher.

1963   Stafne EC: Oral roentgenographic diagnosis including an appendix on roentgenographic technic, ed 2, Philadelphia, 1963, WB Saunders Co.

1964   Egan RL: Mammography, Springfield, Ill, 1964, Charles C Thomas Publisher.

Etter LE et al: Roentgenography and roentgenology of the middle ear and mastoid process, Springfield, Ill, 1964, Charles C Thomas Publisher.

Taveras JM and Wood EH: Diagnostic neuroradiology, Baltimore, 1964, Williams & Wilkins.

1967   Merrill V: Atlas of roentgenographic positions, ed 3, St Louis, 1967, Mosby.

1972   Saxton HM and Strickland B: Practical procedures in diagnostic radiology, New York, 1972, Grune & Stratton.

1973   Greenfield GB: A manual of radiographic positioning, 1973.

1975   Merrill V: Atlas of roetgenographic positions and standard radiologic procedures, ed 4, St Louis, 1975, Mosby.

1977   Gyll C: A handbook of paediatric radiography, London, England, 1977, Blackwell Scientific Publications.

1978   Meschan I: Radiologic positioning and related anatomy, ed 2, Philadelphia, 1978, WB Saunders.

1979   Griffiths HJ and Sarno RC: Contemporary radiology, Philadelphia, 1979, WB Saunders.

Kreel L and Steiner RE, editors: Medical imaging, St Louis, 1979, Mosby.

Lodge T and Steiner RE, editors: Recent advances in radiology and medical imaging, New York, 1979, Churchill Livingstone.

1982   Ballinger PW: Merrill's atlas of radiographic positions and radiologic procedures, ed 5, St Louis, 1982, Mosby.

Bontrager KL and Anthony BT: Textbook of radiographic positioning and related anatomy, Denver, 1982, Multi-Media Publishing.

Tortorici MR: Fundamentals of angiography, St Louis, 1982, Mosby.

Wick L: Atlas of radiographic anatomy, Baltimore, 1982, Urban & Schwarzenberg.

1983   Marlow JE: Surgical radiography, Baltimore, 1983, University Park Press.

Paris DQ: Craniographic positioning with comparison studies, Philadelphia, 1983, FA Davis.

1984   Cahill DR and Orland MJ: Atlas of human cross sectional anatomy, Philadelphia, 1984, Lea & Febiger.

1986 Ballinger PW: Merrill's atlas of radiographic positions and radiologic procedures, ed 6, St Louis, 1986, Mosby.

Bell GA and Finlay DBL: Basic radiographic positioning and anatomy, London, England, 1986, Bailliere Tindall.

Swallow RA and Naylor E, editors: Clark's positioning in radiography, ed 11, Rockville, Md, 1986, Aspen Publishers.

1987 Bontrager KA and Anthony BT: Textbook of radiographic positioning and related anatomy, ed 2, St Louis, 1987, Mosby.

Wicke L: Atlas of radiologic anatomy, ed 4, Baltimore, 1987, Urban & Schwarzenberg.

1988 Jaeger SA: Atlas of radiographic positioning: normal anatomy and developmental variants, Norwalk, CN, 1988, Appleton & Lange.

1989 Ballinger PW: Pocket guide to radiography, St Louis, 1989, Mosby.

Eisenberg RL, Dennis CA, and May CR: Radiographic positioning, Boston, 1989, Little, Brown & Co.

1991 Ballinger PW: Merrill's atlas of radiographic positions and radiologic procedures, ed 7, St Louis, 1991, Mosby.

1992 Ballinger PW: Pocket guide to radiography, ed 2, St Louis, 1992, Mosby.

Snopek AM: Fundamentals of special radiographic procedures, ed 3, Philadelphia, 1992, WB Saunders.

1993 Bontrager KA: Textbook of radiographic positioning and related anatomy, ed 3, St Louis, 1993, Mosby.

Hagler MJ: The pocket rad tech, Philadelphia, 1993, WB Saunders.

NURSING PROCEDURES AND PATIENT CARE

For bibliographic citations before 1964, please see the fifth edition of this atlas. For citations from 1964 through 1974, see the sixth or seventh edition.

1976 Laws PW: How patients view the efficient use of diagnostic radiology, Radiol Technol 47:245-249, 1976.

Sweeney RJ: System designed to improve the communication process between patient and technologist, Radiol Technol 47:295-297, 1976.

1978 Bell ME: Patient-radiologic technologist interpersonal relationship and how it can be improved, Radiol Technol 50:41-44, 1978.

Chesney DN and Chesney MO: Care of the patient in diagnostic radiography, Oxford, 1978, Blackwell Scientific Publications.

Fengler K: The patient-care gap, Radiol Technol 49:599-600, 1978.

Neuhaus B: Our professional image: as we are seen, Radiol Technol 49:485-489, 1978.

Wedel CS: Patient communication: the final step towards professionalism, Radiol Technol 50:27-31, 1978.

Wilson-Barnett J: Patients' responses to barium x-ray studies, Br Med J 1:1324, 1978.

1979 Goldin GJ: Psychodynamic components in the role of the radiologic technologist, Radiol Technol 51:193-197, 1979.

Quinn BC: Improving patient cooperation, Radiol Technol 51:68-71, 1979.

Torres LS and Moore CM: Basic medical techniques and patient care for radiologic technologists, Philadelphia, 1979, JB Lippincott.

1980 Wilkinson DS: Patients, paper, and people, Radiography 46:76-78, 1980.

1981 Hunt L: Employing the success vector in geriatric radiology, Radiol Technol 53:279-280, 1981.

Warner SL: Code of ethics: professional and legal implications, Radiol Technol 52:485-494, 1981.

1982 Jost RG et al: A computer system to monitor radiology department activity: a management tool to improve patient care, Radiology 145:347-350, 1982.

1983 Adams PE: Patient care and the development of the clinical assistant in interventional radiology, Radiol Technol 54:223-225, 1983.

Bryan GJ: Caring for elderly patients, Radiography 49:169-172, 1983.

Dowd SB: Radiographers' knowledge of aging, Radiol Technol 54:192-196, 1983.

Edwards MJ: Effective inservice education in radiography, Radiol Technol 54:206-214, 1983.

Whittaker LR: More active participation by radiographers in the radiography of trauma, Radiography 49:125-129, 1983.

Worrell J: Radiologic examination requisition procedures: a study of their effectiveness in a community hospital, South Med J 76:216-217, 1983.

1988 Duquette AM and Tieuli J: Systematic monitoring: review of nursing care in a radiology department, J Nurs Qual Assur 2:59-67, 1988.

Leads from the MMWR. Update: universal precautions for prevention of transmission of human immunodeficiency virus, hepatitis B virus, and other bloodborne pathogens in health-care settings, JAMA 260:462-465, 1988.

Loth TS and Jones DE: Extravasations of radiographic contrast material in the upper extremity, J Hand Surg Am 13:395-398, 1988.

1989 AIDS: problem solving in infection control. Universal precautions: Part 2, Am J Infect Control 17:39-41, 1989.

Bence L: Disease-specific isolation: the alternate method, Nurs Manage 20:16-18, 1989.

Borgatta L, Fisher M and Robbins N: Hand protection and protection from hands: hand-washing, germicides and gloves, Women Health 15:77-92, 1989.

Guidelines for prevention of transmission of human immunodeficiency virus and hepatitis B virus to health-care and public-safety workers, MMWR 38 (Suppl) 6:1-37, 1989.

Kelly WH: Radiographic asepsis in endodontic practice, Gen Dent 37:302-303, 1989.

Stein RE: Strategies for dealing with AIDS disputes in the workplace, Radiol Technol 61:49-56, 1989.

1990 Adams MP: Attitudes of selected radiographers toward AIDS, Radiol Technol 62:122-129, 1990.

Adler AM: High technology: miracle or malady for patient care, Radiol Technol 61:478-481, 1990.

Cooperstein LA et al: The effect of clinical history on chest radiograph interpretations in a PACS environment, Invest Radiol 25:670-674, 1990.

Field MA: Testing for AIDS: uses and abuses, Am J Law Med 16:33-106, 1990.

Graham M: Frequency and duration of handwashing in an intensive care unit, Am J Infect Control 18:77-81, 1990.

Hadler SC: Hepatitis B virus infection and health care workers, Vaccine 8 (Suppl): S24-S28, 1990.

Lowdermilk DL: Nursing care update: internal radiation therapy, NAACOGS Clin Issu Perinat Women's Health Nurs 1:532-540, 1990.

Morrison R: Interrelationship of the mind, body and emotions in the cancer fight, Radiol Technol 62:28-31, 1990.

1991 Bates BF and Rowe JE: Radiography of patients who don't speak English, Radiol Technol 63:110-112, 1991.

Dowd SB: AIDS, the technologist and universal precautions, Radiol Technol 62:280-283, 1991.

Gerberding JL: Does knowledge of human immunodeficiency virus infection decrease the frequency of occupational exposure to blood? Am J Med 91:308S-311S, 1991.

Goldberg MA et al: Importance of daily rounds by the radiologist after interventional procedures of the abdomen and chest, Radiology 180:767-770, 1991.

Golden DG: Medical ethics courses for student technologists, Radiol Technol 62:452-457, 1991.

Johns CM and Sumkin JH: US-guided venipuncture for venography in the edematous leg, Radiology 180:573, 1991.

Kaczmarek RG et al: Glove use by health care workers: results of a tristate investigation, Am J Infect Control 19:228-232, 1991.

Kelly TJ: Mechanics and treatment of vasovagal syncope, Radiol Technol 62:216-218, 1991.

Linnemann CC Jr et al: Effect of educational programs, rigid sharps containers, and universal precautions on reported needlestick injuries in healthcare workers, Infect Control Hosp Epidemiol 12:214-219, 1991.

Mitchell NJ and Hunt S: Surgical face masks in modern operating rooms—a costly and unnecessary ritual? J Hosp Infect 18:239-242, 1991.

Wall SD, Olcott EW and Gerberding JL: AIDS risk and risk reduction in the radiology department, AJR 157:911-917, 1991.

1992 Barlow R and Handelman E: OSHA's final bloodborne pathogens standard. Part I. AAOHN J 40:562-567, 1992.

Coates D: Disinfectants and spills of body fluids, Nurs RSA 7:25-27, 1992.

Curnes JT: Modification of the standard myelography tray for universal precautions: technical note, Neurosurgery 31:158-159, 1992.

DeFilippo VC, Bowen RW and Ingbar DH: A universal precautions monitoring system adaptable to any health care department, Am J Infect Control 20:159-163, 1992.

Dixon C et al: Another view to blood and body substance precaution: 1988-91, Can J Infect Control 7:107-110, 1992.

Dowd SB: The radiographer's role: part scientist, part humanist, Radiol Technol 63:240-243, 1992.

Helget VM et al: Advances in hospital infection control programs, Nebr Med J 77:105-108, 1992.

Hopper KD et al: Patients' attitudes toward informed consent for intravenous contrast media, Invest Radiol 27:362-366, 1992.

Hudson T, Eubanks P and Lumsdon K: HIV-positive health care workers pose legal, safety challenges for hospitals, Hospitals 66:24-30, 32, 1992.

Hull JE, Hunter CS and Luiken GA: The Groshong catheter: initial experience and early results of imaging-guided placement, Radiology 185:803-807, 1992.

Krain LS: Some thoughts about the importance of x-ray exposure histories for patients, Med Hypotheses 37:225-231, 1992.

Piazza DL: HIV testing: an ethical analysis, Insight 17:17-19, 1992.

Thompson G: Current issues related to the transmission of blood-borne pathogens, Can J Infect Control 7:17-18, 1992.

1993 Greenbaum DM: History, general overview, and protection of health care workers, Crit Care Clin 9:1-11, 1993.

OSHA's bloodborne pathogens standard: analysis and recommendations, Health Devices 22:35-92, 1993.

Roup BJ: OSHA's new standard: exposure to bloodborne pathogens, AAOHN 41:136-142, 1993.

Tyrrell PN, McHugo JM and Hale M: Patients' perception of the hysterosalpingogram: the initial stages of the audit cycle, Br J Radiol 66:103-107, 1993.

Wicher CP: AIDS & HIV: the dilemma of the health care worker, J Neurosci Nurs 25:118-124, 1993.

RADIATION PROTECTION

For bibliographic citations before 1964, please see the fifth edition of this atlas. For citations from 1964 through 1974, see the sixth or seventh edition.

1975 Purdy JA et al: Gonadal shield, Radiology 117:226, 1975.

Ryer FH: The new health and safety act as it relates to occupational radiation exposure, Health Phys 29:207-212, 1975.

1976 Douglas SJ: Protection of patients against the harmful effects of ionizing radiation, Ir Med J 69:475-476, 1976.

Hinds LM: Reducing radiation exposure to patient and operator, J Natl Med Assoc 68:115-116, 152, 1976.

Johnson NE: Radiation protective shield for use during arthrography, Radiol Technol 48:35-38, 1976.

1977 Bergström K, Jorulf H and Löfroth PO: Eye lens protection for radiological personnel, Radiology 124:839-840, 1977.

Gross GP et al: Radiation protection requirements for a whole-body CT scanner, Radiology 122:825-826, 1977.

Seeram E: Protecting patients from radiation, Dimens Health Serv 54:40, 42, 1977.

Ziehm DJ: Guidelines for the diagnostic x-ray examination of fertile women, Ariz Med 34:762-763, 1977.

Bryant TH and Julian WL: Reduction of radiation dose to patients in xeroradiography, Br J Radiol 51:974-980, 1978.

1978 Hemmingsson A and Löfroth PO: Radiation protection in fluoroscopy with an image intensifier, Acta Radiol 19:1007-1013, 1978.

ICRU submits new radiation unit system and reports, Radiol Technol 50:50-51, 1978.

Littleton JT, Durizch ML and Perry N: Radiation protection of the lens for patients and users, Radiology 129:795-798, 1978.

1979 Manny EF, Brown RF and Shaver JW: Gonad shielding in diagnostic radiology: recommendation of the FDA and ACR, Postgrad Med 65:207-211, 1979.

Noz ME and Maguire GQ: Radiation protection in the radiologic and health sciences, Philadelphia, 1979, Lea & Febiger.

1980 Allison JD and Teeslink CR: A special procedures screen, Radiology 136:233-234, 1980.

Beck G: What's next? Rev Interam Radiol 5:93-94, 1980.

Bistline RW, Yoder RE and Hunt DC: Radiation: what do we know about it? Colo Med 77:58-59, 1980.

Caprio ML, Jr: The pregnant x-ray technologist—providing adequate radiation safety for the fetus, Radiol Technol 52:161-163, 1980.

Carlton R: Establishing a total quality assurance program in diagnostic radiology, Radiol Technol 52:23-38, 1980.

Diagnostic radiography: what are the risks? Drug Ther Bull 18:49-51, 1980.

Gloag D: Radiation exposure and the protection of the community, Br Med J 281:1545-1548, 1980.

Leonidas JC: Avoiding unnecessary x-ray exposure in children, Compr Ther 6:46-54, 1980.

Martin EC and Olson A: Radiation exposure to the pediatric patient from cardiac catheterization and angiocardiography, Br J Radiol 53:100-106, 1980.

Moore WE, Ferguson G and Rohrmann C: Physical factors determining the utility of radiation safety glasses, Med Phys 7:8-12, 1980.

Pochin EE: Risk assessment for radiation protection purposes, At Energy Rev 18:779-802, 1980.

Pritchard C: Radiation protection of personnel during pediatric radiodiagnostic examination, Radiography 46:165-169, 1980.

Radiation safety program for diagnostic radiology departments, Radiol Technol 52:321-327, 1980.

1981 Bednarek DR et al: A protocol for exposure limitation in radiography, Radiol Technol 53:229-234, 1981.

DeSmet AA, Fritz SL and Asher MA: A method for minimizing the radiation exposure from scoliosis radiographs, J Bone Joint Surg 63-A:156-161, 1981.

Dunster HJ: Some common questions on ICRP recommendations, Radiography 47:205-206, 1981.

Harrison RM: Central-axis depth-dose data for diagnostic radiology, Phys Med Biol 26:657-670, 1981.

Linton OW: Federal radiation initiatives wane in Reagan administration, AJR 137:1278-1283, 1981.

Oudiz A, Lombard J and Fagnani F: A multi-attribute approach to the rationalization of radiological protection, Health Phys 40:783-799, 1981.

Photochromic sunglasses for radiation protection of the eyes, Radiol Technol 52:448-449, 1981.

Sinclair WK: Effects of low level radiation and comparative risk, Radiology 138:1-9, 1981.

Sinclair WK: Radiation protection: the NCRP guidelines and some considerations for the future, Yale J Biol Med 54:471-484, 1981.

The radiation hazard in hospitals—a reappraisal, J Can Assoc Radiol 32:77-78, 1981.

1982 Anderson PE Jr, Anderson PE and Van-der-Kooy P: Dose reduction in radiography of the spine in scoliosis, Acta Radiol 23:251-253, 1982.

Franz KH: Radiation protection in radiologic technology: apathy versus active involvement, Radiol Technol 54(2)119-122, 1982.

Benson JM: Radiation safety, J Fam Pract 15:435-439, 1982.

Gertz EW et al: Improved radiation protection for physicians performing cardiac catheterization, Am J Cardiol 50:1283-1286, 1982.

Maillie HD, Segal A and Lemkin J: Effect of patient size on doses received by patients in diagnostic radiology, Health Phys 42:665-670, 1982.

Robinson T, Becker JA and Olson AP: Clinical comparison of high-speed rare-earth screen and par-speed screen for diagnostic efficacy and radiation dosage, Radiology 145:214-216, 1982.

Rudin S, Bednarek DR and Wong R: Design of rotating aperture cones for radiographic scatter reduction, Med Phys 9:385-393, 1982.

White SC: Radiation safety for children, Int Dent J 32:259-264, 1982.

1983 Bednarek DR et al: Reduction of fluoroscopic exposure for the air-contrast barium enema, Br J Radiol 56:823-828, 1983.

Drummond D et al: Radiation hazards in scoliosis management, Spine 8:741-748, 1983.

Fitzgerald RH, Reines HD and Wise J: Diagnostic radiation exposure in trauma patients, South Med J 76:1511-1514, 1983.

Frank ED and Kuntz JI: A simple method of protecting the breasts during upright lateral radiography for spine deformities, Radiol Technol 55(1)532-535, 1983.

Frank ED et al: Use of the posteroanterior projection: a method of reducing x-ray exposure to specific radiosensitive organs, Radiol Technol 54:343-347, 1983.

Gray JE, Hoffman AD and Peterson HA: Reduction of radiation exposure during radiography for scoliosis, J Bone Joint Surg 65-A:5-12, 1983.

Gray JE, Stears JG and Frank ED: Shaped, lead-loaded acrylic filters for patient exposure reduction and image-quality improvement, Radiology 146:825-828, 1983.

Harrison RM et al: A survey of radiation doses to patients in five common diagnostic examinations, Br J Radiol 56:383-395, 1983.

Malott JC and Fodor J III: An effective fluoroscopic shield for angiographic equipment, Radiol Technol 54:216-219, 1983.

McGuire EL, Baker ML and Vandergrift JF: Evaluation of radiation exposures to personnel in fluoroscopic x-ray facilities, Health Phys 45:975-980, 1983.

Moilanen A, Kokko ML and Pitkanen M: Gonadal dose reduction in lumbar spine radiography, Skeletal Radiol 9:153-156, 1983.

Thomas SR et al: Characteristics of extrafocal radiation and its potential significance in pediatric radiology, Radiology 146:793-799, 1983.

Wagner HN: Radiation: the risks and the benefits, AJR 140:595-603, 1983.

Weatherburn GC: Reducing radiation doses to the breast, thyroid and gonads during diagnostic radiography, Radiography 49:151-156, 1983.

1984 Proposed recommended practices, Radiation safety in the operating room, AORN 40:881-886, 1984.

Barry TP: Radiation exposure to an orthopedic surgeon, Clin Orthop 182:160-164, 1984.

Bradley WG, Opel W and Kassabian JP: Magnetic resonance installation: siting and economic considerations, Radiology 151:719-721, 1984.

Chakeres DW and Wiatrowski W: Cerebral angiography: a device to reduce exposure to the eye lens, Radiology 152:534-535, 1984.

Cohen G et al: Dose efficiency of screen-film systems used in pediatric radiography, Radiology 152:187-193, 1984.

Glaze S, LeBlanc AD and Bushong SC: Defects in new protective aprons, Radiology 152:217-218, 1984.

Jankowski J: Organ doses in diagnostic x-ray procedures, Health Phys 46:228-234, 1984.

Judkins MP: Guidelines for radiation protection in the cardiac catheterization laboratory, Cathet Cardiovasc Diagn 10:87-92, 1984.

Kelsey CA, Lane RG and Somers JW: Radiation exposure during fluoroscopically controlled percutaneous transhepatic examinations, J Urol 132:1254-1255, 1984.

Miotto D, Feltrin G and Calamosca M: A radiation protection device for use during percutaneous transhepatic examinations, Radiology 151:799-799, 1984.

Servomaa A, Toivonen M and Kiuru A: Mailed TL dosimeters for monitoring the output from diagnostic x-ray equipment, Med Phys 11:75-77, 1984.

Smathers RL et al: Radiation dose reduction in the neonatal intensive care unit: comparison of three gadolinium oxysulfide screen-film combinations, Invest Radiol 19:578-582, 1984.

Spiers FW: 40 years of development in radiation protection, Phys Med Biol 29:145-151, 1984.

Witrak BJ and Sprawls P: Maternity lead apron, Radiology 150:597, 1984.

1985 Miller DL, Vucich JJ and Cope C: A flexible shield to protect personnel during interventional procedures, Radiology 155: 825-825, 1985.

Miller SW and Castronovo FP Jr: Radiation exposure and protection in cardiac catheterization laboratories, Am J Cardiol 55:171-176, 1985.

1986 Butler PF et al: Simple methods to reduce patient exposure during scoliosis radiography, Radiol Technol 57:411-417, 1986.

Campbell JM, Kuntzler CM, and Nikesch W: Exposure reduction using yttrium filters in a cardiac catheterization unit, Cathet Cardiovasc Diagn 12:202-204, 1986.

Cupstid GB: Breast protection during intravenous pyelography, Radiol Technol 57:347-348, 1986.

Doust C: Personal monitoring period for radiographers, Radiography 52:109-112, 1986.

Gerard P and Lefkovitz Z: The optical push device: an aid to the angiographer, Cardiovasc Intervent Radiol 9:111-112, 1986.

Hufton AP and Russell JG: The use of carbon fibre material in table tops, cassette fronts and grid covers: magnitude of possible reduction, Br J Radiol 59:157-163, 1986.

McGuire EL and Dickson PA: Exposure and organ dose estimation in diagnostic radiology, Med Phys 13:913-916, 1986.

Tyndall DA and Washburn DB: Rare-earth filters in panoramic radiography: a means of reducing exposure, Dentomaxillofac Radiol 15:19-25, 1986.

Young AT et al: Surface shield: device to reduce personnel radiation exposure, Radiology 159:801-803, 1986.

1987 Cousin AJ et al: The case for radioprotective eyewear/facewear: practical implications and suggestions, Invest Radiol 22:688-692, 1987.

Herman MW, Mak HK and Lachman RS: Radiation exposure reduction by use of Kevlar cassettes in the neonatal nursery, AJR 148:969-972, 1987.

Lemley AA, Hedl JJ and Griffin EE: A study of radiation safety education practices in acute care Texas hospitals, Radiol Technol 58:323-331, 1987.

Thind KS: Extremity dose: its definition, standards and regulatory limits, radiobiological significance, measurement and practical considerations, Health Phys 52:695-705, 1987.

Tyndall DA and Bedsole SM: Exposure reduction and image quality for pantomographic radiography, Radiol Technol 59:51-53, 1987.

Wesenberg RL et al: Ultra-low-dose routine pediatric radiography utilizing a rare-earth, J Can Assoc Radiol 38:158-164, 1987.

Yoshizumi TT et al: Radiation safety and protection of neonates in radiological examinations, Radiol Technol 58:405-408, 1987.

1988 Britton CA and Wholey MH: Radiation exposure of personnel during digital subtraction angiography, Cardiovasc Intervent Radiol 11:108-110, 1988.

Burton EM et al: Evaluation of a low-dose neonatal chest radiographic system, AJR 151:999-1002, 1988.

Chintapalli K, Wentworth W and Wilson CR: Simple radiation protection device for CT, AJR 150:199-200, 1988.

Davis JP: The future of the de minimis concept, Health Phys 55:379-382, 1988.

Elder JA et al: Nonionizing radiation protection. Radiofrequency radiation, WHO Reg Publ Eur Ser 25:117-173, 1988.

Faulkner K and Harrison RM: Estimation of effective dose equivalent to staff in diagnostic radiology, Phys Med Biol 33:83-91, 1988.

Fearon T et al: Scoliosis examinations: organ dose and image quality with rare-earth screen-film systems, AJR 150:359-362, 1988.

Green P: The response of the International Commission on Radiological Protection to calls for a reduction in the dose limits for radiation workers and members of the public, Int J Radiat Biol Relat Stud Phys Chem Med 53:679-682, 1988.

Gyll C: Gonad protection for the pediatric patient, Radiography 54:9-11, 1988.

Hahn FF et al: Future development of biological understanding of radiation protection: implications of nonstochastic effects, Health Phys 55:303-313, 1988.

Healy JW: H.M. Parker lecture. Radiation protection standards: a historical perspective, Health Phys 55:125-130, 1988.

Kennedy WE Jr and Corley JP: Application of the ICRP recommendations to revised secondary radiation protection standards, Health Phys 55:427-431, 1988.

Kogutt MS, Jones JP and Perkins DD: Low-dose digital computed radiography in pediatric chest imaging, AJR 151:775-779, 1988.

Kohn ML, Gooch AW Jr and Keller WS: Filters for radiation reduction: a comparison, Radiology 167:255-257, 1988.

Lindell B: Radiation protection—a look to the future: ICRP perceptions, Health Phys 55:145-147, 1988.

Manninen H et al: Reduction of radiation dose and imaging costs in scoliosis radiography. Application of large-screen image intensifier photofluorography, Spine 13:409-412, 1988.

Nickoloff EL and Donnelly EM: Use of gypsum drywall as shielding material for mammography, Health Phys 54:465-468, 1988.

Paretzke HG: The impact of the Chernobyl accident on radiation protection, Health Phys 55:139-143, 1988.

Russell JG and Hufton AP: Lead thickness in shielding in the protection of radiodiagnostic staff, Br J Radiol 61:128-132, 1988.

Shrimpton PC, Jones DG and Wall BF: The influence of tube filtration and potential on patient dose during x-ray examinations, Phys Med Biol 33:1205-1212, 1988.

Sinclair WK: Trends in radiation protection—a view from the national Council on Radiation Protection and Measurements (NCRP), Health Phys 55:149-157, 1988.

Stears JG, Gray JG and Frank ED: The variable filter dial, Radiol Technol 59:245-246, 1988.

Taylor LS: Will radiation control be by reason or regulation? Health Phys 55:133-138, 1988.

Underhill TE et al: Radiobiologic risk estimation from dental radiology. Part I. Absorbed doses to critical organs, Oral Surg Oral Med Oral Pathol 66:111-120, 1988.

Upton AC: Evolving perspectives on the concept of dose in radiobiology and radiation protection, Health Phys 55:605-614, 1988.

Vallario EJ: Regulatory perceptions of the future: a view from the United States, Health Phys 55:385-389, 1988.

1989 Brodsky A and Kathren RL: Historical development of radiation safety practices in radiology, Radiographics 9:1267-1275, 1989.

Faulkner K, Barry JL and Smalley P: Radiation dose to neonates on a Special Care Baby Unit, Br J Radiol 62:230-233, 1989.

Gibbs SJ: Influence of organs in the ICRP's remainder on effective dose equivalent computed for diagnostic radiation exposures, Health Phys 56:515-520, 1989.

Huda W et al: Radiation doses and detriment from chest x-ray examinations, Phys Med Biol 34:1477-1492, 1989.

Janssen JH and Wellens HJ: What do medical students know about in-hospital radiation hazards? Angiology 40:36-38, 1989.

Kelsey CA et al: Scattered radiation levels from a portable fluoroscopic/angiographic unit, Health Phys 57:817-818, 1989.

Mountford PJ and Coakley AJ: Radioactive patients, BMJ 298:1538-1539, 1989.

Riley SA: Radiation exposure from fluoroscopy during orthopedic surgical procedures, Clin Orthop 257-260, 1989.

Singer CM et al: Exposure of emergency medicine personnel to ionizing radiation during cervical spine radiography, Ann Emerg Med 18:822-825, 1989.

Walker JS: The controversy over radiation safety. A historical overview, JAMA 262:664-668, 1989.

1990 Bagley DH and Cubler-Goodman A: Radiation exposure during ureteroscopy, J Urol 144:1356-1358, 1990.

Fabrikant JI: Public health regulation and control of population exposures to ionizing radiation, Prev Med 19:705-722, 1990.

Fry RJ and Fry SA: Health effects of ionizing radiation, Med Clin North Am 74:475-488, 1990.

Harding LK et al: The radiation dose to accompanying nurses, relatives and other patients in a nuclear medicine department waiting room, Nucl Med Commun 11:17-22, 1990.

Hendee WR and Edwards FM: Trends in radiation protection of medical workers, Health Phys 58:251-257, 1990.

Kapa SF and Platin E: Exposure reduction in panoramic radiography, Radiol Technol 62:130-133, 1990.

Kling TF Jr et al: Digital radiography can reduce scoliosis x-ray exposure, Spine 15:880-885, 1990.

Kwong LM et al: Shielding of the patient's gonads during intramedullary interlocking femoral nailing, J Bone Joint Surg Am 72:1523-1526, 1990.

Marugg S et al: Additive filtering, Br J Radiol 63:800-801, 1990.

Radiation protection: sense or nonsense? Br J Radiol 63:373-376, 1990.

Rothenberg LN: AAPM tutorial. Patient dose in mammography, Radiographics 10:739-746, 1990.

Rueter FG et al: Average radiation exposure values for three diagnostic radiographic examinations, Radiology 177:341-345, 1990.

Saini T, Manoharan V and al-Agil IA: Radiation doses to the gonadal area in dental radiography, Odonto-Stomatologie Tropicale 13:67-71, 1990.

Wells PN: Technologic advances in radiation protection and other diagnostic topics, Curr Opin Radiol 2:559-564, 1990.

1991 1990 Recommendations of the International Commission on Radiological Protection, Ann ICRP 21:1-201, 1991.

Batchelor S et al: Radiation dose to the hands in nuclear medicine, Nucl Med Commun 12:439-444, 1991.

Edwards M: development of radiation protection standards, Radiographics 11:699-712, 1991.

Jones LW: Port film dosage in radiation therapy, Radiol Technol 62:362-368, 1991.

Kazuo K et al: Organ doses received by atomic bomb survivors during radiological examinations at the Radiation Effects Research Foundation, Br J Radiol 64:720-727, 1991.

Kebart RC and James CD: Benefits of increasing focal film distance, Radiol Technol 62:434-442, 1991.

Nowak B and Jankowski J: Occupational exposure in operational radiology, Pol J Occup Med 4:169-174, 1991.

Oftedal P: Biological low-dose radiation effects, Mutat Res 258:191-205, 1991.

Ruiz MJ et al: Measurement of radiation doses in the most frequent simple examinations in paediatric radiology and its dependence on patient age, Br J Radiol 64:929-933, 1991.

Thierens H et al: Evaluation of the use of a niobium filter for patient dose reduction in chest radiography, Br J Radiol 64:334-340, 1991.

Vehmas T: Finger doses during interventional radiology: the value of flexible protective gloves, ROFO Fortschr Geb Rontgenstr Nuklearmed 154:555-559, 1991.

Velders XL, van Aken J and van der Stelt PF: Absorbed dose to organs in the head and neck from bitewing radiography, Dentomaxillofac Radiol 20:161-165, 1991.

Vijayakumar S et al: Estimation of doses to heart, coronary arteries, and spinal cord in mediastinal irradiation for Hodgkin's disease, Med Dosim 16:237-241, 1991.

Wu JR et al: Radiation exposure of pediatric patients and physicians during cardiac catheterization and balloon pulmonary valvuloplasty, Am J Cardiol 68:221-225, 1991.

Yaffe MJ et al: Composite materials for x-ray protection, Health Phys 60:661-664, 1991.

1992 Broadbent MV and Hubbard LB: Science and perception of radiation risk, Radiographics 12:381-392, 1992.

Burns CB et al: Niobium/aluminum filters reduce patient exposure, Radiol Technol 63:170-175, 1992.

Geleijns J et al: AMBER and conventional chest radiography: comparison of radiation dose and image quality, Radiology 185:719-723, 1992.

Johansson L et al: Effective dose from radiopharmaceuticals, Eur J Nucl Med 19:933-938, 1992.

Kenny N and Hill J: Gonad protection in young orthopaedic patients, BMJ 304:1411-1413, 1992.

Krain LS: Some thoughts about the importance of x-ray exposure histories for patients, Med Hypotheses 37:225-231, 1992.

Mand FF: Radiation safety for beginners, J Nucl Med 33:167-169, 1992.

Marx MV, Niklason L and Mauger EA: Occupational radiation exposure to interventional radiologists: a prospective study, J Vasc Interv Radiol 3:597-606, 1992.

Moore B et al: The relationship between back pain and lead apron use in radiologists, AJR 158:191-193, 1992.

Rudin S and Bednarek DR: Minimizing radiation dose to patient and staff during fluoroscopic, nasoenteral tube insertions, Br J Radiol 65:162-166, 1992.

Silini G: Ethical issues in radiation protection—the 1992 Sievert Lecture, Health Phys 63:139-148, 1992.

Zoeller G et al: Digital radiography in urologic imaging: radiation dose reduction on urethrocystography, Urol Radiol 14:56-58, 1992.

1993 Chotas HG et al: Digital chest radiography with photostimulable storage phosphors: signal-to-noise ratio as a function of kilovoltage with matched exposure risk, Radiology 186:395-398, 1993.

Mayo JR, Jackson SA and Muller NL: High-resolution CT of the chest: radiation dose, AJR 160:479-481, 1993.

Murphy PH, Wu Y and Glaze SA: Attenuation properties of lead composite aprons, Radiology 186:269-272, 1993.

Sanders R et al: Exposure of the orthopaedic surgeon to radiation, J Bone Joint Surg Am 75:326-330, 1993.

ANATOMY

For bibliographic citations before 1964, please see the fifth edition of this atlas.

1975 McInnes J: Radiographic anatomy, New York, 1975, Appleton-Century-Crofts.

1976 Snell RS and Wyman AC: An atlas of normal radiographic anatomy, Boston, 1976, Little Brown & Co.

1979 Wicke L: Atlas of radiologic anatomy, Baltimore, 1979, Urban & Schwarzenberg.

1980 Swinburne K: Medical education and the x-ray department, J R Coll Physicians Lond 14:245-246, 1980.

Weir J and Abrahams P: X-ray anatomy, Nurs Times 76:1-7, 1980.

1982 Bottomlet PA and Edelstein WA: NMR imaging applications in medicine and biology, Curr Probl Cancer 7:20-31, 1982.

1983 McNiesh LM, Madewell JE and Allman RM: Cadaver radiography in the teaching of gross anatomy, Radiology 148:73-74, 1983.

Proto AV, Simmons JD and Zylak CJ: The anterior junction anatomy, CRC Crit Rev Diagn Imaging 19:111-173, 1983.

Proto AV, Simmons JD and Zylak CJ: The posterior junction anatomy, CRC Crit Rev Diagn Imaging 20:121-173, 1983.

1984 Totty WG and Vannier MW: Complex musculoskeletal anatomy: analysis using three dimensional surface reconstruction, Radiology 150:173-177, 1984.

1987 Goldberg I and Nathan H: Anatomy and pathology of the sesamoid bones. The hand compared to the foot, Int Orthop 11:141-147, 1987.

Sartoris DJ and Resnick D: Pictorial review: cross-sectional imaging of the foot and ankle, Foot Ankle 8:59-80, 1987.

1988 Cronier P et al: Scanographic study of the calcaneus: normal anatomy and clinical applications, Surg Radiol Anat 10:303-310, 1988.

Czervionke LF and Daniels DL: Cervical spine anatomy and pathologic processes. Applications of new MR imaging techniques, Radiol Clin North Am 26:921-947, 1988.

Karssemeijer N, van Erning LJ and Eijkman EG: Recognition of organs in CT-image sequences: a model guided approach, Comput Biomed Res 21:434-448, 1988.

Sartoris DJ and Resnick D: Cross-sectional imaging of the foot: test of anatomical knowledge, J Foot Surg 27:374-383, 1988.

Zlatkin MB et al: Cross-sectional imaging of the capsular mechanism of the glenohumeral joint, AJR 150:151-158, 1988.

1989 Collins JD et al: Anatomy of the abdomen, back, and pelvis as displayed by magnetic resonance imaging. Part III. J Natl Med Assoc 81:857-861, 1989.

Johnson ND et al: MR imaging anatomy of the infant hip, AJR 153:127-133, 1989.

Neri M and Querin F: CT scan in a study of the normal anatomy of the hindfoot and midfoot, Ital J Orthop Traumatol 15:507-520, 1989.

1990 Bhalla M et al: Counting ribs on chest CT, J Comput Assist Tomogr 14:590-594, 1990.

Dhawan AP and Juvvadi S: Knowledge-based analysis and understanding of medical images, Comput Methods Programs Biomed 33:221-239, 1990.

Erkonen WE et al: Gross anatomy instruction with diagnostic images, Invest Radiol 25:292-294, 1990.

Logan BM, Liles RP and Bolton I: A photographic technique for teaching topographical anatomy from whole body transverse sections, J Audiov Media Med 13:45-48, 1990.

Mano I et al: Computerized three-dimensional normal atlas, Radiat Med 8:50-54, 1990.

Pinsky WW and Arciniegas E: Tetralogy of Fallot, Pediatr Clin North Am 37:179-192, 1990.

Raider L, Landry BA and Brogdon BG: The retrotracheal triangle, Radiographics 10:1055-1079, 1990.

1991 Chevallier JM et al: The thoracic esophagus: sectional anatomy and radiosurgical applications, Surg Radiol Anat 13:313-321, 1991.

Collins JD et al: Anatomy of the thorax and shoulder girdle displayed by magnetic resonance imaging, J Natl Med Assoc 83:26-32, 1991.

Conway WF et al: Cross-sectional imaging of the patellofemoral joint and surrounding structures, Radiographics 11:195-217, 1991.

Ferkel RD, flannigan BD and Elkins BS: Magnetic resonance imaging of the foot and ankle: correlation of normal anatomy with pathologic conditions, Foot Ankle 11:289-305, 1991.

Greitz T et al: A computerized brain atlas: construction, anatomical content, and some applications, J Comput Assist Tomogr 15:26-38, 1991.

Krasny R et al: MR anatomy of infants hip: comparison to anatomical preparations, Pediatr Radiol 21:211-215, 1991.

McCracken TO and Spurgeon TL: The Vesalius Project: interactive computers in anatomical instruction, J Biocommun 18:40-44, 1991.

Spring BI and Schiebler ML: Normal anatomy of the thoracic inlet as seen on transaxial MR images, AJR 157:707-710, 1991.

Yu S, Haughton VM and Rosenbaum AE: Magnetic resonance imaging and anatomy of the spine, Radiol Clin North Am 29:691-710, 1991.

1992 Cobb TK et al: The carpal tunnel as a compartment. An anatomic perspective, Orthop Rev 21:451-453, 1992.

Desai S and Chan O: Interpretation of a normal chest x-ray, Nurs Stand 7:38-39, 1992.

Doby T: Leonardo da Vinci's anatomy revisited, Caduceus 8:23-38, 1992.

Erkonen WE et al: Cardiac anatomy instruction by ultrafast computed tomography versus cadaver dissection, Invest Radiol 27:744-747, 1992.

Erkonen WE et al: Effectiveness of teaching radiologic image interpretation in gross anatomy. A long-term follow-up, Invest Radiol 27:264-266, 1992.

Mallon WJ et al: Radiographic and geometric anatomy of the scapula, Clin Orthop 142-154, 1992.

Michelson JD et al: Examination of the pathologic anatomy of ankle fractures, J Trauma 32:65-70, 1992.

Ney DR et al: Comparison of helical and serial CT with regard to three-dimensional imaging of musculoskeletal anatomy, Radiology 185:865-869, 1992.

Proto AV: Conventional chest radiographs: anatomic understanding of newer observations, Radiology 183:593-603, 1992.

Rathe R, Lanier L and Seymour J: Radiologic Anatomy: an interactive system for first year medical students, Proc Annu Symp Comput Appl Med Care 802-803, 1992.

Sartoris DJ: Diagnostic imaging insight: cross-sectional imaging of the foot (computed tomography-magnetic resonance), J Foot Surg 31:190-202, 1992.

Scatliff JH and Clark JK: How the brain got its names and numbers, AJNR 13:241-248, 1992.

Schatzki SC: Anatomical lectures by Dr. William W. Keen, AJR 158:1210, 1992.

Sofranik RM, Gross BH and Spizarny DL: Radiology of the pleural fissures, Clin Imaging 16:221-229, 1992.

1993   Bonadio WA: Cervical spine trauma in children. Part I. General concepts, normal anatomy, radiographic evaluation, Am J Emerg Med 11:158-165, 1993.

el-Khoury GY and Whitten CG: Trauma to the upper thoracic spine: anatomy, biomechanics, and unique imaging features, AJR 160:95-102, 1993.

Erickson SJ and Rosengarten JL: MR imaging of the forefoot: normal anatomic findings, AJR 160:565-571, 1993.

Klein MA and Spreitzer AM: MR imaging of the tarsal sinus and canal: normal anatomy, pathologic findings, and features of the sinus tarsi syndrome, Radiology 186:233-240, 1993.

Upper limb

For bibliographic citations before 1964, please see the fifth edition of this atlas. For citations from 1964 through 1974, see the sixth or seventh edition.

1975   Eto RT, Anderson PW and Harley JD: Elbow arthrography with the application of tomography, Radiology 115:283-288, 1975.

Resnick D: Roentgenographic anatomy of the tendon sheaths of the hand and wrist: tenography, AJR 124:44-51, 1975.

1976   Rapport AS, Sosman JL and Weissman BN: Spontaneous fractures of the olecranon process in rheumatoid arthritis, Radiology 119:83-84, 1976.

1977   Horsman A et al: Effect of rotation on radiographic dimensions of the humerus and femur, Br J Radiol 50:23-28, 1977.

Murphy WA and Siegel MJ: Elbow fat pads with new signs and extended differential diagnosis, Radiology 124:659-665, 1977.

Yeh HC and Wolf BS: Radiographic anatomical landmarks of the metacarpophalangeal joints, Radiology 122:353-355, 1977.

1978   Hayes N, Gerard FM and Burkhalter WE: Air gap magnification techniques in upper extremity fractures, Clin Orthop 131:173-175, 1978.

Kaye JJ: Fractures and dislocations of the hand and wrist, Semin Roentgenol 13:109-116, 1978.

Kaye JJ and Lister GD: Another use for the Brewerton view, J Hand Surg 3:603, 1978.

Rogers LF: Fractures and dislocations of the elbow, Semin Roentgenol 13:97-107, 1978.

1979   Khanna KK and Kiran S: Radiological study at wrist and elbow-epiphyseal fusion with diaphysis, Indian J Med Sci 33:121-125, 1979.

Silberstein MJ, Brodeur AE and Graviss ER: Some vagaries of the capitellum, J Bone and Joint Surg 61:244-247, 1979.

1980   Danzig LA, Greenway G and Resnick D: The Hill-Sachs lesion: an experimental study, Am J Sports Med 8:328-332, 1980.

Desaultels JE, Radomsky JW and Erickson LM: Evaluation of mammography unit and rare earth screens for high resolution hand radiography, J Can Assoc Radiol 31:185-186, 1980.

Fodor J and Malott JC: Radiography of the carpal navicular, Radiol Technol 52:175-180, 1980.

Jones RP and Leach RE: Fracture of the ulnar sesamoid bone of the thumb, Am J Sports Med 8:446-447, 1980.

Rosenthal D, Murray WT and Smith RJ: Finger arthrography, Radiology 147:647-651, 1980.

1981   Dalinka MK and Bonavita JA: Injury to the shoulder, elbow, and forearm, Bull NY Acad Med 57:113-126, 1981.

De Smet AA et al: Radiographic projections for the diagnosis of the hands and wrists, Radiology 139:577-581, 1981.

Zbrodowski A, Gajisin S and Grodecki J: The anatomy of the digitopalmar arches, J Bone and Joint Surg 63-B:108-113, 1981.

Zucker-Pinchoff B, Hermann G and Srinivasan R: Computed tomography of the carpal tunnel: a radioanatomical study, J Comput Assist Tomogr 5:525-528, 1981.

1982   Brady TJ et al: NMR imaging of forearms in healthy volunteers and patients with giant-cell tumor of the bone, Radiology 144:549-552, 1982.

Greenspan A and Norman A: The radial head, capitellum view: useful technique in elbow trauma, AJR 138:1186-1188, 1982.

1983   Cone RO, Szabo R and Resnick D: Computed tomography of the normal radioulnar joints, Invest Radiol 18:541-545, 1983.

Dalinka MK, Osterman AL and Albert AS: Arthrography of the wrist and shoulder, Orthop Clin North Am 14:193-215, 1983.

Gilula LA, Totty WG and Weeks PM: Wrist arthrography: the value of fluoroscopic spot viewing, Radiology 146:555-556, 1983.

John V et al: CT of carpal tunnel syndrome, AJNR 4:770-772, 1983.

1984   Ahovuo J, Paavolainen P and Slatis P: The diagnostic value of arthrography and plain radiography in rotator cuff tears, Acta Orthop Scand 55:220-223, 1984.

Buckland-Wright JC: Microfocal radiographic examination of erosions in the wrist and hand of patients with rheumatoid arthritis, Ann Rheum Dis 43:160-171, 1984.

Curtis DJ et al: Importance of soft-tissue evaluation in hand and wrist trauma: statistical evaluation, AJR 142:781-788, 1984.

Himes JH: An early hand-wrist atlas and its implications for secular change in bone age, Ann Hum Biol 11:71-75, 1984.

Katch FI and Behnke AR: Arm x-ray assessment of percent body fat in men and women, Med Sci Sports Exerc 16:316-321, 1984.

Mikic ZD: Arthrography of the wrist joint, J Bone Joint Surg 66-A:371-378, 1984.

Patel RB, Barton P and Green L: CT of isolated elbow in evaluation of trauma: a modified technique, Comput Radiology 8:1-4, 1984.

1986   Belsole RJ: Radiography of the wrist, Clin Orthop 50-56, 1986.

Bresina SJ: Three-dimensional wrist imaging: evaluation of functional and pathologic anatomy by computer, Clin Plast Surg 13:389-405, 1986.

Finke M: Dynamic imaging of the wrist, Radiol Technol 57(3):225-231, 1986.

Singson RD, Feldman F and Rosenberg ZS: Elbow joint: assessment with double-contrast CT arthrography, Radiology 160:167-173, 1986.

Tornvall AH et al: Radiologic examination and measurement of the wrist and distal radioulnar joint: new aspects, Acta Radiol [diagn] (Stockh) 27:581-588, 1986.

1987   Abbitt PL and Riddervold HO: The carpal tunnel view: helpful adjuvant for unrecognized fractures of the carpus, Skeletal Radiol 16:45-47, 1987.

Biondetti PR et al: Wrist: coronal and transaxial CT scanning, Radiology 163:149-151, 1987.

Bush CH, Gillespy T and Dell PC: High-resolution CT of the wrist: initial experience with scaphoid disorders and surgical fusions, AJR 149:757-760, 1987.

Cassel J: A technique to control hand position for intraoperative radiography, J Hand Surg Am 12:148-149, 1987.

De-Beer JD and Hudson DA: Fractures of the triquetrum, J Hand Surg Br 12:52-53, 1987.

Engel J et al: The role of three dimension computerized imaging in hand surgery, J Hand Surg Br 12:349-352, 1987.

Fodor J, Malott J and Merhar G: Carpal tunnel syndrome: the role of radiography, Radiol Technol 58(6), 1987.

Greenspan A and Norman A: Radial head-capitellum view: an expanded imaging approach to elbow, Radiology 164:272-274, 1987.

Hardy DC et al: Posteroanterior wrist radiography: importance of arm positioning, J Hand Surg Am 12:504-508, 1987.

Jessurun W et al: Anatomical relations in the carpal tunnel: a computed tomographic study, J Hand Surg Br 12:64-67, 1987.

Levinsohn EM et al: Wrist arthrography: the value of the three compartment injection, Skeletal Radiol 16:539-544, 1987.

Newberg AH: The radiographic evaluation of shoulder and elbow pain in the athlete, Clin Sports Med 6:785-809, 1987.

Porter M and Stockley I: Fractures of the distal radius. Intermediate and end results in relation to radiologic parameters, Clin Orthop 241:252, 1987.

Recht MP, Burk DL Jr and Dalinka MK: Radiology of wrist and hand injuries in athletes, Clin Sports Med 6:811-828, 1987.

Sartoris DJ and Resnick D: MR imaging of the musculoskeletal system: current and future status, AJR 149:457-467, 1987.

1988   Alexander JE and Holder JC: Fat pad signs in the diagnosis of subtle fractures, Am Fam Physician 37:93-102, 1988.

Biondetti PR et al: Three-dimensional surface reconstruction of the carpal bones from CT scans: transaxial versus coronal technique, Comput Med Imaging Graph 12:67-73, 1988.

Bishop AT and Beckenbaugh RD: Fracture of the hamate hook, J Hand Surg Am 13:135-139, 1988.

Brismar J: Skeletal scintigraphy of the wrist in suggested scaphoid fracture, Acta Radiol 29:101-107, 1988.

De-flaviis L et al: Ultrasonography of the hand in rheumatoid arthritis, Acta Radiol 29:457-460, 1988.

Fornage BD and Rifkin MD: Ultrasound examination of the hand and foot, Radiol Clin North Am 26:109-129, 1988.

Franklin PD et al: Computed tomography of the normal and traumatized elbow, J Comput Assist Tomogr 12:817-823, 1988.

Gilula LA, Hardy DC and Totty WG: Distal radioulnar joint arthrography, AJR 150:864-866, 1988.

Horsfield D: The bicipital groove: a simple technique, Radiography 54:109-110, 1988.

Imamura T and Miura T: The carpal bones in congenital hand anomalies: a radiographic study in patients older than ten years, J Hand Surg Am 13:650-656, 1988.

Lewis S: New angles on the radiographic examination of the hand—I, Radiogr Today 54:44-45, 1988.

Lewis S: New angles on the radiographic examination of the hand—II, Radiogr Today 54:29, 1988.

Lewis S: New angles on the radiographic examination of the hand—III, Radiogr Today 54:47-48, 1988.

Margles SW: Intra-articular fractures of the metacarpophalangeal and proximal interphalangeal joints, Hand Clin 4:67-74, 1988.

Minakuchi K et al: Diagnosis and evaluation of diseases of the hand by intravenous digital subtraction angiography done by an improved method, Osaka City Med J 34:191-200, 1988.

Ngo C and Yaghmai I: The value of immersion hand radiography in soft tissue changes of musculoskeletal disorders, Skeletal Radiol 17:259-263, 1988.

Posner MA and Greenspan A: Trispiral tomography for the evaluation of wrist problems, J Hand Surg Am 13:175-181, 1988.

Quinn SF et al: Digital subtraction wrist arthrography: evaluation of the multiple-compartment technique, AJR 151:1173-1174, 1988.

Simmons BP and Lovallo JL: Hand and wrist injuries in children, Clin Sports Med 7:495-512, 1988.

Walker JL, Greene TL and Lunseth PA: Fractures of the body of the trapezium, J Orthop Trauma 2:22-28, 1988.

Zammit-Maempel I et al: The value of soft tissue signs in wrist trauma, Clin Radiol 39:664-668, 1988.

Zinberg EM et al: The triple-injection wrist arthrogram, J Hand Surg Am 13:803-809, 1988.

1989   Ahovuo J, Paavolainen P and Bjorkenheim JM: Fractures of the proximal humerus involving the intertubercular groove, Acta Radiol 30:373-374, 1989.

Bodell LS and Martin ML: Hand and wrist fractures in occupational medicine, Occup Med 4:497-524, 1989.

Bramble JM et al: Image data compression in magnification hand radiographs, Radiology 170:133-136, 1989.

Corfitsen M, Christensen SE and Cetti R: The anatomical fat pad and the radiological "scaphoid fat stripe", J Hand Surg Br 14:326-328, 1989.

Erickson SJ et al: MR imaging of the finger: correlation with normal anatomic sections, AJR 152:1013-1019, 1989.

Hindman BW et al: Occult fractures of the carpals and metacarpals: demonstration by CT, AJR 153:529-532, 1989.

Jarry G et al: In vivo transillumination of the hand using near infrared laser pulses and differential spectroscopy, J Biomed Eng 11:293-299, 1989.

Kerr R: Diagnostic imaging of the upper extremity trauma, Radiol Clin North Am 27:891-908, 1989.

Marquis GP: Radiolucent foreign bodies in the hand: case report, J Trauma 29:403-404, 1989.

Nakamura R et al: Three-dimensional CT imaging for wrist disorders, J Hand Surg Br 14:53-58, 1989.

Propp DA and Chin H: Forearm and wrist radiology. Part II. J Emerg Med 7:491-496, 1989.

Stahelin A et al: Determining carpal collapse. An improved method, J Bone Joint Surg Am 71:1400-1405, 1989.

Stark HH et al: Fracture of the hook of the hamate, J Bone Joint Surg Am 71:1202-1207, 1989.

Subin GD, Mallon WJ and Urbaniak JR: Diagnosis of ganglion in Guyon's canal by magnetic resonance imaging, J Hand Surg Am 14:640-643, 1989.

Ueba Y et al: Computed radiography (Fuji) as a diagnostic tool for carpal disease, J Hand Surg Am 14:408-410, 1989.

Zeiss J et al: Anatomic relations between the median nerve and flexor tendons in the carpal tunnel: MR evaluation in normal volunteers, AJR 153:533-536, 1989.

1990   Balfour GW: Diagnosis of oblique fractures of the distal ulna using an extended pronated view of the wrist, Orthopedics 13:247-250, 1990.

Boulas HJ and Milek MA: Hook of the hamate fractures. Diagnosis, treatment, and complications, Orthop Rev 19:518-529, 1990.

Cole PR et al: High resolution, high field magnetic resonance imaging of joints: unexpected features in proton images of cartilage, Br J Radiol 63:907-909, 1990.

Courtenay BG and Bowers DM: Stress fractures: clinical features and investigation, Med J Aust 153:155-156, 1990.

Davies AM et al: Real-time digital contrast enhancement and magnification in the assessment of scaphoid and other wrist injuries, Br J Radiol 63:934-939, 1990.

Frahm R, Saul O and Mannerfelt L: Diagnostic applications of wrist arthrography, Arch Orthop Trauma Surg 109:39-42, 1990.

Friedman L, Johnston GH and Yong-Hing K: Computed tomography of wrist trauma, Can Assoc Radiol J 41:141-145, 1990.

Herndon JH: Radiology review: the wrist, Orthop Nurs 9:61-63, 1990.

Jeneson JA et al: 1H MR imaging of anatomical compartments within the finger flexor muscles of the human forearm, Magn Reson Med 15:491-496, 1990.

Kursunoglu-Brahme S, Gundry CR and Resnick D: Advanced imaging of the wrist, Radiol Clin North Am 28:307-320, 1990.

Larsen CF et al: Radiography of the wrist. A new device for standardized radiographs, Acta Radiol 31:459-462, 1990.

Lawson JP: Not-so-normal variants, Orthop Clin North Am 21:483-495, 1990.

Linn MR, Mann FA and Gilula LA: Imaging the symptomatic wrist, Orthop Clin North Am 21:515-543, 1990.

Marshall J and Davies R: Imaging the carpal tunnel, Radiogr Today 56:11-13, 1990.

McGeorge DD and McGeorge S: Diagnostic medical ultrasound in the management of hand injuries, J Hand Surg Br 15:256-261, 1990.

Mehta M and Brautigan MW: Fracture of the carpal navicular—efficacy of clinical findings and improved diagnosis with six-view radiography, Ann Emerg Med 19:255-257, 1990.

Moreland LW, Daniel WW and Alarcon GS: The value of the Norgaard view in the evaluation of erosive arthritis, J Rheumatol 17:614-617, 1990.

Schernberg F: Roentgenographic examination of the wrist: a systematic study of the normal, lax and injured wrist. Part I. The standard and positional views, J Hand Surg Br 15:210-219, 1990.

Schernberg F: Roentgenographic examination of the wrist: a systematic study of the normal, lax and injured wrist. Part II. Stress views, J Hand Surg Br 15:220-228, 1990.

Scotter E and Ignotus P: Wrist arthrography, Radiogr Today 56:15-18, 1990.

Smith DK et al: Radiographic features of hand and wrist arthroplasties, Eur J Radiol 10:3-8, 1990.

Smith DK et al: Radiographic features of hand and wrist surgery excluding arthroplasties, Eur J Radiol 10:85-91, 1990.

van der Voort JH and Kon M: Chronic painful sesamoids of the thumb, Arch Orthop Trauma Surg 110:22-23, 1990.

Wilson AJ, Mann FA and Gilula LA: Imaging the hand and wrist, J Hand Surg Br 15:153-167, 1990.

1991 Ahovuo J et al: Bone malalignment in acute injuries of the wrist, Ann Chir Gynaecol 80:282-284, 1991.

Atar D et al: Ilizarov technique in treatment of congenital hand anomalies. Two case reports, Clin Orthop 268-274, 1991.

Bond JR and Berquist TH: Radiologic evaluation of hand and wrist motion, Hand Clin 7:113-123, 1991.

Brahme SK and Resnick D: Magnetic resonance imaging of the wrist, Rheum Dis Clin North Am 17:721-739, 1991.

Buckwalter KA, Swan JS and Braunstein EM: Evaluation of joint disease in the adult hand and wrist, Hand Clin 7:135-151, 1991.

Burk DL Jr, Karasick D and Wechsler RJ: Imaging of the distal radioulnar joint, Hand Clin 7:263-275, 1991.

Clements RW and Nakayama HK: Technique for detecting early rheumatoid arthritis, Radiol Technol 62:443-451, 1991.

Donaldson JS: Radiographic imaging of foreign bodies in the hand, Hand Clin 7:125-134, 1991.

Evans S: Radiological appearances of a dorsal fracture dislocation of the lunate, Radiogr Today 57:30, 1991.

Feinstein KA and Poznanski AK: Evaluation of joint disease in the pediatric hand, Hand Clin 7:167-182, 1991.

FitzRandolph RL et al: Radiographic and orthopedic evaluation of wrist trauma, Curr Probl Diagn Radiol 20:1-42, 1991.

Foley-Nolan D et al: Magnetic resonance imaging in the assessment of rheumatoid arthritis—a comparison with plain film radiographs, Br J Rheumatol 30:101-106, 1991.

Fry ME et al: High-resolution magnetic resonance imaging of the interphalangeal joints of the hand, Skeletal Radiol 20:273-277, 1991.

Gruber L: Practical approaches to obtaining hand radiographs and special techniques in hand radiology, Hand Clin 7:1-20, 1991.

Gupta A: The treatment of Colles' fracture. Immobilisation with the wrist dorsiflexed, J Bone Joint Surg Br 73:312-315, 1991.

Hawkes DJ et al: Registration and display of the combined bone scan and radiograph in the diagnosis and management of wrist injuries, Eur J Nucl Med 18:752-756, 1991.

Hawksworth CR and Freeland P: Inability to fully extend the injured elbow: an indicator of significant injury, Arch Emerg Med 8:253-256, 1991.

Ho CP and Sartoris DJ: Magnetic resonance imaging of the elbow, Rheum Dis Clin North Am 17:705-720, 1991.

Imaging of the hand, Hand Clin 7:1-238, 1991.

Jarvik JG, Dalinka MK and Kneeland JB: Hand injuries in adults, Semin Roentgenol 26:282-299, 1991.

Jupiter JB: Fractures of the distal end of the radius, J Bone Joint Surg Am 73:461-469, 1991.

Karasick D, Burk DL Jr and Gross GW: Trauma to the elbow and forearm, Semin Roentgenol 26:318-330, 1991.

Keats TE: Normal variants of the hand and wrist, Hand Clin 7:153-166, 1991.

Koch J and Rahimi F: Nutcracker fractures of the cuboid, J Foot Surg 30:336-339, 1991.

Langhoff O, Andersen K and Kjaer-Petersen K: Rolando's fracture, J Hand Surg Br 16:454-459, 1991.

Macfarlane DG et al: Comparison of clinical, radionuclide, and radiographic features of osteoarthritis of the hands, Ann Rheum Dis 50:623-626, 1991.

Magid D, Thompson JS and Fishman EK: Computed tomography of the hand and wrist, Hand Clin 7:219-233, 1991.

Meyer S: Radiographic evaluation of wrist trauma, Semin Roentgenol 26:300-317, 1991.

Mortensson W and Thonell S: Left side dominance of upper extremity fracture in children, Acta Orthop Scand 62:154-155, 1991.

Pirela Cruz MA et al: Stress computed tomography analysis of the distal radioulnar joint: a diagnostic tool for determining translational motion, J Hand Surg Am 16:75-82, 1991.

Poznanski AK: Useful measurements in the evaluation of hand radiographs, Hand Clin 7:21-36, 1991.

Rafert JA and Long BW: Technique for diagnosis of scaphoid fractures, Radiol Technol 63:16-20, 1991.

Russell RC et al: Detection of foreign bodies in the hand, J Hand Surg Am 16:2-11, 1991.

Schiller MG, af-Ekenstam F and Kirsch PT: Volar dislocation of the distal radio-ulnar joint. A case report, J Bone Joint Surg Am 73:617-619, 1991.

Stapczynski JS: Fracture of the base of the little finger metacarpal: importance of the "ball-catcher" radiographic view, J Emerg Med 9:145-149, 1991.

Sullivan PP and Berquist TH: Magnetic resonance imaging of the hand, wrist, and forearm: utility in patients with pain and dysfunction as a result of trauma, Mayo Clin Proc 66:1217-1221, 1991.

Wolfe SW and Dick HM: Articular fractures of the hand. Part I. Guidelines for assessment, Orthop Rev 20:27-32, 1991.

Wong EC, Jesmanowicz A and Hyde JS: High-resolution, short echo time MR imaging of the fingers and wrist with a local gradient coil, Radiology 181:393-397, 1991.

Zerin JM and Hernandez RJ: Approach to skeletal maturation, Hand Clin 7:53-62, 1991.

Zoltie N: Fractures of the body of the hamate, Injury 22:459-462, 1991.

1992 Abdel-Salam A, Eyres KS and Cleary J: Detecting fractures of the scaphoid: the value of comparative x-rays of the uninjured wrist, J Hand Surg Br 17:28-32, 1992.

Barnaby W: Fractures and dislocations of the wrist, Emerg Med Clin North Am 10:133-149, 1992.

Beaty JH: Fractures and dislocations about the elbow in children, Instr Course Lect 41:373-384, 1992.

Botte MJ: Fracture of the trapezial ridge, Clin Orthop 202-205, 1992.

Braun RM: The distal joint of the radius and ulna. Diagnostic studies and treatment rationale, Clin Orthop 74-78, 1992.

Bruckner JD, Lichtman DM and Alexander AH: Complex dislocations of the distal radioulnar joint. Recognition and management, Clin Orthop 90-103, 1992.

Buchberger W et al: Carpal tunnel syndrome: diagnosis with high-resolution sonography, AJR 159:793-798, 1992.

Cavanagh S: The true 'boxer's fracture,' Injury 23:204-205, 1992.

Chacon D et al: Use of comparison radiographs in the diagnosis of traumatic injuries of the elbow, Ann Emerg Med 21:895-899, 1992.

Cobb TK et al: The carpal tunnel as a compartment. An anatomic perspective, Orthop Rev 21:451-453, 1992.

Corvetta A et al: MR imaging of rheumatoid hand lesions: comparison with conventional radiology in 31 patients, Clin Exp Rheumatol 10:217-222, 1992.

Daffner RH, Emmerling EW and Buterbaugh GA: Proximal and distal oblique radiography of the wrist: value in occult injuries, J Hand Surg Am 17:499-503, 1992.

Foo TK et al: High-resolution MR imaging of the wrist and eye with short TR, short TE, and partial-echo acquisition, Radiology 183:277-281, 1992.

Giordano N: Telethermographic assessment of carpal tunnel syndrome, Scand J Rheumatol 21:42-45, 1992.

Glickel SZ, Kornstein AN and Eaton RG: Long-term follow-up of trapeziometacarpal arthroplasty with coexisting scapho-trapezial disease, J Hand Surg Am 17:612-620, 1992.

Goldberg HD et al: Double injuries of the forearm: a common occurrence, Radiology 185:223-227, 1992.

Imaeda T et al: Magnetic resonance imaging in scaphoid fractures, J Hand Surg Br 17:20-27, 1992.

James SE, Richards R and McGrouther DA: Three-dimensional CT imaging of the wrist. A practical system, J Hand Surg Br 17:504-506, 1992.

Johnston GH, Friedman L and Kriegler JC: Computerized tomographic evaluation of acute distal radial fractures, J Hand Surg Am 17:738-744, 1992.

Lane CS, Kennedy JF and Kuschner SH: The reverse oblique x-ray film: metacarpal fractures revealed, J Hand Surg Am 17:504-506, 1992.

Larsen CF, Lindequist S and Bellstrom T: Lack of correlation between ulnar variance and carpal bone angles on lateral radiographs in normal wrists, Acta Radiol 33:275-276, 1992.

Maggi G et al: Pure traumatic dislocation of the elbow, Chir Organi Mov 77:195-198, 1992.

Mann FA, Wilson AJ and Gilula LA: Radiographic evaluation of the wrist: what does the hand surgeon want to know? Radiology 184:15-24, 1992.

Munk PL: Current status of magnetic resonance imaging of the wrist, Can Assoc Radiol J 43:8-18, 1992.

Murphy BJ: MR imaging of the elbow, Radiology 184:525-529, 1992.

Oberlin C et al: Three-dimensional reconstruction of the carpus and its vasculature: an anatomic study, J Hand Surg Am 17:767-772, 1992.

Parkinson RW and Paton RW: Carpometacarpal dislocation: an aid to diagnosis, Injury 23:187-188, 1992.

Patten RM et al: Nondisplaced fractures of the greater tuberosity of the humerus: sonographic detection, Radiology 182:201-204, 1992.

Regan W and Morrey BF: Classification and treatment of coronoid process fractures, Orthopedics 15:845-848, 1992.

Richmond BJ et al: Diagnostic efficacy of digitized images vs plain films: a study of the joints of the fingers, AJR 158:437-441, 1992.

Riddervold HO: Easily missed fractures, Radiol Clin North Am 30:475-494, 1992.

Sach R: The injured hand, Aust Fam Physician 21:920-924, 927-930, 1992.

Savage R and Nathdwarawala Y: Role of CT scan in clicking forearm, Injury 23:356-357, 1992.

Schweitzer ME et al: Chronic wrist pain: spin-echo and short tau inversion recovery MR imaging and conventional and MR arthrography, Radiology 182:205-211, 1992.

Stewart NR and Gilula LA: CT of the wrist: a tailored approach, Radiology 183:13-20, 1992.

Tehranzadeh J, Kerr R and Amster J: Magnetic resonance imaging of tendon and ligament abnormalities. Part I. Spine and upper extremities, Skeletal Radiol 21:1-9, 1992.

Thomas D et al: Computerized infrared thermography and isotopic bone scanning in tennis elbow, Ann Rheum Dis 51:103-107, 1992.

Tiel-van-Buul MM et al: Diagnosing scaphoid fractures: radiographs cannot be used as a gold standard! Injury 23:77-79, 1992.

Tiernan E: The syringe plunger in intraoperative hand surgery radiography, Br J Plast Surg 45:616, 1992.

Zeiss J et al: The ulnar tunnel at the wrist (Guyon's canal): normal MR anatomy and variants, AJR 158:1081-1085, 1992.

Zlatkin MB and Greenan T: Magnetic resonance imaging of the wrist, Magn Reson Q 8:65-96, 1992.

1993 Atar D et al: Ilizarov technique in treatment of congenital hand anomalies. Two case reports, Clin Orthop 268-274, 1993.

Donaldson JS: Radiographic imaging of foreign bodies in the hand, Hand Clin 7:125-134, 1993.

Feinstein KA and Poznandki AK: Evaluation of joint disease in the pediatric hand, Hand Clin 7:167-182, 1993.

Gupta A: The treatment of Colles' fracture. Immobilization with the wrist dosiflexed, J Bone Joint Surg Br 73:312-315, 1993.

Jarvik JG, Dalinka MK and Kneeland JB: Hand injuries in adults, Semin Roentgenol 26:282-299, 1993.

Levine WN and Leslie BM: The use of ultrasonography to detect a radiolucent foreign body in the hand: a case report, J Hand Surg Am 18:218-220, 1993.

Mortensson W and Thonell S: Left-side dominance of upper extremity fracture in children, Acta Orthop (Scand) 62:154-155, 1993.

Okubo S, Lehtinen K and Isomaki H: Sensitivity of radiographic changes of hand and foot joints as a diagnostic criterion in patients with rheumatoid arthritis, Scand J Rheumatol 21:145-147, 1993.

Parkinson RW and Paton RW: Carpometacarpal dislocation: an aid to diagnosis, Injury 23:187-188, 1993.

Poznandki AK: Useful measurements in the evaluation of hand radiographs, Hand Clin 7:21-36, 1993.

Sach R: The injured hand, Aust Fam Physician 21:920-924, 1993.

Lower limb

For bibliographic citations before 1964, please see the fifth edition of this ATLAS. For citations from 1964 through 1974, see the sixth or seventh edition.

1975 Flynn M, Moulton A and Rose GK: A simple method of obtaining a lateral radiograph of the head and neck of the femur, Injury 6:246-247, 1975.

Gamble FO and Yale I: Clinical foot roentgenology, Huntington, NY, 1975, RE Krieger Publishing Co, Inc.

Resnick D: The interphalangeal joint of the great toe in rheumatoid arthritis, J Can Assoc Radiol 26:255-262, 1975.

1976 Cobey JC: Posterior roentgenogram of the foot, Clin Orthop 118:202-207, 1976.

Elstrom J et al: The use of tomography in the assessment of fractures of the tibial plateau, J Bone Joint Surg 58:551-555, 1976.

1977 Goergen TG et al: Roentgenographic evaluation of the tibiotalar joint, J Bone Joint Surg 59:874-877, 1977.

Horsman A et al: Effect of rotation on radiographic dimensions of the humerus and femur, Br J Radiol 50:23-28, 1977.

McCrea JD et al: Effects of radiographic technique on the metatarsophalangeal joints, J Am Podiatr Med Assoc 67:837-840, 1977.

Moore TH and Meyers MH: Apparatus to position knees for varus-valgus stress roentgenograms, J Bone Joint Surg 59:984, 1977.

Winiecki DG and Biggs EW: Xeroradiography and its application in podiatry, J Am Podiatr Med Assoc 67:393-400, 1977.

1978 Diamond MJ: The upright lateral exposure: a new view for podiatric radiology, J Am Podiatr Med Assoc 68:47-52, 1978.

Edeiken J and Cotler JM: Ankle injury: the need for stress films, JAMA 240:1182-1184, 1978.

Kehr LE: Radiology: a simplified axial view, J Am Podiatr Med Assoc 68:130-131, 1978.

Rogers LF and Campbell RE: Fractures and dislocations of the foot, Semin Roentgenol 13:157-166, 1978.

Throckmorton JK and Gudas CJ: Radiographic axial sesamoid projection in the diagnosis of sesamoid fractures: two case reports, J Am Podiatr Med Assoc 68:96-100, 1978.

1979 Laurin CA, Dussault R and Levesque HP: The tangential x-ray investigation of the patello-femoral joint x-ray technique, diagnostic criteria, and their interpretation, Clin Orthop 144:16-26, 1979.

1980 Laursen K and Reiter S: Computed tomography in soft tissue disorders of the lower extremities, Acta Orthop Scand 51:881-885, 1980.

Newberg AH and Seligson D: The patellofemoral joint: 30 degrees, 60 degrees, and 90 degrees views, Radiology 137:57-61, 1980.

Norfray JF, et al: Common calcaneal avulsion fracture, AJR 134:119-123, 1980.

1981 Bradley WG and Ominsky SH: Mountain view of the patella, AJR 136:53-58, 1981.

Byron TJ: Foreign bodies found in the foot, J Am Podiatr Med Assoc 71:30-35, 1981.

Clancy WB Jr: The role of arthrography and arthroscopy in the acutely injured knee, Med Times 109:22s-27s, 1981.

Crystal L and Orminski D: Axial views and angle and base of gait, J Am Podiatr Med Assoc 71:331-332, 1981.

Danzig LA et al: Osseous landmarks of the normal knee, Clin Orthop 156:201-206, 1981.

Engelstad BL, Friedman EM and Murphy WA: Diagnosis of joint effusion on lateral and axial projections of the knee, Invest Radiol 16:188-192, 1981.

Fernbach SK and Wilkinson RH: Avulsion injuries of the pelvis and proximal femur, AJR 137:581-584, 1981.

Goldman F et al: Sinography in the diagnosis of foot infections, J Am Podiatr Med Assoc 71:497-502, 1981.

Hendrix RW and Anderson TM: Arthrographic and radiologic evaluation of prosthetic joints, Radiol Clin North Am 19:349-364, 1981.

Hernandez RJ et al: CT determination of femoral torsion, AJR 137:97-101, 1981.

Protas JM and Kornblatt BA: Fractures of the lateral margins of the distal tibia: the Tillaux fracture, Radiology 138:55-57, 1981.

Scranton PE Jr.: Pathologic anatomic variations in the sesamoids, Foot Ankle 1:321-326, 1981.

1982 Boven F et al: A comparative study of the patello-femoral joint on axial roentgenogram, axial arthrogram, and computed tomography following arthrography, Skeletal Radiol 8:179-181, 1982.

De Smet AA, Reckling FW and McNamara GR: Radiographic classification of ankle injuries, J Can Assoc Radiol 33:142-147, 1982.

Fodor J III, Malott JC and Weinberg S: Accurate radiography of the patellofemoral joint, Radiol Technol 53(7):570-579, 1982.

Reinherz RP: Contrast media in the foot, J Am Podiatr Med Assoc 72:569-571, 1982.

Turner GW and Burns CB: Erect position/ tangential projection of the patellofemoral joint, Radiol Technol 54:11-21, 1982.

1983 Butt WP, Lederman H and Chuang S: Radiology of the suprapatellar region, Clin Radiol 34:511-522, 1983.

Fam AG et al: Stress fractures in rheumatoid arthritis, J Rheumatol 10:722-726, 1983.

Goldman F, Manzi JA and Medawar S: A radiopaque-labeling technique to visualize the distribution of local anesthesia, J Foot Surg 22:329-331, 1983.

Martinez S et al: Computed tomography of the normal patellofemoral joint, Invest Radiol 18:249-253, 1983.

Passariello R et al: Computed tomography of the knee joint: clinical results, J Comput Assist Tomogr 7:1043-1049, 1983.

Passariello R et al: Computed tomography of the knee joint: technique of study and normal anatomy, J Comput Assist Tomogr 7:1035-1042, 1983.

Patel RB et al: Computed tomography demonstration of distal femoral (trochlear) articular groove: a normal variant, Skeletal Radiol 10:170-172, 1983.

Sauser DD et al: Acute injuries of the lateral ligaments of the ankle: comparison of stress radiography and arthrography, Radiology 148:653-657, 1983.

Shereff MJ and Johnson KA: Radiographic anatomy of the hindfoot, Clin Orthop 177:16-22, 1983.

Turner GW, Burns CB and Previtte RG Jr: Erect positions for "tunnel" views of the knee, Radiol Technol 55:640-642, 1983.

1984 Beals RK and Skyhar M: Growth and development of the tibia, fibula, and ankle joint, Clin Orthop 182:289-292, 1984.

Carson WG et al: Patellofemoral disorders: physical and radiographic evaluation, Clin Orthop 185:178-186, 1984.

Firooznia H et al: Computed tomography in localization of foreign bodies lodged in the extremities, Comput Radiol 8:237-239, 1984.

Floyd EJ, Ransom RA and Dailey JM: Computed tomography scanning of the subtalar joint, J Am Podiatr Med Assoc 74:533-537, 1984.

Spinner SM, Lipsman S and Spector F: Radiographic criteria in the assessment of hallux abductus deformities, J Foot Surg 23:25-30, 1984.

Wolfgang GL: Complex congenital anomalies of the lower extremities: femoral bifurcation, tibial hemimelia, and diastasis of the ankle, J Bone Joint Surg 66-A:453-458, 1984.

1985 Aitken AG et al: Leg length determination by CT digital radiography, AJR 144:613-615, 1985.

Fodor J, Malott JC and Mencini R: The radiographic appearance of a ceramic total hip replacement, Radiol Technol 56(4):222-225, 1985.

Singer AM et al: Comparison of overhead and cross-table lateral views for detection of knee joint effusion, AJR 144:973-975, 1985.

Turula KB et al: Weight-bearing radiography in total hip replacement, Skeletal Radiol 14:200-204, 1985.

Woolson ST et al: Three-dimensional imaging of the ankle joint from computerized tomography, Foot Ankle 6:2-6, 1985.

1986 Gersten K et al: Crossed-leg technique for digital subtraction angiography, AJR 146:843-844, 1986.

Reinherz RP, Zawada SJ and Sheldon DP: Tenography around the ankle and introduction of a new technique, J Foot Surg 25:357-363, 1986.

1987 Bone LB: Fractures of the tibial plafond. The pilon fracture, Orthop Clin North Am 18:95-104, 1987.

Bouysset M et al: Deformation of the adult rheumatoid rearfoot. A radiographic study, Clin Rheumatol 6:539-544, 1987.

Chioros PG, Frankel SL and Sidlow CJ: Unusual osteochondroma of the foot and ankle, J Foot Surg 26:407-411, 1987.

Daffner RH and Tabas JH: Trauma oblique radiographs of the knee, J Bone Joint Surg 69-A:568-572, 1987.

Jacobs AM et al: Magnetic resonance imaging of the foot and ankle, Clin Podiatr Med Surg 4:903-924, 1987.

Kravette MA: Medical imaging of the foot and leg. An overview, J Am Podiatr Med Assoc 77:462-466, 1987.

Marchisello PJ: The use of computerized axial tomography for the evaluation of talocalcaneal coalition. A case study, J Bone Joint Surg Am 69:609-611, 1987.

Petersen TD and Rohr W Jr: Improved assessment of lower extremity alignment using new roentgenographic techniques, Clin Orthop 112-119, 1987.

Sartoris DJ and Resnick D: Pictorial review: cross-sectional imaging of the foot and ankle, Foot Ankle 8:59-80, 1987.

Sartoris DJ and Resnick D: Magnetic resonance imaging of the foot: technical aspects, J Foot Surg 26:351-358, 1987.

Wilson AJ and Ramsby GR: Skeletal measurements using a flying spot digital imaging device, AJR 149:339-43, 1987.

1988 Adler SJ et al: Three-dimensional computed tomography of the foot: optimizing the image, Comput Med Imaging Graph 12:59-66, 1988.

Ahovuo J, Kaartinen E and Slatis P: Diagnostic value of stress radiography in lesions of the lateral ligaments of the ankle, Acta Radiol 29:711-714, 1988.

Cronier P et al: Scanographic study of the calcaneus: normal anatomy and clinical applications, Surg Radiol Anat 10:303-310, 1988.

Egund N, Lundin A and Wallengren NO: The vertical position of the patella: a new radiographic method for routine use, Acta Radiol 29:555-558, 1988.

Fornage BD and Rifkin MD: Ultrasound examination of the hand and foot, Radiol Clin North Am 26:109-129, 1988.

Freiberger RH and Pavlov H: Knee arthrography, Radiology 166:489-492, 1988.

Haller J et al: Arthrography, tenography, bursography of the ankle and foot, Clin Podiatr Med Surg 5:893-908, 1988.

Hampton S, Read B and Nixon W: Diagnosis of congenital dislocated hips (CDH), Radiol Technol 59(3):211-219, 1988.

Hirose K et al: Antenatal ultrasound diagnosis of the femur-fibula-ulna syndrome, JCU J Clin Ultrasound 16:199-203, 1988.

Karpman RR and MacCollum MS III: Arthrography of the metatarsophalangeal joint, Foot Ankle 9:125-129, 1988.

Kaschak TJ and Laine W: Surgical radiology, Clin Podiatr Med Surg 5:797-829, 1988.

Keyser CK et al: Soft-tissue abnormalities of the foot and ankle: CT diagnosis, AJR 150:845-850, 1988.

Kingston S: Magnetic resonance imaging of the ankle and foot, Clin Sports Med 7:15-28, 1988.

Kirby KA, Loendorf AJ and Greforio R: Anterior axial projection of the foot, J Am Podiatr Med Assoc 78:159-170, 1988.

Mainwaring BL, Daffner RH and Riemer BL: Pylon fractures of the ankle: a distinct clinical and radiologic entity, Radiology 168:215-218, 1988.

McManama GBJ: Ankle injuries in the young athlete, Clin Sports Med 7:547-562, 1988.

Mudge B et al: Multiplanar imaging of the hip: a systematic approach, Radiol Technol 59:307-311, 1988.

Oloff-Solomon J and Solomon MA: Computed tomographic scanning of the foot and ankle, Clin Podiatr Med Surg 5:931-944, 1988.

Perlman MD: Usage of radiopaque contrast media in the foot and ankle, J Foot Surg 27:3-29, 1988.

Romash MM: Calcaneal fractures: three-dimensional treatment, Foot Ankle 8:180-197, 1988.

Rosenberg TD et al: The forty-five–degree posteroanterior flexion weight-bearing radiograph of the knee, J Bone Joint Surg 70-A:1479-1483, 1988.

Sartoris DJ and Resnick D: Cross-sectional imaging of the foot: test of anatomical knowledge, J Foot Surg 27:374-383, 1988.

Sartoris DJ and Resnick D: Pictorial analysis—computed tomography of trauma to the ankle and hindfoot, J Foot Surg 27:80-91, 1988.

Solomon MA and Oloff-Solomon J: Magnetic resonance imaging in the foot and ankle, Clin Podiatr Med Surg 5:945-965, 1988.

Stevens PM: Effect of ankle valgus on radiographic appearance of the hindfoot, J Pediatr Orthop 8:184-186, 1988.

van der Werken C and Zeegers EV: Fracture of the lower leg with involvement of the posterior malleolus: a neglected combination? Injury 19:241-243, 1988.

Weissman S: Standard radiographic techniques for the foot and ankle, Clin Podiatr Med Surg 5:767-775, 1988.

1989   An HS et al: The value of internal oblique radiographs for posterolateral bone grafting of the tibia, Clin Orthop 209-210, 1989.

Blair VP et al: Closed shortening of the femur, J Bone Joint Surg Am 71:1440-1447, 1989.

Crim JR et al: Magnetic resonance imaging of the hindfoot, Foot Ankle 10:1-7, 1989.

David HG: Value of radiographs in managing common foot injuries, BMJ 298:1492-1493, 1989.

Gavant ML: Digital subtraction angiography of the foot in atherosclerotic occlusive disease, South Med J 82:328-334, 1989.

Goossens M et al: Posterior subtalar joint arthrography. A useful tool in the diagnosis of hindfoot disorders, Clin Orthop 248-255, 1989.

Hirsh BE, Udupa JK and Roberts D: Three-dimensional reconstruction of the foot from computed tomography scans, J Am Podiatr Med Assoc 79:384-394, 1989.

Keene JS: Diagnosis of undetected knee injuries. Interpreting subtle clinical and radiologic findings, Postgrad Med 85:153-156, 161, 1989.

Keigley BA et al: Primary tumors of the foot: MR imaging, Radiology 171:755-759, 1989.

Malghem J and Maldague B: Patellofemoral joint: 30 degrees axial radiograph with lateral rotation of the leg, Radiology 170:566-567, 1989.

Mitchell MJ et al: Diagnostic imaging of trauma to the ankle and foot. Part II. J Foot Surg 28:266-271, 1989.

Mitchell MJ et al: Diagnostic imaging of trauma to the ankle and foot. Part III. Fractures and dislocations of the talus, J Foot Surg 28:378-383, 1989.

Mitchell MJ et al: Diagnostic imaging of trauma to the ankle and foot. Part IV. Fractures of the calcaneus, J Foot Surg 28:479-484, 1989.

Mitchell MJ et al: Diagnostic imaging of trauma to the ankle and foot. Part V. Midfoot injuries, J Foot Surg 28:591-596, 1989.

Mitchell MJ, Sartoris DJ and Resnick D: The foot and ankle, Top Magn Reson Imaging 1:57-73, 1989.

Murari TM et al: Primary benign and malignant osseous neoplasms of the foot, Foot Ankle 10:68-80, 1989.

Neri M and Querin F: CT scan in a study of the normal anatomy of the hindfoot and midfoot, Ital J Orthop Traumatol 15:507-520, 1989.

Nyska M et al: Fractures of the body of the tarsal navicular bone: case reports and literature review, J Trauma 29:1448-1451, 1989.

Sartoris DJ and Resnick D: Magnetic resonance imaging of tendons in the foot and ankle, J Foot Surg 28:370-377, 1989.

Sartoris DJ and Resnick D: Magnetic resonance imaging of the diabetic foot, J Foot Surg 28:485-491, 1989.

Williamson BR et al: Computed tomography as a diagnostic aid in diabetic and other problem feet, Clin Imaging 13:159-163, 1989.

1990   Adelaar RS: Fractures of the talus, Instr Course Lect 39:147-156, 1990.

Berquist TH: Magnetic resonance imaging of the foot and ankle, Semin Ultrasound CT MR 11:327-345, 1990.

Canale ST: Fractures of the neck of the talus, Orthopedics 13:1105-1115, 1990.

Forrester DM and Kerr R: Trauma to the foot, Radiol Clin North Am 28:423-433, 1990.

Johnson EE: Intraarticular fractures of the calcaneus: diagnosis and surgical management, Orthopedics 13:1091-1100, 1990.

Kerr R and Forrester DM: Magnetic resonance imaging of foot and ankle trauma, Orthop Clin North Am 21:591-601, 1990.

Magid D et al: Adult ankle fractures: comparison of plain films and interactive two- and three-dimensional CT scans, AJR 154:1017-1023, 1990.

Martensen KM: A consistent method to produce lateral knee radiographs, Radiol Technol 62:24-27, 1990.

Mitchell MJ et al: Diagnostic imaging of trauma to the ankle and foot. Part VI. Forefoot injuries, J Foot Surg 29:188-194, 1990.

Pavlov H: Imaging of the foot and ankle, Radiol Clin North Am 28:991-1018, 1990.

Porter RW, Roy A and Rippstein J: Assessment in congenital talipes equinovarus, Foot Ankle 11:16-21, 1990.

Sartoris DJ and Resnick D: Magnetic resonance imaging of pediatric foot and ankle disorders, J Foot Surg 29:489-494, 1990.

Shereff MJ: Fractures of the forefoot, Instr Course Lect 39:133-140, 1990.

1991   Auletta AG et al: Indications for radiography in patients with acute ankle injuries: role of the physical examination, AJR 157:789-791, 1991.

Bresnahan PJ and Fung J: Magnetic resonance imaging of the foot and ankle in the pediatric patient, J Am Podiatr Med Assoc 81:112-118, 1991.

Camasta CA, Pontious J and Boyd RB: Quantifying magnification in pedal radiographs, J Am Podiatr Med Assoc 81:545-548, 1991.

Cameron J: Using Doppler to diagnose leg ulcers, Nurs Stand 5:25-27, 1991.

Conway WF et al: Cross-sectional imaging of the patellofemoral joint and surrounding structures, Radiographics 11:195-217, 1991.

Deconinck K, Bellemans M and Van-Herreweghe W: CT of the heel and midfoot, J Belge Radiol 74:1-9, 1991.

Dickson KF and Sartoris DJ: Injuries to the talus-neck fractures and osteochondral lesions (osteochondritis dissecans), J Foot Surg 30:310-318, 1991.

Dixon AM: Demonstration of lateral patellar subluxation: the 30 degrees LR projection lateral rotation, Radiogr Today 57:20-21, 1991.

Ebraheim NA et al: Radiological evaluation of peroneal tendon pathology associated with calcaneal fractures, J Orthop Trauma 5:365-369, 1991.

Everson LI et al: Radiologic case study. Cuboid subluxation, Orthopedics 14:1037-1048, 1991.

Feldman F, Staron RB and Haramati N: Magnetic resonance imaging of the foot and ankle, Rheum Dis Clin North Am 17:617-636, 1991.

Ferkel RD, Flannigan BD and Elkins BS: Magnetic resonance imaging of the foot and ankle: correlation of normal anatomy with pathologic conditions, Foot Ankle 11:289-305, 1991.

Frank ED et al: Radiography of the ankle mortise, Radiol Technol 62:354-359, 1991.

Hirsch BE: Structural biomechanics of the foot bones, J Am Podiatr Med Assoc 81:338-343, 1991.

Kerr R and Frey C: MR imaging in tarsal tunnel syndrome, J Comput Assist Tomogr 15:280-286, 1991.

Koch J and Rahimi F: Nutcracker fractures of the cuboid, J Foot Surg 30:336-339, 1991.

Macaulay KE, Sartoris DJ and Resnick D: Diseases of the foot: test of radiographic interpretation, J Foot Surg 30:419-427, 1991.

McDonald JF, Pruzansky JD and Meltzer RM: Evaluation of recurrent macrodactyly with three-dimensional imaging, J Am Podiatr Med Assoc 81:84-87, 1991.

Patel DV, Ferris BD and Aichroth PM: Radiological study of alignment after total knee replacement. Short radiographs or long radiographs? Int Orthop 15:209-210, 1991.

Pearse MF, Fowler JL and Bracey DJ: Fracture of the body of the talus, Injury 22:155-156, 1991.

Rafert JA and Long BW: Showing acetabular trauma with more clarity, less pain, Radiol Technol 63:92-97, 1991.

Rijke AM et al: Graded stress radiography of injured anterior cruciate ligaments, Invest Radiol 26:926-933, 1991.

Santi M and Sartoris DJ: Diagnostic imaging approach to stress fractures of the foot, J Foot Surg 30:85-97, 1991.

Urman M et al: The role of bone scintigraphy in the evaluation of talar dome fractures, J Nucl Med 32:2241-2244, 1991.

Williamson S: A comparison of imaging techniques for leg lengthening osteotomies, Radiogr Today 57:20-21, 1991.

1992   Armstrong PF: Serious fractures and joint injuries involving the foot and ankle, Instr Course Lect 41:413-420, 1992.

Aspelin P et al: Ultrasound examination of soft tissue injury of the lower limb in athletes, Am J Sports Med 20:601-603, 1992.

Bailey MM and Michalski J: Close-up on calcaneal fracture, Nursing 22:57, 1992.

Bellon RJ and Horwitz SM: Three-dimensional computed tomography studies of the tendons of the foot and ankle, J Digit Imaging 5:46-49, 1992.

Bradley SA and Davies AM: Computed tomographic assessment of soft tissue abnormalities following calcaneal fractures, Br J Radiol 65:105-111, 1992.

Briggs TW, Orr MM and Lightowler CD: Isolated tibial fractures in children, Injury 23:308-310, 1992.

Burton PD and Page BJ II: Fracture of the neck of the talus associated with a trimalleolar ankle fracture and ruptured tibialis posterior tendon, J Orthop Trauma 6:248-251, 1992.

Downey DJ, Drennan JC and Garcia JF: Magnetic resonance image findings in congenital talipes equinovarus, J Pediatr Orthop 12:224-228, 1992.

Ebraheim NA et al: Marginal fractures of the lateral malleolus in association with other fractures in the ankle region, Foot Ankle 13:171-175, 1992.

Grogan DP and Ogden JA: Knee and ankle injuries in children, Pediatr Rev 13:429-434, 1992.

Harcke HT et al: Growth plate of the normal knee: evaluation with MR imaging, Radiology 183:119-123, 1992.

Harper MC: Stress radiographs in the diagnosis of lateral instability of the ankle and hindfoot, Foot Ankle 13:435-438, 1992.

Herzog RJ: Imaging of the knee, Orthop Rev 21:1409-1417, 1992.

Janzen DL et al: Intra-articular fractures of the calcaneus: value of CT findings in determining prognosis, AJR 158:1271-1274, 1992.

Kneeland JB and Dalinka MK: Magnetic resonance imaging of the foot and ankle, Magn Reson Q 8:97-115, 1992.

Levy AS et al: Magnetic resonance imaging evaluation of calcaneal fat pads in patients with os calcis fractures, Foot Ankle 13:57-62, 1992.

Macaulay KE, Beim GM and Sartoris DJ: Classics in conventional radiography of the foot, J Foot Surg 31:519-526, 1992.

Martensen KM: Alternate AP knee method assures open joint space, Radiol Technol 64:19-23, 1992.

Mayer DP, et al: Magnetic resonance arthrography of the ankle, J Foot Surg 31:584-587, 1992.

Michelson JD et al: Examination of the pathologic anatomy of ankle fractures, J Trauma 32:65-70, 1992.

Milants WP et al: CT imaging of soft tissue pathology of the ankle. A pictorial essay, J Belge Radiol 75:410-415, 1992.

Munk PL et al: Current status of magnetic resonance imaging of the ankle and the hindfoot, Can Assoc Radiol J 43:19-30, 1992.

Nguyen VD: The radiologic spectrum of abnormalities of the foot in diabetic patients, Can Assoc Radiol J 43:333-339, 1992.

Plecha DM, Plecha FM and King TA: Invasive diagnostic imaging of the lower extremities, Clin Podiatr Med Surg 9:57-68, 1992.

Richardson ML et al: CT measurement of the calcaneal varus angle in the normal and fractured hindfoot, J Comput Assist Tomogr 16:261-264, 1992.

Riddervold HO: Easily missed fractures, Radiol Clin North Am 30:475-494, 1992.

Romash MM: Fracture of the calcaneus: an unusual fracture pattern with subtalar joint interposition of the flexor hallucis longus. A report of two cases, Foot Ankle 13:32-41, 1992.

Rosenberg ZS et al: Osgood-Schlatter lesion: fracture or tendinitis? Scintigraphic, CT, and MR imaging features, Radiology 185:853-858, 1992.

Sanders R: Intra-articular fractures of the calcaneus: present state of the art, J Orthop Trauma 6:252-265, 1992.

Sartoris DJ: Diagnostic imaging insight: cross-sectional imaging of the foot (computed tomography-magnetic resonance), J Foot Surg 31:190-202, 1992.

Shahabpour M et al: Magnetic resonance imaging (MRI) of the ankle and hindfoot, Acta Orthop Belg 58 (Suppl) 1:5-14, 1992.

Steiner GM and Sprigg A: The value of ultrasound in the assessment of bone, Br J Radiol 65:589-593, 1992.

Stiell IG et al: Use of radiography in acute ankle injuries: physicians' attitudes and practice, Can Med Assoc J 147:1671-1678, 1992.

Tehranzadeh J, Kerr R and Amster J: Magnetic resonance imaging of tendon and ligament abnormalities. Part II. Pelvis and lower extremities, Skeletal Radiol 21:79-86, 1992.

Watanabe H, Fujita S and Ika I: Polydactyly of the foot: an analysis of 265 cases and a morphological classification, Plast Reconstr Surg 89:856-877, 1992.

Wechsler RJ, Karasick D and Schweitzer ME: Computed tomography of talocalcaneal coalition: imaging techniques, Skeletal Radiol 21:353-358, 1992.

1993   Biedert R: Which investigations are required in stress fracture of the great toe sesamoids? Arch Orthop Trauma Surg 112:94-95, 1993.

Burdeaux BDJ: The medical approach for calcaneal fractures, Clin Orthop 96-107, 1993.

Christman RA and Zulli LP: Radiologic aspects of aging in the foot, Clin Podiatr Med Surg 10:97-112, 1993.

Erickson SJ and Rosengarten JL: MR imaging of the forefoot: normal anatomic findings, AJR 160:565-571, 1993.

Kier R: MR imaging of foot and ankle tumors, Magn Reson Imaging 11:149-162, 1993.

Klein MA and Spreitzer AM: MR imaging of the tarsal sinus and canal: normal anatomy, pathologic findings, and features of the sinus tarsi syndrome, Radiology 186:233-240, 1993.

Koval KJ and Sanders R: The radiologic evaluation of calcaneal fractures, Clin Orthop 41-46, 1993.

Martin SD et al: Stress fracture MRI, Orthopedics 16:75-78, 1993.

Okubo S, Lehtinen K, Isomaki H: Sensitivity of radiographic changes of hand and foot joints as a diagnostic criterion in patients with rheumatoid arthritis, Scand J Rheumatol 21:145-147, 1993.

Schenck RC Jr and Heckman JD: Injuries of the knee, Clin Symp 45:1-32, 1993.

Thometz JG and Simons GW: Deformity of the calcaneocuboid joint in patients who have talipes equinovarus, J Bone Joint Surg Am 75:190-195, 1993.

Winalski CS et al: Enhancement of joint fluid with intravenously administered gadopentetate dimeglumine: technique, rationale, and implications, Radiology 187:179-185, 1993.

Limbs (extremities): general

For bibliographic citations before 1964, please see the fifth edition of this atlas. For citations from 1964 through 1974, see the sixth or seventh edition.

1975 Genant HK, Doi K and Mall JC: Optical versus radiographic magnification for fine-detail skeletal radiography, Invest Radiol 10:160-172, 1975.

1976 Genant HK, Doi K and Mall JC: Comparison of non-screen techniques (medical vs. industrial film) for fine detail skeletal radiography, Invest Radiol 11:486-500, 1976.

1977 Genant HK et al: Direct radiographic magnification for skeletal radiology: an assessment of image quality and clinical application, Radiology 123:47-55, 1977.

Goodman DA, Wells CA and Weston PJ: An evaluation of some screen film combinations for use in radiography of the extremities, Radiography 43(515):253-255, 1977.

1978 Resnick D: Skeletal aches and pains, Radiol Clin North Am 16:37-47, 1978.

1979 Spencer JD and Hill ID: Imaging factors for xeroradiography of the extremities, Br J Radiol 52:51-55, 1979.

1980 Murray RO: Orthopaedic radiology: an expanding discipline, J R Soc Med 73:320-323, 1980.

1981 Bernardino ME et al: The extremity soft-tissue lesion: a comparative study of ultrasound, computed tomography, and xeroradiography, Radiology 139:53-59, 1981.

Paling MR: The computed tomography of normal long bone anatomy and its simulation of disease, CT 5:201-213, 1981.

1982 Brand DA et al: A protocol for selecting patients with injured extremities who need x-rays, N Engl J Med 306:333-339, 1982.

Ekelund L, Herrlin K and Rydholm A: Comparison of computed tomography and angiography in the evaluation of soft tissue tumors of the extremities, Acta Radiol 23:15-27, 1982.

Soye I et al: Computed tomography in the preoperative evaluation of masses arising in or near the joints of extremities, Radiology 143:727-732, 1982.

Yeh HC and Rabinowitz JG: Ultrasonography of the extremities and pelvic girdle and correlation with computed tomography, Radiology 143:519-525, 1982.

1983 Whittaker LR: More active participation by radiographers in the radiography of trauma, Radiography 49:125-129, 1983.

1984 Firooznia H et al: Computed tomography in localization of foreign bodies lodged in the extremities, Comput Radiol 8:237-239, 1984.

Heiken JP et al: CT of benign soft-tissue masses of the extremities, AJR 142:575-580, 1984.

Hermann G, Yeh HC and Schwartz I: Computed tomography of soft-tissue lesions of the extremities, pelvic and shoulder girdles: sonographic and pathological correlations, Clin Radiol 35:193-202, 1984.

1985 McCorkell SJ et al: Indications for angiography in extremity trauma, AJR 145:1245-1247, 1985.

1987 Charny MC et al: Can the use of radiography of arms and legs in accident and emergency units be made more efficient? Br Med J [clin res] 294:291-293, 1987.

Fodor J and Malott JC: Magnification radiography, Radiol Technol 58:313-319, 1987.

Goldberg I and Nathan H: Anatomy and pathology of the sesamoid bones. The hand compared to the foot, Int Orthop 11:141-147, 1987.

Gratale P, Burns CB and Murray J: Advantages of a 400 speed image receptor system for cast radiography, Radiol Technol 58:401-403, 1987.

1988 Oloff-Solomon J and Solomon MA: Special radiographic techniques in the evaluation of arthritic disease, Clin Podiatr Med Surg 5:25-36, 1988.

1990 Radiographic imaging in orthopedics, Orthop Clin North Am 21:405-624, 1990.

Brower AC: Use of the radiograph to measure the course of rheumatoid arthritis. The gold standard versus fool's gold, Arthritis Rheum 33:316-324, 1990.

Gratale P, Wright DL and Daughtry L: Using the anode heel effect for extremity radiography, Radiol Technol 61:195-198, 1990.

Jones R and Adler AM: The saline solution bag as a compensating filter, Radiol Technol 62:134-138, 1990.

1991 Banerjee B and Das RK: Sonographic detection of foreign bodies of the extremities, Br J Radiol 64:107-112, 1991.

Ledesma-Medina J, Bender TM and Oh KS: Radiographic manifestations of anomalies of the limbs, Radiol Clin North Am 29:383-405, 1991.

Mandell GA, Harcke HT and Kumar SJ: Congenital disorders of the extremities, Top Magn Reson Imaging 4:1-20, 1991.

Mandell GA, Harcke HT and Kumar SJ: Developmental disorders of the extremities, Top Magn Reson Imaging 4:21-30, 1991.

Minami M et al: MR study of normal joint function using a low field strength system, J Comput Assist Tomogr 15:1017-1023, 1991.

1992 Buckwalter KA and Braunstein EM: Digital skeletal radiography, AJR 158:1071-1080, 1992.

Davies AM and Wellings RM: Imaging of bone tumors, Curr Opin Radiol 4:32-38, 1992.

Edeiken-Monroe BS and Edeiken J: Imaging of the normal spine, developmental anomalies, and trauma of the spine and extremities, Curr Opin Radiol 4:95-102, 1992.

Ney DR et al: Comparison of helical and serial CT with regard to three-dimensional imaging of musculoskeletal anatomy, Radiology 185:865-869, 1992.

Oestreich AE: Imaging of the skeleton and soft tissues in children, Curr Opin Radiol 4:55-61, 1992.

Pope CF: Radiologic evaluation of tendon injuries, Clin Sports Med 11:579-599, 1992.

1993 Hughes TH, Maffulli N and Fixsen JA: Ultrasonographic appearance of regenerate bone in limb lengthening, J R Soc Med 86:18-20, 1993.

Leventhal JM et al: Fractures in young children. Distinguishing child abuse from unintentional injuries, Am J Dis Child 147:87-92, 1993.

Malloy PC, Scott WW Jr and Hruban RH: Case report 769. Fibrous dysplasia, Skeletal Radiol 22:66-69, 1993.

McLennan MK and Margolis M: Radiology rounds. Fibrous dysplasia, Can Fam Physician Med Fam Can 39:29, 217, 1993.

Quirk R: Stress fractures, Aust Fam Physician 22:300-304, 307, 1993.

Zerin JM and Hernandez RJ: Approach to skeletal maturation, Hand Clin 7:53-62, 1993.

Long bone measurement

For bibliographic citations before 1964, please see the fifth edition of this atlas. For citations from 1964 through 1974, see the sixth or seventh edition.

1977 Gore DR et al: Roentgenographic measurement after Muller total hip replacement, J Bone Joint Surg 59:948-953, 1977.

Horsman A et al: Effect of rotation on radiographic dimensions of the humerus and femur, Br J Radiol 50:23-28, 1977.

1979 Ogata K and Goldsand EM: A simple, biplanar method of measuring femoral anteversion and neck-shaft angle, J Bone Joint Surg 61:846-851, 1979.

1980 Korbuly D, Moore R and Formanek A: Scanography with rotation of the radiographic tube: a new method, Radiology 135:495-499, 1980.

Scheuer JL, Musgrave JH and Evans SP: The estimation of late fetal and perinatal age from limb bone length by linear and logarithmic regression, Ann Hum Biol 7:257-265, 1980.

Strop MA and Moreland MS: A radiographic method of measuring axial rotation of bone in vivo, Med Res Eng 13:11-16, 1980.

Weiner DS and Cook AJ: Practical considerations in the use of computed tomography in the measurement of femoral anteversion, Ir J Med Sci 16:288-294, 1980.

1981 Burr DB et al: Measurement accuracy of proximal femoral geometry using biplanar radiography, J Pediatr Orthop 1:171-179, 1981.

1982 Moulton A and Upadhyay SS: A direct method of measuring femoral anteversion using ultrasound, J Bone Joint Surg 64-B:469-472, 1982.

Robinow M and Chumlea WC: Standards for limb bone length ratios in children, Radiology 143:433-436, 1982.

1987 Temme JB, Chu W and Anderson JC: CT scanograms compared with conventional orthoroentgenograms in long bone measurement, Radiol Technol 59(3):233-237, 1987.

Wilson AJ and Ramsby GR: Skeletal measurements using a flying spot digital imaging device, AJR 149:339-343, 1987.

1989 Blair V et al: Closed shortening of the femur, J Bone Joint Surg Am 71:1440-1447, 1989.

1991 Osterman K and Merikanto J: Diaphyseal bone lengthening in children using Wagner device: long term results, J Pediatr Orthop 11:449-451, 1991.

Williamson S: A comparison of imaging techniques for leg lengthening osteotomies, Radiogr Today 57:20-21, 1991.

1992 Aaron A et al: Comparison of orthoroentgenography and computed tomography in the measurement of limb-length discrepancy, J Bone Joint Surg Am 74:897-902, 1992.

Kane TJ, Henry G and Furry D: A simple roentgenographic measurement of femoral anteversion. A short note, J Bone Joint Surg Am 74:1540-1542, 1992.

Lee DY, Lee CK and Cho TJ: A new method for measurement of femoral anteversion. A comparative study with other radiographic methods, Int Orthop 16:277-281, 1992.

Steiner GM and Sprigg A: The value of ultrasound in the assessment of bone, Br J Radiol 65:589-593, 1992.

Tjernstrom B, Thoumas KA and Pech P: Bone remodeling after leg lengthening: evaluation with plain radiographs, and computed tomography and magnetic resonance imaging scans, J Pediatr Orthop 12:751-755, 1992.

1993 Ensley NJ, Green NE and Barnes WP: Femoral lengthening with the Barnes device, J Pediatr Orthop 13:57-62, 1993.

Hughes TH, Maffulli N and Fixsen JA: Ultrasonographic appearance of regenerate bone in limb lengthening, J R Soc Med 86:18-20, 1993.

Arthrography, contrast

For bibliographic citations before 1964, please see the fifth edition of this atlas. For citations from 1964 through 1974, see the sixth or seventh edition.

1975 Clark JM: Arthrography in the diagnosis of synovial cysts of the knee, Radiology 115:480-481, 1975.

Eto RT, Anderson PW and Harley JD: Elbow arthrography with the application of tomography, Radiology 115:283-288, 1975.

Neviaser JS: Arthrography of the shoulder, Springfield, Ill, 1975, Charles C Thomas Publisher.

Wershba M et al: Double contrast knee arthrography in the evaluation of osteochondritis dissecans, Clin Orthop 107:81-86, 1975.

1976 Katzberg RW, Burgener PA and Fischer HW: Evaluation of various contrast agents for arthrography, Invest Radiol 11:528-533, 1976.

Wilson ES: Positive contrast shoulder arthrography, J Med Soc NJ 73:933-938, 1976.

1977 Dalinka MK: A simple aid to the performance of shoulder arthrography, AJR 129:942, 1977.

Dirkheimer Y, Ramsheyi A and Reolon M: Positive arthrography of the craniocervical joints, Neuroradiology 12:257-260, 1977.

1978 Lee KR and Sanders WF: A practical stress device for knee arthrography, Radiology 127:542, 1978.

Lindholmer E, Foged N and Jensen JT: Arthrography of the ankle: value in diagnosis of rupture of the lateral ligaments, Acta Radiol 19:585-598, 1978.

Spataro RF et al: Evaluation of epinephrine for arthrography, Invest Radiol 13:286-390, 1978.

1979 Katzberg RW et al: Arthrotomography of the temporomandibular joint: new technique and preliminary observations, AJR 132:949-955, 1979.

Pavlov H, Ghelman B and Warren RF: Double-contrast arthrography of the elbow, Radiology 130:87-95, 1979.

Silverbach S: Simple method for marking knee arthrograms, AJR 133:155, 1979.

Ward MD: Fluoroscopic technique for double contrast knee arthrography, Radiol Technol 50:675-681, 1979.

1980 Arida EJ and Mooken TT: Arthrography of the knee using remote-control fluororadiography, AJR 135:1295-1297, 1980.

Baird M: Double contrast arthrography of the knee, Radiography 46:206-208, 1980.

Blaschke DD, Solberg WK and Sanders B: Arthrography of the temporomandibular joint: review of current status, J Am Dent Assoc 100:388-395, 1980.

Dalinka MK, editor: Arthrography, New York, 1980, Springer-Verlag New York, Inc.

Frede TE and Lee JK: The "overturned lateral" view in arthrography of the knee, Radiology 134:249-250, 1980.

Freiberger RH and Kaye JJ: Arthrography, New York, 1980, Appleton-Century-Crofts.

Garcia JF: Arthrography, Curr Probl Diagn Radiol 9:1-37, 1980.

Goldman AB: Arthrography of the hip joint, CRC Crit Rev Diagn Imaging 13:111-171, 1980.

Mink JH and Dickerson R: Air or CO_2.MDNM/ for knee arthrography? AJR 134:991-993, 1980.

Neviaser TJ: Arthrography of the shoulder, Orthop Clin North Am 11:205-217, 1980.

Rosenthal D, Murray WT and Smith RJ: Finger arthrography, Radiology 137:647-651, 1980.

Watt I and Tasker T: Pitfalls in double contrast knee arthrography, Br J Radiol 53:754-759, 1980.

1981 Wrist arthrography, Radiol Clin North Am 19:217-226, 1981.

Farren J: Double contrast shoulder arthrography, Radiography 47:159-161, 1981.

Franji SM: New radiographic technique utilizing arthrotomography for studying shoulder derangements, Radiol Technol 52:384, 1981.

Goldberg RP, Hall FM and Wyshak G: Pain in knee arthrography: comparison of air vs CO_2.MDNM/ and reaspiration vs no reaspiration, AJR 136:377-379, 1981.

Hall FM: Methodology in knee arthrography, Radiol Clin North Am 19:269-275, 1981.

Hall FM et al: Morbidity from shoulder arthrography: etiology, incidence, and prevention, AJR 136:59-62, 1981.

Hudson TM: Elbow arthrography, Radiol Clin North Am 19:227-241, 1981.

Murphy WA: Arthrography of the temporomandibular joint, Radiol Clin North Am 19:365-378, 1981.

Olson RW: Ankle arthrography, Radiol Clin North Am 19:255-268, 1981.

Resnick D: Shoulder arthrography, Radiol Clin North Am 19:243-253, 1981.

Symposium on arthrography, Radiol Clin North Am 19:215-395, 1981.

Weissman BN: Arthrography in arthritis, Radiol Clin North Am 19:379-392, 1981.

1982 Braunstein EM and O'Connor G: Double-contrast arthrotomography of the shoulder, J Bone Joint Surg 64-A:192-195, 1982.

Crawford AH and Carothers TA: Hip arthrography in the skeletally immature, Clin Orthop 162:54-60, 1982.

Weaver JW: Stereoscopic spot filming in arthrography, AJR 138:172-174, 1982.

1983 Campbell RL and Alexander JM: Temporomandibular joint arthrography: negative pressure, nontomographic techniques, Oral Surg Oral Med Oral Pathol 55:121-126, 1983.

Delinka MK et al: Arthrography of the wrist and shoulder, Orthop Clin North Am 14:193-215, 1983.

Doyle T: Arthrography of the temporomandibular joint: a simple technique, Clin Radiol 34:147-151, 1983.

Gilula LA, Totty WG and Weeks PM: Wrist arthrography: the value of fluoroscopic spot viewing, Radiology 146:555-556, 1983.

Laasonen EM and Lindholm A: Double contrast arthrography of the knee. Comparison between three contrast media, Acta Radiol 24:225-229, 1983.

Lindholmer E et al: Arthrography of the ankle. Value in diagnosis of rupture of the calcaneofibular ligament, Acta Radiol 24:217-223, 1983.

Palmer AK, Levinsohn EM and Kuzma GR: Arthrography of the wrist, J Hand Surg 8:15-23, 1983.

Salazar JE, Sebes JI and Scott RL: The supine view in double-contrast knee arthrography, AJR 141:585-586, 1983.

Tielbeck AV and van Horn JR: Double-contrast arthrography of the shoulder, Diagn. Imaging 52:154-162, 1983.

Westesson PL: Double-contrast arthrotomography of the temporomandibular joint: introduction of an arthrographic technique for visualization of the disk and articular surfaces, J Oral Maxillofac Surg 41:163-172, 1983.

1984 Ahovuo J: Single and double contrast arthrography in lesions of the glenohumeral joint, Eur J Radiol 4:237-240, 1984.

Doyle T: A simplified method for temporomandibular joint arthrography, Australas Radiol 28:12-15, 1984.

Fars-Nielsen F, deCarvalho A and Hjllund-Madsen E: Omnipaque and urografin in arthrography of the knee, Acta Radiol [diagn] (Stockh) 25:151-154, 1984.

Garcia JF: Arthrographic visualization of rotator cuff tears, Optimal Radiology 150:595-595, 1984.

1984 Kleinman PK et al: Axillary arthrotomography of the glenoid labrum, AJR 142:993-999, 1984.

Mekic ZD: Arthrography of the wrist joint: an experimental study, J Bone Joint Surg 66-A:371-378, 1984.

Thijn CJ and Hillen B: Arthrography and the medial compartment of the patellofemoral joint, Skeletal Radiol 11:183-190, 1984.

1985 Apple JS et al: A comparison of Hexabrix and Renografin-60 in knee arthrography, AJR 145:139-142, 1985.

Gasparini D et al: Shoulder arthrography, Rays 10:23-30, 1985.

Kaplan P et al: Temporomandibular joint arthrography of normal subjects: prevalence, Radiology 156:825-826, 1985.

Katzberg RW et al: Temporomandibular joint arthrography: comparison of morbidity with ionic and low osmolality contrast media, Radiology 155:245-246, 1985.

Mink JH, Harris E and Rappaport M: Rotator cuff tears: evaluation using double-contrast shoulder arthrography, Radiology 157:621-623, 1985.

Vezina JA and Beauregard CG: An update on the technique of double-contrast arthrotomography of the shoulder, J Can Assoc Radiol 36:176-182, 1985.

1986 Gillespy T III and Helms CA: Oblique head position in temporomandibular joint arthrography, Radiology 158:541-543, 1986.

Singson RD, Feldman F and Rosenberg ZS: Elbow joint: assessment with double-contrast CT arthrography, Radiology 160:167-173, 1986.

Willetts PG: Arthrography of the temporomandibular joint, Radiography 52:229-231, 1986.

1987 Fukuda H, Mikasa M and Yamanaka K: Incomplete thickness rotator cuff tears diagnosed by subacromial bursography, Clin Orthop 51-58, 1987.

Levinsohn EM et al: Wrist arthrography: the value of the three compartment injection, Skeletal Radiol 16:539-544, 1987.

Neviaser RJ: Radiologic assessment of the shoulder: plain and arthrographic, Orthop Clin North Am 18:343-349, 1987.

Reinus WR et al: Arthrographic evaluation of the carpal triangular fibrocartilage complex, J Hand Surg Am 12:495-503, 1987.

Westesson PL and Bronstein SL: Temporomandibular joint: comparison of single- and double-contrast, Radiology 164:65-70, 1987.

1988 Ahovuo J, Paavolainen P and Jaaskinen J: Arthrotomography of the unstable shoulder, Acta Orthop Scand 59:681-683, 1988.

Benhamou CL et al: Costo-vertebral arthropathy. Diagnostic and therapeutic value of arthrography, Clin Rheumatol 7:220-223, 1988.

Bonamo JJ and Shulman G: Double contrast arthrography of the knee. A comparison to clinical diagnosis and arthroscopic findings, Orthopedics 11:1041-1046, 1988.

Evancho AM et al: MR imaging diagnosis of rotator cuff tears, AJR 151:751-754, 1988.

Faithfull GR and Sonnabend DH: Computerised arthrotomography of the glenohumeral joint, Australas Radiol 32:111-116, 1988.

Freiberger RH and Pavlov H: Knee arthrography, Radiology 166:489-492, 1988.

Gilula LA, Hardy DC and Totty WG: Distal radioulnar joint arthrography, AJR 150:864-866, 1988.

Haller J et al: Arthrography, tenography, bursography of the ankle and foot, Clin Podiatr Med Surg 5:893-908, 1988.

Heffez L, Mafee MF and Langer B: Double-contrast arthrography of the temporomandibular joint, Oral Surg Oral Med Oral Pathol 65:511-514, 1988.

Karpman RR and MacCollum MS: Arthrography of the metatarsophalangeal joint, Foot Ankle 9:125-129, 1988.

Lott CW, Wilson DJ and Juniper RP: Temporomandibular joint arthrography: dynamic study by videorecording, Clin Radiol 39:73-76, 1988.

Paille P et al: Computed arthrography: its role in the screening of joint diseases in pediatric radiology, Pediatr Radiol 18:386-390, 1988.

Pittman CC et al: Digital subtraction wrist arthrography: use of double contrast technique as a supplement to single contrast arthrography, Skeletal Radiol 17:119-122, 1988.

Quinn SF et al: Digital subtraction wrist arthrography: evaluation of the multiple-compartment technique, AJR 151:1173-1174, 1988.

Reed DP and Heys J: Computerised arthrotomography of the shoulder joint, Radiography 54:49-51, 1988.

Stiles RG et al: Rotator cuff disruption: diagnosis with digital arthrography, Radiology 168:705-707, 1988.

Zinberg EM et al: The triple-injection wrist arthrogram, J Hand Surg 13:803-809, 1988.

1989 Conway WF and Hayes CW: Three-compartment wrist arthrography: use of a low-iodine-concentration contrast agent to decrease study time, Radiology 173:569-570, 1989.

Cook JV and Tayar R: Double-contrast computed tomographic arthrography of the shoulder joint, Br J Radiol 62:1043-1049, 1989.

Drummond DS et al: Arthrography in the evaluation of congenital dislocation of the hip, Clin Orthop 148-156, 1989.

Goossens M et al: Posterior subtalar joint arthrography. A useful tool in the diagnosis of hindfoot disorders, Clin Orthop 248-255, 1989.

Jones A and Watt I: Diagnostic imaging of the shoulder joint, Baillieres Clin Rheumatol 3:475-510, 1989.

Mespreuve M and Coenen L: Three-point arthrography of the wrist, Acta Orthop Belg 55:197-202, 1989.

Peh W and Hoe J: Using a curved cassette for the axial view in double contrast shoulder arthrography, Radiogr Today 55:26, 1989.

Schmidt M and Papassotiriou V: Arthrography with iotrolan: double-blind comparison between nonionic, monomeric (iohexol 300) and nonionic, dimeric (iotrolan 300) contrast media, Fortschr Geb Rontgenstr Nuklearmed Erganzungsbd 128:182-189, 1989.

Shigematsu S et al: Arthrography of the normal and posttraumatic wrist, J Hand Surg Am 14:410-412, 1989.

1990 Atar D et al: Intra-operative arthrography in open reduction of congenital hip dislocation, J Bone Joint Surg Br 72:526, 1990.

Belsole RJ et al: Digital subtraction arthrography of the wrist, J Bone Joint Surg Am 72:846-851, 1990.

Duvoisin B, Klaus E and Schnyder P: Coronal radiographs and videofluoroscopy improve the diagnostic quality of temporomandibular joint arthrography, AJR 155:105-107, 1990.

Ekstrom JE: Arthrography. Where does it fit in? Clin Sports Med 9:561-566, 1990.

Flannigan B et al: MR arthrography of the shoulder: comparison with conventional MR imaging, AJR 155:829-832, 1990.

Frahm R, Saul O and Mannerfelt L: Diagnostic applications of wrist arthrography, Arch Orthop Trauma Surg 109:39-42, 1990.

Gundry CR et al: Is MR better than arthrography for evaluating the ligaments of the wrist? In vitro study, AJR 54:337-341, 1990.

Helms CA and Kaplan P: Diagnostic imaging of the temporomandibular joint: recommendations for use of the various techniques, AJR 154:319-322, 1990.

Herbert TJ et al: Bilateral arthrography of the wrist, J Hand Surg Br 15:233-235, 1990.

Horsfield D and Phillips RR: The zero projection, Radiogr Today 56:14-16, 1990.

Hove B and Gyldensted C: Cervical analgesic facet joint arthrography, Neuroradiology 32:456-459, 1990.

Kaplan PA and Walker CW: Contrast radiology, Curr Opin Rheumatol 2:355-360, 1990.

Nance EP Jr and Powers TA: Imaging of the temporomandibular joint, Radiol Clin North Am 28:1019-1031, 1990.

Radiographic imaging in orthopedics, Orthop Clin North Am 21:405-624, 1990.

Scotter E and Ignotus P: Wrist arthrography, Radiogr Today 56:15-18, 1990.

Stoker DJ: Arthrography: time for reappraisal or the end of the road? Clin Radiol 41:371-372, 1990.

1991 Bradley SA and Chandy J: Air aspiration after double-contrast knee arthrography: a worthwhile exercise? Br J Radiol 64:796-797, 1991.

Burk DL Jr, Karasick D and Wechsler RJ: Imaging of the distal radioulnar joint, Hand Clin 7:263-275, 1991.

Davies AM: The current role of computed tomographic arthrography of the shoulder, Clin Radiol 44:369-375, 1991.

Dixon DC: Diagnostic imaging of the temporomandibular joint, Dent Clin North Am 35:53-74, 1991.

Huylebroek J et al: Correlation of computed arthrotomography with arthroscopy of the glenohumeral joint, Acta Orthop Belg 57:83-88, 1991.

Katzberg RW: Imaging of the temporomandibular joint, Curr Opin Dent 1:476-479, 1991.

Levinsohn EM, Rosen ID and Palmer AK: Wrist arthrography: value of the three-compartment injection method, Radiology 179:231-239, 1991.

Lupi L et al: Diagnostic potential of double contrast arthrography of the knee with the digital technique, Skeletal Radiol 20:5-8, 1991.

Manaster BJ: The clinical efficacy of triple-injection wrist arthrography, Radiology 178:267-270, 1991.

Mrose HE and Rosenthal DI: Arthrography of the hand and wrist, Hand Clin 7:201-217, 1991.

Reiskin AB: Digital subtraction arthrography, Cranio Clin Int 1:79-91, 1991.

Walker CW et al: Arthrography of painful hips following arthroplasty: digital versus plain film subtraction, Skeletal Radiol 20:403-407, 1991.

Westesson PL: Double contrast arthrography, Cranio Clin Int 1:53-77, 1991.

1992 Ando M, Gotoh E and Matsuura J: Tangential view arthrogram at closed reduction in congenital dislocation of the hip, J Pediatr Orthop 12:390-395, 1992.

Cicak N, Matasovic T and Bajraktarevic T: Ultrasonographic guidance of needle placement for shoulder arthrography, J Ultrasound Med 11:135-137, 1992.

Harcke HT: Imaging in congenital dislocation and dysplasia of the hip, Clin Orthop 22-28, 1992.

Jahnke AH Jr et al: A prospective comparison of computerized arthrotomography and magnetic resonance imaging of the glenohumeral joint, Am J Sports Med 20:695-700, 1992.

Jim YF et al: Shoulder impingement syndrome: impingement view and arthrography study based on 100 cases, Skeletal Radiol 21:449-451, 1992.

Mayer DP et al: Magnetic resonance arthrography of the ankle, J Foot Surg 31:584-587, 1992.

1993 Fransson SG: Wrist arthrography, Acta Radiol 34:111-116, 1993.

Snyder SJ: Evaluation and treatment of the rotator cuff, Orthop Clin North Am 24:173-192, 1993.

Winalski CS et al: Enhancement of joint fluid with intravenously administered gadopentetate dimeglumine: technique, rationale, and implications, Radiology 187:179-185, 1993.

Shoulder girdle

For bibliographic citations before 1964, please see the fifth edition of this atlas. For citations from 1964 through 1974, see the sixth or seventh edition.

1975 Protass JJ, Stampfli FV and Osmer JC: Coracoid process fracture diagnosis in acromioclavicular separation, Radiology 116:61-64, 1975.

Reichmann S et al: Soft tissue xeroradiography of the shoulder joint, Acta Radiol 16:572-576, 1975.

1976 Wilson ES: Positive contrast shoulder arthrography, J Med Soc NJ 73:993-938, 1976.

1978 Froimson AI: Fracture of the coracoid process of the scapula, J Bone Joint Surg 60:710-711, 1978.

Pavlov H and Freiberger RH: Fractures and dislocations about the shoulder, Semin Roentgenol 13:85-96, 1978.

1979 Cockshott WP: The coracoclavicular joint, Radiology 131:313-316, 1979.

Slivka J and Resnick D: An improved radiographic view of the glenohumeral joint, J Can Assoc Radiol 30:83-85, 1979.

1980 DeSmet AA: Anterior oblique projection in radiography of the traumatized shoulder, AJR 134:515-518, 1980.

DeSmet AA: Axillary projection in radiography of the non-traumatized shoulder, AJR 134:511-514, 1980.

Franji SM and El-Khoury GY: A new radiographic technique utilizing multidirectional tomography with double contrast arthrography for studying the glenoidal labrum, Radiol Technol 52:143-147, 1980.

Horsfield D and Renton P: The "other view" in the radiography of shoulder trauma, Radiography 46:213-214, 1980.

McGahan JP, Rab GT and Dublin A: Fractures of the scapula, J Trauma 20:880-883, 1980.

Neviaser RJ: Anatomic considerations and examination of the shoulder, Orthop Clin North Am 11(2):187-195, 1980.

Neviaser RJ: Arthrography of the shoulder, Orthop Clin North Am 11(2):205-217, 1980.

1981 Brandt TL and LeClair RG: A tangential projection or a lateral view of the scapula, Radiol Technol 52:631-634, 1981.

Fagerlund M and Ahlgren O: Axial projection of the humeroscapular joint, Acta Radiol 22:203-205, 1981.

Farren J: Double contrast shoulder arthrography, Radiography 47:159-161, 1981.

1982 Danzig L, Resnick D and Greenway G: Evaluation of unstable shoulders by computed tomography, a preliminary study, Am J Sports Med 10:138-141, 1982.

Greenway GD et al: The painful shoulder, Med Radiogr Photogr 58:21-67, 1982.

Heberling F and Bickel W: Performing shoulder arthrography without image converters in the field of orthopedic accident surgery, Arch Orthop Trauma Surg 100:123-126, 1982.

Lamm CR, Zachrisson BE and Korner L: Radiography of the shoulder after Bristow repair, Acta Radiol [diagn] (Stockh) 23:523-528, 1982.

Lie S and Mast WA: Subacromial bursography: technical and clinical application, Radiology 144:626-630, 1982.

Nussbaum AJ and Doppman JL: Shoulder arthropathy in primary hyperparathyroidism, Skeletal Radiol 9:98-102, 1982.

1983 Dalinka MK et al: Arthrography of the wrist and shoulder, Orthop Clin North Am 14:193-215, 1983.

Flinn RM et al: Optimal radiography of the acutely injured shoulder, J Can Assoc Radiol 34:128-132, 1983.

Goldberg RP and Vicks B: Oblique angled view for coracoid fracture, Skeletal Radiol 9:195-197, 1983.

Kahan A, Amor B and Benhamou CL: Rapidly progressive idiopathic chondrolysis simulating tuberculosis of the shoulder, J Rheumatol 10:291-293, 1983.

Kilcoyne RF and Matsen FA III: Rotator cuff tear measurement by arthropneumotomography, AJR 140:315-318, 1983.

Kinnard P et al: Assessment of the unstable shoulder by computed arthrography, Am J Sports Med 11:157-159, 1983.

Miller KD and Moore ME: Tuberculous arthritis of the shoulder: delayed diagnosis aided, Clin Rheumatol 2:61-64, 1983.

Paavolainen P et al: Surgical treatment of acromioclavicular dislocation: a review, Injury 14:415-420, 1983.

Petersson CJ and Redlund-Johnell I: Radiographic joint space in normal acromioclavicular joints, Acta Orthop Scand 54:431-433, 1983.

Petersson CJ and Redlund-Johnell I: Joint space in normal gleno-humeral radiographs, Acta Orthop Scand 54:274-276, 1983.

Quinn SF and Glass TA: Posttraumatic osteolysis of the clavicle, South Med J 76:307-308, 1983.

Resnick D: Shoulder pain, Orthop Clin North Am 14:81-97, 1983.

Shuman WP et al: Double-contrast computed tomography of the glenoid labrum, AJR 141:581-584, 1983.

Tielbeek AV and van Horn JR: Double-contrast arthrography of the shoulder, Diagn Imaging 52:154-162, 1983.

Wallace WA and Hellier M: Improving radiographs of the injured shoulder, Radiography 49:229-233, 1983.

Wing PC and Tredwell SJ: The weight-bearing shoulder, Paraplegia 21:107-113, 1983.

1984 Adler H and Lohmann B: The stability of the shoulder joint in stress radiography, Arch Orthop Trauma 103:83-4, 1984.

Ahovuo J, Paavolainen P and Slatis P: The diagnostic value of arthrography and plain radiography in rotator cuff tears, Acta Orthop Scand 55:220-223, 1984.

Cofield RH and Simonet WT: The shoulder in sports, Mayo Clin Proc 59:157-164, 1984.

Cone RO and Resnick D: Degenerative disease of the shoulder, Australas Radiol 28:232-239, 1984.

Cone RO III, Resnick D and Danzig L: Shoulder impingement syndrome: radiographic evaluation, Radiology 159:29-33, 1984.

Dorwart RH et al: Pigmented villonodular synovitis of the shoulder: radiologic-pathologic assessment, AJR 143:886-888, 1984.

Fodor J III and Malott JC: The radiographic evaluation of the dislocated shoulder, Radiol Technol 55:154-160, 1984.

Garcia JF: Arthrographic visualization of rotator cuff tears: optimal application of stress to the shoulder, Radiology 150: 595-595, 1984.

Garth WP Jr, Slappey CE and Ochs CW: Roentgenographic demonstration of instability of the shoulder, J Bone Joint Surg 66-A:1450-1453, 1984.

Hakuno A et al: Arthrographic findings in hemiplegic shoulders, Arch Phys Med Rehabil 65:706-711, 1984.

Kinnard P et al: Computerized arthrotomography in recurring shoulder, Can J Surg 27:487-488, 1984.

Kleinman PK et al: Axillary arthrotomography of the glenoid labrum, AJR 142:993-999, 1984.

Petersson CJ and Redlund-Johnell I: The subacromial space in normal shoulder radiographs, Acta Orthop Scand 55:57-58, 1984.

Resnik CS et al: Intra-articular pressure determination during glenohumeral joint arthrography, Invest Radiol 19:45-50, 1984.

Rizk TE et al: Arthrographic studies in painful hemiplegic shoulders, Arch Phys Med Rehabil 65:254-256, 1984.

Szalay EA and Rockwood CA Jr: Injuries of the shoulder and arm, Emerg Med Clin North Am 2:279-294, 1984.

1985 Deutsch AL, Resnick D and Mink JH: Computed tomography of the glenohumeral and sternoclavicular joints, Orthop Clin North Am 16:497-511, 1985.

Gasparini D et al: Shoulder arthrography, Rays 10:23-30, 1985.

Gould R, Rosenfield AT and Friedlaender GE: Loose body within the glenohumeral joint in recurrent anterior dislocation: CT demonstration, J Comput Assist Tomogr 9:404-406, 1985.

Hall FM et al: Shoulder arthrography: comparison of morbidity after use of various contrast media, Radiology 154:339-341, 1985.

Lahde S and Putkonen M: Positioning of the painful patient for the axial view of the shoulder, Rontgenblatter 38:380-382, 1985.

Mink JH, Harris E and Rappaport M: Rotator cuff tears: evaluation using double-contrast shoulder arthrography, Radiology 157:621-623, 1985.

Pavlov H et al: The roentgenographic evaluation of anterior shoulder, Clin Orthop 153-158, 1985.

Post M: Current concepts in the diagnosis and management of acromioclavicular dislocations. Clin Orthop 234-247, 1985.

Tallroth K and Vankka E: Iohexol and meglumine iothalamate in shoulder arthrography: a double-blind investigation, Acta Radiol [diagn] (Stockh) 26:1985.

Vandekerckhove B, van Meirhaeghe J and van Steenkiste M: Surgical treatment of acromioclavicular dislocations, Acta Orthop Belg 51:66-79, 1985.

1986 Beltran J et al: Rotator cuff lesions of the shoulder: evaluation by direct sagittal CT arthrography, Radiology 160:161-165, 1986.

Calvert PT et al: Arthrography of the shoulder after operative repair of the torn rotator cuff, J Bone Joint Surg 68-B:147-150, 1986.

Feldman F: The radiology of total shoulder prostheses, Semin Roentgenol 21:47-65, 1986.

Rozing PM, de Bakker HM and Obermann WR: Radiographic views in recurrent anterior shoulder dislocation: comparison of six methods for identification of typical lesions, Acta Orthop Scand 57:328-330, 1986.

1987 Fukuda H, Mikasa M and Yamanaka K: Incomplete thickness rotator cuff tears diagnosed by subacromial bursography, Clin Orthop 51-58, 1987.

Gerber C et al: The subcoracoid space. An anatomic study, Clin Orthop 132-138, 1987.

Gerber C and Rockwood CA Jr: Subcoracoid dislocation of the lateral end of the clavicle: a report of three cases, J Bone Joint Surg 69-A:924-927, 1987.

Horsfield D and Jones SN: A useful projection in radiography of the shoulder, J Bone Joint Surg 69-B: 338-338, 1987.

Morgan JP, Pool RR and Miyabayashi T: Primary degenerative joint disease of the shoulder in a colony, J Am Vet Med Assoc 190:531-540, 1987.

Newberg AH: The radiographic evaluation of shoulder and elbow pain in the athlete, Clin Sports Med 6:785-809, 1987.

Petersson CJ: The acromioclavicular joint in rheumatoid arthritis, Clin Orthop 86-93, 1987.

1988 Bossart PJ et al: Lack of efficacy of 'weighted' radiographs in diagnosing acute acromioclavicular separation, Ann Emerg Med 17:20-24, 1988.

Crass JR: Current concepts in the radiographic evaluation of the rotator cuff, CRC Crit Rev Diagn Imaging 28:23-73, 1988.

Ebraheim NA et al: Scapulothoracic dissociation, J Bone Joint Surg 70-B:428-432, 1988.

Evancho AM et al: MR imaging diagnosis of rotator cuff tears, AJR 151:751-754, 1988.

Faithfull GR and Sonnabend DH: Computerised arthrotomography of the glenohumeral joint, Acta Radiol 32:111-116, 1988.

Guttentag IJ and Rechtine GR: Fractures of the scapula. A review of the literature, Orthop Rev 17:147-158, 1988.

Harris RD and Harris JHJ: The prevalence and significance of missed scapular fractures in blunt chest trauma, AJR 151:747-750, 1988.

Horsfield D and Stutley J: The unstable shoulder—a problem solved, Radiography 54:74-76, 1988.

Keats TE and Pope TL Jr: The acromioclavicular joint: normal variation and the diagnosis of dislocation, Skeletal Radiol 17:159-162, 1988.

Kieft GJ et al: Rotator cuff impingement syndrome: MR imaging, Radiology 166:211-214, 1988.

Kirkland S et al: Chronic unreduced dislocations of the glenohumeral joint: imaging strategy and pathologic correlation, J Trauma 28:1622-1631, 1988.

Kneisl JS, Sweeney HJ and Paige ML: Correlation of pathology observed in double contrast arthrotomography and arthroscopy of the shoulder, Arthroscopy 4:21-24, 1988.

Maki NJ: Cineradiographic studies with shoulder instabilities, Am J Sports Med 16:362-364, 1988.

Putkonen M et al: The value of axial view in the radiography of shoulder girdle—experiences with a new modification of positioning, Rontgen-Blatter 41:158-62, 1988.

Rafii M et al: Computed tomography (CT) arthrography of shoulder, Am J Sports Med 16:352-361, 1988.

Reed DP and Heys J: Computerised arthrotomography of the shoulder joint, Radiography 54:49-51, 1988.

Seeger LL, Gold RH and Bassett LW: Shoulder instability: evaluation with MR imaging, Radiology 168:695-697, 1988.

Stiles RG et al: Rotator cuff disruption: diagnosis with digital arthrography, Radiology 168:705-707, 1988.

Thomas D and Moody A: The acromioclavicular joint: an alternative view, Radiography 54:119-120, 1988.

Treble NJ: Normal variations in radiographs of the clavicle: brief report, J Bone Joint Surg Br 70:490, 1988.

Zlatkin MB et al: Cross-sectional imaging of the capsular mechanism of the glenohumeral joint, AJR 150:151-158, 1988.

Zlatkin MB et al: The painful shoulder: MR imaging of the glenohumeral joint, J Comput Assist Tomogr 12:995-1001, 1988.

1989   Fronek J, Warren RF and Bowen M: Posterior subluxation of the glenohumeral joint, J Bone Joint Surg Am 71:205-216, 1989.

Jones A and Watt I: Diagnostic imaging of the shoulder joint, Baillieres Clin Rheumatol 3:475-510, 1989.

Kumar R et al: The clavicle: normal and abnormal, Radiographics 9:677-706, 1989.

Zlatkin MB and Dalinka MK: The glenohumeral joint, Top Magn Reson Imaging 1:1-13, 1989.

1990   Hamada K et al: Roentgenographic findings in massive rotator cuff tears. A long-term observation, Clin Orthop 92-96, 1990.

Horsfield D and Phillips RR: The zero projection, Radiogr Today 56:14-16, 1990.

Martin-Herrero T et al: Fractures of the coracoid process: presentation of seven cases and review of the literature, J Trauma 30:1597-1599, 1990.

Rafert JA et al: Axillary shoulder with exaggerated rotation: the Hill-Sachs defect, Radiol Technol 62:18-21, 1990.

1991   Chan TW et al: Biceps tendon dislocation: evaluation with MR imaging, Radiology 179:649-652, 1991.

Collins JD et al: Anatomy of the thorax and shoulder girdle displayed by magnetic resonance imaging, J Natl Med Assoc 83:26-32, 1991.

Davies AM: The current role of computed tomographic arthrography of the shoulder, Clin Radiol 44:369-375, 1991.

Garneau RA: Glenoid labrum: evaluation with MR imaging, Radiology 179:519-522, 1991.

Levinsohn EM and Santelli ED: Bicipital groove dysplasia and medial dislocation of the biceps brachii tendon, Skeletal Radiol 20:419-423, 1991.

Neustadter LM and Weiss MJ: Trauma to the shoulder girdle, Semin Roentgenol 26:331-343, 1991.

Nguyer V, Williams G and Rockwood C: Radiography of acromioclavicular dislocation and associated injuries, Crit Rev Diagn Imaging 32:191-228, 1991.

Riemer BL et al: The abduction lordotic view of the clavicle: a new technique for radiographic visualization, J Orthop Trauma 5:392-394, 1991.

Vaatainen U, Pirinen A and Makela A: Radiological evaluation of the acromioclavicular joint, Skeletal Radiol 20:115-116, 1991.

Vellet AD, Munk PL and Marks P: Imaging techniques of the shoulder: present perspectives, Clin Sports Med 10:721-756, 1991.

Weinberg B, Seife B and Alonso P: The apical oblique view of the clavicle: its usefulness in neonatal and childhood trauma, Skeletal Radiol 20:201-203, 1991.

1992   Bannister GC et al: A classification of acute acromioclavicular dislocation: a clinical, radiological and anatomical study, Injury 23:194-196, 1992.

Cockshott WP: The geography of coracoclavicular joints, Skeletal Radiol 21:225-227, 1992.

Coumas JM et al: CT and MR evaluation of the labral capsular ligamentous complex of the shoulder, AJR 158:591-597, 1992.

Gudinchet F et al: Magnetic resonance imaging of nontraumatic shoulder instability in children, Skeletal Radiol 21:19-21, 1992.

Harvey RA, Trabulsy ME and Roe L: Are postreduction anteroposterior and scapular Y views useful in anterior shoulder dislocations, Am J Emerg Med 10:149-151, 1992.

Jahnke AH Jr et al: A prospective comparison of computerized arthrotomography and magnetic resonance imaging of the glenohumeral joint, Am J Sports Med 20:695-700, 1992.

Jalovaara P, Myllyla V and Paivansalo M: Autotraction stress roentgenography for demonstration of anterior and inferior instability of the shoulder joint, Clin Orthop 136-143, 1992.

Jim YF et al: Shoulder impingement syndrome: impingement view and arthrography study based on 100 cases, Skeletal Radiol 21:449-451, 1992.

Kaplan PA et al: MR imaging of the normal shoulder: variants and pitfalls, Radiology 184:519-524, 1992.

Mallon WJ et al: Radiographic and geometric anatomy of the scapula, Clin Orthop 142-154, 1992.

Olive JR Jr and Marsh HO: Ultrasonography of rotator cuff tears, Clin Orthop 110-113, 1992.

Papilion JA and Shall LM: Fluoroscopic evaluation for subtle shoulder instability, Am J Sports Med 20:548-552, 1992.

Riddervold HO: Easily missed fractures, Radiol Clin North Am 30:475-494, 1992.

Stenlund B, Goldie I and Marions O: Diminished space in the acromioclavicular joint in forced arm adduction as a radiographic sign of degeneration and osteoarthrosis, Skeletal Radiol 21:529-533, 1992.

Vahlensieck M, Resendes M and Genant HK: MRI of the shoulder, Bildgebung 59:123-132, 1992.

Vecchio PC et al: Thermography of frozen shoulder and rotator cuff tendinitis, Clin Rheumatol 11:382-384, 1992.

Workman TL et al: Hill-Sachs lesion: comparison of detection with MR imaging, radiography, and arthroscopy, Radiology 185:847-852, 1992.

1993   Snyder SJ: Evaluation and treatment of the rotator cuff, Orthop Clin North Am 24:173-192, 1993.

Bony thorax
Sternum

For bibliographic citations before 1964, please see the fifth edition of this atlas.

1981   Destouet JM et al: Computed tomography of the sternoclavicular joint and sternum, Radiology 138:123-128, 1981.

Sanders RC and Knight RW: Radiological appearances of the xyphoid process presenting as an upper abdominal mass, Radiology 141:489-490, 1981.

1982   Markowitz RI: The radiographic recognition of sternal retraction in infants, Clin Radiol 33:307-311, 1982.

1983   Goodman LR, Teplick SK and Kay H: Computed tomography of the normal sternum, AJR 141:219-223, 1983.

Scher AT: Associated sternal and spinal fractures: case reports, S Afr Med J 64:98-100, 1983.

Sebes JI, and Salazar JE: The manubriosternal joint in rheumatoid disease, AJR 140:117-121, 1983.

1984   Hatfield MK et al: Computed tomography of the sternum and its articulations, Skeletal Radiol 11:197-203, 1984.

1987   Stark P: Computed tomography of the sternum, CRC Crit Rev Diagn Imaging 27:321-349, 1987.

1988   Arnold M and Mills P: The oblique sternum: an alternative projection, Radiography 54:159-161, 1988.

Cooper KL: Insufficiency fractures of the sternum: a consequence of thoracic kyphosis? Radiology 167:471-472, 1988.

Moore TF: An alternative to the standard radiographic position for the sternum, Radiol Technol 60:133-134, 1988.

Nicholson AA, Holt ME and Jessop JD: Dislocation of the manubriosternal joint: detection on frontal chest radiographs, Br J Radiol 61:643-645, 1988.

Bibliography

1989   Ward CS, Halpin SF and Wilson AG: The posteroanterior chest radiograph in depressed sternum, Clin Radiol 40:139-143, 1989.

1992   Kai CH et al: Pulmonary scintigraphic findings in children with pectus excavatum by the comparison of chest radiograph indices, Clin Nucl Med 17:874-876, 1992.

Lee JD, Kim SM and Park CH: Tc-99m MIBI uptake in the sternum, Clin Nucl Med 17:819, 1992.

Sternoclavicular articulation

For bibliographic citations before 1964, please see the fifth edition of this atlas. For citations from 1964 through 1974, see the sixth or seventh edition.

1975   Morag B and Shahin N: The value of tomography of the sterno-clavicular region, Clin Radiol 26:57-62, 1975.

1979   Abel MS: Symmetrical anteroposterior projections of the sternoclavicular joints with motion studies, Radiology 132:757-759, 1979.

Levinsohn EM, Bunnell WP and Yuan HA: Computed tomography in the diagnosis of dislocations of the sternoclavicular joint, Clin Orthop 140:12-16, 1979.

1980   Lourie JA: Tomography in the diagnosis of posterior dislocation of the sterno-clavicular joint, Acta Orthop Scand 51:579-580, 1980.

Resnick D: Sternoclavicular hyperostosis, AJR 135:1278-1280, 1980.

1981   Destouet JM et al: Computed tomography of the sternoclavicular joint and sternum, Radiology 138:123-128, 1981.

1983   Hermann G, Rothenberg RR and Spiera H: The value of tomography in diagnosing infection of the sternoclavicular joint, Mt Sinai J Med 50:52-55, 1983.

1985   Deutsch AL, Resnick D and Mink JH: Computed tomography of the glenohumeral and sternoclavicular joints, Orthop Clin North Am 16:497-511, 1985.

1989   Leighton D, Oudjhane K and Ben-Mohammed H: The sternoclavicular joint in trauma: retrosternal dislocation versus epiphyseal fracture, Pediatr Radiol 20:126-127, 1989.

1992   van Holsbeeck M et al: Radiographic findings of spontaneous subluxation of the sternoclavicular joint, Clin Rheumatol 11:376-381, 1992.

Ribs

For bibliographic citations before 1964, please refer to the fifth edition of this atlas. For citations from 1964 through 1974, see the sixth or seventh edition.

1980   Brown TS: Tuberculosis of the ribs, Clin Radiol 31:681-684, 1980.

Christensen EE and Dietz GW: Injuries of the first costovertebral articulation, Radiology 134:41-43, 1980.

Kattan KR: What to look for in rib fractures and how, JAMA 243:262-264, 1980.

Paling MR and Dwyer A: The first rib as the cause of a "pulmonary nodule" on chest computed tomography, J Comput Assist Tomogr 4:847-848, 1980.

1981   Dixon AK and Wylie IG: Rib artifact in computed tomography, Br J Radiol 54:78-79, 1981.

McKendry RJ and Hogan DB: Superior margin rib defects in rheumatoid arthritis, J Rheumatol 8:673-678, 1981.

1982   DeLuca SA, Rhea JT and O'Malley T: Radiologic evaluation of rib fractures, AJR 138:91-92, 1982.

1983   Dwivedi SC and Varma AN: Bilateral fracture of the first ribs, J Trauma 23:538, 1983.

1989   Poole GV: Fracture of the upper ribs and injury to the great vessels, Surg Gynecol Obstet 169:275-282, 1989.

1991   Sanada S, Doi K and MacMahon H: Image feature analysis and computer-aided diagnosis in digital radiography: automated delineation of posterior ribs in chest images, Med Phys 18:964-971, 1991.

1992   Edwards PR, Moody AP and Harris PL: First rib abnormalities in association with cervical ribs: a cause for postoperative failure in the thoracic outlet syndrome, Eur J Vasc Surg 6:677-681, 1992.

Mehta MH et al: Congenital absence of ribs, Indian Pediatr 29:1149-1152, 1992.

1993   Faro SH, Mahboubi S and Ortega W: CT diagnosis of rib anomalies, tumors, and infection in children, Clin Imaging 17:1-7, 1993.

Malloy PC, Scott WW Jr and Hruban RH: Case report 769. Fibrous dysplasia, Skeletal Radiol 22:66-69, 1993.

McLennan MK and Margolis M: Radiology rounds. Fibrous dysplasia, Can Fam Physician Med Fam Can 39:29, 217, 1993.

Thorax: general

1980   Carilli AD et al: Clinical usefulness of computerized tomography of the thorax, J Med Soc NJ 77:883-888, 1980.

Veiga-Pires JA and Kaiser MC: Preliminary report on a new mode of CT-scanning of the thorax, CT 4:139-143, 1980.

1981   de Gautard R et al: Contribution of CT in thoracic bony lesions, J Can Assoc Radiol 32:39-41, 1981.

Heitzman ER: Fleischner Lecture. Computed tomography of the thorax: current perspectives AJR 136:2-12, 1981.

Pugatch RD and Faling LJ: Computed tomography of the thorax: a status report, Chest 80:618-626, 1981.

Shin MS, Ho KJ and Witten DM: Application of computed tomography in differential diagnosis of radiographic opacities in the lower thorax and upper abdomen, CT 5:519-528, 1981.

1982   Munro CJ: Computerized tomography of the thorax, Radiography 48:95-101, 1982.

Sones PJ Jr et al: Effectiveness of CT in evaluating intrathoracic masses, AJR 139:469-475, 1982.

Spiro SG et al: Computed tomography of the thorax in the diagnosis and management of malignant disease, Br J Dis Chest 76:209-222, 1982.

1983   Brown LR and Muhm JR: Computed tomography of the thorax: current perspectives, Chest 83:806-813, 1983.

Scholten ET: Computed multiplanar reconstructions of the thorax using thin transverse-axial slices: a preliminary study, Eur J Radiol 3:85-91, 1983.

Webb WR: Advances in computed tomography of the thorax, Radiol Clin North Am 21:723-739, 1983.

1984   Brasch RC et al: Magnetic resonance imaging of the thorax in childhood: work in progress, Radiology 150:463-467, 1984.

Strickland B: Computed tomography of the thorax, Postgrad Med J 60:208-212, 1984.

1988   Batra P et al: MR imaging of the thorax: a comparison of axial, coronal, and sagittal imaging planes, J Comput Assist Tomogr 12:75-81, 1988.

Edwards DK, Berry CC and Hilton SW: Trisomy 21 in newborn infants: chest radiographic diagnosis, Radiology 167:317-318, 1988.

Harris RD and Harris JHJ: The prevalence and significance of missed scapular fractures in blunt chest trauma, AJR 151:747-750, 1988.

Verschakelen J et al: Ultrasound of the chest, J Belge Radiol 71:615-621, 1988.

1989   Bisset GS: Pediatric thoracic applications of magnetic resonance imaging, J Thorac Imaging 4:51-57, 1989.

Gamsu G and Sostman D: Magnetic resonance imaging of the thorax, Am Rev Respir Dis 139:254-274, 1989.

Heare MM, Heare TC and Gillespy T: Diagnostic imaging of pelvic and chest wall trauma, Radiol Clin North Am 27:873-889, 1989.

MRI of the thorax. State of the art, J Thorac Imaging 4:1-92, 1989.

Spritzer C, Gamsu G and Sostman HD: Magnetic resonance imaging of the thorax: techniques, current applications, and future directions, J Thorac Imaging 4:1-18, 1989.

Swensen SJ, Ehman RL and Brown LR: Magnetic resonance imaging of the thorax, J Thorac Imaging 4:19-33, 1989.

The diaphragm, chest wall, and pleura, J Thorac Imaging 4:1-94, 1989.

1990   Bhalla M et al: Counting ribs on chest CT, J Comput Assist Tomogr 14:590-594, 1990.

Hehir MD, Hollands MJ and Deane SA: The accuracy of the first chest x-ray in the trauma patient, Aust N Z J Surg 60:529-532, 1990.

Stark P: Radiology of thoracic trauma, Invest Radiol 25:1265-1275, 1990.

1991   Collins JD et al: Anatomy of the thorax and shoulder girdle displayed by magnetic resonance imaging, J Natl Med Assoc 83:26-32, 1991.

MacMahon H et al: The nature and subtlety of abnormal findings in chest radiographs, Med Phys 18:206-210, 1991.

Spring BI and Schiebler ML: Normal anatomy of the thoracic inlet as seen on transaxial MR images, AJR 157:707-710, 1991.

1992 Castellino RA: Diagnostic imaging studies in patients with newly diagnosed Hodgkin's disease, Ann Oncol 3 Suppl 4:45-47, 1992.

Kono M, Kusumoto M and Adachi S: Thoracic magnetic resonance imaging, Curr Opin Radiol 4:62-68, 1992.

Mirvis SE and Templeton P: Imaging in acute thoracic trauma, Semin Roentgenol 27:184-210, 1992.

Schiebler ML and Listerud J: Common artifacts encountered in thoracic magnetic resonance imaging: recognition, derivation, and solutions, Top Magn Reson Imaging 4:1-17, 1992.

Stark P and Jacobson F: Radiology of thoracic trauma, Curr Opin Radiol 4:87-93, 1992.

van Sonnenberg E et al: Interventional radiology in the chest, Chest 102:608-612, 1992.

1993 Dumoulin CL et al: Reduction of artifacts from breathing and peristalsis in phase-contrast MRA of the chest and abdomen, J Comput Assist Tomogr 17:328-332, 1993.

Manson D et al: CT of blunt chest trauma in children, Pediatr Radiol 23:1-5, 1993.

Padovani B et al: Chest wall invasion by bronchogenic carcinoma: evaluation with MR imaging, Radiology 187:33-38, 1993.

Randall PA et al: MR imaging in the evaluation of the chest after uncomplicated median sternotomy, Radiographics 13:329-340, 1993.

Pulmonary apices

For bibliographic citations before 1964, please see the fifth edition of this atlas. For citations from 1964 through 1974, see the sixth or seventh edition.

1992 Proto AV: Conventional chest radiographs: anatomic understanding of newer observations, Radiology 183:593-603, 1992.

Lungs

For bibliographic citations before 1964, please see the fifth edition of this atlas. For citations from 1964 through 1974, see the sixth or seventh edition.

1975 McLoud TC and Putman CE: Radiology of the Swan-Ganz catheter and associated pulmonary complications, Radiology 116:19-22, 1975.

Reed JC and Reeder MM: Honeycomb lung (interstitial fibrosis), JAMA 231:646-647, 1975.

Simonds B, Friedman PJ and Sokoloff J: The prone chest film, Radiology 116:11-17, 1975.

1976 Polga JP and Watnick M: Whole lung tomography in metastatic disease, Clin Radiol 27:53-56, 1976.

Riggs W Jr and Parvey L: Differences between right and left lateral chest radiographs, AJR 127:997-1000, 1976.

1978 Bachman DM, Ellis K and Austin JH: The effects of minor degrees of obliquity on the lateral chest radiograph, Radiol Clin North Am 16:465-485, 1978.

Beeckman P et al: A radiological study of the effects of body position and respiration on regional differences in the lung, J Belge Radiol 61:229-236, 1978.

Rosenblum LJ et al: Computed tomography of the lung, Radiology 129:521-524, 1978.

Savoca CJ, Gamsu G and Rohlfing BM: Chest radiography in intensive care units, West J Med 129:469-474, 1978.

Stitik FP and Tockman MS: Radiographic screening in the early detection of lung cancer, Radiol Clin North Am 16:347-366, 1978.

1979 Forrest JV and Sagel SS: The lateral radiograph for early diagnosis of lung cancer, Radiology 131:309-310, 1979.

Golden WA and Myers J: A case of hyperlucent lung, JAMA 242:1079-1080, 1979.

Kanemoto N et al: Chest roentgenograms in primary pulmonary hypertension, Chest 76:45-49, 1979.

Proto AV and Speckman JM: The left lateral radiograph of the chest, Med Radiogr Photogr 55:30-74, 1979.

Wesenberg RL and Blumhagen JD: Assisted expiratory chest radiography: an effective technique for the diagnosis of foreign-body aspiration, Radiology 130:538-539, 1979.

1980 Maltby JD: Post-trauma chest film, CRC Crit Rev Diagn Imaging 14:1-36, 1980.

1981 Bein ME and Stone DN: Full lung linear and pluridirectional tomography: a preliminary evaluation of nodule detection, AJR 136:1013-1015, 1981.

Naidich DP et al: Computed tomography of the pulmonary hila, J Comput Assist Tomogr 5:459-475, 1981.

Schnur MJ et al: Thickening of the posterior wall of the bronchus intermedius: a sign on lateral chest radiographs of congestive heart failure, lymph node enlargement, and neoplastic infiltration, Radiology 139:551-559, 1981.

Webb WR, Glazer G and Gamsu G: Computed tomography of the normal pulmonary hilum, J Comput Assist Tomogr 5:476-484, 1981.

1982 Frija J et al: Computed tomography of the pulmonary fissures: normal anatomy, J Comput Assist Tomogr 6:1069-1074, 1982.

Herrera M et al: The significance of efficient scatter removal in chest radiography, ROFO 137:711-717, 1982.

Vock P and Owens A: Computed tomography of the normal and pathological thoracic inlet, Eur J Radiol 2:187-193, 1982.

1983 Chasen MH and Yrizarry JM: Tomography of the pulmonary hila. Anatomical reassessment of the conventional 55 degrees posterior oblique, Radiology 149:365-369, 1983.

Glazer GM et al: Evaluation of the pulmonary hilum: comparison of conventional radiography, 55 degrees posterior oblique tomography, and dynamic computed tomography, J Comput Assist Tomogr 7:983-989, 1983.

Gyll C: Preventing lordotic projection of the chest, Radiography 49:291-293, 1983.

Hedlund LW, Vock P and Effmann EL: Computed tomography of the lungs: densitometric studies, Radiol Clin North Am 21:775-788, 1983.

Huebener KH: Scanned projection radiography of the chest versus standard film, Radiology 148:363-368, 1983.

Proto AV and Ball JB: The superolateral major fissures, AJR 140:431-437, 1983.

Proto AV and Ball JB: Computed tomography of the major and minor fissures, AJR 140:439-448, 1983.

Williford ME and Godwin JD: Computed tomography of lung abscess and empyema, Radiol Clin North Am 21:575-583, 1983.

1984 Proto AV: The chest radiograph: anatomic considerations, Clin Chest Med 5:213-246, 1984.

Webb WR and LaBerge JM: Radiographic recognition of chest tube malposition in the major fissure, Chest 85:81-83, 1984.

Woodring JH: Recognition of pleural effusion on supine radiographs: how much fluid is required? AJR 142:59-64, 1984.

1985 Butler PF et al: Chest radiography: a survey of techniques and exposure levels currently used, Radiology 156:533-536, 1985.

1986 Minagi H and Jeffrey RB Jr: Radiologic techniques in the treatment of the critically ill trauma patient, Crit Care Clin 2:821-838, 1986.

Strickland B, Brennan J and Denison DM: Computed tomography in diffuse lung disease: improving the image, Clin Radiol 37:335-338, 1986.

1987 Batra P, Brown K and Steckel R: Diagnostic imaging techniques in lung carcinoma, Am J Surg 153:517-524, 1987.

Bressler EL et al: Bolus contrast medium enhancement for distinguishing pleural from parenchymal lung disease, J Comput Assist Tomogr 11:436-440, 1987.

Mayo JR et al: High-resolution CT of the lungs: an optimal approach, Radiology 163:507-510, 1987.

Norman S: Radiographic appearances of common lung pathology, Radiography 53:153-159, 1987.

Siafakas NM et al: Radiographic determination of total lung capacity in patients with acromegaly, Br J Dis Chest 81:280-286, 1987.

1988 Batra P et al: Evaluation of intrathoracic extent of lung cancer by plain chest radiography, computed tomography, and magnetic resonance imaging, Am Rev Respir Dis 137:1456-1462, 1988.

Casola G et al: Pneumothorax: radiologic treatment with small catheters, Radiology 166:89-91, 1988.

Collins JD, Graves WA and Shaver ML: The importance of the "sloping rib" in interventional radiology procedures of the chest, J Natl Med Assoc 80:1293-1296, 1988.

Edwards DK, Berry CC and Hilton SW: Trisomy 21 in newborn infants: chest radiographic diagnosis, Radiology 167:317-318, 1988.

Eggleston DE, Slovis TL and Watts FB: Update on pediatric chest imaging, Pediatr Pulmonol 5:158-175, 1988.

Gefter WB and Conant EF: Issues and controversies in the plain-film diagnosis of asbestos-related disorders in the chest, J Thorac Imaging 3:11-28, 1988.

Giger ML, Doi K and MacMahon H: Image feature analysis and computer-aided diagnosis in digital radiography. 3. Automated detection of nodules in peripheral lung fields, Med Phys 15:158-166, 1988.

Goodman LR et al: Pneumothorax and other lung diseases: effect of altered resolution and edge enhancement on diagnosis with digitized radiographs, Radiology 167:83-88, 1988.

Guilbeau JC et al: Chest radiography with a shaped filter at 140 kVp: its diagnostic accuracy compared with that of standard radiographs, AJR 150:1007-1010, 1988.

Hayt DB: Angulated fluoroscopy with light localizer in percutaneous lung biopsy, Chest 93:642-643, 1988.

Katsuragawa S, Doi K and MacMahon H: Image feature analysis and computer-aided diagnosis in digital radiography: detection and characterization of interstitial lung disease in digital chest radiographs, Med Phys 15:311-319, 1988.

Kogutt MS, Jones JP and Perkins DD: Low-dose digital computed radiography in pediatric chest imaging, AJR 151:775-779, 1988.

Kool LJ et al: Advanced multiple-beam equalization radiography in chest radiology: a simulated nodule detection study, Radiology 169:35-39, 1988.

MacMahon H et al: Digital chest radiography: effect on diagnostic accuracy of hard copy, conventional video, and reversed gray scale video display formats, Radiology 168:669-673, 1988.

Markowitz RI: The anterior junction line: a radiographic sign of bilateral pneumothorax in neonates, Radiology 167:717-719, 1988.

Muller NL et al: "Density mask." An objective method to quantitate emphysema using computed tomography, Chest 94:782-787, 1988.

Murata K et al: Optimization of computed tomography technique to demonstrate the fine structure of the lung, Invest Radiol 23:170-175, 1988.

Oestmann JW et al: Subtle lung cancers: impact of edge enhancement and gray scale reversal on detection with digitized chest radiographs, Radiology 167:657-658, 1988.

Peruzzi W et al: Portable chest roentgenography and computed tomography in critically ill patients, Chest 93:722-726, 1988.

Pugh P, Brenner M and Milne EN: Splenic size on routine chest films in AIDS: diagnostic and prognostic significance, J Thorac Imaging 3:40-51, 1988.

Remy-Jardin M and Remy J: Comparison of vertical and oblique CT in evaluation of bronchial tree, J Comput Assist Tomogr 12:956-962, 1988.

Sherman CB, Barnhart S and Rosenstock L: Use of oblique chest roentgenograms in detecting pleural disease in asbestos-exposed workers, J Occup Med 30:681-683, 1988.

Shih WJ et al: Application of I-123 HIPDM as a lung imaging agent, Eur J Nucl Med 14:21-24, 1988.

Spirn PW et al: Radiology of the chest after thoracic surgery, Semin Roentgenol 23:9-31, 1988.

Vlasbloem H and Kool LJ: AMBER: a scanning multiple-beam equalization system for chest radiography, Radiology 169:29-34, 1988.

Wandtke JC, Plewes DB and McFaul JA: Improved pulmonary nodule detection with scanning equalization radiography, Radiology 169:23-27, 1988.

Zylak CJ, Littleton JT and Durizch ML: Illusory consolidation of the left lower lobe: a pitfall of portable, Radiology 167:653-655, 1988.

1989
Barker EJ: An old problem seen again, Radiol Technol 60:427-428, 1989.

Dobbins JT and Powell AO: Variable compensation technique for digital radiography of the chest, Radiology 173:451-458, 1989.

Fisher MR: Magnetic resonance for evaluation of the thorax, Chest 95:166-173, 1989.

Glasier CM et al: Extracardiac chest ultrasonography in infants and children: radiographic and clinical implications, J Pediatr 114:540-544, 1989.

Glazer HS et al: Pneumothorax: appearance on lateral chest radiographs, Radiology 173:707-711, 1989.

Hollman AS and Adams FG: The influence of the lordotic projection on the interpretation of the chest radiograph, Clin Radiol 40:360-364, 1989.

Huda W et al: Radiation doses and detriment from chest x-ray examinations, Phys Med Biol 34:1477-1492, 1989.

Kaplan IL and Swayne LC: Composite SPECT-CT images: technique and potential applications in chest and abdominal imaging, AJR 152:865-866, 1989.

McCleane GJ: Routine preoperative chest x-rays, Ir J Med Sci 158:67-68, 1989.

Rosengarten PL, Tuxen DV and Weeks AM: Whole lung pulmonary angiography in the intensive care unit with two portable chest x-rays, Crit Care Med 17:274-278, 1989.

Sivit CJ et al: Efficacy of chest radiography in pediatric intensive care, AJR 152:575-577, 1989.

Stern RL et al: Three-dimensional imaging of the thoracic cavity, Invest Radiol 24:282-288, 1989.

Svedstrom E, Puhakka H and Kero P: How accurate is chest radiography in the diagnosis of tracheobronchial foreign bodies in children? Pediatr Radiol 19:520-522, 1989.

1990
Cohn M, Trefler M and Young TY: Enhancement and compression of digital chest radiographs, J Thorac Imaging 5:92-95, 1990.

Connett R and Paris A: Low cost equipment for rapid throughput chest radiography, Radiogr Today 56:25-26, 1990.

Cooperstein LA et al: The effect of clinical history on chest radiograph interpretations in a PACS environment, Invest Radiol 25:670-674, 1990.

Gagner M and Chiasson A: Preoperative chest x-ray films in elective surgery: a valid screening tool, Can J Surg 33:271-274, 1990.

Geijer M, Jensen C and Schlossman D: Chest radiography in the intensive care unit. Indications for radiography and effects of selective archiving of films, Acta Radiol 31:321-323, 1990.

Hedlund GL and Kirks DR: Emergency radiology of the pediatric chest, Curr Probl Diagn Radiol 19:133-164, 1990.

Hehir MD, Hollands MJ and Deane SA: The accuracy of the first chest x-ray in the trauma patient, Aust N Z J Surg 60:529-532, 1990.

Landay MJ, Mootz AR and Estrera AS: Apparatus seen on chest radiographs after cardiac surgery in adults, Radiology 174:477-482, 1990.

Mann H: Common errors in evaluating chest radiographs, Postgrad Med 87:275-278, 281, 1990.

Newman B, Bowen A and Oh KS: A practical approach to the newborn chest, Curr Probl Diagn Radiol 19:41-84, 1990.

Siegel MJ: Chest applications of magnetic resonance imaging in children, Top Magn Reson Imaging 3:1-23, 1990.

Snow N, Bergin KT and Horrigan TP: Thoracic CT scanning in critically ill patients. Information obtained frequently alters management, Chest 97:1467-1470, 1990.

Tarver RD et al: Pediatric digital chest imaging, J Thorac Imaging 5:31-35, 1990.

Wandtke JC: Newer imaging methods in chest radiography, J Thorac Imaging 5:1-9, 1990.

1991
Chotas HG et al: Small object contrast in AMBER and conventional chest radiography, Radiology 180:853-859, 1991.

Hansell DM: Digital chest radiology, Curr Opin Radiol 3:364-371, 1991.

Kavanagh G, McNulty J and Fielding JF: Complications of liver biopsy: the incidence of pneumothorax and role of post biopsy chest x-ray, Ir J Med Sci 160:387-388, 1991.

MacMahon H et al: The nature and subtlety of abnormal findings in chest radiographs, Med Phys 18:206-210, 1991.

MacMahon H and Doi K: Digital chest radiography, Clin Chest Med 12:19-32, 1991.

Swensen SJ et al: Radiology in the intensive-care unit, Mayo Clin Proc 66:396-410, 1991.

Thierens H et al: Evaluation of the use of a niobium filter for patient dose reduction in chest radiography, Br J Radiol 64:334-340, 1991.

Weinreb JC and Naidich DP: Thoracic magnetic resonance imaging, Clin Chest Med 12:33-54, 1991.

Wiener MD et al: Imaging of the intensive care unit patient, Clin Chest Med 12:169-198, 1991.

1992 Blume H and Jost RG: Chest imaging within the radiology department by means of photostimulable phosphor computed radiography: a review, J Digit Imaging 5:67-78, 1992.

Chest radiology, Curr Opin Radiol 4:161-172, 1992.

Costello P et al: Spiral CT of the thorax with reduced volume of contrast material: a comparative study, Radiology 183:663-666, 1992.

Davis SD and Umlas SL: Radiology of congenital abnormalities of the chest, Curr Opin Radiol 4:25-35, 1992.

Dee PM: The radiology of chest trauma, Radiol Clin North Am 30:291-306, 1992.

Desai S and Chan O: Interpretation of a normal chest x-ray, Nurs Stand 7:38-39, 1992.

Geleijns J et al: AMBER and conventional chest radiography: comparison of radiation dose and image quality, Radiology 185:719-723, 1992.

Graham NJ and Muller NL: The diaphragm, Can Assoc Radiol J 43:250-257, 1992.

Gray P et al: Value of postprocedural chest radiographs in the adult intensive care unit, Crit Care Med 20:1513-1518, 1992.

Gross GW: Pediatric chest imaging, Curr Opin Radiol 4:36-43, 1992.

Grossglauser L: Assessment of the quality of the neonatal chest x-ray film, Neonatal Netw 11:69-72, 1992.

Grum CM and Lynch JP: Chest radiographic findings in cystic fibrosis, Semin Respir Infect 7:193-209, 1992.

Henschke CI: Image selection for computed tomography of the chest. A sampling approach, Invest Radiol 27:908-911, 1992.

Jennings P, Padley SP and Hansell DM: Portable chest radiography in intensive care: a comparison of computed and conventional radiography, Br J Radiol 65:852-856, 1992.

Klein JS and Schultz S: Interventional chest radiology, Curr Probl Diagn Radiol 21:219-277, 1992.

Klein JS: Thoracic intervention, Curr Opin Radiol 4:94-103, 1992.

LaBelle VS and Spock A: Hair artifacts that may simulate disease, N C Med J 53:170-171, 1992.

Lyn BE et al: Chest radiography or computed tomography in the assessment of lung cancer prior to radiography, Clin Oncol R Coll Radiol 4:148-153, 1992.

Moskovic E, Parsons C and Baum M: Chest radiography in the management of breast cancer, Br J Radiol 65:30-32, 1992.

Murray JG and Breatnach E: Imaging of the mediastinum and hila, Curr Opin Radiol 4:44-52, 1992.

Pietka E, Huang HK: Orientation correction for chest images, J Digit Imaging 5:185-189, 1992.

Pirronti T et al: Digital radiography in chest imaging, Rays 17:469-481, 1992.

Proto AV: Conventional chest radiographs: anatomic understanding of newer observations, Radiology 183:593-603, 1992.

Sanada S, Doi K and MacMahon H: Image feature analysis and computer-aided diagnosis in digital radiography: automated detection of pneumothorax in chest images, Med Phys 19:1153-1160, 1992.

Sofranik RM, Gross BH and Spizarny DL: Radiology of the pleural fissures, Clin Imaging 16:221-229, 1992.

Stapakis JC and Thickman D: Diagnosis of pneumoperitoneum: abdominal CT vs. upright chest film, J Comput Assist Tomogr 16:713-716, 1992.

Stark P and Jacobson F: Radiology of thoracic trauma, Curr Opin Radiol 4:87-93, 1992.

Trulzsch DV et al: Gastrografin-induced aspiration pneumonia: a lethal complication of computed tomography, South Med J 85:1255-1256, 1992.

Umezawa T et al: A computerized automatic exposure device for chest radiography in infants, Clin Pediatr Phila 31:751-752, 1992.

Whalen E: Thoracic imaging, 1992, AJR 158:1391-1398, 1992.

1993 Beres RA and Goodman LR: Pneumothorax: detection with upright versus decubitus radiography, Radiology 186:19-22, 1993.

Caceres J et al: Increased density of the azygos lobe on frontal chest radiographs simulating disease: CT findings in seven patients, AJR 160:245-248, 1993.

Chotas HG et al: Digital chest radiography with photostimulable storage phosphors: signal-to-noise ratio as a function of kilovoltage with matched exposure risk, Radiology 186:395-398, 1993.

Engdahl O, Toft T and Boe J: Chest radiograph—a poor method for determining the size of a pneumothorax, Chest 103:26-29, 1993.

Figa FH et al: Horseshoe lung— a case report with unusual bronchial and pleural anomalies and a proposed new classification, Pediatr Radiol 23:44-47, 1993.

Goodman LR, Wilson CR and Kim CS: Computed equalization radiography: preliminary clinical evaluation, Radiology 186:399-404, 1993.

Hansell DM: Digital chest radiography, Br J Hosp Med 49:117-120, 1993.

Hubbell FA et al: The value of baseline chest radiograph reports in the care of elderly patients in an emergency department, Am J Med Sci 305:145-149, 1993.

Saifuddin A and Arthur RJ: Congenital diaphragmatic hernia—a review of pre- and postoperative chest radiology, Clin Radiol 47:104-110, 1993.

Strauss GM, Gleason RE and Sugarbaker DJ: Screening for lung cancer re-examined. A reinterpretation of the Mayo Lung Project randomized trial on lung cancer screening, Chest 103:337S-341S, 1993.

Swensen SJ et al: A new asymmetric screen-film combination for conventional chest radiography: evaluation in 50 patients, AJR 160:483-486, 1993.

Heart and mediastinum

For bibliographic citations before 1964, please see the fifth edition of this atlas. For citations from 1964 through 1974, see the sixth or seventh edition.

1976 Beeckman P et al: Critical evaluation of different x-ray methods in exploration of mediastinal lymphadenopathy, J Belge Radiol 59:459-465, 1976.

Galvin PG and Devlin HB: Outpatient thyrography: its value in the diagnosis of thyroid and mediastinal lesions, Proc R Soc Med 69:848-851, 1976.

1977 Blank N and Castellino RA: Mediastinal lymphadenopathy, Semin Roentgenol 12:215-223, 1977.

Goldwin RL, Heitzman ER and Proto AV: Computed tomography of the mediastinum: normal anatomy and indications for the use of CT, Radiology 124:235-241, 1977.

Sharov BK: Pneumomediastinography: techniques for studying intrathoracic lymphadenitis, Lymphology 10:120-125, 1977.

Webster RV and Viamonte M: Some aspects of mediastinal anatomy and radiology, CRC Crit Rev Diagn Imaging 10:1-16, 1977.

1978 Maher JT et al: Radiographic changes in cardiac dimensions during exhaustive exercise in man, J Sports Med Phys Fitness 18:263-269, 1978.

Stiner RM and Morse D: The radiology of cardiac pacemakers, JAMA 240:2574-2576, 1978.

1979 Guthaner DF, Wexler L and Harrell G: CT demonstration of cardiac structures, AJR 133:75-81, 1979.

Hyson EA and Ravin CE: Radiographic features of mediastinal anatomy, Chest 75:609-613, 1979.

Kruger RA et al: Computerized fluoroscopy in real time for noninvasive visualization of the cardiovascular system, Radiology 130:49-57, 1979.

Sos TA et al: Cinefluoroscopy in evaluating left ventricular contractility and aneurysms, Radiology 133:31-37, 1979.

1980 Formanek A et al: Selective coronary angiography in children, Circulation 61:84-95, 1980.

Green CE and Kelley MJ: A renewed role for fluoroscopy in the evaluation of cardiac disease, Radiol Clin North Am 18:345-357, 1980.

Pridie RB: The importance of magnification in left ventriculography, Br J Radiol 53:642-646, 1980.

Raphael MJ, Hawtin DR and Allwork SP: The angiographic anatomy of the coronary arteries, Br J Surg 67:181-187, 1980.

Sone S et al: Normal anatomy of thymus and anterior mediastinum by pneumomediastinum, AJR 134:81-89, 1980.

1981 Ceballos R, Soto B and Bargeron LM Jr: Angiographic anatomy of the normal heart through axial angiography, Circulation 64:351-359, 1981.

Rose JS: Radiologic analysis of the mediastinum, Ear Nose Throat J 60:170-184, 1981.

Schwarten DE: Radiologic examination of the heart, Cardiovasc Clin 12:75-93, 1981.

1982 Alderman EL et al: Anatomically flexible, computer-assisted reporting system for coronary angiography, Am J Cardiol 49:1208-1215, 1982.

Brundage BH and Lipton MJ: The emergence of computed tomography as a cardiovascular diagnostic technique, Am Heart J 103:313-316, 1982.

Weikl A and Hubmann M: A survey of contrast media used in coronary angiography, Cardiovasc Intervent Radiol 5:202-210, 1982.

1983 Barter SJ et al: Computed tomography of the heart: initial experience, Clin Radiol 34:693-699, 1983.

Dreslinski GR: Identification of left ventricular hypertrophy: chest roentgenography, echocardiography, electrocardiography, Am J Med 75:47-50, 1983.

Elliott LP, Bargeron LM Jr and Green CE: Angled angiography: general approach and findings, Cardiol Clin 1:361-385, 1983.

Higgins CB and Buonocore E: Digital subtraction angiography: techniques and applications for evaluating cardiac anatomy and function, Cardiol Clin 1:413-425, 1983.

Rodgers H: Rapid sequence computed tomography of the heart, Radiography 49:55-58, 1983.

Selin K and Bjork L: Two new contrast media in coronary angiography, Acta Radiol 24:37-41, 1983.

1984 Brandt PW: Axially angled angiocardiography, Cardiovasc Intervent Radiol 7:166-169, 1984.

Cragg AH et al: Rotational kymography: technique for automated analysis of cine, Radiology 150:260-262, 1984.

Greenbaum RA and Evans TR: Investigation of left ventricular function by digital subtraction angiography, Br Heart J 51:163-167, 1984.

Gwilt DJ and Nagle RE: Contrast media for left ventricular angiography. A comparison between Cardio-Conray and iopamidol, Br Heart J 51:427-430, 1984.

Higgins CB et al: Multiplane magnetic resonance imaging of the heart and major vessels: studies in normal volunteers, AJR 142:661-667, 1984.

McInerney JJ et al: The measurement of multidimensional myocardial dynamics using scattered radiation fields, Invest Radiol 19:385-393, 1984.

Sinak LJ, Hoffman EA and Ritman EL: Subtraction gated computed tomography with the dynamic spatial reconstructor: simultaneous evaluation of left and right heart from single right-sided bolus contrast media injection, J Comput Assist Tomogr 8:1-9, 1984.

Soto B, Coghlan CH and Bargeron LM: Present status of axially angled angiocardiography, Cardiovasc Intervent Radiol 7:156-165, 1984.

Woodring JH and Dillon ML: Radiographic manifestations of mediastinal hemorrhage from blunt chest trauma, Ann Thorac Surg 37:171-178, 1984.

1985 Garrett JS, Higgins CB and Lipton MJ: Computed axial tomography of the heart, Int J Card Imaging 1:113-126, 1985.

Perry NM et al: Heart size in high-kilovoltage chest radiography, Clin Radiol 36:335-339, 1985.

1986 Farmer D et al: High-speed (cine) computed tomography of the heart, Cardiovasc Clin 17:345-356, 1986.

Feldman L: Digital vascular imaging of the great vessels and heart, Cardiovasc Clin 17:357-384, 1986.

Rees MR et al: Heart evaluation by cine CT: use of two new oblique views, Radiology 159:804-806, 1986.

1987 Lipton MJ: Cine computerized tomography, Int J Card Imaging 2:209-221, 1987.

Pietras RJ, Kondos GT and Juska J: Quantitative validation of cineangiographic axial oblique biplane, Cathet Cardiovasc Diagn 13:157-161, 1987.

1988 Florence SH et al: Cardiac transplantation: postoperative chest radiographs, Can Assoc Radiol J 39:115-117, 1988.

Milne EN et al: Assessment of cardiac size on portable chest films, J Thorac Imaging 3:64-72, 1988.

Peruzzi W et al: Portable chest roentgenography and computed tomography in critically ill patients, Chest 93:722-726, 1988.

Piao ZE et al: Contrast media-induced ventricular fibrillation. A comparison of Hypaque-76, Hexabrix, and Omnipaque, Invest Radiol 23:466-470, 1988.

Reed DH and Morgan S: The changing mediastinum, Br J Radiol 61:695-696, 1988.

Seward JB et al: Transesophageal echocardiography: technique, anatomic correlations, implementation, and clinical applications, Mayo Clin Proc 63:649-680, 1988.

Toomey FB et al: Chest radiography in infant cardiac allotransplantation, AJR 150:369-372, 1988.

Tsai FY et al: Aberrant placement of a Kimray-Greenfield filter in the right atrium: percutaneous retrieval, Radiology 167:423-424, 1988.

Vogel RA: Left ventricular imaging by digital subtraction angiography, Int J Card Imaging 3:29-38, 1988.

1989 Felson B: Aortic arch anomalies: a few facts and a lot of speculation, Semin Roentgenol 24:69-74, 1989.

Glasier CM et al: Extracardiac chest ultrasonography in infants and children: radiographic and clinical implications, J Pediatr 114:540-544, 1989.

Holt WW, Wong E and Lipton MJ: Conventional and ultrafast cine-computed tomography in cardiac imaging, Current Opinion in Radiology 1:159-165, 1989.

Newell JD Jr: Conventional and digital radiography of the heart, aorta, and pulmonary vascularity, Current Opinion in Radiology 1:179-182, 1989.

Stanford W and Galvin JR: The radiology of right heart dysfunction: chest roentgenogram and computed tomography, J Thorac Imaging 4:7-19, 1989.

Steiner RM et al: Clinical experience with rapid acquisition cardiovascular CT imaging (cine CT) in the adult patient, Radiographics 9:283-305, 1989.

1990 Brinker JA: Selection of a contrast agent in the cardiac catheterization laboratory, American Journal of Cardiology 66:26F-33F, 1990.

Chen JT: Plain radiographic evaluation of the aorta, J Thorac Imaging 5:1-17, 1990.

Henriksson L et al: Assessment of congestive heart failure in chest radiographs. Observer performance with two common film-screen systems, Acta Radiol 31:469-471, 1990.

Pinsky WW and Arciniegas E: Tetralogy of Fallot, Pediatr Clin North Am 37:179-192, 1990.

Ritman EL: Fast computed tomography for quantitative cardiac analysis—state of the art and future perspectives, Mayo Clinic Proceedings 65:1336-1349, 1990.

Siegel MJ: Chest applications of magnetic resonance imaging in children, Top Magn Reson Imaging 3:1-23, 1990.

Swensen SJ and Brown LR: Conventional radiography of the hilum and mediastinum in bronchogenic carcinoma, Radiol Clin North Am 28:521-538, 1990.

1991   Aguirre FV et al: The effects of high (sodium meglumine diatrizoate, Renografin-76) and low osmolar (sodium meglumine ioxaglate, Hexabrix) radiographic contrast media on diastolic function during left ventriculography in patients, American Heart Journal 121:848-857, 1991.

Bruggemann A, Greie A and Lepsien G: Real-time sonography of the mediastinum in adults: a study in 100 healthy volunteers, Surg Endosc 5:150-153, 1991.

Chevallier JM et al: The thoracic esophagus: sectional anatomy and radiosurgical applications, Surg Radiol Anat 13:313-321, 1991.

Dreesen RG et al: Apicoaortic valved conduits in a canine model, Radiol Technol 62:228-230, 1991.

Manninen H et al: Evaluation of heart size and pulmonary vasculature. Conventional chest roentgenography and image intensifier photofluorography compared, Acta Radiol 32:226-231, 1991.

Patel A and Cholankeril J: Case of the migrating embolic filter, Hospital Practice 26:129-132, 1991.

Richardson P et al: Value of CT in determining the need for angiography when findings of mediastinal hemorrhage on chest radiographs are equivocal, AJR 156:273-279, 1991.

Weinreb JC and Naidich DP: Thoracic magnetic resonance imaging, Clin Chest Med 12:33-54, 1991.

1992   Bleiweis MS, Georgiou D and Brundage BH: Ultrafast CT and the cardiovascular system, International Journal of Cardiac Imaging 8:289-302, 1992.

Bogaert J et al: Pictorial essay: right aortic arch, J Belge Radiol 75:406-409, 1992.

Davis SD and Umlas SL: Radiology of congenital abnormalities of the chest, Curr Opin Radiol 4:25-35, 1992.

Dyet JF et al: Digital cardiac imaging—the death knell of cineangiography? Br J Radiol 65:818-821, 1992.

Erkonen WE et al: Cardiac anatomy instruction by ultrafast computed tomography versus cadaver dissection, Invest Radiol 27:744-747, 1992.

Kawashima A, Fishman EK and Kuhlman JE: CT and MR evaluation of posterior mediastinal masses, Crit Rev Diagn Imaging 33:311-367, 1992.

Mousseaux E and Gaux JC: Ultrafast computed tomography of the heart, Curr Opin Radiol 4:34-40, 1992.

Murray JG and Breatnach E: Imaging of the mediastinum and hila, Curr Opin Radiol 4:44-52, 1992.

Proto AV: Conventional chest radiographs: anatomic understanding of newer observations, Radiology 183:593-603, 1992.

Souto M et al: Enhancement of chest images by automatic adaptive spatial filtering, J Digit Imaging 5:223-229, 1992.

Stark P and Jacobson F: Radiology of thoracic trauma, Curr Opin Radiol 4:87-93, 1992.

van der Jagt EJ and Smits HJ: Cardiac size in the supine chestfilm, Eur J Radiol 14:173-177, 1992.

1993   Erdkamp FL et al: The reliability and value of determining mediastinal involvement and width on chest radiographs in patients with Hodgkin's disease, Eur J Radiol 16:143-146, 1993.

Fransson SG: Pacemaker wires. Difference in performance between AMBER and conventional chest radiography, Acta Radiol 34:419-421, 1993.

Goldberg BB et al: Sonographically guided laparoscopy and mediastinoscopy using miniature catheter-based transducers, J Ultrasound Med 12:49-54, 1993.

Link KM: Magnetic resonance imaging of the mediastinum, J Thorac Imaging 8:34-53, 1993.

Mayo JR: Thoracic magnetic resonance imaging: physics and pulse sequences, J Thorac Imaging 8:1-11, 1993.

Vargo L: Evaluation of cardiac size on the neonatal chest x-ray, Neonatal Netw 12:65-67, 1993.

Weintraub WS et al: Long-term clinical follow-up in patients with angiographic restudy after successful angioplasty, Circulation 87:831-840, 1993.

White RD, Boxt LM and Wexler L: Cardiac radiology. An asset to radiology? Invest Radiol 28:550-556, 1993.

White RD, Boxt LM and Wexler L: Cardiac radiology. A survey of its current status, Invest Radiol 28:545-549, 1993.

Pelvic bones and upper femora

For bibliographic citations before 1964, please see the fifth edition of this atlas. For citations from 1964 through 1974, see the sixth or seventh edition.

1975   Hooper AC and Ormond DJ: A radiographic study of hip rotation, Ir J Med Sci 144:25-29, 1975.

Rogers LF, Novy SB and Harris NF: Occult central fractures of the acetabulum, AJR 124:96-101, 1975.

1976   Salvati EA et al: Radiology of total hip replacements, Clin Orthop 121:74-82, 1976.

1978   Armbuster TG et al: The adult hip: an anatomic study. Part I. The bony landmarks, Radiology 128:1-10, 1978.

Chuinard EG: Lateral roentgenography in the diagnosis and treatment of dysplasia/dislocation of the hip, Orthopedics 1:130-140, 1978.

Fredensborg N and Nilsson BE: The joint space in normal hip radiographs, Radiology 126:325-326, 1978.

Thaggard A III, Harle TS and Carlson V: Fractures and dislocations of bony pelvis and hip, Semin Roentgenol 13:117-134, 1978.

Whitehouse GH: Radiological aspects of posterior dislocation of the hip, Clin Radiol 29:431-441, 1978.

1979   Katz JF: Precise identification of radiographic acetabular landmarks, Clin Orthop 141:166-168, 1979.

Naimark A, Kossoff J and Schepsis A: Intertrochanteric fractures: current concepts of an old subject, AJR 133:889-894, 1979.

1980   Clements RW and Nakayama HK: Radiographic methods in total hip arthroplasty, Radiol Technol 51:589-600, 1980.

Naidich DP et al: Ten section approach to computed tomography of the pelvis, Skeletal Radiol 5:213-217, 1980.

Osborn AG et al: Direct sagittal computed tomographic scans in the radiographic evaluation of the pelvis, Radiology 134:25-257, 1980.

Resnick D and Guerra J Jr: Stress fractures of the inferior pubic ramus following hip surgery, Radiology 137:35-338, 1980.

Sauser DD et al: CT evaluation of hip trauma, AJR 135:269-274, 1980.

Visser JD and Jonkers A: A method for calculating acetabular anteversion, femur anteversion and the instability index of the hip joint, Neth J Surg 32:146-149, 1980.

1981   Dubowitz B et al: Normal axial anatomy of the hip as demonstrated by computed tomography, Clin Radiol 32:663-668, 1981.

Eisenberg RL, Hedgecock MW and Akin JR: The 40° cephalad view of the hip, AJR 136:835-836, 1981.

Fernbach SK and Wilkinson RH: Avulsion injuries of the pelvis and proximal femur, AJR 137:581-584, 1981.

Hamlin DJ and Burgener FA: Positive and negative contrast agents in CT evaluation of the abdomen and pelvis, CT 5:82-90, 1981.

1982   Bowerman JW, Sena JM and Chang R: The teardrop shadow of the pelvis; anatomy and clinical significance, Radiology 143:659-662, 1982.

Harley JD, Mack LA and Winquist RA: CT of acetabular fractures: comparison with conventional radiography, AJR 138:413-417, 1982.

Klein A et al: Combined CT-arthrography in recurrent traumatic hip dislocation, AJR 138:963-964, 1982.

Walker RH and Burton DS: Computerized tomography in assessment of acetabular fractures, J Trauma 22:227-234, 1982.

1983   Dunn EL, Berry PH and Connally JD: Computed tomography of the pelvis in patients with multiple injuries, J Trauma 23:378-383, 1983.

Eid EM: Fractures of the pelvis, Postgrad Med J 59:560-565, 1983.

Hricak H et al: Anatomy and pathology of the male pelvis by magnetic resonance imaging, AJR 141:1101-1110, 1983.

Rubenstein JD: Radiographic assessment of pelvic trauma, J Can Assoc Radiol 34:228-236, 1983.

Rubenstein J, Kellam J and McGonigal D: Cross-sectional anatomy of the adult bony acetabulum, J Can Assoc Radiol 34:16-18, 1983.

Siegel MJ: Computed tomography of the pediatric pelvis, CT 7:7-83, 1983.

1984 Burk DL Jr et al: Pelvic and acetabular fractures: examination by CT scanning, Radiology 153:548, 1984.

Chandler DR et al: Radiographic assessment of acetabular cup orientation. A new design concept, Clin Orthop 186:60-64, 1984.

Gill K and Bucholz RW: The role of computerized tomographic scanning in the evaluation of major pelvic fractures, J Bone Joint Surg 66-A:34-39, 1984.

Goldberg HI et al: Device for performing direct coronal CT scanning of the pelvis, AJR 143:900-902, 1984.

1985 Turula KB et al: Weight-bearing radiography in total hip replacement, Skeletal Radiol 14:200-204, 1985.

1986 Amstutz HC et al: The grid radiograph: a simple technique for consistent high-resolution visualization of the hip, J Bone Joint Surg 68-A:1052-1056, 1986.

1987 Scott WW Jr, Fishman EK and Magid D: Acetabular fractures: optimal imaging, Radiology 165:537-539, 1987.

West JD, Mayor MB and Collier JP: Potential errors inherent in quantitative densitometric analysis of orthopaedic radiographs. A study after total hip arthroplasty, J Bone Joint Surg Am 69:58-64, 1987.

1988 Magid D et al: 2D and 3D computed tomography of the pediatric hip, Radiographics 8:901-933, 1988.

Mudge B et al: Multiplanar imaging of the hip: a systematic approach, Radiol Technol 59:307-311, 1988.

Sundram SR: Direct coronal imaging of the abdomen and pelvis, Radiography 54:86-92, 1988.

Sutherland CJ: Radiographic evaluation of acetabular bone stock in failed total hip arthroplasty, J Arthroplasty 3:73-79, 1988.

1989 Edeiken-Monroe BS, Browner BD and Jackson H: The role of standard roentgenograms in the evaluation of instability of pelvic ring disruption, Clin Orthop 63-76, 1989.

Johnson ND et al: MR imaging anatomy of the infant hip, AJR 153:127-133, 1989.

Ragnarsson JI et al: Low field magnetic resonance imaging of femoral neck fractures, Acta Radiol 30:247-252, 1989.

1990 O'Brien T and Barry C: The importance of standardised radiographs when assessing hip dysplasia, Ir Med J 83:159-161, 1990.

1991 Ebraheim NA et al: Percutaneous computed tomography stabilization of moderate to severe slipped capital femoral epiphysis, Orthopedics 859-863, 1991.

Krasny R et al: MR anatomy of infants hip: comparison to anatomical preparations, Pediatr Radiol 21:211-215, 1991.

Lindaman LM et al: A fluoroscopic technique for determining the incision site for percutaneous fixation of slipped capital femoral epiphysis, J Pediatr Orthop 11:397-401, 1991.

Nelson DW and Duwelius PJ: CT-guided fixation of sacral fractures and sacroiliac joint disruptions, Radiology 180:527-532, 1991.

Rafert JA and Long BW: Showing acetabular trauma with more clarity, less pain, Radiol Technol 63:92-97, 1991.

1992 Ablin DS, Greenspan A and Reinhart MA: Pelvic injuries in child abuse, Pediatr Radiol 22:454-457, 1992.

Apuzzio JJ et al: Prenatal ultrasonographic fetal iliac bone measurement. Correlation with gestational age, J Reprod Med 37:348-350, 1992.

Cardinal E and White SJ: Imaging pediatric hip disorders and residual dysplasia of adult hips, Curr Opin Radiol 4:83-89, 1992.

Castellino RA: Diagnostic imaging studies in patients with newly diagnosed Hodgkin's disease, Ann Oncol 3 Suppl 4:45-47, 1992.

Crawford HV, Unwin PS and Walker PS: The CADCAM contribution to customized orthopaedic implants, Proc Inst Mech Eng H 206:43-46, 1992.

Eich GF, Babyn P and Giedion A: Pediatric pelvis: radiographic appearance in various congenital disorders, Radiographics 12:467-484, 1992.

Farber JM: A helpful radiographic sign in CDH, Orthopedics 15:1072-1074, 1992.

Harcke HT: Imaging in congenital dislocation and dysplasia of the hip, Clin Orthop 22-28, 1992.

Kane TJ, Henry G and Furry D: A simple roentgenographic measurement of femoral anteversion. A short note, J Bone Joint Surg Am 74:1540-1542, 1992.

Lang P et al: Imaging of the hip joint. Computed tomography versus magnetic resonance imaging, Clin Orthop 135-153, 1992.

Lee DY, Lee CK and Cho TJ: A new method for measurement of femoral anteversion. A comparative study with other radiographic methods, Int Orthop 16:277-281, 1992.

McCauley TR et al: Effect of prone versus supine patient positioning on pelvic magnetic resonance image quality, Invest Radiol 27:1005-1008, 1992.

Pitt MJ, Ruth JT and Benjamin JB: Trauma to the pelvic ring and acetabulum, Semin Roentgenol 27:299-318, 1992.

Resnik CS et al: Diagnosis of pelvic fractures in patients with acute pelvic trauma: efficacy of plain radiographs, AJR 158:109-112, 1992.

Tehranzadeh J, Kerr R and Amster J: Magnetic resonance imaging of tendon and ligament abnormalities. Part II. Pelvis and lower extremities, Skeletal Radiol 21:79-86, 1992.

Wirth T, LeQuesne GW and Paterson DC: Ultrasonography in Legg-Calve-Perthes disease, Pediatr Radiol 22:498-504, 1992.

1993 Jerrard DA: Pelvic fractures, Emerg Med Clin North Am 11:147-163, 1993.

Koury HI, Peschiera JL and Welling RE: Selective use of pelvic roentgenograms in blunt trauma patients, J Trauma 34:236-237, 1993.

Lang P et al: Acute fracture of the femoral neck: assessment of femoral head perfusion with gadopentetate dimeglumine-enhanced MR imaging, AJR 160:335-341, 1993.

Patel K and Chapman S: Normal symphysis pubis width in children, Clin Radiol 47:56-57, 1993.

Rizzo PF et al: Diagnosis of occult fractures about the hip. Magnetic resonance imaging compared with bone-scanning, J Bone Joint Surg Am 75:395-401, 1993.

Roffi RP and Matta JM: Unrecognized posterior dislocation of the hip associated with transverse and T-type fractures of the acetabulum, J Orthop Trauma 7:23-27, 1993.

Terjesen T, Anda S and Ronningen H: Ultrasound examination for measurement of femoral anteversion in children, Skeletal Radiol 22:33-36, 1993.

Vertebral column
Occipitocervical articulations

For bibliographic citations before 1964, please see the fifth edition of this atlas. For citations from 1964 through 1974, see the sixth or seventh edition.

1977 Dirkheimer Y, Ramsheyi A and Reolon M: Positive arthrography of the craniocervical joints, Neuroradiology 12:257-260, 1977.

1980 Dunsker SB, Brown O and Thomson N: Craniovertebral anomalies, Clin Neurosurg 27:430-439, 1980.

1981 Burrows EH: Clinical relevance of radiological abnormalities of the craniovertebral junction, Br J Radiol 54:195-202, 1981.

1983 Agnoli L and Hildebrandt G: Computer-tomographic investigations in malformations of the occipitocervical junction, Neurosurg Rev 6:177-185, 1983.

Coria F et al: Craniocervical abnormalities in Down's syndrome, Dev Med Child Neurol 25:252-255, 1983.

Osborne D et al: Assessment of craniocervical junction and atlantoaxial relation using metrizamide-enhanced CT in flexion and extension, AJNR 4:843-845, 1983.

1989 Fezoulidis I et al: Diagnostic imaging of the occipito-cervical junction in patients with rheumatoid arthritis. Plain films, computed tomography, magnetic resonance imaging, Acta Radiol 9:5-11, 1989.

1991 Ellis JH et al: Magnetic resonance imaging of the normal craniovertebral junction, Spine 16:105-111, 1991.

1992 Menezes AH and Ryken TC: Craniovertebral abnormalities in Down's syndrome, Pediatr Neurosurg 18:24-33, 1992.

Atlas and axis

For bibliographic citations before 1964, please see the fifth edition of this atlas. For citations from 1964 through 1974, see the sixth or seventh edition.

1978 Apuzzo ML, Weiss MH and Heiden JS: Transoral exposure of the atlantoaxial region, Neurosurgery 3:201-207, 1978.

1979 Farman AG, Nortjé CJ and Joubert JJ: Radiographic profile of the first cervical vertebra, J Anat 128:595-600, 1979.

Kattan KR: Two features of the atlas vertebra simulating fractures by tomography, AJR 132:963-965, 1979.

1980 Flournoy JG et al: Jefferson fracture: presentation of a new diagnostic sign, Radiology 134:88, 1980.

Harrison RB et al: Pseudosubluxation of the axis in young adults, J Can Assoc Radiol 31:176-177, 1980.

Mellstrom A, Grepe A and Levander B: Atlantoaxial arthrography. A postmortem study, Neuroradiology 20:135-144, 1980.

Whaley WJ and Gray WD: Atlantoaxial dislocation and Down's syndrome, Can Med Assoc J 123:35-37, 1980.

1981 Pueschel SM et al: Atlanto-axial instability in children with Down's syndrome, Pediatr Radiol 10:129-132, 1981.

1982 Clyburn TA, Lionberger DR and Tullos HS: Bilateral fracture of the transverse process of the atlas, J Bone Joint Surg 64-A:948, 1982.

Ryan MD and Taylor TK: Odontoid fractures. A rational approach to treatment, J Bone Joint Surg 64-B:416-421, 1982.

1983 Gerlock AJ Jr. and Mirfakhraee M: Computed tomography and hangman's fracture, South Med J 76:727-728, 1983.

Osborne D et al: Assessment of craniocervical junction and atlantoaxial relation, AJNR 4:843-845, 1983.

Osborne D et al: Assessment of craniocervical junction and atlantoaxial relation using metrizamide-enhanced CT in flexion and extension, AJNR 4:843-845, 1983.

Sinh G: Congenital atlanto-axial dislocation, Neurosurg Rev 6:211-220, 1983.

Swartz JD and Puleo S: Fractures of the C1 vertebra: report of two cases documented with computed tomography, CT 7:311-314, 1983.

1984 Nicolet V et al: C2 "target": composite shadow, AJNR 5:331-332, 1984.

Turns JE, Shaffer MA and Doris PE: The modified odontoid view: an alternative visualization of the atlantoaxial joint, J Emerg Med 1:321-325, 1984.

1988 Jagjivan B, Spencer PA and Hosking G: Radiological screening for atlanto-axial instability in Down's syndrome, Clin Radiol 39:661-663, 1988.

1989 Barton D, Redmond HP and Quinlan W: Radiological assessment of atlanto-axial injuries, Injury 20:42-45, 1989.

Burke JT and Harris JH Jr: Acute injuries of the axis vertebra, Skeletal Radiol 18:335-346, 1989.

Ducker TB: C1-C2 subluxation, J Spinal Disord 2:301-302, 1989.

1991 Levine AM and Edwards CC: Fractures of the atlas, J Bone Joint Surg Am 73:680-691, 1991.

Selby KA et al: Clinical predictors and radiological reliability in atlantoaxial subluxation in Down's syndrome, Arch Dis Child 66:876-878, 1991.

1992 Ehara S, el-Khoury GY and Clark CR: Radiologic evaluation of dens fracture. Role of plain radiography and tomography, Spine 17:475-479, 1992.

Forlin E, Herscovici D and Bowern JR: Understanding the os odontoideum, Orthop Rev 21:1441-1447, 1992.

Pueschel SM, Moon AC and Scola FH: Computerized tomography in persons with Down syndrome and atlantoaxial instability, Spine 17:735-737, 1992.

Pueshel SM, Scola FH and Pezzullo JC: A longitudinal study of atlanto-dens relationships in asymptomatic individuals with Down syndrome, Pediatrics 89:1194-1198, 1992.

Reijnierse M et al: The signal intensity of the normal odontoid process (dens) displayed on magnetic resonance images, Skeletal Radiol 21:519-521, 1992.

Van-Harem RS and Yaron M: The ring of C2 and evaluation of the cross-table lateral view of the cervical spine, Arch Emerg Med 21:733-735, 1992.

Cervical vertebrae

For bibliographic citations before 1964, please see the fifth edition of this atlas. For citations from 1964 through 1974, see the sixth or seventh edition.

1975 Smith GR and Abel MS: Visualization of the posterolateral elements of the upper cervical vertebrae in the anteroposterior projection, Radiology 115:219-220, 1975.

1976 Kattan KR: The notched articular process of C7, AJR 126:612-616, 1976.

1977 Dolan KD: Cervical spine injuries below the axis, Radiol Clin North Am 15:247-259, 1977.

Furuse M et al: Orthopantomography of the cervical spine, Radiology 124:517-520, 1977.

Jergens ME, Morgan MT and McElroy CE: Selective use of radiography of the skull and cervical spine, West J Med 127:1-4, 1977.

Tenney RF and Kerekes ES: Cervical spine lateral horizontal beam technique, Radiology 124:520, 1977.

1979 Braun JP et al: The transverse cervical canal: anatomical-radiological comparison with a review of the values and limitations of different radiographic techniques, J Neuroradiol 6:327-334, 1979.

Park WM, O'Neill M and McCall IW: The radiology of rheumatoid involvement of the cervical spine, Skeletal Radiol 4:1-7, 1979.

Yelton R: Cervical spine protocol for emergency room use, Radiol Technol 50:693-698, 1979.

1980 Austin CJ: A technique of examining the cervical spine and neck using a CT 5005 body scanner, Radiography 46:125-127, 1980.

Cerisoli M, Vernizzi E and Giulioni M: Cervical spine changes following laminectomy: clinico-radiological study, J Neurosurg Sci 24:63-70, 1980.

Cloward RB: Acute cervical spine injuries, Clin Symp 32:1-32, 1980.

DeLuca SA and Rhea JA: Radiographic anatomy of the cervical vertebrae, Med Radiogr Photogr 56:18-24, 1980.

Dolan KD: Radiological determination of cervical spine fracture and stability, Clin Neurosurg 27:368-384, 1980.

Riddervold HO and Gandee RW: Diagnostic value of tomography for cervical spine injuries, Va Med 107:630-632, 1980.

Scher AT: The value of erect radiographs in cervical spine injury, S Afr Med J 58:574-575, 1980.

Shmueli G and Herold ZH: Prevertebral shadow in cervical trauma, Isr J Med Sci 16:698-700, 1980.

1981 Boger D and Ralls PW: New traction device for radiography of the lower cervical spine, AJR 137:1202-1204, 1981.

Pope TL Jr, Riddervold HO and Frankel CJ: Right or left intervertebral foramina? A simple method, J Can Assoc Radiol 32:236-237, 1981.

Scher AT: Articular pillar fractures of the cervical spine: diagnosis on the anteroposterior radiograph, S Afr Med J 60:968-969, 1981.

Shaffer MA and Doris PE: Limitation of the cross table lateral view in detecting cervical spine injuries: a retrospective analysis, Ann Emerg Med 10:508-513, 1981.

Williams CF, Bernstein TM and Jelenko C III: Essentiality of the lateral cervical spine radiograph, Ann Emerg Med 10:198-204, 1981.

1982 Abel MS: The exaggerated supine oblique view of the cervical spine, Skeletal Radiol 8:213-219, 1982.

Anderson LD et al: The role of polytomography in the diagnosis and treatment of cervical spine injuries, Clin Orthop 165:64-67, 1982.

Farman AG and Escobar V: Radiographic appearance of the cervical vertebrae in normal and abnormal development, Br J Oral Surg 20:264-274, 1982.

Foley MJ et al: Radiologic evaluation of surgical cervical spine fusion, AJR 138:79-89, 1982.

Orrison WW et al: Optimal computed-tomographic techniques for cervical spine imaging, Radiology 144:180-182, 1982.

Sarant G and Chipman C: Early management of cervical spine injuries, Postgrad Med 71:164-171, 1982.

Scher AT: Rotation of the head—a hazardous procedure in the injured patient, S Afr Med J 62:526-528, 1982.

Scher AT: Radiographic indicators of traumatic cervical spine instability, S Afr Med J 62:562-565, 1982.

Bibliography

Sherk HH, Pasquariello PS and Watters WC: Multiple dislocations of the cervical spine in a patient with juvenile rheumatoid arthritis and Down's syndrome, Clin Orthop 162:37-40, 1982.

1983 Evans DK: Dislocations at the cervicothoracic junction, J Bone Joint Surg 65-B:124-127, 1983.

Heller CA et al: Value of x-ray examinations of the cervical spine, Br Med J 287:1276-1278, 1983.

Le Floch-Prigent P: Computed-tomographical biometry of the cervical spine on horizontal cross-sections every 6 mm, Morphol Med 3:135-141, 1983.

Streitwieser DR et al: Accuracy of standard radiographic views in detecting cervical spine fractures, Ann Emerg Med 12:538-542, 1983.

Vibhakar SD, Eckhauser C and Bellon EM: Computed tomography of the nasopharynx and neck, CT 7:259-265, 1983.

1985 Mayer ET et al: Functional radiographs of the craniocervical region and the cervical spine: a new computer-aided technique, Cephalalgia 5:237-243, 1985.

1986 Boger DC: Traction device to improve CT imaging of lower cervical spine, AJNR 7:719-721, 1986.

1987 Stimac GK et al: A device for maintaining cervical spine stabilization and traction, AJR 149:345-346, 1987.

Tihansky DP and Augustine G: Magnified axial-oblique projection of cervical articular facets, Radiol Technol 58:426-430, 1987.

1988 Berquist TH: Imaging of adult cervical spine trauma, Radiographics 8:667-694, 1988.

Bryan AS: A review of cervical spine x-rays from a casualty department, J R Coll Surg Edinb 33:143-145, 1988.

Clark CR et al: Radiographic evaluation of cervical spine injuries, Spine 13:742-747, 1988.

Czervionke LF and Daniels DL: Cervical spine anatomy and pathologic processes. Applications of new MR imaging techniques, Radiol Clin North Am 26:921-947, 1988.

Goldberg AL et al: The impact of magnetic resonance on the diagnostic evaluation of acute cervicothoracic spinal trauma, Skeletal Radiol 17:89-95, 1988.

Horsfield D and Page J: Acute injury to the cervical spine, Radiography 54:32-36, 1988.

Karnaze MG et al: Comparison of MR and CT myelography in imaging the cervical and thoracic spine, AJR 150:397-403, 1988.

Neifeld GL et al: Cervical injury in head trauma, J Emerg Med 6:203-207, 1988.

Ramthun SK and Bender CE: Tomography of the posterior cervical spine fusion: a new concept, Radiol Technol 60:27-31, 1988.

Ringerberg BJ et al: Rational ordering of cervical spine radiographs following trauma, Arch Emerg Med 17:792-796, 1988.

Roberge RJ et al: Selective application of cervical spine radiography in alert victims of blunt trauma: a prospective study, J Trauma 28:784-788, 1988.

Simon JE and Lukin RR: Diskogenic disease of the cervical spine, Semin Roentgenol 23:118-124, 1988.

Walker J et al: Water-soluble contrast medium for intraoperative evaluation of anterior cervical discectomy, J Neurosurg 68:491-492, 1988.

1989 Davis JW: Cervical injuries—perils of the swimmer's view: case report, J Trauma 29:891-893, 1989.

Evand DL and Bethem D: Cervical spine injuries in children, J Pediatr Orthop 9:563-568, 1989.

Fesmire FM and Luten RC: The pediatric cervical spine: developmental anatomy and clinical aspects, J Emerg Med 7:133-142, 1989.

Freemyer B et al: Comparison of five-view and three-view cervical spine series in the evaluation of patients with cervical trauma, Arch Emerg Med 18:818-821, 1989.

Lally KP et al: Utility of the cervical spine radiograph in pediatric trauma, Am J Surg 158:540-541, 1989.

Modic MT, Ross JS and Masaryk TJ: Imaging of degenerative disease of the cervical spine, Clin Orthop 109-120, 1989.

Rosa L: Missed fractures of the cervical spine, Mil Med 154:39-41, 1989.

Singer CM et al: Exposure of emergency medicine personnel to ionizing radiation during cervical spine radiography, Ann Emerg Med 18:822-825, 1989.

Spielmann RP et al: Radiological diagnosis of cervical trauma at the level C7/T1, Arch Orthop Trauma Surg 108:122-124, 1989.

1990 Bohn D et al: Cervical spine injuries in children, J Trauma 30:463-469, 1990.

Bohrer SP, Chen YM and Sayers DG: Cervical spine flexion patterns, Skeletal Radiol 19:521-525, 1990.

Clayman DA, Murakami ME and Vines FS: Compatibility of cervical spine braces with MR imaging: a study of nine nonferrous devices, AJNR 11:385-390, 1990.

Hove B and Gyldensted C: Cervical analgesic facet joint arthrography, Neuroradiology 32:456-459, 1990.

Kaye JJ and Nance EP Jr: Cervical spine trauma, Orthop Clin North Am 21:449-462, 1990.

Kreipke DL et al: Readability of cervical spine imaging: digital versus film/screen radiographs, Comput Med Imaging Graph 14:119-125, 1990.

MacDonald RL et al: Diagnosis of cervical spine injury in motor vehicle crash victims: how many x-rays are enough? J Trauma 30:392-397, 1990.

Pueschel SM et al: Skeletal anomalies of the upper cervical spine in children with Down syndrome, J Pediatr Orthop 10:607-611, 1990.

Russell EJ: Cervical disk disease, Radiology 177:313-352, 1990.

Smith MD and Kim SS: A herniated cervical disc resulting from discography: an unusual complication, J Spinal Disord 3:392-394, 1990.

Tredwell SJ, Newman DE and Lockitch G: Instability of the upper cervical spine in Down syndrome, J Pediatr Orthop 10:602-606, 1990.

Tress BM and Hare WS: CT of the spine: are plain spine radiographs necessary? Clin Radiol 41:317-320, 1990.

Vandemark RM: Radiology of the cervical spine in trauma patients: practice pitfalls and recommendations for improving efficiency and communication, AJR 155:465-472, 1990.

Vanden-Hoek T and Propp D: Cervicothoracic junction injury, Am J Emerg Med 8:30-33, 1990.

1991 Bell GR and Stearns KL: Flexion-extension MRI of the upper rheumatoid cervical spine, Orthopedics 14:969-973, 1991.

Camins MB and Rosenblum BR: Osseous lesions of the cervical spine, Clin Neurosurg 37:722-739, 1991.

Haug RH et al: Cervical spine fractures and maxillofacial trauma, J Oral Maxillofac Surg 49:725-729, 1991.

Hoffman JR and Mower W: When to image cervical spine injuries, West J Med 155:290, 1991.

Holliman CJ et al: Is the anteroposterior cervical spine radiograph necessary in initial trauma screening? Am J Emerg Med 9:421-425, 1991.

Hudgins PA and Hudgins RJ: Radiology of cervical spine trauma, Clin Neurosurg 37:571-595, 1991.

Jonsson H Jr et al: Hidden cervical spine injuries in traffic accident victims with skull fractures, J Spinal Disord 4:251-263, 1991.

Kettner NW and Guebert GM: The radiology of cervical spine injury, J Manipulative Physiol Ther 14:518-526, 1991.

Lee C and Woodring JH: Sagittally oriented fractures of the lateral masses of the cervical vertebrae, J Trauma 31:1638-1643, 1991.

Lewis LM: Flexion-extension views in the evaluation of cervical-spine injuries, Arch Emerg Med 20:117-121, 1991.

Roberge RJ: Facilitating cervical spine radiography in blunt trauma, Emerg Med Clin North Am 9:733-742, 1991.

Saddison D, Vanek VW and Racanelli JL: Clinical indications for cervical spine radiographs in alert trauma patients, Am Surg 57:366-369, 1991.

1992 Andrew CT: Is routine cervical spine radiographic evaluation indicated in patients with mandibular fractures? Arch Surg 58:369-372, 1992.

Bonneville JF: Plain radiography in the evaluation of cervicobrachial neuralgia, J Neuroradiol 19:160-166, 1992.

Chandler DR et al: Emergency cervical-spine immobilization, Arch Emerg Med 21: 1185-1188, 1992.

Daffner RH: Evaluation of cervical vertebral injuries, Semin Roentgenol 27:239-253, 1992.

Diliberti T and Lindsey RW: Evaluation of the cervical spine in the emergency setting: who does not need an x-ray? Orthopedics 15:179-183, 1992.

Fallone BG, Evans MD and Parmar D: Technique to improve lateral cervico-thoracic radiographs, Radiol Technol 64:104-107, 1992.

Hoffman JR et al: Low-risk criteria for cervical-spine radiography in blunt trauma: a prospective study, Arch Emerg Med 21:1454-1460, 1992.

Larsson EM: Magnetic resonance imaging of the cervical and thoracic spine and the spinal cord. A study using a 0.3 T vertical magnetic field, Acta Radiol Suppl Stockh 378:71-92, 1992.

Levine AM et al: Benign tumors of the cervical spine, Spine 17:399-406, 1992.

Perneczky G et al: Diagnosis of cervical disc disease. MRI versus cervical myelography, Acta Neurochir Wien 116:44-48, 1992.

Rahim KA and Stambough JL: Radiographic evaluation of the degenerative cervical spine, Orthop Clin North Am 23:395-403, 1992.

Ross JS: MR imaging of the cervical spine: techniques for two- and three-dimensional imaging, AJR 159:779-786, 1992.

Silberstein M, Tress BM and Hennessy O: Prevertebral swelling in cervical spine injury: identification of ligament injury with magnetic resonance imaging, Clin Radiol 46:318-323, 1992.

Sweeney JF et al: Is the cervical spine clear? Undetected cervical fractures diagnosed only at autopsy, Arch Emerg Med 21:1288-1290, 1992.

Wober-Bingol C et al: Tension headache and the cervical spine—plain x-ray findings, Cephalalgia 12:152-154, 1992.

Woodring JH and Lee C: The role and limitations of computed tomographic scanning in the evaluation of cervical trauma, J Trauma 33:698-708, 1992.

Yoshino MT et al: Diagnostic performance of teleradiology in cervical spine fracture detection, Invest Radiol 27:55-59, 1992.

1993   Bonadio WA: Cervical spine trauma in children. Part I. General concepts, normal anatomy, radiographic evaluation, Am J Emerg Med 11:158-165, 1993.

Davidorf J, Hoyt D and Rosen P: Distal cervical spine evaluation using swimmer's flexion-extension radiographs, J Emerg Med 11:55-59, 1993.

Page JE, Olliff JF and Dundas DD: Value of anteroposterior radiography in cervical pain of non-traumatic origin, BMJ, 1993.

Turetsky DB et al: Technique and use of supine oblique views in acute cervical spine trauma, Ann Emerg Med 22:685-689, 1993.

Woodring JH and Lee C: Limitations of cervical radiography in the evaluation of acute cervical trauma, J Trauma 34:32-39, 1993.

Thoracic vertebrae

For bibliographic citations before 1964, please see the fifth edition of this atlas.

1976   McAllister VL and Sage MR: The radiology of thoracic disc protrusion, Clin Radiol 27:291-299, 1976.

1980   Fon GT, Pitt MJ and Thies AC Jr: Thoracic kyphosis: range in normal subjects, AJR 134:979-983, 1980.

Scher AT: The diagnostic value of the anteroposterior radiograph for thoracolumbar spinal injuries, S Afr Med J 58:415-117, 1980.

1981   Handelberg F et al: The use of computerised tomographs in the diagnosis of thoracolumbar injury, J Bone Joint Surg 63-B:337-341, 1981.

1982   Brant-Zawadzki M et al: High resolution CT of thoracolumbar fractures, AJR 138:699-704, 1982.

Jelsma RK et al: The radiographic description of thoracolumbar fractures, Surg Neurol 18:230-236, 1982.

Williams F et al: Severe kyphosis due to congenital dorsal hemivertebrae, Clin Radiol 33:445-452, 1982.

1983   Herrlin K, Ekelund L and Sunden G: Radiologic and clinical evaluation of Harrington instrumentation in the injured dorsolumbar spine, Acta Radiol 24:289-295, 1983.

Scher AT: Radiological assessment of thoracolumbar spinal injuries, S Afr Med J 64:384-387, 1983.

1984   Young JW, Andersen BL and Reinig JW: Oblique chest film: value in routine and selective use, AJR 142:69-72, 1984.

1986   Harris JH Jr: Radiographic evaluation of spinal trauma, Orthop Clin North Am 17:75-86, 1986.

1987   Francavilla TL et al: MR imaging of thoracic disk herniations, J Comput Assist Tomogr 11:1062-1065, 1987.

1988   Blumenkopf B and Juneau PA III: Magnetic resonance imaging (MRI) of thoracolumbar fractures, J Spinal Disord 1:144-150, 1988.

Karnaze MG et al: Comparison of MR and CT myelography in imaging the cervical and thoracic spine, AJR 150:397-403, 1988.

1989   Charles R and Govender S: Anterior approach to the upper thoracic vertebrae, J Bone Joint Surg 71-B:81-84, 1989.

Hanley EN and Eskay ML: Thoracic spine fractures, Orthopedics 12:689-696, 1989.

Kupferschmid JP et al: Thoracic spine injuries in victims of motorcycle accidents, J Trauma 29:593-596, 1989.

1990   Daffner RH: Thoracic and lumbar vertebral trauma, Orthop Clin North Am 21:463-482, 1990.

DeLuca SA: Thoracic spine fractures, Am Fam Physician 42:419-421, 1990.

Kaye JJ and Nance EP Jr: Thoracic and lumbar spine trauma, Radiol Clin North Am 28:361-377, 1990.

Keluca SA: Thoracic spine fractures, Aust Fam Physician 42:419-421, 1990.

1992   el-Khoury GY, Moore TE and Kathol MH: Radiology of the thoracic spine, Clin Neurosurg 38:261-295, 1992.

Larsson EM: Magnetic resonance imaging of the cervical and thoracic spine and the spinal cord. A study using a 0.3 T vertical magnetic field, Acta Radiol Suppl Stockh 378:71-92, 1992.

Martin DS et al: Current imaging concepts of thoracic intervertebral disks, Crit Rev Diagn Imaging 33:109-181, 1992.

Meyer S: Thoracic spine trauma, Semin Roentgenol 27:254-261, 1992.

Perrin RG, McBroom RJ: Thoracic spine tumors, Clin Neurosurg 28:353-372, 1992.

Wilson TA and Branch CL Jr: Thoracic disk herniation, Aust Fam Physician 45:2162-2168, 1992.

1993   Baldor RA, Quirk ME and Dohan D: Magnetic resonance imaging use by primary care physicians, J Fam Pract 36:281-285, 1993.

el-Khoury GY and Whitten CG: Trauma to the upper thoracic spine: anatomy, biomechanics, and unique imaging features, AJR 160:95-102, 1993.

Samuels LE and Kerstein MD: 'Routine' radiologic evaluation of the thoracolumbar spine in blunt trauma patients: a reappraisal, J Trauma 34:85-89, 1993.

Lumbar vertebrae

For bibliographic citations before 1964, please see the fifth edition of this atlas. For citations from 1964 through 1974, see the sixth or seventh edition.

1976   Hanley EN, Matteri RE and Frymoyer JW: Accurate roentgenographic determination of lumbar flexion-extension, Clin Orthop 115:145-148, 1976.

1978   Rosomoff HL, Post MJ and Quencer RM: Axial radiology of the lumbar spine, Clin Neurosurg 25:251-265, 1978.

1979   MacGibbon B and Farfan HF: A radiologic survey of various configurations of the lumbar spine, Spine 4:258, 266, 1979.

1980   Carrera GF et al: Computed tomography in sciatica, Radiology 137:433-437, 1980.

Rhea JT et al: The oblique view: an unnecessary component of the initial adult lumbar spine examination, Radiology 134:45-47, 1980.

Wagner AC: "Spurious" defect of the lumbar vertebral body, AJR 135:1095-1096, 1980.

Wigh RE: The thoracolumbar and lumbosacral transition junctions, Spine 5:215-222, 1980.

1981   Heithoff KB: High resolution computed tomography of the lumbar spine, Postgrad Med 70:193-199, 202-206, 208 passim, 1981.

Jones MA and Gonzalez AC: Ultrasonic determination of lumbar spine angulation, Anat Rec 199:281-286, 1981.

Scavone JG, Latshaw RF and Roher GV: Use of lumbar spine films. Statistical evaluation at a university teaching hospital, JAMA 246:1105-1108, 1981.

Scavone JG, Latshaw RF and Weidner WA: Anteroposterior and lateral radiographs: an adequate lumbar spine examination, AJR 136:715-717, 1981.

Weitz EM: The lateral bending sign, Spine 6:388-397, 1981.

1982   Pearcy MJ and Whittle MW: Movements of the lumbar spine measured by three-dimensional x-ray analysis, J Biomed Eng 4:107-112, 1982.

1983   Lau LS et al: High resolution CT scanning of the lumbar spine. Technique and anatomy, Med J Aust 2:21-25, 1983.

Patrick JD et al: Lumbar spine x-rays: a multihospital study, Ann Emerg Med 12:84-87, 1983.

Quinnell RC and Stockdale HL: Flexion and extension radiography of the lumbar spine: a comparison with lumbar diskography, Clin Radiol 34:405-411, 1983.

Resnik CS et al: The two-eyed Scotty dog: a normal anatomic variant, Radiology 149:680, 1983.

Stratemeier PH: Evaluation of the lumbar spine; a comparison between computed tomography and myelography, Radiol Clin North Am 21:221-257, 1983.

1984   Dorwart RH: Computed tomography of the lumbar spine: techniques, normal anatomy, CRC Crit Rev Diagn Imaging 22:1-42, 1984.

Korber J and Bloch B: The "normal" lumbar spine, Med J Aust 140:70-72, 1984.

Libson E et al: Oblique lumbar spine radiographs: importance in young patients, Radiology 151:89-90, 1984.

Libson E et al: Oblique lumbar spine radiographs: importance in young patients, Radiology 151:89-90, 1984.

Pearcy M, Portek I and Shepherd J: Three-dimensional x-ray analysis of normal movement in the lumbar spine, Spine 9:294-297, 1984.

Tehranzadeh J and Gabriele OF: The prone position for CT of the lumbar spine, Radiology 152:817-818, 1984.

Witt I, Vestergaard A and Rosenklint A: A comparative analysis of x-ray findings of the lumbar spine in patients with and without lumbar pain, Spine 9:298-300, 1984.

1986   Schnyder P, Mansouri B and Uske A: Direct coronal computed tomography of the lumbar spine: a new technical approach in supine position, Eur J Radiol 6:248-251, 1986.

1987   Dubowitz B, Friedman L and Papert B: The oblique cranial tilt view for spondylolysis, J Bone Joint Surg 69-B:421-421, 1987.

Friberg O: Lumbar instability: a dynamic approach by traction-compression radiography, Spine 12:119-129, 1987.

Gower DJ, Culp P and Ball M: Lateral lumbar spine roentgenograms: potential role in complications, Surg Neurol 27:316-318, 1987.

1988   Eriksson S, Isberg B and Lindgren U: Vertebral bone mineral measurement using dual photon absorptiometry, Acta Radiol 29:89-94, 1988.

Kelly TL et al: Quantitative digital radiography versus dual photon absorptiometry, J Clin Endocrinol Metab 67:839-844, 1988.

1990   Daffner RH: Thoracic and lumbar vertebral trauma, Orthop Clin North Am 21:463-482, 1990.

Kaye JJ and Nance EP Jr: Thoracic and lumbar spine trauma, Radiol Clin North Am 28:361-377, 1990.

1992   Gennuso R et al: Lumbar intervertebral disc disease in the pediatric population, Pediatr Neurosurg 18:282-286, 1992.

Kricun ME and Kricun R: Fractures of the lumbar spine, Semin Roentgenol 27:262-270, 1992.

1993   Davies AM et al: Detection of significant abnormalities on lumbar spine radiographs, Br J Radiol 66:37-43, 1993.

Even-Sapir E et al: Role of SPECT in differentiating malignant from benign lesions in the lower thoracic and lumbar vertebrae, Radiology 187:193-198, 1993.

Fischgrund JS and Montgomery DM: Diagnosis and treatment of discogenic low back pain, Orthop Rev 22:311-318, 1993.

Francis C: Centering technique for posterior obliques of the lumbar vertebrae, Radiog Today 59(669): 20, 1993.

Hecht ST and Greenspan A: Digital subtraction lumbar diskography: technical note, J Spinal Disord 6:68-70, 1993.

Holtas S: Radiology of the degenerative lumbar spine, Acta Orthop Scand Suppl 251:16-18, 1993.

Thornbury JR et al: Disk-caused nerve compression in patients with acute low-back pain: diagnosis with MR, CT myelography, and plain CT, Radiology 186:731-738, 1993.

Lumbosacral region

For bibliographic citations before 1964, please see the fifth edition of this atlas.

1975   Curran JT: New approach to positioning for lumbosacral junction in lateral projection, Radiol Technol 46:294-297, 1975.

1979   Eisenberg RL, Akin JR and Hedgcock MW: Single, well-centered lateral view of lumbosacral spine: is coned view necessary? AJR 133:711-713, 1979.

1980   Federle MP, Moss AA and Margolin FR: Role of computed tomography in patients with "sciatica," J Comput Assist Tomogr 4:335-341, 1980.

1981   Hirschy JC et al: CT of the lumbosacral spine: importance of tomographic planes parallel to vertebral end plate, AJR 136:47-52, 1981.

Panagiotacopulos ND: Digital image processing, a potential noninvasive technique in the diagnosis of diseased intervertebral discs, Spine 7:506-511, 1982.

1983   Dorwart RH and Genant HK: Anatomy of the lumbosacral spine, Radiol Clin North Am 21:201-220, 1983.

Leonardi M et al: CT evaluation of the lumbosacral spine, AJNR 4:846-847, 1983.

1992   Francis C: Method improves consistency in L5-S1 joint space films, Radiol Technol 63:302-305, 1992.

Sacroiliac joints

For bibliographic citations before 1964, please see the fifth edition of this atlas. For citations from 1964 through 1974, see the sixth or seventh edition.

1978   Dory MA and Francois RJ: Craniocaudal axial view of the sacroiliac joint, AJR 130:1125-1131, 1978.

1980   De Carvalho A and Graudal H: Sacroiliac involvement in classical or definite rheumatoid arthritis, Acta Radiol 21:417-423, 1980.

1981   Borlaza GS et al: Computed tomography in the evaluation of sacroiliac arthritis, Radiology 139:437-440, 1981.

Carrera GF et al: CT of sacroiliitis, AJR 136:41-46, 1981.

1982   Lawson TL et al: The sacroiliac joints: anatomic, plain roentgenographic, and computed tomographic analysis, J Comput Assist Tomogr 6:307-314, 1982.

1983   Ryan LM et al: The radiographic diagnosis of sacroiliitis; a comparison of different views with computed tomograms of the sacroiliac joint, Arthritis Rheum 26:760-763, 1983.

1984   Firooznia H et al: Computed tomography of the sacroiliac joints: comparison with complex-motion tomography, CT 8:31-39, 1984.

1989   Edeiken-Monroe BS, Browner BD and Jackson H: The role of standard roentgenograms in the evaluation of instability of pelvic ring disruption, Clin Orthop 63-76, 1989.

1991   Nelson DW and Duwelius PJ: CT-guided fixation of sacral fractures and sacroiliac joint disruptions, Radiology 180:527-532, 1991.

1992   Resnik CS et al: Diagnosis of pelvic fractures in patients with acute pelvic trauma: efficacy of plain radiographs, AJR 158:109-112, 1992.

Verlooy H et al: Quantitative scintigraphy of the sacroiliac joints, Clin Imaging 16:230-233, 1992.

Sacrum and coccyx

For bibliographic citations before 1964, please see the fifth edition of this atlas.

1975   Northrop CH, Eto RT and Loop JW: Vertical fracture of the sacral ala: significance of the noncontinuity of the anterior superior sacral foraminal line, AJR 124:102-106, 1975.

1976 Bucknill TM and Blackburne JS: Fracture-dislocations of the sacrum, J Bone Joint Surg 58-B(4):467-470, 1976.

1977 Fountain SS, Hamilton RD and Jameson RM: Transverse fractures of the sacrum, J Bone Joint Surg 59:486-489, 1977.

1981 Turner ML, Mulhern CB and Dalinka MK: Lesions of the sacrum: differential diagnosis and radiological evaluation, JAMA 245:275-277, 1981.

1982 Soye I et al: Computed tomography of sacral and presacral lesions, Neuroradiology 24:71-76, 1982.

Whelan MA and Gold RP: Computed tomography of the sacrum, AJR 139:1183-1195, 1982.

1983 Postacchini F and Massobrio M: Idiopathic coccygodynia: analysis of fifty-one operative cases and a radiographic study of the normal coccyx, J Bone Joint Surg 65-A:1116-1124, 1983.

1984 Moed BR and Morawa LG: Displaced midline longitudinal fracture of the sacrum, J Trauma 24:435-437, 1984.

Shirkhoda A et al: Sacral abnormalities—computed tomography versus conventional radiography, CT 8:41-51, 1984.

1988 Fishman EK, Magrid D, Brooker AF and Siegelman SS: Fractures of the sacrum and sacroiliac joint: evaluation by computerized tomography with multiplaner reconstruction, South Med J 81:171-177, 1988.

1989 Edeiken-Monroe BS, Browner BD and Jackson H: The role of standard roentgenograms in the evaluation of instability of pelvic ring disruption, Clin Orthop 63-76, 1989.

1991 Nelson DW and Duwelius PJ: CT-guided fixation of sacral fractures and sacroiliac joint disruptions, Radiology 180:527-532, 1991.

1992 Eich GF, Babyn P and Giedion A: Pediatric pelvis: radiographic appearance in various congenital disorders, Radiographics 12:467-484, 1992.

Resnik CS et al: Diagnosis of pelvic fractures in patients with acute pelvic trauma: efficacy of plain radiographs, AJR 158:109-112, 1992.

Schils J and Hauzeur JP: Stress fracture of the sacrum, Am J Sports Med 20:769-770, 1992.

Vertebral column: entire

For bibliographic citations before 1964, please see the fifth edition of this atlas. For citations from 1964 through 1974, see the sixth or seventh edition.

1980 Ghoshhajra K and Rao KC: CT in spinal trauma, CT 4:309-318, 1980.

Ritter EM et al: Use of a gradient intensifying screen for scoliosis radiography, Radiology 135:230-232, 1980.

Wigh RE: Classification of the human vertebral column: phylogeretic departures and junctional anomalies, Med Radiogr Photogr 56:2-11, 1980.

1981 Bhatnagar JP: X-ray doses to patients undergoing full-spine radiographic examination, Radiology 138:231-233, 1981.

Faren J: Routine radiographic assessment of the scoliotic spine, Radiography 47:92-96, 1981.

Handel SF and Lee YY: Computed tomography of spinal fractures, Radiol Clin North Am 19:69-89, 1981.

1982 de Graaf RJ, Matricali B and Hamburger HL: Butterfly vertebra, Clin Neurol Neurosurg 84:163-169, 1982.

Friedmann G and Promper C: CT examination of the spine and the spinal canal, Eur J Radiol 2:60-65, 1982.

Keene JS et al: Diagnosis of vertebral fractures. A comparison of conventional radiography, conventional tomography, and computed axial tomography, J Bone Joint Surg 64-A:586-594, 1982.

Quiroga O et al: Normal CT anatomy of the spine: anatomo-radiological correlations, Neuroradiology 24:1-6, 1982.

1983 Foley MJ et al: Thoracic and lumbar spine fusion: postoperative radiologic evaluation, AJR 141:373-380, 1983.

Libson E and Bloom RA: Anteroposterior angulated view: a new radiographic technique for the evaluation of spondylolysis, Radiology 149:315-316, 1983.

Modic MT et al: Nuclear magnetic resonance imaging of the spine, Radiology 148:757-762, 1983.

Post MJ and Green BA: The use of computed tomography in spinal trauma, Radiol Clin North Am 21:327-375, 1983.

Suomalainen O, Kettunen K and Saari T: Computed tomography of spinal and pelvic fractures, Ann Chir Gynaecol 72:337-341, 1983.

Verbout AJ, Falke TH and Tinkelenberg J: A three-dimensional graphic reconstruction method of the vertebral column, Eur J Radiol 3:167-170, 1983.

1984 Golimbu C et al: Computed tomography of thoracic and lumbar spine fractures that have been treated with Harrington instrumentation, Radiology 151:731-733, 1984.

Svensson O, Aaro S, and Ohlen G: Harrington instrumentation for thoracic and lumbar vertebral fractures, Acta Orthop Scand 55:38-47, 1984.

1986 Virapongse C et al: Three-dimensional computed tomographic reformation of the spine, Neurosurgery 18:53-58, 1986.

Harris JH Jr: Radiographic evaluation of spinal trauma, Orthop Clin North Am 17:75-86, 1986.

1987 Kruger RA: Dual-energy electronic scanning-slit fluorography for the determination of vertebral bone mineral content, Med Phys 14:562-566, 1987.

1988 Benhamou CL et al: Costo-vertebral arthropathy. Diagnostic and therapeutic value of arthrography, Clin Rheumatol 7:220-223, 1988.

Benson DR: Unstable thoracolumbar fractures, with emphasis on the burst fracture, Clin Orthop 14-29, 1988.

Butt WP: Interpreting the spinal x-ray: 1, Br J Hosp Med 40:46-49, 51, 1988.

Fearon T et al: Scoliosis examinations: organ dose and image quality with rare-earth screen-film systems, AJR 150:359-362, 1988.

Fodor J and Malott JC: Chemonucleolysis, Radiol Technol 59:233-237, 1988.

Manninen H et al: Reduction of radiation dose and imaging costs in scoliosis radiography. Application of large-screen image intensifier photofluorography, Spine 13:409-412, 1988.

Pettersson H et al: Digital radiography of the spine, large bones and joints using stimulable phosphor: Early clinical experience, Acta Radiol 29:267-271, 1988.

Stonelake PS, Burwell RG and Webb JK: Variation in vertebral levels of the vertebra prominens and sacral dimples in subjects with scoliosis, J Anat 159:165-172, 1988.

1990 Kling TF Jr et al: Digital radiography can reduce scoliosis x-ray exposure, Spine 15:880-885, 1990.

1991 Giles LG: Review of tethered cord syndrome with a radiological and anatomical study: case report, Surg Radiol Anat 13:339-343, 1991.

Pathria MN and Petersilge CA: Spinal trauma, Radiol Clin North Am 29:847-865, 1991.

Yu S, Haughton VM and Rosenbaum AE: Magnetic resonance imaging and anatomy of the spine, Radiol Clin North Am 29:691-710, 1991.

1992 Andre B, Dansereau J and Labelle H: Effect of radiographic landmark identification errors on the accuracy of three-dimensional reconstruction of the human spine, Med Biol Eng Comput 30:569-575, 1992.

Ballock RT et al: Can burst fractures be predicted from plain radiographs? J Bone Joint Surg Br 74:147-150, 1992.

Dickson RA: The etiology and pathogenesis of idiopathic scoliosis, Acta Orthop Belg 58 Suppl 1:21-25, 1992.

Drerup B and Hierholzer E: Evaluation of frontal radiographs of scoliotic spines. Part II. Relations between lateral deviation, lateral tilt and axial rotation of vertebrae, J Biomech 25:1443-1450, 1992.

Edeiken-Monroe BS and Edeiken J: Imaging of the normal spine, developmental anomalies, and trauma of the spine and extremities, Curr Opin Radiol 4:95-102, 1992.

Harrison LA, Pretorius DH and Budorick NE: Abnormal spinal curvature in the fetus, J Ultrasound Med 11:473-479, 1992.

Ho EK et al: A comparative study of computed tomographic and plain radiographic methods to measure vertebral rotation in adolescent idiopathic scoliosis, Spine 17:771-774, 1992.

Hobson DA and Tooms RE: Seated lumbar/pelvic alignment. A comparison between spinal cord-injured and noninjured groups, Spine 17:293-298, 1992.

Hu SS and Pashman RS: Spinal instrumentation. Evolution and state of the art, Invest Radiol 27:632-647, 1992.

Karasick D, Huettl EA and Cotler JM: Value of polydirectional tomography in the assessment of the postoperative spine after anterior decompression and vertebral body autografting, Skeletal Radiol 21:359-363, 1992.

Riddervold HO: Easily missed fractures, Radiol Clin North Am 30:475-494, 1992.

Rumball K, Jarvis J: Seat-belt injuries of the spine in young children, J Bone Joint Surg Br 74:571-574, 1992.

Schmidt J, Gassel F and Naughton S: Calculation of 3-D deformity in scoliosis by standard roentgenograms, Acta Orthop Belg 58 Suppl 1:60-65, 1992.

Shuren N et al: Reevaluation of the use of the Risser sign in idiopathic scoliosis, Spine 17:359-361, 1992.

Tehranzadeh J, Kerr R and Amster J: Magnetic resonance imaging of tendon and ligament abnormalities. Part I. Spine and upper extremities, Skeletal Radiol 21:1-9, 1992.

1993 Barnes PD et al: Atypical idiopathic scoliosis: MR imaging evaluation, Radiology 186:247-253, 1993.

Garcia FF et al: Diagnostic imaging of childhood spinal infection, Orthop Rev 22:321-327, 1993.

Samuels LE and Kerstein MD: 'Routine' radiologic evaluation of the thoracolumbar spine in blunt trauma patients: a reappraisal, J Trauma 34:85-89, 1993.

BRONCHOGRAPHY

For bibliographic citations before 1964, please see the fifth edition of this atlas. For citations from 1964 through 1974, see the sixth or seventh edition.

1975 Reed JC and Madewell JE: The air bronchogram is interstitial disease of the lungs: a radiological-pathological correlation, Radiology 116:1-9, 1975.

1976 Moore DH: A simple technique for performing bronchography, J Miss State Med Assoc 17:303-305, 1976.

Smith JC, Stitik FP and Swift DL: Airway visualization by tantalum inhalation bronchography, Am Rev Respir Dis 113:515-529, 1976.

1978 Stitik FP et al: Tantalum tracheography in upper airway obstruction: 100 experiences in adults, AJR 130:35-41, 1978.

1979 Strecker EP et al: Inhalation bronchography using powdered calcium ioglycamic acid, Radiology 130:303-309, 1979.

1980 Ryan DR: Anaesthesia for bronchography in small children, Ann J Coll Surg Engl 62:223-227, 1980.

1981 Kogutt MS: Pediatric bronchography: simplified method for selective visualization, AJR 136:1249-1250, 1981.

1982 Furlonger BJ: High kV filtered beam technique for demonstrating bronchial situs, Radiography 48:197-199, 1982.

Lundgren R, Hietala SO and Adelroth E: Diagnosis of bronchial lesions by fiberoptic bronchoscopy combined, Acta Radiol [diagn] (Stockh) 23:231-234, 1982.

1983 Gamsu G and Webb WR: Computed tomography of the trachea and mainstem bronchi, Semin Roentgenol 18:51-60, 1983.

Levy M et al: Bronchoscopy and bronchography in children. Experience with 110 investigations, Am J Dis Child 137:14-16, 1983.

1984 Proto AV: Evaluation of the bronchi with CT, Semin Roentgenol 19:199-210, 1984.

Young JW, Andersen BL and Reinig JW: Oblique chest film: value in routine and selective use, AJR 142:69-72, 1984.

1985 Lau LS, Simpson L and Murphy F: High resolution CT scanning of the bronchial tree. CT bronchography: technique and clinical application, Australas Radiol 29:323-331, 1985.

1987 Koval JC et al: Fiberoptic bronchoscopy combined with selective bronchography, Chest 91:776-778, 1987.

1989 McAlister WH: Death associated with bronchography. Question role of heating the contrast agent, Pediatr Radiol 19:458-460, 1989.

Morcos SK et al: Iotrolan in selective bronchography via the fibreoptic bronchoscope, Br J Radiol 62:383-385, 1989.

1990 Morcos SK et al: Suitability of and tolerance to Iotrolan 300 in bronchography via the fibreoptic bronchoscope, Thorax 45:628-629, 1990.

Riebel T and Wartner R: Use of non-ionic contrast media for tracheobronchography in neonates and young infants, Eur J Radiol 11:120-124, 1990.

1991 Buschman DL: Barium sulfate bronchography. Report of a complication, Chest 99:747-749, 1991.

Szmigielski W et al: Powdered diatrizoic acid for radiography of the respiratory tract. Part I. Experimental investigation, Acta Radiol 32:415-420, 1991.

Szmigielski W et al: Powdered diatrizoic acid for radiography of the respiratory tract. Part II. Clinical application, Acta Radiol 32:467-473, 1991.

Takasugi JE and Godwin JD: The airway, Semin Roentgenol 26:175-190, 1991.

1992 Davis SD and Umlas SL: Radiology of congenital abnormalities of the chest, Curr Opin Radiol 4:25-35, 1992.

1993 Bramson RT, Sherman JM and Blickman JG: Pediatric bronchography performed through the flexible bronchoscope, Eur J Radiol 16:158-161, 1993.

BEDSIDE RADIOGRAPHY

For bibliographic citations before 1964, please see the fifth edition of this atlas.

1978 Barnhard HJ: The bedside examination: a time for analysis and appropriate action, Radiology 129:539-540, 1978.

Cantwell KG, Press HC and Anderson JE: Bedside radiographic examinations: indications and contraindications, Radiology 129:383-384, 1978.

1979 Colley DP: Device for improving quality of bedside decubitus examinations, Radiol Technol 51:88-89, 1979.

1980 Dougherty JE, LaSala AF and Fieldman A: Bedside pulmonary angiography utilizing an existing Swan-Ganz catheter, Chest 77:43-46, 1980.

Eisenberg RL, Akin JR and Hedgecock MW: Optimal use of portable and stat examination, AJR 134:523-524, 1980.

Tabrisky J et al: Mobile 240 kVp phototimed chest radiography, AJR 135:295-300, 1980.

1981 Robinson DR: Port-Clamp—an aid in portable radiography, Radiol Technol 53:267-268, 1981.

1982 Fisher MR et al: Evaluation of a new mobile automatic exposure control device, AJR 139:1055-1059, 1982.

Shaffer MA and Doris PE: Increasing the diagnostic yield of portable skull films, Ann Emerg Med 11:303-306, 1982.

1983 Henschke CI et al: Bedside chest radiography: diagnostic efficacy, Radiology 149:23-26, 1983.

Lewis DW: Double film radiography, Radiol Technol 54:388-390, 1983.

1984 Markowitz RI: Radiologic assessment in the pediatric intensive care unit, Yale J Biol Med 57:49-82, 1984.

1986 Foley KT, Cahan LD and Hieshima GB: Intraoperative angiography using a portable digital subtraction unit, J Neurosurg 64:816-818, 1986.

1988 Milne EN et al: Assessment of cardiac size on portable chest films, J Thorac Imaging 3:64-72, 1988.

Peruzzi W et al: Portable chest roentgenography and computed tomography in critically ill patients, Chest 93:722-726, 1988.

Saito H et al: Digital radiography in an intensive care unit, Clin Radiol 39:127-130, 1988.

Zylak CJ, Littleton JT and Durizch ML: Illusory consolidation of the left lower lobe: a pitfall of portable radiography, Radiology 167:653-655, 1988.

1989 Cohen MD et al: Digital imaging of the newborn chest, Clin Radiol 40:365-368, 1989.

Hauser GJ et al: Routine chest radiographs in pediatric intensive care: a prospective study, Pediatrics 83:465-470, 1989.

Rosengarten PL, Tuxen DV and Weeks AM: Whole lung pulmonary angiography in the intensive care unit with two portable chest x-rays, Crit Care Med 17:274-278, 1989.

Schaefer CM et al: Improved control of image optical density with low-dose digital and conventional radiography in bedside imaging, Radiology 173:713-716, 1989.

Sivit CJ et al: Efficacy of chest radiography in pediatric intensive care, AJR 152:575-577, 1989.

1990 Geijer M, Jensen C and Schlossman D: Chest radiography in the intensive care unit. Indications for radiography and effects of selective archiving of films, Acta Radiol 31:321-323, 1990.

Marglin SI, Rowberg AH and Godwin JD: Preliminary experience with portable digital imaging for intensive care radiography, J Thorac Imaging 5:49-54, 1990.

Sagel SS et al: Digital mobile radiography, J Thorac Imaging 5:36-48, 1990.

Tarver RD et al: Pediatric digital chest imaging, J Thorac Imaging 5:31-35, 1990.

1991 MacMahon H and Doi K: Digital chest radiography, Clin Chest Med 12:19-32, 1991.

Moller A: Radiography transculcitam: technique and devices to simplify bedside radiography, Radiology 179:283-284, 1991.

Rose CC, Delbridge TR and Mosesso VNJ: The portable chest film, Emerg Med Clin North Am 9:767-788, 1991.

Swensen SJ et al: Radiology in the intensive care unit, Mayo Clin Proc 66:396-410, 1991.

Wiener MD et al: Imaging of the intensive care unit patient, Clin Chest Med 12:169-198, 1991.

1992 Broderick NJ et al: Comparison of computerized digital and film-screen radiography: response to variation in imaging kVp, Pediatr Radiol 22:346-349, 1992.

Gray P et al: Value of postprocedural chest radiographs in the adult intensive care unit, Crit Care Med 20:1513-1518, 1992.

Jennings P, Padley SP and Hansell DM: Portable chest radiography in intensive care: a comparison of computed and conventional radiography, Br J Radiol 65:852-856, 1992.

Lam RW and Price SC: Pitfalls of rare earth imaging: conquering the three Ps, Radiol Technol 63:248-251, 1992.

Lyttkens K et al: Bedside chest radiography using digital luminescence. A comparison between digital radiographs reviewed on a personal computer and as hard-copies, Acta Radiol 33:427-430, 1992.

O'Donovan PB et al: Device for facilitating precise alignment in bedside radiography, Radiology 184:284-285, 1992.

Yu CJ et al: Diagnostic and therapeutic use of chest sonography: value in critically ill patients, AJR 159:695-701, 1992.

1993 Frank MS et al: High-resolution computer display of portable, digital, chest radiographs of adults: suitability for primary interpretation, AJR 160:473-477, 1993.

Niklason LT et al: Portable chest imaging: comparison of storage phosphor digital, asymmetric screen-film, and conventional screen-film systems, Radiology 186:387-393, 1993.

OPERATING ROOM RADIOGRAPHY

For bibliographic citations before 1964, please see the fifth edition of this atlas. For citations from 1964 through 1974, see the sixth or seventh edition.

1976 Berci G and Zheutlin N: Improving radiology in surgery, Med Instrum 10:110-114, 1976.

Carter PR: Brief note: simple method of obtaining intraoperative x-rays of the hand, J Bone Joint Surg 58:576, 1976.

1977 Pochaczevsky R: Kidney cassettes for intraoperative radiography, Radiology 123:237-238, 1977.

1978 Berci G et al: Operative fluoroscopy and cholangiography: the use of modern radiologic technics during surgery, Am J Surg 135:32-35, 1978.

1979 Forster IW and Lindsay JA: Image intensifier as an aid to insertion of the Zickel nail apparatus for proximal femoral fractures, Injury 11:148-154, 1979.

1980 Giachino AA and Cheng M: Irradiation of the surgeon during pinning of femoral fractures, J Bone Joint Surg 62-B:227-229, 1980.

Konnak JW and Wedemeyer G: The use of a portable dental x-ray unit for intraoperative renal roentgenograms, J Urol 124:768-769, 1980.

Linos DA, Gray JE and McIlrath DC: Radiation hazard to operating room personnel during operative cholangiography, Arch Surg 115:1431-1433, 1980.

Sigel B et al: Sterile, portable radiation shield for the operating room, Arch Surg 115:347-348, 1980.

1981 Pietila K, Pukkila O and Slatis P: Reduced radiation exposure in orthopaedic surgery: experience with video disk recording in nailing of fractured hips, Eur J Radiol 1:152-154, 1981.

1982 Coelho JC et al: Detection of experimental arterial defects by portable and serial biplanar operative arteriography, Invest Radiol 17:259-264, 1982.

1983 Machi J et al: Critical factors in the image clarity of operative cholangiography, J Surg Res 35:480-489, 1983.

Roth D and Griffith DP: Operative renal radiography, Urology 21:60-61, 1983.

1984 Proposed recommended practices: radiation safety in the operating room, AORN J 40:881-886, 1984.

1986 Foley KT, Cahan LD and Hieshima GB: Intraoperative angiography using a portable digital subtraction unit, J Neurosurg 64:816-818, 1986.

1987 Cassel J: A technique to control hand position for intraoperative radiography, J Hand Surg Am 12:148-149, 1987.

Levin PE, Schoen RW Jr and Browner BD: Radiation exposure to the surgeon during closed interlocking intramedullary nailing, J Bone Joint Surg Am 69:761-766, 1987.

1989 Pond GD et al: Intraoperative arteriography: comparison of conventional screen-film with photostimulable imaging plate radiographs, Radiology 170:367-370, 1989.

Riley SA: Radiation exposure from fluoroscopy during orthopedic surgical procedures, Clin Orthop 257-260, 1989.

1990 Baagley DH and Cubler-Goodman A: Radiation exposure during ureteroscopy, J Urol 144:1356-1358, 1990.

Croft MJ: Stereotactic radiosurgery of arteriovenous malformations, Radiol Technol 61:375-379, 1990.

Hariz MI and Bergenheim AT: A comparative study on ventriculographic and computerized tomography-guided determinations of brain targets in functional stereotaxis, Journal of Neurosurgery 73:565-571, 1990.

Kwong LM et al: Shielding of the patient's gonads during intramedullary interlocking femoral nailing, J Bone Joint Surg Am 72:1523-1526, 1990.

1991 Mitchell NJ and Hunt S: Surgical face masks in modern operating rooms—a costly and unnecessary ritual? J Hosp Infect 18:239-242, 1991.

Nowak B and Jankowski J: Occupational exposure in operational radiology, Pol J Occup Med 4:169-174, 1991.

1992 Abdul-Karim FW et al: Case report 736: Retained surgical sponge (gossypiboma) with a foreign body reaction and remote and organizing hematoma, Skeletal Radiol 21:466-469, 1992.

Machi J and Sigel B: Intraoperative ultrasonography, Radiol Clin North Am 30:1085-1103, 1992.

Mughmaw SB: An overview of methods in stereotactic radiosurgery, Radiol Technol 63:402-405, 1992.

Waldron VD: Improving the C-arm image of small bones, Orthop Rev 21:887-888, 1992.

1993 Kuster GG, Gilroy S and Graefen M: Intraoperative cholangiography for laparoscopic cholecystectomy, Surg Gynecol Obstet 176:411-417, 1993.

Sanders R et al: Exposure of the orthopaedic surgeon to radiation, J Bone Joint Surg Am 75:326-330, 1993.

ANESTHETICS IN RADIOLOGY

For bibliographic citations before 1964, please see the fifth edition of this atlas.

1976 Aidinis SJ et al: Anesthesia for brain computer tomography, Anesthesiology 44:420-425, 1976.

1977 Korten K: Anesthesia for diagnostic procedures, Am Fam Physician 15:103-107, 1977.

1980 Ryan DW: Anaesthesia for bronchography in small children, Ann R Coll Surg Engl 62:223-227, 1980.

Spigos DG et al: Epidural anesthesia: effective analgesia in aortoiliofemoral arteriography, AJR 134:335-337, 1980.

1983 Wenz W et al: Anaesthesia problems in angiography with special reference to modern contrast media, Fortschr Geb Rontgenstr Nuklearmed Erganzungsbund 118:92-101, 1983.

1985 Weston G, Strunin L and Amundson GM: Imaging for anaesthetists: a review of the methods and anaesthetic, Can Anaesth Soc J 32:552-561, 1985.

1987 Nilsson P: Addition of local anesthetics to contrast media. Part I. Effects on, Acta Radiol 128:209-214, 1987.

1988 Akber SF: Influence of anesthetics on relaxation times, Anesthesiology 69:290-291, 1988.

Hedenstierna G: Causes of gas exchange impairment during general anaesthesia, Eur J Anaesthesiol 5:221-231, 1988.

Karlik SJ et al: Patient anesthesia and monitoring at a 1.5-T MRI installation, Magn Reson Med 7:21-221, 1988.

Nahata MC: Sedation in pediatric patients undergoing diagnostic procedures, Drug Intell Clin Pharm 22:711-715, 1988.

FOREIGN BODY LOCALIZATION

For bibliographic citations before 1964, please see the fifth edition of this atlas. For citations from 1964 through 1974, see the sixth or seventh edition.

1975   McArthur DR and Taylor DF: A determination of the minimum radiopacification necessary for radiographic detection of an aspirated or swallowed object, Oral Surg 39:329-338, 1975.

Meyer WG: Sequel technique for localization and extraction of radiopaque foreign bodies in various anatomic sites, Ohio State Med J 71:15-18, 1975.

Taupman RE and Martin JE: The detection of non-opaque foreign bodies by xeroradiography, South Med J 68:1186-1187, 1975.

1977   Bowers DG Jr and Lynch JB: Xeroradiography for non-metallic foreign bodies, Plast Reconstr Surg 60:470-471, 1977.

1978   Thompson DH, Stasney CR and Miller T: Xeroradiographic detection of foreign bodies, Laryngoscope 88:254-259, 1978.

1979   Kjhns LR et al: An in vitro comparison of computed tomography, xeroradiography, and radiography in the detection of soft-tissue foreign bodies, Radiology 132: 218-219, 1979.

1980   Berger PE, Kuhn JP and Kuhns LR: Computed tomography and the occult tracheobronchial foreign body, Radiology 134: 133-135, 1980.

Gaster RN and Duda EE: Localization of intraocular foreign bodies by computed tomography, Ophthalmic Surg 11:25-29, 1980.

Grasso L: Foreign body localization by computed tomography, Radiol Technol 51: 668, 1980.

Healy JF: Computed tomography of a cranial wooden foreign body, J Comput Assist Tomogr 4:555-556, 1980.

1981   Pick RY: The roentgenographic appearance of lead paint as a foreign body, Clin Orthop 155:305-306, 1981.

1982   Moskowitz D, Gardiner LJ and Sasaki CT: Foreign-body aspiration. Potential misdiagnosis, Arch Otolaryngol 108:806-807, 1982.

Tandberg D: Glass in the hand and foot: will an x-ray film show it? JAMA 248:1872-1874, 1982.

1983   Fodor J III and Malott JC: The radiographic detection of foreign bodies, Radiol Technol 54:361-370, 1983.

Kulig K et al: Disk battery ingestion; elevated urine mercury levels and enema removal of battery fragments, JAMA 249:2502-2504, 1983.

Weisman RA et al: Computed tomography in penetrating wounds of the orbit with retained foreign bodies, Arch Otolaryngol 109:265-268, 1983.

Xeroradiography for foreign body detection, Radiography 49:33, 1983.

1984   Firooznia H et al: Computed tomography in localization of foreign bodies lodged in the extremities, Comput Radiol 8:237-239, 1984.

Fodor J III and Malott JC: The Min-R system: an alternative to xeroradiography, Radiol Technol 55:41-43, 1984.

Griffiths DM and Freeman NV: Expiratory chest x ray examination in the diagnosis of inhaled foreign bodies, Br Med J [Clin Res] 288:1074-1075, 1984.

1984   Sassani JW et al: Combined use of A-scan ultrasound, plain roentgenograms, and computerized axial tomography in the evaluation of a pseudo-intraocular foreign body, JCU 12:171-173, 1984.

Selivanov V et al: Management of foreign body ingestion, Ann Surg 199:187-191, 1984.

Watson A and Hartley DE: Alternative method of intraocular foreign-body localization, AJR 142:789-790, 1984.

1985   de Lacey G, Evans R and Sandin B: Penetrating injuries: how easy is it to see glass (and plastic) on radiographs? Br J Radiol 58:27-30, 1985.

1986   Charney DB et al: Nonmetallic foreign bodies in the foot: radiography versus xeroradiography, J Foot Surg 25:44-49, 1986.

Grn P, Andersen K and Vraa A: Detection of glass foreign bodies by radiography, Injury 17:404-406, 1986.

Pamilo M, Suoranta H and Suramo I: Narcotic smuggling and radiography of the gastrointestinal tract, Acta Radiol [diagn] (Stockh) 27:213-216, 1986.

Zigler J et al: Localization of foreign bodies in the spinal canal by computer-assisted biplanar digitizer, Spine 11:892-894, 1986.

Zinreich SJ et al: Computed tomographic three-dimensional localization and compositional evaluation of intraocular and orbital foreign bodies, Arch Ophthalmol 104:1477-1482, 1986.

1987   Boothroyd AE, Carty HM and Robson WJ: 'Hunt the thimble': a study of the radiology of ingested foreign bodies, Arch Emerg Med 4:33-38, 1987.

Brandt C: A shot in the dark: foreign body localization, Radiography 53:26-26, 1987.

Lindahl S: Computed tomography of intraorbital foreign bodies, Acta Radiol 28:235-240, 1987.

Myllyla V et al: CT detection and location of intraorbital foreign bodies: experiments with wood and glass, ROFO 146:639-643, 1987.

1988   Bronstein AD, Kilcoyne RF and Moe RE: Complications of needle localization of foreign bodies and nonpalpable breast lesions, Arch Surg 123:775-779, 1988.

Galuten A and Austin JH: Permanent subcutaneous acupuncture needles: radiographic manifestations, J Can Assoc Radiol 39:54-56, 1988.

Laks Y and Barzilay Z: Foreign body aspiration in childhood, Pediatr Emerg Care 4:102-106, 1988.

O'Driscoll SW: Glass is detectable on plain radiographs, Can Med Assoc J 139:643-644, 1988.

Savitt DL and Wason S: Delayed diagnosis of coin ingestion in children, Am J Emerg Med 6:378-381, 1988.

1989   Svedstrom E, Puhakka H and Kero P: How accurate is chest radiography in the diagnosis of tracheobronchial foreign bodies in children? Pediatr Radiol 19:520-522, 1989.

1990   Blyme PJ et al: Ultrasonographic detection of foreign bodies in soft tissue. A human cadaver study, Arch Orthop Trauma Surg 110:24-25, 1990.

Hedlund GL and Kirks DR: Emergency radiology of the pediatric chest, Curr Probl Diagn Radiol 19:133-164, 1990.

1992   Abdul-Karim FW et al: Case report 736: Retained surgical sponge (gossypiboma) with a foreign body reaction and remote and organizing hematoma, Skeletal Radiol 21:466-469, 1992.

1993   Donaldson JS: Radiographic imaging of foreign bodies in the hand, Hand Clin 7:125-134, 1993.

Levine WN and Leslie BM: The use of ultrasonography to detect a radiolucent foreign body in the hand: a case report, J Hand Surg Am 18:218-220, 1993.

EXPOSURE TECHNIQUES

For bibliographic citations before 1964, please see the fifth edition of this atlas. For citations from 1964 through 1974, see the sixth or seventh edition.

1975   Eastman TR: Technique charts: the key to radiographic quality, Radiol Technol 46:365-368, 1975.

Hiss SS: Technique management, Radiol Technol 46:369-375, 1975.

Stein JA: X-ray imaging with a scanning beam, Radiology 117:713-716, 1975.

Sweeney RJ: Some factors affecting image clarity and detail perception in the radiograph, Radiol Technol 46:443-451, 1975.

1976   Genant HK, Doi K and Mall JC: Comparison of non-screen techniques (medical vs industrial film) for fine detail skeletal radiography, Invest Radiol 11:486-500, 1976.

Rossi RP, Hendee WR and Athrens CR: An evaluation of rare earth screen/film combinations, Radiology 121:465-471, 1976.

1977   Castle JW: Sensitivity of radiographic screens to scattered radiation and its relationship to image contrast, Radiology 122:805-809, 1977.

Harms AA and Zeilinger A: A new formulation of total unsharpness in radiography, Phys Med Biol 22:70-80, 1977.

Moyer RF: The mysterious wall around exposure, Radiol Technol 48:707-710, 1977.

Stables DP et al: The application of fast screen-film systems to excretory urography, AJR 128:617-619, 1977.

1978 Amplatz K, Moore R and Korbuly D: The "swinging" tube: a new concept, Radiology 128:783-785, 1978.

Newlin N: Reduction in radiation exposure: the rare-earth screen, AJR 130:1195-1196, 1978.

Rao GU, Fatouros PP and James AE Jr: Physical characteristics of modern radiographic screen-film systems, Invest Radiol 13:460-469, 1978.

Weaver KE, Barone GJ and Fewell TR: Selection of technique factors for mobile capacitor energy storage x-ray equipment, Radiology 128:223-228, 1978.

1979 Stopford JE: Log$_{10}$.MDNM/ technique charts, Radiol Technol 51:331-333, 1979.

Venema HW: X-ray absorption, speed, and luminescent efficiency of rare-earth and other intensifying screens, Radiology 130:765-771, 1979.

1980 Barnes GT et al: The scanning grid: a novel and effective bucky movement, Radiology 135:765-767, 1980.

Duck FA, Starrett HC and Davies AR: Errors in measurement of kVp and exposure time from the presence of a premagnetization pulse, Br J Radiol 53:716-718, 1980.

Hill SJ, O'Brian AR and Watkins RA: A multiple exposure penetrameter cassette for measurement of effective kilovoltage, Br J Radiol 53:358-360, 1980.

Ritter EM et al: Use of a gradient intensifying screen for scoliosis radiography, Radiology 135:230-232, 1980.

Skucas J and Gorski J: Application of modern intensifying screens in diagnostic radiology, Med Radiogr Photogr 56:25-36, 1980.

Vyborny CJ, Metz CE and Doi K: Relative efficiencies of energy to photographic density conversions in typical screen-film systems, Radiology 136:465-471, 1980.

Yester MV, Barnes GT and King MA: Kilovoltage bootstrap sensitometry, Radiology 136:785-786, 1980.

1981 Brodeur AE et al: Three-tier rare-earth imaging system, AJR 136:755-758, 1981.

Franji SM and El-Koury GY: Applications of double screen roentgenography, Appl Radiol 10:59-61, 1981.

McDaniel SJ: High- and normal-speed rotors: effect on focal spot size, resolution and density, Radiol Technol 53:47-49, 1981.

Posada FP: Clinical applications of rare earth imaging in diagnostic radiology, Radiol Technol 53:49-52, 1981.

1982 Burgess AE and Hicken P: Comparative performance of x-ray-intensifying screens, Radiology 143:551-556, 1982.

Fisher MR et al: Evaluation of a new mobile automatic exposure control device, AJR 139:1055-1059, 1982.

Kruger RA et al: Digital subtraction angiography using a temporal bandpass filter, Radiology 145:315-320, 1982.

Moseley RD and Kelsey CA: Evaluating imaging methods, AJR 138:977-999, 1982.

Robinson T, Becker JA and Olson AP: Clinical comparison of high-speed rare-earth screen and par-speed, Radiology 145:214-216, 1982.

1983 Carroll C: Geometric fallacies, Radiol Technol 54:297-301, 1983.

De Smet AA et al: Comparison of two detail screen-film systems using a rheumatoid erosion model, Invest Radiol 18:359-363, 1983.

Feczko PJ et al: Compensation filtration for decubitus radiography during double-contrast barium enema examinations, Radiology 149:848-850, 1983.

James N: High kilovoltage radiography using the Cincinnati filter, Radiography 49:210-214, 1983.

1984 Malott JC: Light fog: picture of a problem, Radiol Technol 55:105-106, 1984.

1985 Burgess AE: Scatter radiation from abdominal CT examinations, J Comput Assist Tomogr 9:926-930, 1985.

Butler PF et al: Chest radiography: a survey of techniques and exposure levels currently used, Radiology 156:533-536, 1985.

Fodor J III et al: Indications for the use of high kVp in the plain film examination of the abdomen, Radiol Technol 57:159-161, 1985.

Pahira JJ and Pollack HM: New self-developing film for intraoperative renal stone localization, Urology 25:418-424, 1985.

Perry NM et al: Heart size in high-kilovoltage chest radiography, Clin Radiol 36:335-339, 1985.

1986 Nielsen B and Fagerberg G: Image quality in mammography with special reference to anti-scatter, Acta Radiol [diagn] (Stockh) 27:467-479, 1986.

1987 Compton SC: Bit conversion of technical factors in vascular procedures, Radiol Technol 58:413-416, 1987.

Fodor J and Malott JC: Magnification radiography, Radiol Technol 58:313-319, 1987.

Gratale P, Burns CB and Murray J: Advantages of a 400 speed image receptor system for cast radiography, Radiol Technol 58:401-403, 1987.

Kimme-Smith C, Bassett LW and Gold RH: Evaluation of radiation dose, focal spot, and automatic exposure of newer film-screen mammography units, AJR 149:913-917, 1987.

Neufang KF, Zanella FE and Ewen K: Radiation doses to the eye lenses in computed tomography of the orbit and the petrous bone, Eur J Radiol 7:203-205, 1987.

Olson DL et al: Efficacy of an intracassette filter for improved pneumocolon decubitus radiographs, AJR 148:547-549, 1987.

Pruneau D et al: A practical approach to direct magnification radiography, Radiol Technol 59:121-127, 1987.

Weeks LA: Static film/screen imaging terminology: the need to standardize, Radiol Technol 58:203-209, 1987.

1988 Burton EM et al: Evaluation of a low-dose neonatal chest radiographic system, AJR 151:999-1002, 1988.

Dailey JC and Furue T: A photographic technique for the restoration of damaged radiographs, J Forensic Sci 33:1273-1277, 1988.

Fodor J: Recent advances in x-ray tube design, Radiol Technol 60:33-35, 1988.

Fuhrman CR et al: Storage phosphor radiographs vs conventional films: interpreters' perceptions of diagnostic quality, AJR 150:1011-1014, 1988.

Guilbeau JC et al: Chest radiography with a shaped filter at 140 kVp: its diagnostic accuracy compared with that of standard radiographs, AJR 150:1007-1010, 1988.

Kruger RA: Medical imaging strategies, J Digit Imaging 1:13-17, 1988.

LaFrance R, Gelskey DE and Barnes GT: A circuit modification that improves mammographic phototimer performance, Radiology 166:773-776, 1988.

Manninen H et al: Image-intensifier photofluorography and conventional chest radiography: comparison of diagnostic efficacy, AJR 150:539-544, 1988.

Sterling S: Automatic exposure control: a primer, Radiol Technol 59:421-427, 1988.

1989 Barker EJ: An old problem seen again, Radiol Technol 60:427-428, 1989.

Chakraborty DP and Barnes GT: An energy sensitive cassette for dual-energy mammography, Med Phys 16:7-13, 1989.

Conlogue G et al: Dr. Leidy's soap lady: imaging the past, Radiol Technol 60:411-415, 1989.

Lam RW and Price SC: The influence of film-screen color sensitivity and type of measurement device on kVp measurements, Radiol Technol 60:319-321, 1989.

Stevens PM: Radiographic distortion of bones: a marker study, Orthopedics 12:1457-1463, 1989.

1990 Gratale P, Wright DL and Daughtry L: Using the anode heel effect for extremity radiography, Radiol Technol 61:195-198, 1990.

Henriksson L et al: Assessment of congestive heart failure in chest radiographs. Observer performance with two common film-screen systems, Acta Radiol 31:469-471, 1990.

Jones R and Adler AM: The saline solution bag as a compensating filter, Radiol Technol 62:134-138, 1990.

Kruger RA, Reinecke DR and Power RL: Light equalization radiography, Med Phys 17:696-700, 1990.

Plewes DB, McFaul J and Ivanovic M: Maximizing film contrast for scanning equalization radiography, Med Phys 17:357-361, 1990.

1991 David G and Price SC: Improved calibrations using personal computers, Radiol Technol 63:32-39, 1991.

David G: Worksheets simplify use of Wisconsin Test Cassette, Radiol Technol 63:106-109, 1991.

Kebart RC and James CD: Benefits of increasing focal film distance, Radiol Technol 62:434-442, 1991.

Siegel EL, Cook LT and Parsa MB: Conventional screen/film vs reduced exposure photostimulable phosphor plate imaging in lower extremity venography: an ROC analysis, AJR 156:1095-1099, 1991.

Yester MV: Radiologic equipment, Curr Opin Radiol 3:233-239, 1991.

1992 Broderick NJ et al: Comparison of computerized digital and film-screen radiography: response to variation in imaging kVp, Pediatr Radiol 22:346-349, 1992.

Lam RW and Price SC: Pitfalls of rare earth imaging: conquering the three Ps, Radiol Technol 63:248-251, 1992.

Umezawa T et al: A computerized automatic exposure device for chest radiography in infants, Clin Pediatr Phila 31:751-752, 1992.

1993 Dobbins JT et al: Variable compensation chest radiography performed with a computed radiography system: design considerations and initial clinical experience, Radiology 187:55-63, 1993.

Ito W et al: Improvement of detection in computed radiography by new single-exposure dual-energy subtraction, J Digit Imaging 6:42-47, 1993.

Kido S et al: Interpretation of subtle interstitial lung abnormalities: conventional versus storage phosphor radiography, Radiology 187:527-533, 1993.

Pirtle OL: Study shows inconsistency in film processing quality, Radiol Technol 64:154-159, 1993.

Prokop M et al: Improved parameters for unsharp mask filtering of digital chest radiographs, Radiology 187:521-526, 1993.

Swensen SJ et al: A new asymmetric screen-film combination for conventional chest radiography: evaluation in 50 patients, AJR 160:483-486, 1993.

Yoshimura H et al: Development of a high quality film duplication system using a laser digitizer: comparison with computed radiography, Med Phys 20:51-58, 1993.

CONTRAST MEDIA

For bibliographic citations before 1964, please see the fifth edition of this atlas. For citations from 1964 through 1974, see the sixth or seventh edition.

1975 Jekell K, Ohlson T and Widebeck J: Physical characteristics of barium contrast media and their influence on roentgen image information, Acta Radiol [diagn] 16:263-272, 175.

Sargent NE et al: A new contrast medium for cholangio-cholecystography: meglumine iodoxamate, AJR 125:251-258, 1975.

Shehadi WH: Adverse reactions to intravascularly administered contrast media, AJR 124:145-152, 1975.

1976 Andrews EJ: The vagus reaction as a possible cause of severe complications of radiological procedures, Radiology 121:1-4, 1976.

Bentson JR and Wilson GH: Clinical comparison of three contrast agents used in cerebral angiography, Invest Radiol 11:602-604, 1976.

Berk RN and Loeb RM: Pharmacology and physiology of the biliary radiographic contrast materials, Semin Roentgenol 11:147-156, 1976.

Robbins AH et al: Double-blind comparison of meglumine iodoxamate (Cholevue) and meglumine iodipamide (Cholegrafin), AJR 127:257-260, 1976.

1977 Grepe A: Cisternography with metrizamide of the posterior fossa following lateral C1-C2 puncture, Acta Radiol (Stockh) 355(suppl):257-268, 1977.

Hekster RE, Prins HJ and Pennings-Braun AG: Lumbar myelography with metrizamide, Acta Radiol (Stockh) 355(suppl):38-41, 1977.

Lindgren E, editor: Metrizamide—Amipaque: the non-ionic water-soluble contrast medium, Acta Radiol 355(suppl):1-432, 1977.

Loeb PM, Barnhart JL and Berk RN: Iotroxamide—a new intravenous cholangiographic agent, Radiology 125:323-329, 1977.

Miller RE and Skucas J: Radiographic contrast agents, Baltimore, 1977, University Park Press.

Potts DG, Gomez DG and Abbott GF: Possible causes of complications of myelography with water-soluble contrast media, Acta Radiol (Stockh) 355(suppl):390-402, 1977.

Roberson GH et al: Cisternography with metrizamide and hypocycloidal tomography, Acta Radiol (Stockh) 355(suppl):314-322, 1977.

Shehadi WH: Contrast media in diagnostic radiology: recommendations for labels, package inserts, and dosage determination, AJR 129:167-170, 1977.

Skalpe IO: Adverse effects of water-soluble contrast media in myelography, reference to metrizamide, Acta Radiol (Stockh) 355(suppl):359-370, 1977.

Skalpe IO and Sortland O: Thoracic myelography with metrizamide: technical and diagnostic aspects, Acta Radiol (Stockh) 355(suppl):57-64, 1977.

Sortland O, Magnaes B and Hauge T: Functional myelography with metrizamide in the diagnosis of lumbar spinal stenosis, Acta Radiol (Stockh) 355(suppl):42-54, 1977.

1978 Johansen JG: Assessment of a nonionic contrast medium (Amipaque) in the gastrointestinal tract, Invest Radiol 13:523-527, 1978.

Kieffer AA et al: Contrast agents for myelography: clinical and radiological evaluation of Amipaque and Pantopaque, Radiology 129:695-705, 1978.

Miller ES: Reactions to intravenous pyelography contrast media, Radiol Technol 50:269-273, 1978.

Pizzolato NF, Arcomano JP and Baum AE: A new contrast agent for oral cholecystography: iopronic acid (Oravue), AJR 130:845-847, 1978.

1979 Gelmers HJ: Adverse side effects of metrizamide in myelography, Neuroradiology 18:119-123, 1979.

1980 Bush WH, Mullarky MF and Webb DR: Adverse reactions to radiographic contrast material, Western J Med 132:95-98, 1980.

Dean PB: Contrast media in body computed tomography: experimental and theoretical background, present limitations, and proposals for improved diagnostic efficacy, Invest Radiol 15:S164-169, 1980.

Fischer HW: The need for more study of gastrointestinal contrast media, Invest Radiol 15:S148-150, 1980.

Grainger RG: Osmality of intravascular radiological contrast media, Br J Radiol 53:739-746, 1980.

Harnish PP et al: Drugs providing protection from severe contrast media reactions, Invest Radiol 15:248-259, 1980.

Violante MR, Fischer HW and Mahoney JA: New media. Particulate contrast media, Invest Radiol 15:S329-334, 1980.

Virkkunen P, Retulainen M and Keto P: Observations on the behavior of barium sulfate contrast media in vitro, Invest Radiol 15:346-349, 1980.

1981 Rubin DL, Carroll BA and Snow HD: The harmful effects of aqueous contrast agents on the gastrointestinal tract: a study of mechanism and means of counteraction, Invest Radiol 16:50-58, 1981.

Virkkunen P: Variation in the quality of barium sulfate contrast media, Radiology 140:833-834, 1981.

1982 Chrzanowski R: The contrast media used for myelography, Eur Neurol 21:194-197, 1982.

Kallehauge HE and Praestholm J: Iopamidol, a new nonionic contrast medium in peripheral angiography, Cardiovasc Intervent Radiol 5:325-328, 1982.

Levorstad K et al: Tolerability and diagnostic usefulness of iohexol in urography; an open multicentre clinical trial, Acta Radiol 23:491-496, 1982.

Macpherson P: Comparison of iopamidol with three other contrast media in orbital venography/cavernous sinography, Br J Radiol 55:539-540, 1982.

Siegle RL, Davies P and Fullerton GD: Urography with metrizamide in children, AJR 139:927-930, 1982.

Suzuki S, Mine H and Iwai T: Clinical experience of iozaglate in femoral angiography, Acta Radiol 23:87-92, 1982.

Thompson WM et al: Gallbladder density and iodine concentration in humans during oral cholecystography, Invest Radiol 17:621-628, 1982.

Whitehouse GH and Snowdon SL: An assessment of iopamidol, a non-ionic contrast medium, in aoro-femoral angiography, Clin Radiol 33:231-234, 1982.

1983 Alenghat JP, Kim HS and Duda EE: Cervical and lumbar metrizamide myelography: split-dose technique, Radiology 149:852-853, 1983.

Antes G and Lissner J: Double-contrast small-bowel examination with barium and methylcellulose, Radiology 148:37-40, 1983.

Bannon KR et al: Comparison of radiographic quality and adverse reactions in myelography with iopamidol and metrizamide, AJNR 4:312-313, 1983.

Burgener FA and Hamlin DJ: Contrast enhancement of hepatic tumors in CT: comparison between bolus and infusion techniques, AJR 140:291-295, 1983.

Cacayorin ED et al: Intravenous digital subtraction angiography with iohexol, AJNR 4:329-332, 1983.

Davis GR and Smith HJ: Double-contrast examination of the colon after preparation with Golytely (a balanced lavage solution), Gastrointest Radiol 8:173-176, 1983.

Diament MJ and Kangarloo H: Dosage schedule for pediatric urography based on body surface, AJR 140:815-816, 1983.

Foord KD, Morcos SK and Ward P: A comparison of mannitol and magnesium citrate preparations for double-contrast barium enema, Clin Radiol 34:309-312, 1983.

Fraser GM and Preston PG: The small bowel barium follow-through enhanced with an oral effervescent agent, Clin Radiol 34:673-679, 1983.

Gronnerod TA et al: Documentation of a new contrast medium for the subarachnoid space; demands, design, and results from the first multicentre trial with iohexol, Acta Radiol 24:487-491, 1983.

Hada M et al: Double-contrast cervical esophagography: use of a specially designed cup to aid double-contrast cervical esophagography, Radiat Med 1:211-215, 1983.

Hindmarsh T et al: Comparative double-blind investigation of meglumine metrizoate, metrizamide, and iohexol in carotid angiography, AJNR 4:347-349, 1983.

Kerber CW et al: Iotrol, a new myelographic agent: 1. Radiography, CT, CSF clearance, and brain penetration, AJNR 4:317-318, 1983.

Kormano M et al: Dynamic contrast enhancement of the upper abdomen: effect of contrast medium and body weight, Invest Radiol 18:364-367, 1983.

Laasonen EM and Lindholm A: Double contrast arthrography of the knee. Comparison between three contrast medium, Acta Radiol 24:225-229, 1983.

Laitakari K, Suonpaa J and Kortekangas AE: Radiography of the maxillary sinus mucosal surface with Tantalum, Acta Otolaryngol 95:454-459, 1983.

Levorstad K, Kolbenstvedt A and Lyning EW: Iohexol compared with metrizoate in urography, Acta-Radiol [diagn] (Stockh) 24:337-342, 1983.

Maglinte DD and Miller RE: A simplified method for imaging the anterior gastroduodenal wall by double-contrast study, AJR 141:971-972, 1983.

Mancini GB et al: Hemodynamic and electrocardiographic effects in man of a new nonionic contrast agent (iohexol): advantages over standard ionic agents, Am J Cardiol 51:1218-1222, 1983.

Miller DL et al: Experimental evaluation of five liver-spleen specific CT contrast agents, J Comput Assist Tomogr 7:1022-1028, 1983.

Moschini L et al: Iopamidol and metrizamide in cervical myelography: side effect, EEG, and CSF changes, AJNR 4:848-850, 1983.

Ott DJ and Gelfand DW: Gastrointestinal contrast agents: indications, uses, and risks, JAMA 249:2380-2384, 1983.

Owen JP et al: Comparative study of the sodium salts of iodamide and iothalimate in clinical urology, Clin Radiol 34:353-357, 1983.

Parvey LS, Grizzard M and Coburn TP: Use of infusion pump for intravenous enhanced computed tomography, J Comput Assist Tomogr 7:175-176, 1983.

Sacks BA et al: A comparison of hexabrix and Renografin 60 in peripheral arteriography, AJR 140:975-977, 1983.

Selin K and Bjork L: Two new contrast media in coronary angiography, Acta Radiol [diagn] (Stockh) 24:37-41, 1983.

Skalpe IO and Hordvik M: Comparison of side effects during cerebral computed tomography with a nonionic (iohexol) and an ionic (metrizoate) contrast medium, AJNR 4:326-328, 1983.

Thomsen HS: Pressures during retrograde pyelography, Acta Radiol [diagn] (Stockh) 24:171-175, 1983.

Thron A et al: Iohexol and ioxaglate in cerebral angiography, Fortschr Geb Rontgenstr Nuklearmed Erganzungsband 118:115-119, 1983.

Tylen U: Iohexol in cardioangiography: survey and present state, Acta Radiol (Stockh) 366(suppl):94-100, 1983.

1984 Bartram CI, Mootoosamy IM and Lim IK: Washout versus non-washout (Picolax) preparation for double-contrast, Clin Radiol 35:143-146, 1984.

Bell JM et al: A comparison of two high-density barium sulphate preparations for double-contrast barium meals, Clin Radiol 35:367-368, 1984.

Bolz KD, Skalpe IO and Gutteberg TJ: Iohexol and metrizoate in urography in children: comparison, Acta Radiol [diagn] (Stockh) 25:155-158, 1984.

Chambers SE and Best JJ: A comparison of dilute barium and dilute water-soluble contrast in opacification of the bowel for abdominal computed tomography, Clin Radiol 35:463-464, 1984.

Culp WC: Buoyancy of gallstones in varying concentrations of contrast media, AJR 143:79-81, 1984.

Dawson P, Bradshaw A and Hill C: Iopromide: a new non-ionic contrast medium, Acta Radiol [diagn] (Stockh) 25:253-256, 1984.

Dawson P: Contrast agents: a review of 'low osmolarity' media, Radiography 50:142-145, 1984.

Fars-Nielsen F, deCarvalho A and Hjllund-Madsen E: Omnipaque and Urografin in arthrography of the knee, Acta Radiol [diagn] (Stockh) 25:151-154, 1984.

Gabrielsen TO et al: Iohexol versus metrizamide for lumbar myelography: double-blind trial, AJR 142:1047-1049, 1984.

Hunter DW et al: Carbon dioxide as a lighter-than-urine contrast medium for percutaneous nephrostomy, Radiology 152:211-212, 1984.

Katzberg RW: Preliminary evaluation of Hexabrix for temporomandibular joint arthrography, Invest Radiol 19:S387-S388, 1984.

Kieffer SA et al: Lumbar myelography with iohexol and metrizamide: a comparative multicenter prospective study, Radiology 151:665-670, 1984.

Mintz MC and Seltzer SE: Oral administration of contrast medium for rectal opacification in pelvic computed tomography, J Comput Tomogr 8:73-74, 1984.

Malott JC and Fodor J: Advantages of non-ionic contrast media in vascular applications, Radiol Technol 56(2):95-98, 1984.

Nakstad P et al: Cervical myelography with iohexol, Neuroradiology 26:123-129, 1984.

Ott DJ et al: Cold barium suspensions in the clinical evaluation of the esophagus, Gastrointest Radiol 9:193-196, 1984.

Partanen K et al: Comparison of iohexol and metrizamide in dynamic CT of the upper abdomen, Eur J Radiol 4:227-228, 1984.

Reiser UJ: Study of bolus geometry after intravenous contrast medium injection: dynamic and qualitative measurements (Chronogram) using an x-ray CT device, J Comput Assist Tomogr 8:251-262, 1984.

Robey G et al: Pediatric urography: comparison of metrizamide and methylglucamine, Radiology 150:61-63, 1984.

Smith W and Franken EA: Metrizamide as a contrast medium for visualization of the tracheobronchial tree: its drawbacks and possible advantages, Pediatr Radiol 14:158-160, 1984.

Spataro RF: Newer contrast agents for urography, Radiol Clin North Am 22:365-380, 1984.

Sullivan ID et al: Comparative trial of iohexol 350, a non-ionic contrast medium, with diatrizoate (Urographin 370) in left ventriculography and coronary arteriography, Br Heart J 51:643-647, 1984.

Svenson RH: Comparison of the hemodynamic effects of Hexabrix and Renografin-76, Invest Radiol 19:S333-S334, 1984.

Thompson WM et al: Iopamidol: new, nonionic contrast agent for excretory urography, AJR 142:329-332, 1984.

Vermess M: New contrast material improves detection of liver and spleen metastases, JAMA 251:707-708, 1984.

Whitehouse GH and Snowdon SL: A comparison between iohexol and metrizamide, two nonionic contrast media, in aortofemoral angiography, Br J Radiol 57:39-42, 1984.

Winfield AC et al: Hexabrix as a contrast agent for hysterosalpingography, Radiology 152:232-233, 1984.

1985 Apple JS et al: A comparison of Hexabrix and Renografin-60 in knee arthrography, AJR 145:139-142, 1985.

Carlsson EC et al: Pediatric angiocardiography with iohexol, Invest Radiol 20:75-78, 1985.

Carr DH and Banks LM: Comparison of barium and diatrizoate bowel labelling agents in computed tomography, Br J Radiol 58:393-394, 1985.

Cayea PD and Seltzer SE: A new barium paste for computed tomography of the esophagus, J Comput Assist Tomogr 9:214-216, 1985.

Davies P et al: The old and the new: a study of five contrast media for urography, Br J Radiol 58:593-597, 1985.

de Lange EE and Shaffer HA Jr: Barium suspension formulation for use with the bubbly barium method, Radiology 154:825-825, 1985.

Denardo SJ et al: Feasibility, reliability, and advantage of utilizing low contrast dose digital subtraction, Am Heart J 110:631-636, 1985.

Hammer B and Deisenhammer E: Iotrol, a new water-soluble non-ionic dimeric contrast medium, Neuroradiology 27:337-341, 1985.

Hosoki T and Mori S: Use of meglumine iotroxate in the detection of liver tumors by computed tomography, Comput Radiol 9:387-393, 1985.

Kawada TK: Iohexol and iopamidol: second-generation nonionic radiographic contrast media, Drug Intell Clin Pharm 19:525-529, 1985.

Mitchell DG et al: Gastrografin versus dilute barium for colonic CT examination: a blind, randomized study, J Comput Assist Tomogr 9:451-453, 1985.

Nakstad P et al: Functional cervical myelography with iohexol, Neuroradiology 27:220-225, 1985.

Passariello R: Angio CT techniques, Eur J Radiol 5:193-198, 1985.

Phillips VM, Erwin EC and Bernardino ME: Delayed iodine scanning of the liver: a promising CT, J Comput Assist Tomogr 9:415-416, 1985.

Postacchini F and Massobrio M: Outpatient lumbar myelography: analysis of complications after myelography comparing outpatients with inpatients, Spine 10:567-570, 1985.

Rigler RG: A simple pressure injector for contrast material, Radiology 154:248-248, 1985.

Saddekni S et al: Contrast administration and techniques of digital subtraction angiography performance, Radiol Clin North Am 23:275-291, 1985.

Smith HJ et al: High dose urography in patients with renal failure: a double blind study, Acta Radiol [diagn] (Stockh) 26:213-220, 1985.

Stake G and Smevik B: Iohexol and metrizamide for urography in infants and children, Invest Radiol 20:115-116, 1985.

Stork J: Intraperitoneal contrast agents for computed tomography, AJR 145:300-300, 1985.

Tallroth K and Vankka E: Iohexol and meglumine iothalamate in shoulder arthrography: a double-blind investigation, Acta Radiol [diagn] (Stockh) 26: 1985.

Wisneski JA, Gertz EW and Neese RA: Absence of myocardial biochemical toxicity with a nonionic contrast medium, Am Heart J 110:609-617, 1985.

1986 Alper MM et al: Pregnancy rates after hysterosalpingography with oil- and water-soluble contrast media, Obstet Gynecol 68:6-9, 1986.

Ball DS et al: Contrast medium precipitation during abdominal CT, Radiology 158:258-260, 1986.

Bettmann MA and Morris TW: Recent advances in contrast agents, Radiol Clin North Am 24:347-357, 1986.

Fader M: Preheated contrast media: the advantage of intravenous injection, Radiol Technol 58(2):117-119, 1986.

Grainger RG: The optimal concentration of contrast medium for aortography, Clin Radiol 37:281-284, 1986.

Hoe JW, Ng AM and Tan LK: A comparison of iohexol and iopamidol for lumbar myelography, Clin Radiol 37:505-507, 1986.

Lilleas F, Bach-Gansmo T and Weber H: Lumbar myelography with Omnipaque (iohexol), Neuroradiology 28:344-346, 1986.

McKee MW and Jurgens RW Jr: Barium sulfate products for roentgenographic examination of the gastrointestinal tract, Am J Hosp Pharm 43:145-148, 1986.

Morewood DJ and Whitehouse GH: A comparison of three methods for performing barium follow-through, Br J Radiol 59:971-973, 1986.

Nakstad P et al: Intra-arterial digital subtraction angiography of the carotid artery, Neuroradiology 28:195-198, 1986.

Niendorf HP et al: Some aspects of the use of contrast agents in magnetic resonance, Diagn Imaging Clin Med 55:25-36, 1986.

Nilson AE: The layering phenomenon and boundary formation in radiographs, Acta Radiol [diagn] (Stockh) 27: 1986.

Panto PN and Davies P: Delayed reactions to urographic contrast media, Br J Radiol 59:41-44, 1986.

Peeters F: Myelography using iohexol (Omnipaque), Diagn Imaging Clin Med 55:348-351, 1986.

Revel D: Gd-DTPA contrast enhancement and tissue, Radiology 158:319-323, 1986.

Tash RR, Weingarten M and Geller M: An alternative technique for double-contrast esophagography (technical note), AJR 147:266-267, 1986.

Tash RR, Weingarten M and Geller M: An alternative technique for double-contrast esophagography, AJR 147:266-267, 1986.

Wang H et al: Low dose cervical CT myelography. How acceptable are adverse effects at this juncture? Acta Radiol Suppl Stockh 369:539-541, 1986.

1987 Bateman BG et al: Utility of the 24-hour delay hysterosalpingogram film, Fertil Steril 47:613-617, 1987.

Cohen MD: Choosing contrast media for the evaluation of the gastrointestinal tract of neonates and infants, Radiology 162:447-456, 1987.

Doyon D et al: Comparative trial of Hexabrix (320 mg iodine/ml), iohexol (300 mg iodine/ml) and iopamiron (300 mg iodine/ml) in cerebral and spinal angiography: a preliminary report, Br J Radiol 60:671-675, 1987.

Hajek PC et al: Potential contrast agents for MR arthrography: in vitro evaluation, AJR 149:97-104, 1987.

Halsell RD: Heating contrast media in a microwave oven, Radiology 163:279-280, 1987.

Hodges SD and Berasi CC: Complications of myelography after partial metrizamide withdrawal, Spine 12:53-5, 1987.

McClennan BL: Low-osmolality contrast media: premises and promises, Radiology 162:1-8, 1987.

Miller K: Advantages of a low-osmolality ionic contrast medium in intra-arterial applications, Radiol Technol 59:43-48, 1987.

Nunley WC Jr et al: Intravasation during hysterosalpingography using oil-base contrast, Obstet Gynecol 70:309-312, 1987.

Payne NI and Whitehouse GH: Delineation of the spleen by a combination of proliposomes with, Br J Radiol 60:535-541, 1987.

Pochaczevsky R: Double-contrast examination of the colon with carbon dioxide, AJR 149:502-504, 1987.

Raptopoulos V et al: Fat-density oral contrast agent for abdominal CT, Radiology 164:653-656, 1987.

Trewhella M et al: Dehydration, antidiuretic hormone and the intravenous urogram, Br J Radiol 60:445-447, 1987.

Valenti RM: Lumber myelography: contrast agents used in the past, present, and future, Radiol Technol 58(6):493-496, 1987.

Vogelzang RL and Gore RM: Bolus-rapid infusion of contrast medium: simplified technique, J Comput Tomogr 11:1-3, 1987.

1988   Angelelli G and Macarini L: CT of the bowel: use of water to enhance depiction, Radiology 169:848-849, 1988.

Back SE, Krutzen E and Nilsson-Ehle P: Contrast media and glomerular filtration: dose dependence of clearance for three agents, J Pharm Sci 77:765-767, 1988.

Benotti JR: The comparative effects of ionic versus non-ionic agents in cardiac catheterization, Invest Radiol 23:366-373, 1988.

Bird CR et al: Gd-DTPA-enhanced MR imaging in pediatric patients after brain tumor, Radiology 169:123-126, 1988.

Conces DJ Jr, Tarver RD and Lappas JC: The value of opacification of the esophagus by low density barium, J Comput Assist Tomogr 12:202-205, 1988.

de Boer AD et al: Oil or aqueous contrast media for hysterosalpingography: a prospective, randomized, clinical study, Eur J Obstet Gynecol Reprod Biol 28:65-68, 1988.

Feldman RL et al: Contrast media-related complications during cardiac catheterization, Am J Cardiol 61:1334-1337, 1988.

Gibby WA: MR contrast agents: an overview, Radiol Clin North Am 26:1047-1058, 1988.

Hopkins AL et al: Oxygen-17 contrast agents: fast imaging techniques, Invest Radiol 23:240-242, 1988.

Jacobsson BF: Nonionic versus ionic contrast media in intravenous urography, Radiology 167:601-605, 1988.

Kaye B et al: Comparison of the image quality of intravenous urograms using low-osmolar contrast media, Br J Radiol 61:589-591, 1988.

Keidan RD, Unger EC and Weese JL: MRI of thorotrastoma, Magn Reson Imaging 6:717-720, 1988.

Listinsky JJ and Bryant RG: Gastrointestinal contrast agents: a diamagnetic approach, Magn Reson Med 8:285-292, 1988.

Muller RN: The importance of nuclear magnetic relaxation dispersion (NMRD), Invest Radiol 23:229-231, 1988.

Nestvold K and Sortland O: Lumbar myelography with iohexol: adverse effects compared with spinal puncture, Acta Radiol 29:637-640, 1988.

Ohnesorgen EG: Selective use of low osmolality contrast agents; cost and benefits, Radiol Technol 59(6):499-502, 1988.

Perlman MD: Usage of radiopaque contrast media in the foot and ankle, J Foot Surg 27:3-29, 1988.

Piao ZE et al: Hemodynamic effects of contrast media during coronary angiography: a comparison of three nonionic agents to Hypaque-76, Cathet Cardiovasc Diagn 14:53-58, 1988.

Piao ZE et al: Contrast media-induced ventricular fibrillation. A comparison of Hypaque-76, Hexabrix, and Omnipaque, Invest Radiol 23:466-470, 1988.

Platt JF and Glazer GM: IV contrast material for abdominal CT comparison of three methods, AJR 151:275-277, 1988.

Raptopoulos V et al: CT of the pancreas with a fat-density oral contrast regimen, AJR 150:1303-1306, 1988.

Robertson HJ: Nonionic contrast media in radiology: procedural considerations, Invest Radiol 23:S374-S377, 1988.

Sharma S, Mishra NK and Rajani M: Evaluation of the central injection technique for intravenous digital subtraction angiography—a preliminary report, Indian Heart J 40:12-16, 1988.

Slappendel R et al: Spread of radiopaque dye in the thoracic epidural space, Anaesthesia 43:939-942, 1988.

Stordahl A et al: Water-soluble contrast media in radiography of small bowel obstruction: comparison of ionic and non-ionic contrast media, Acta Radiol 29:53-56, 1988.

Takeda T et al: Intraarterial digital subtraction angiography with carbon dioxide, Cardiovasc Intervent Radiol 11:101-107, 1988.

Walker J et al: Water-soluble contrast medium for intraoperative evaluation of anterior cervical discectomy: technical note, J Neurosurg 68:491-492, 1988.

1989   Benamor M et al: Ioversol clinical safety summary, Invest Radiol 24 Suppl 1:S67-S72, 1989.

Bettmann MA: Guidelines for use of low-osmolality contrast agents, Radiology 172:901-903, 1989.

Bisset GS: Evaluation of potential practical oral contrast agents for pediatric magnetic resonance imaging. Preliminary observations, Pediatr Radiol 20:61-66, 1989.

Brown RC: Ionic and non-ionic contrast media and reactions, Iowa Medicine 79:244-246, 1989.

Campbell JB: Contrast media in intussusception, Pediatr Radiol 19:293-296, 1989.

Cho YD, Yum HY and Park YH: Hepatocellular carcinoma with skeletal metastasis: management with intraarterial radioactive iodine, J Belge Radiol 72:267-271, 1989.

Dawson P: Contrast media for urography, Curr Opin Radiol 1:283-289, 1989.

Dawson P and Allison DJ: Safer contrast agents? Br J Hosp Med 42:406-407, 1989.

Desaga JF: Visualization of the mucosal villi on double-contrast barium studies, Gastrointest Radiol 14:25-30, 1989.

Gomes AS et al: Acute renal dysfunction in high-risk patients after angiography: comparison of ionic and nonionic contrast media, Radiology 170:65-68, 1989.

Hwang MH et al: The potential risk of thrombosis during coronary angiography using non-ionic contrast media, Cathet Cardiovasc Diagn 16:209-213, 1989.

Jakobsen JA et al: Safety and toleration of the non-ionic contrast medium iopentol. An intravenous phase I trial, Eur J Radiol 9:203-207, 1989.

Lasser EC, Berry CC: Nonionic vs ionic contrast media: what do the data tell us? AJR 152:945-946, 1989.

Lemansky E: Contrast agents used for myelography: an historical perspective, Radiol Technol 60:489-496, 1989.

Loy RA, Weinstein FS and Seibel MM: Hysterosalpingography in perspective: the predictive value of oil-soluble versus water-soluble contrast media, Fertil Steril 51:170-172, 1989.

Mattrey RF: Potential role of perfluorooctylbromide in the detection and characterization of liver lesions with CT, Radiology 170:18-20, 1989.

Mattrey RF: Perfluorooctylbromide: a new contrast agent for CT, and sonography, AJR 152:247-252, 1989.

McAlister WH: Death associated with bronchography. Question role of heating the contrast agent, Pediatr Radiol 19:458-460, 1989.

Millen SJ, Daniels DL and Meyer GA: Gadolinium-enhanced magnetic resonance imaging in the temporal bone, Laryngoscope 99:257-260, 1989.

Moore RD et al: Frequency and determinants of adverse reactions induced by high-osmolality contrast media, Radiology 170:727-732, 1989.

Morcos SK et al: Iotrolan in selective bronchography via the fibreoptic bronchoscope, Br J Radiol 62:383-385, 1989.

Schmidt M and Papassotiriou V: Arthrography with iotrolan: double-blind comparison between nonionic, monomeric (iohexol 300) and nonionic, dimeric (iotrolan 300) contrast media, Fortschr Geb Rontgenstr Nuklearmed Erganzungsbd 128:182-189, 1989.

Sutherland JB and Huda W: Costs and benefits of low-osmolality contrast agents in radiology, Can Assoc Radiol J 40:18-21, 1989.

Swensen SJ, Ehman RL and Brown LR: Magnetic resonance imaging of the thorax, J Thorac Imaging 4:19-33, 1989.

Wolf GL, Arenson RL and Cross AP: A prospective trial of ionic vs nonionic contrast agents in routine clinical practice: comparison of adverse effects, AJR 152:939-944, 1989.

1990   Altschuler EM and Segal R: Generalized seizures following myelography with iohexol (Omnipaque), J Spinal Disord 3:59-61, 1990.

Belanger JG et al: Adult myelography with iohexol, Can Assoc Radiol J 41:191-194, 1990.

Bergqvist D and Bergentz SE: Diagnosis of deep vein thrombosis, World J Surg 14:679-687, 1990.

Bettmann MA, Holzer JF and Trombly ST: Risk management issues related to the use of contrast agents, Radiology 175:629-631, 1990.

Brinker JA: Selection of a contrast agent in the cardiac catheterization laboratory, Am J Cardiol 66:26F-33F, 1990.

Buck BA: Ethical issues of randomized clinical trials, Radiol Technol 61:202-205, 1990.

Cohan RH et al: Extravascular extravasation of radiographic contrast media. Effects of conventional and low-osmolar agents in the rat thigh, Invest Radiol 25:504-510, 1990.

Dawson P: Iodinated intravascular contrast agents past and present. Toxicity considerations, Invest Radiol 25 Suppl 1:S11, 1990.

Duddy MJ, Manns RA and Wormald SA: Injection rate: a factor in contrast reactions, Clin Radiol 41:42-43, 1990.

Gluck BS and Mitty HA: Reactions to iodinated radiographic contrast agents. How to identify and manage patients at risk, Postgrad Med 88:187-189, 193-194, 1990.

Grainger RG and Dawson P: Low osmolar contrast media: an appraisal, Clin Radiol 42:1-5, 1990.

Kaplan PA and Walker CW: Contrast radiology, Curr Opin Rheumatol 2:355-360, 1990.

Katayama H: Survey of safety of clinical contrast media, Invest Radiol 25 Suppl 1:S7-S10, 1990.

Katayama H: Adverse reactions to contrast media. What are the risk factors? Invest Radiol 25 Suppl 1:S16-S17, 1990.

Langer M et al: Analysis of renal and hepatic impairment by ionic and nonionic contrast media, Invest Radiol 25 Suppl 1:S125-S126, 1990.

Lasser EC: Contrast reactions. Eked data from contrast-reaction surveys, Invest Radiol 25 Suppl 1:S14-S15, 1990.

McAlister WH and Kissane JM: Comparison of soft tissue effects of conventional ionic, low osmolar ionic and nonionic iodine containing contrast material in experimental animals, Pediatr Radiol 20:170-174, 1990.

Mishkin MM: Contrast media safety: what do we know and how do we know it, Am J Cardiol 66:34F-36F, 1990.

Morcos SK et al: Suitability of and tolerance to Iotrolan 300 in bronchography via the fibreoptic bronchoscope, Thorax 45:628-629, 1990.

Nicholson DA: Contrast media in sialography: a comparison of Lipiodol Ultra Fluid and Urografin 290, Clin Radiol 42:423-426, 1990.

Palmer J: Morbidity and mortality with intravenous contrast media. Ionic and nonionic, Invest Radiol 25 Suppl 1:S18-S19, 1990.

Riebel T and Wartner R: Use of non-ionic contrast media for tracheobronchography in neonates and young infants, Eur J Radiol 11:120-124, 1990.

Wolf GL and Silvay-Mandeau O: Adverse reactions to intravenous contrast media in routine clinical practice, Invest Radiol 25 Suppl 1:S20-S21, 1990.

Yamaguchi K et al: Pretesting as a predictor of severe adverse reactions to contrast media, Invest Radiol 25 Suppl 1:S22-S23, 1990.

1991   Aguirre FV et al: The effects of high (sodium meglumine diatrizoate, Renografin-76) and low osmolar (sodium meglumine ioxaglate, Hexabrix) radiographic contrast media on diastolic function during left ventriculography in patients, Am Heart J 121:848-857, 1991.

Bernard MS, Hourihan MD and Adams H: Computed tomography of the brain: does contrast enhancement really help? Clin Radiol 44:161-164, 1991.

Bolstad B et al: Safety and tolerability of iodixanol. A dimeric, nonionic contrast medium: an emphasis on European clinical phases I and II, Invest Radiol 26 Suppl 1:S201-S204; discuss, 1991.

Buschman DL: Barium sulfate bronchography. Report of a complication, Chest 99:747-749, 1991.

Bush WH and Swanson DP: Acute reactions to intravascular contrast media: types, risk factors, recognition, and specific treatment, AJR 157:1153-1161, 1991.

DeSimone D et al: Evaluation of the safety and efficacy of gadoteridol injection (a low osmolal magnetic resonance contrast agent). Clinical trials report, Invest Radiol 26 Suppl 1:S212-S216; discuss, 1991.

Hughes PM and Bisset R: Non-ionic contrast media: a comparison of iodine delivery rates during manual injection angiography, Br J Radiol 64:417-419, 1991.

Ida M et al: Radiographic quality and patient discomfort in sialography: comparison of iohexol with iothalamate, Dentomaxillofac Radiol 20:81-86, 1991.

Lasser EC and Berry CC: Adverse reactions to contrast media. Ionic and nonionic media and steroids, Invest Radiol 26:402-403, 1991.

Lindequist S et al: Diagnostic quality and complications of hysterosalpingography: oil- versus water-soluble contrast media—a randomized prospective study, Radiology 179:69-74, 1991.

Marshall GD Jr and Lieberman PL: Comparison of three pretreatment protocols to prevent anaphylactoid reactions to radiocontrast media, Annals of Allergy 67:70-74, 1991.

Marzilli M: Contribution of contrast media and technical factors to the safety of invasive procedures, Seminars in Hematology 28:11-14, 1991.

McClennan BL and Stolberg HO: Intravascular contrast media. Ionic versus nonionic: current status, Radiol Clin North Am 29:437-454, 1991.

Sachinwalla T, Godfrey C and Palmer J: A survey of risk factors for adverse reactions to intravascular contrast media, Australas Radiol 35:106-108, 1991.

Steinberg EP et al: Nephrotoxicity of low osmolality contrast media versus high osmolality media, Invest Radiol 26 Suppl 1:S86, 1991.

Szmigielski W et al: Powdered diatrizoic acid for radiography of the respiratory tract. Part I. Experimental investigation, Acta Radiol 32:415-420, 1991.

Szmigielski W et al: Powdered diatrizoic acid for radiography of the respiratory tract. Part II. Clinical application, Acta Radiol 32:467-473, 1991.

Wang H et al: Iohexol cervical myelography in adult outpatients, Spine 16:1356-1358, 1991.

Westhoff-Bleck M, Bleck JS and Jost S: The adverse effects of angiographic radiocontrast media, Drug Safety 6:28-36, 1991.

1992   Ansell G: Epidemiology of adverse reactions to intravascular iodinated contrast media, Toxicology Letters 64-65 Spec No:717-723, 1992.

Barrett BJ et al: Nonionic low-osmolality versus ionic high-osmolality contrast material for intravenous use in patients perceived to be at high risk: randomized trial, Radiology 183:105-110, 1992.

Barrett BJ et al: A comparison of nonionic, low-osmolality radiocontrast agents with ionic, high-osmolality agents during cardiac catheterization, N Engl J Med 326:431-436, 1992.

Caro JJ, Trindade E and McGregor M: the cost-effectiveness of replacing high-osmolality with low-osmolality contrast media, AJR 159:869-874, 1992.

Carvlin MJ, DeSimone DN and Meeks MJ: Phase II clinical trial of gadoteridol injection, a low-osmolal magnetic resonance imaging contrast agent, Invest Radiol 27 Suppl 1:S16-S21, 1992.

Cohen MD et al: Comparison of intravenous contrast agents for CT studies in children, Acta Radiol 33:592-595, 1992.

Gavant ML, Ellis JV and Klesges LM: Diagnostic efficacy of excretory urography with low-dose, nonionic contrast media, Radiology 182:657-660, 1992.

Hopper KD, Lambe H and Matthews YL: Current usage of nonionic contrast, Urol Radiol 14:218-220, 1992.

Hopper KD et al: Patients' attitudes toward informed consent for intravenous contrast media, Invest Radiol 27:362-366, 1992.

Jahn H and Muller-Spath R: Ioversol in intravenous excretory urography. Evaluation of radiographic quality, patient tolerance and safety in four clinical studies, Ann Radiol Paris 35:297-302, 1992.

Kim SH and Han MC: Reversed contrast-urine levels in urinary bladder: CT findings, Urol Radiol 13:249-252, 1992.

Lawrence V, Matthai W and Hartmaier S: Comparative safety of high-osmolality and low-osmolality radiographic contrast agents. Report of a multidisciplinary working group, Invest Radiol 27:2-28, 1992.

Manotti C et al: Variation in hemostatic parameters after intra-arterial and intravenous administration of iodinated contrast media, Invest Radiol 27:1025-1030, 1992.

McCarthy CS and Becker JA: Multiple myeloma and contrast media, Radiology 183:519-521, 1992.

Moore RD et al: Nephrotoxicity of high-osmolality versus low-osmolality contrast media: randomized clinical trial, Radiology 182:649-655, 1992.

Rieser R, Beinborn W and Ney N: A double-blind comparative study on the contrast quality, tolerance and safety of ioversol 300 versus iohexol 300 in central venous angiography (C.V. DSA), Ann Radiol Paris 35:311-314, 1992.

Sortland O et al: Iopentol in urography. A clinical comparison between iopentol and metrizoate including delayed reactions, Acta Radiol 33:368-373, 1992.

Tauber WB: Clinical consequences of Thorotrast in a long-term survivor, Health Phys 63:13-19, 1992.

Trulzsch DV et al: Gastrografin-induced aspiration pneumonia: a lethal complication of computed tomography, South Med J 85:1255-1256, 1992.

1993   Baker ME et al: Contrast material for combined abdominal and pelvic CT: can cost be reduced by increasing the concentration and decreasing the volume, AJR 160:637-641, 1993.

Bulte JW et al: Magnetite as a potent contrast-enhancing agent in magnetic resonance imaging to visualize blood-brain barrier disruption, Acta Neurochir Suppl Wien 57:30-34, 1993.

Hopper KD and Matthews YL: Patient choice and nonionic contrast media, Invest Radiol 28:303-307, 1993.

Hricak H and Kim B: Contrast-enhanced MR imaging of the female pelvis, J Magn Reson Imaging 3:297-306, 1993.

MacVicar D et al: Phase III trial of oral magnetic particles in MRI of abdomen and pelvis, Clin Radiol 47:183-188, 1993.

Montefusco von Kleist CM et al: Comparison of duplex ultrasonography and ascending contrast venography in the diagnosis of venous thrombosis, Angiology 44:169-175, 1993.

Pallan TM et al: Incompatibility of Isovue 370 and papaverine in peripheral arteriography, Radiology 187:257-259, 1993.

Papadaki PJ et al: A modified per os double contrast examination of the colon in the elderly, ROFO Fortschr Geb Rontgenstr Neuen Bildgeb Verfahr 158:320-324, 1993.

Van Wagoner M and Worah D: Gadodiamide injection. First human experience with the nonionic magnetic resonance imaging enhancement agent, Invest Radiol 28 Suppl 1:S44-S48, 1993.

Weese DL, Greenberg HM and Zimmern PE: Contrast media reactions during voiding cystourethrography or retrograde pyelography, Urology 41:81-84, 1993.

Winalski CS et al: Enhancement of joint fluid with intravenously administered gadopentetate dimeglumine: technique, rationale, and implications, Radiology 187:179-185, 1993.

INDEX

Cancer—cont'd
  surgery and/or chemotherapy in, **3**:302
  uterine, **3**:302
Canine fossa, **2**:230
Canthomeatal line, **3**:288, **3**:289
Capillaries, **2**:515
Capitate, **1**:60, **1**:61; *see also* Wrist
Capitellum; *see* Capitulum
Capitulum, **1**:62; *see also* Humerus
Capsule of Bowman; *see* Glomerular capsule
Carcinogen, defined, **3**:295, **3**:303
Carcinoma; *see also* Cancer
  of breast, **2**:464, **2**:469, **2**:492
  of thyroid gland, nuclear medicine and, **3**:271
Cardia of stomach, **2**:85; *see also* Stomach
Cardiac antrum, **2**:84
Cardiac catheterization, **3**:89-103
  ancillary equipment and supplies for, **3**:95
  care after, **3**:102
  catheter introduction in, **3**:96
  contraindications to, **3**:91
  data collection in, **3**:96
  equipment for, **3**:92-94
  exercise tests and, **3**:98
  history of, **3**:90
  indications for, **3**:90-91
  methods and techniques for, **3**:96
  patient positioning for, **3**:95
  precatheterization care for, **3**:96
  procedures for
    interventional manipulative, **3**:99-101
    interventional pharmacologic, **3**:98
    pediatric, **3**:98, **3**:101
  risks of, **3**:91
  studies in, **3**:97-101
    adult, **3**:97-98
    pediatric, **3**:98
  trends in, **3**:102
Cardiac cycle, **1**:12, **2**:517
Cardiac fossa; *see* Cardiac impression
Cardiac gated study
  of blood pool, **3**:268
  of heart wall motion, **3**:261
Cardiac impression, **1**:438
Cardiac incisura; *see* Cardiac notch
Cardiac muscular tissue, **1**:12
Cardiac notch, **2**:85; *see also* Stomach
Cardiac orifice, **2**:85
Cardiac output, **3**:96
  defined, **3**:103
Cardiac sphincter; *see* Esophagogastric junction
Cardiology applications of ultrasound, **3**:239-245
Cardiomyopathy, **3**:91
  defined, **3**:103
Cardiovascular system, nuclear medicine and, **3**:261, **3**:268
C-arm configuration for image intensifier and fluoroscopic tube, **3**:95
Carotid arteries, **2**:594
  angiography of, **2**:543, **2**:544, **2**:546
  sectional anatomy of, **2**:595, **2**:596, **2**:600, **2**:602
Carotid sheath, **2**:596
  sectional anatomy of, **2**:596
Carotid vessels, nuclear medicine and, **3**:267
Carpal bones, **1**:60; *see also* Wrist
  terminology conversion of, **1**:60
Carpal boss, **1**:86
Carpal bridge, **1**:96-97

Carpal canal, **1**:94-95; *see also* Wrist
  anatomy of, **1**:63
  Gaynor-Hart method for, **1**:94
  superoinferior projections for, **1**:95
  tangential projections for, **1**:94-95
Carpal sulcus, **1**:63; *see also* Carpal canal
Carpal tunnel, **1**:63; *see also* Carpal canal; Wrist
Carpometacarpal joint; *see also* Digit, first
  anatomy of, **1**:63
  AP axial projection for, **1**:82
Cartilaginous joints, **1**:44, **1**:45
Cassettes, **1**:9
  quality assurance for, **3**:318
CAT; *see* Computed tomography
Catheter
  folding knifelike blade in, **3**:101
  foreign body removal from, **2**:573
  Gruntzig and Hopff double-lumen balloon-tipped, **2**:561
  pigtail, **2**:526
  for transluminal coronary angioplasty, **3**:99
  urinary drainage, **2**:568
  Vance nephrostomy, **2**:568
Catheterization
  in angiography, **2**:524-526
  cardiac; *see* Cardiac catheterization
  Seldinger technique for angiography, **2**:520
Cathode ray tube, **3**:112, **3**:160, **3**:256
  in computed tomography, **3**:128, **3**:152
  defined, **3**:125, **3**:168, **3**:272
Cauda equina, sectional anatomy of, **2**:618
Caudad as term, **1**:49
Caudal as term, **1**:49
Caudate nucleus, sectional anatomy of, **2**:592, **2**:599
Causton method for sesamoids projection, **1**:196-197
Cavernous sinus, sectional anatomy of, **2**:599
Cavitation
  acoustic, defined, **3**:202, **3**:246
  defined, **3**:212, **3**:246
Cavity
  glenoid, **1**:123
  peritoneal, **2**:32
Cavogram, vena, **2**:535-536
Cecostomy, **2**:148
Cecum, **2**:87; *see also* Intestine, large
  sectional anatomy of, **2**:614
Celiac arteriogram, **2**:531
Celiac trunk, sectional anatomy of, **2**:608
Centers of ossification, **1**:48
Central as term, **1**:49
Central nervous system, **2**:495-511
  anatomy of, **2**:496-498
  chemonucleolysis and, **2**:506
  contrast media and, **2**:500
  diskography and, **2**:506
  examination of, **2**:499
  lumbar diskography and, **2**:506
  magnetic resonance imaging and, **2**:507, **3**:194-195
  myelography and, **2**:500-505
    computed tomographic, **2**:504-505
  nuclear medicine and, **3**:267
  plain radiographic examination of, **2**:499
  pneumonography and, **2**:508
  stereotactic surgery and, **2**:509-510
  ventriculography and, **2**:508

Central processing unit, **3**:109
  defined, **3**:125
Central ray
  in decubitus position, **1**:54
  direction of, **1**:17
Central venography, **2**:535-536
Cephalic as term, **1**:49
Cephalometry, **2**:206
  external landmarks for pelvic inlet plane in, **2**:206
  projections for, AP, **2**:207
Cerebellar peduncles, **2**:594
  sectional anatomy of, **2**:600
Cerebellum, **2**:496
  sectional anatomy of, **2**:594, **2**:598
Cerebral angiography, **2**:543-559
  of anterior circulation, **2**:551-555
  aortic arch, **2**:550
  arteries in; *see* Cerebral arteries
  circulation time and filming program for, **2**:546, **2**:547
  equipment for, **2**:548
  positioning for, **2**:549
  of posterior circulation, **2**:556-558
  preparation of patient and examining room for, **2**:548
  projections for anterior circulation in
    AP axial, **2**:554, **2**:555
    AP axial oblique, **2**:554, **2**:555
    AP axial oblique (supraorbital), **2**:553
    AP axial oblique (transorbital), **2**:554
    AP axial (supraorbital), **2**:552
    AP axial (transorbital), **2**:553
    lateral, **2**:551
  projections for posterior circulation in
    AP axial, **2**:557
    lateral, **2**:556
    submentovertical, **2**:558, **2**:559
  radiation protection in, **2**:549
  technique for, **2**:546
Cerebral aqueduct, **2**:498; *see also* Central nervous system
Cerebral arteries, **2**:543-544, **2**:545, **2**:546
  anomalies of, **2**:544
  chart of, **2**:559
  embolization of, **2**:566
  sectional anatomy of, **2**:595, **2**:599
Cerebral blood flow
  local, **3**:282, **3**:289, **3**:290
  nuclear medicine and, **3**:267
Cerebral hemispheres, **2**:496; *see also* Brain
  sectional anatomy of, **2**:592, **2**:598-599
Cerebral metabolic rate of glucose utilization, local, **3**:283, **3**:289, **3**:290
Cerebral nuclei, sectional anatomy of, **2**:592
Cerebral pneumonography, **2**:508
Cerebral veins, sectional anatomy of, **2**:598
Cerebral ventriculography, **2**:508
Cerebrospinal fluid, **2**:497
  nuclear medicine and, **3**:267
  sectional anatomy and, **2**:592, **2**:598
Cerebrum, **2**:496; *see also* Brain
Cervical esophagus, **2**:84
Cervical intervertebral foramina, **1**:340-343
  Barsóny and Koppenstein's method for, **1**:342-343
  projection for
    axial oblique, **1**:340-341

Index

Iliac artery
    common, **2:**516
    external, **2:**516
    internal, **2:**516
        sectional anatomy of, **2:**614, **2:**618
        transluminal angioplasty and, **2:**563
Iliac fossa, **1:**272, **2:**60
Iliac spines, **1:**272
    sectional anatomy of, **2:**614, **2:**615, **2:**616
Iliac vessels, sectional anatomy of, **2:**614
Iliacus muscle, sectional anatomy of, **2:**614, **2:**616, **2:**618
Iliopectineal eminence, **1:**275
Iliopelvic-abdominoaortic region lymphography, **2:**577
Iliopsoas muscles, sectional anatomy of, **2:**616, **2:**618
Ilium, **1:**308-309; *see also* Hip
    anatomy of, **1:**272
        sectional, **2:**614, **2:**618
    AP and PA oblique projections for, **1:**308-309
    crest of, **1:**272
Illuminators, quality assurance for, **3:**319
IMA; *see* Inferior mesenteric artery
Image
    coregistration of, positron emission tomography and, **3:**277, **3:**289
    misregistration of, in volume computed tomography scanning, **3:**146, **3:**152
    quality of, in computed tomography, **3:**144-145
    zoom of, in digital subtraction angiography, **3:**175
Image intensifier, **2:**91
    defined, **3:**178
    digital radiography based on, **3:**13
    in digital subtraction angiography, **3:**172
    tube for, **3:**94
Image plate reader in computed radiography, **3:**158
    defined, **3:**168
Image processor
    defined, **3:**178
    in digital subtraction angiography, **3:**172
Image receptors, **1:**32
    quality assurance and, **3:**318-319
Imaging time in magnetic resonance imaging, **3:**190, **3:**194
Immobilization
    of child, **3:**14
        in abdominal radiography, **3:**34-35
        in gastrointestinal and genitourinary procedures, **3:**36-37
        head and neck immobilizer in, **3:**39
        in hip radiography, **3:**21
        in limb radiography, **3:**30-31
        octagonal immobilizer in, **3:**36
        tools for, **3:**14
    devices for, **1:**13
    for tomography, **3:**65
Impedance, acoustic, **3:**209, **3:**246
Impedance angle of ultrasound wave, **3:**209
Implant, breast, **2:**479-480
Implant therapy, **3:**297
Implantation
    of ovum, **2:**196
    of permanent pacemaker, **3:**100
In vitro, **3:**272
In vivo, **3:**272
Incisura angularis; *see* Angular notch
Incus, **2:**229

Index in table movement, **3:**137, **3:**152
Indium, **3:**253
Indium 111 Satumomab Pendetide, in inflammation/infection studies, **3:**271
Indium 111-DTPA imaging of cerebral spinal fluid, **3:**267
Indium 111-labeled white blood cells in inflammation/infection studies, **3:**271
Industrial applications of ionizing radiation, **1:**25
Infant
    approach to, **3:**2, **3:**5
    premature, **3:**10
    supine immobilizer method for, **3:**18
Infarction, myocardial, **3:**90
    defined, **3:**103
    perfusion studies in, **3:**268
    single photon emission computed tomography in, **3:**258
Infection, nuclear medicine and, **3:**271
Inferior apophyseal process of vertebrae; *see* Inferior articular process
Inferior articular process, **1:**314; *see also* Lumbar spine
    of cervical vertebrae, **1:**315-316
    of lumbar vertebrae, **1:**320
    of thoracic vertebrae, **1:**318-319
Inferior as term, **1:**49
Inferior constrictor muscle; *see* Neck
Inferior horns, **2:**498
Inferior mesenteric artery, **2:**533
Inferior orbital fissure, **2:**284-285
Inferior vena cava, **2:**515
    cavogram of, **2:**536
    CT axial image of, **3:**130
    in diagnostic ultrasound, **3:**214
    filter placement in, **2:**570-572
    sectional anatomy of, **2:**606, **2:**608, **2:**610
Inflammation, nuclear medicine and, **3:**271
Information and management systems, **3:**123-124
Infraorbitomeatal line, **2:**233
Infrared radiation, **3:**76
    defined, **3:**86
Infrared thermography, **3:**76
Infraspinatus fossa, **1:**123; *see also* Scapula
Infraspinatus muscle, **1:**123
    anatomy of, **1:**125
    insertion of, **1:**152
    sectional anatomy of, **2:**602
Infundibula; *see* Major calyces
Infundibulum of uterine tube, **2:**194
Infusion nephrotomography, **2:**156
Inguinal ligament, sectional anatomy of, **2:**616
Inion; *see* External occipital protuberance
Initial examination general procedures, **1:**8
Injection techniques for angiography, **2:**521
Innominatum; *see* Os coxae
Input, defined, **3:**125
Input devices for computers, **3:**110
Input phosphor, defined, **3:**178
Input/output terminal, defined, **3:**125
Inspiration
    patient instructions and, **1:**15; *see also* Breathing
    in thoracic viscera projections, **1:**444
Inspiratory phonation, **2:**21
Instruction
    defined, **3:**125
    for patient, **1:**13, **1:**15
Insula, **2:**592, **2:**599
Intensifying screens, quality assurance for, **3:**318

Intensity, **3:**208, **3:**247
Interarytenoid folds, **2:**14
Intercondylar eminence, **1:**182; *see also* Tibia
Intercondylar fossa, **1:**250-255
    anatomy of, **1:**183
    Béclére method for, **1:**254-255
    Camp-Coventry method for, **1:**252, **1:**253
    Holmblad method for, **1:**250-251
    projection for
        AP axial, **1:**254-255
        PA axial, **1:**250-251
Intercostal spaces, **1:**402
Interface, defined, **3:**125
Interfacing devices for computers, **3:**115
Interfascial space of Tenon, **2:**288
Interlobar fissures, **1:**439; *see also* Thoracic viscera
Internal as term, **1:**49
Internal conjugate diameter, **2:**206
Internal iliac vein, sectional anatomy of, **2:**614
Internal mammary lymph nodes, **2:**460
Internal oblique muscle, sectional anatomy of, **2:**608
Internal os; *see* Isthmus of uterus
Internally deposited radionuclides, **1:**25
International Standards Organization nomenclature, **1:**17
International system of weights and measures, **1:**23
Interphalangeal articulations
    of toes, **1:**184; *see also* Toes
    of upper limb, **1:**63; *see also* Digit
Interrupt, defined, **3:**125
Intersinus septum, **2:**219
Intertarsal articulations, **1:**184
Intertrochanteric crest, **1:**273
Intertrochanteric line, **1:**273
Intertubercular groove, **1:**124
    of humerus, **1:**124; *see also* Humerus
Intervention, defined, **3:**103
Interventricular foramen, **2:**498
Intervertebral disk, lumbar, sectional anatomy of, **2:**612
Intervertebral disks
    lumbar
        Duncan and Hoen method for, **1:**392-393
        in R and L bending positions, **1:**392-393
        weight-bearing studies of, **1:**392-393
    slipped, **1:**314
Intervertebral foramina, **1:**314
    of cervical vertebrae, **1:**317
    lumbar, **1:**321
        fifth, Kovacs method for, **1:**376-377
    projection for
        PA axial oblique 7, **1:**376-377
        in RAO and LAO positions, **1:**376-377
    of thoracic vertebrae, **1:**319
Intestine
    foreign body localization in, **1:**518
    large, **2:**122-150; *see also* Large intestine
    peristaltic action in, **2:**88
    preparation for examination of, **1:**11
    small; *see* Small intestine
Intraarterial digital subtraction angiography, **3:**176-177
    intravenous injection versus, **3:**171
Intracavitary radiation, **3:**297
Intracerebral circulation, **2:**543-544, **2:**545, **2:**546
    chart for, **2:**559
Intrahepatic portosystemic shunt, transjugular, **2:**573

Index

Notch—cont'd
sciatic, **1**:272
suprasternal, **1**:400
Nuclear magnetic resonance, **3**:182
defined, **3**:203
Nuclear medicine, **3**:249-273
clinical, **3**:261-265
bone and, **3**:262
bone marrow and, **3**:270
brain and; *see* Brain
cardiovascular system in, **3**:261, **3**:268
central nervous system in, **3**:267
endocrine system in, **3**:266
gastrointestinal system in, **3**:268-269
genitourinary system in, **3**:269-270
heart and, **3**:261, **3**:268
hematologic system in, **3**:270
in vitro procedures in, **3**:264-265
in vivo nonimaging in, **3**:264
in vivo procedures in, **3**:261-264
inflammation/infection in, **3**:271
kidney and, **3**:259, **3**:269-270
liver and spleen and, **3**:260, **3**:269
lungs and, **3**:252, **3**:267
musculoskeletal system in, **3**:270
radioimmunoassay in, **3**:265, **3**:268, **3**:271
respiratory system in, **3**:267
thyroid and, **3**:265, **3**:266, **3**:271
tumors in, **3**:271
dynamic imaging in, **3**:263
instrumentation in, **3**:255-260, **3**:261
nuclear pharmacy in, **3**:252-253
in pediatrics, **3**:42
physics of, **3**:250-251
quantitative analysis of, **3**:260, **3**:261
radiation safety in, **3**:254
therapeutic, **3**:265, **3**:271-272
whole body imaging in, **3**:262
Nuclear particle accelerator, **3**:280, **3**:290
Nuclear pharmacy, **3**:252-253
Nuclear reactor, **3**:252
defined, **3**:272
Nucleography, **2**:506
Nucleus, **3**:250
defined, **3**:203, **3**:272
neutron-deficient decay of, **3**:279
Nucleus pulposus, **1**:314
herniated, **1**:314
Nuclide, **3**:251, **3**:272

O

Object distance, **1**:4, **1**:16
Objective, defined, **3**:309, **3**:320
Oblique image plane in ultrasound, **3**:213
Oblique muscles, sectional anatomy of, **2**:608
Oblique plane, **1**:38
Oblique position, **1**:53-54
Oblique projection, **1**:51, **1**:53-54
Obstetrics
diagnostic ultrasound in, **3**:232-237, **3**:238
thermography and, **3**:81
Obstruction, ureteral, nuclear medicine and, **3**:270
Obstructive jaundice, **2**:73
Obturator foramen, **1**:272
Obturator internus muscle, **2**:616
Occipital bone, **2**:216, **2**:217, **2**:224-225
Occipital protuberance, external, **2**:224; *see also*
Skull
Occipitoatlantal joints, **2**:224

Occipitocervical articulations, **1**:323, **1**:324-326;
see also Atlantooccipital articulations
Buetti's method for, **1**:324-325
Occluding coil of Gianturco, **2**:566
Occlusion
defined, **3**:103
of patent ductus arteriosus, **3**:98
Occupancy factor, **1**:35
Occupational exposure, **1**:25
OCG; *see* Cholecystography, oral
Octagonal immobilizer, **3**:36
OD; *see* Object distance
Oddi's sphincter, **2**:33, **2**:35
Odontoid process; *see* Dens
Off-line, defined, **3**:126
Olecranon fossa, **1**:62, **1**:65; *see also* Humerus
Olecranon process, **1**:113
anatomy of, **1**:61
PA axial projection for, **1**:113
Omenta, **2**:32
Omphalocele, **3**:11
Oncologist, defined, **3**:292, **3**:304
Oncology, radiation, **3**:291-304
altering biologic environment in, **3**:302-303
basic physics in, **3**:296-297
in cancer, **3**:294-295
clinical applications of, **3**:298-302
defined, **3**:292, **3**:304
definition of terms in, **3**:303-304
dosimetry in, **3**:298-299
timing and, **3**:303
future trends in, **3**:302-303
history of, **3**:292-293
inverted Y-radiation field in, **3**:299
multifield, **3**:298, **3**:299
opposing ports in, **3**:298, **3**:299
rotational field in, **3**:298
shaped fields in, **3**:299
single field in, **3**:298
theory of, **3**:293-297
timing of treatment in, **3**:302
treatment with, **3**:298
wedge fields in, **3**:298, **3**:299
On-line, defined, **3**:126
Opacified colon; *see* Large intestine, opacified
Opacified renal pelvis, **2**:568
Opaque arthrography, **1**:488
Opaque contrast media, **2**:500
Opaque myelography, **2**:500
Operating room, **1**:11
Operating system for computers, **3**:111
Operator's console for computed tomography,
3:137-139
Oppenheimer method
for thoracic vertebrae, **1**:358
for zygapophyseal articulations, **1**:361
Opposing ports teletherapy, **3**:298
Optic bulb, **2**:286
Optic canal, **2**:222; *see also* Optic foramen
Optic chiasm, **2**:222
sectional anatomy of, **2**:595, **2**:598, **2**:599
Optic foramen, **2**:222, **2**:271, **2**:272-279
Alexander method for, **2**:276-277
anatomy of, **2**:222
Lysholm method for, modified, **2**:278-279
projections for, **2**:271, **2**:272-279
orbitoparietal oblique, **2**:274-277
parieto-orbital oblique, **2**:271, **2**:272-273,
2:278-279

Optic foramen—cont'd
Rhese methods for, **2**:272-275
superior orbital fissure and anterior clinoid
process with, **2**:278-279
Optic groove; *see* Chiasmatic groove
Optic sulcus; *see* Chiasmatic groove
Optical density of radiograph, **1**:2, **1**:3
Optical disk, characteristics of, **3**:161
Optical scanner, **3**:110
defined, **3**:126
Optical storage and retrieval systems, **3**:123
Optical tape, characteristics of, **3**:161
Oragrafin, **2**:53
Oral cavity, **2**:2; *see also* Mouth
cancer of, **3**:301
Oral vestibule, **2**:2
Orbit, **2**:270-298
anatomy of, **2**:219, **2**:270, **2**:271
blow-out fractures of, **2**:270
computed tomography of, **3**:149
eye in, **2**:286-296; *see also* Eye
fissures in, **2**:282-285
localization of foreign body in, **2**:288-296
optic canal and, **2**:272-279
projection for, parieto-orbital oblique, **2**:271
sectional anatomy of, **2**:595
sphenoid strut and, **2**:280, **2**:281
Orbital fissure
inferior, **2**:222, **2**:270
Bertel method for, **2**:284-285
PA axial projection for, **2**:284-285
superior, **2**:222, **2**:280
Lysholm method for, modified, **2**:278-279
PA axial projection for, **2**:282, **2**:283
parieto-orbital oblique projection for, **2**:278-
279
Orbitomeatal line, **2**:233, **2**:271
Organ of hearing, **2**:228-229
Organ dose, **1**:30
Ornaments, **1**:14
Oropharynx, **2**:13
sectional anatomy of, **2**:599
Orthogonal coned magnification, **2**:492
Orthoroentgenography, **1**:482-485
Os calcis; *see* Calcaneus
Os capitatum; *see* Capitate
Os coxae, **1**:272; see also Hip
Os magnum; see Capitate
Ossicles, acoustic, **2**:228
Ossification centers, **1**:48, **3**:38-40
Osteoblasts, **1**:48
Osteogenesis imperfecta, **3**:11
Osteology, **1**:38
Ostium of uterus, **2**:196
Ottonello method for cervical vertebrae, **1**:344-345
Outpatient, pediatric, **3**:7
Output
defined, **3**:126
intensity of, **1**:29
Output device for computer, **3**:112
Output phosphor, defined, **3**:179
Ova, **2**:194
implantation of, **2**:196
Oval window; *see* Fenestra vestibuli
Ovary
anatomy of, **2**:194
fimbria of, **2**:194
pelvic pneumography for, **2**:199, **2**:202
shield, **3**:13

Index

Index

Index

Transjugular intrahepatic portosystemic shunt, **2**:573

Translumbar aortography, **2**:526

Transluminal angioplasty, percutaneous, **2**:561-565
coronary, **3**:99
defined, **3**:103
defined, **2**:587
stent placement in, **2**:564, **2**:565

Transmission scan, **3**:277, **3**:290

Transmission spectroscopy, **3**:83

Transonic, defined, **3**:247

Transposition of great arteries, **3**:101
defined, **3**:103

Transverse abdominis muscle, sectional anatomy of, **2**:608

Transverse atlantal ligament, **1**:315

Transverse colon, sectional anatomy of, **2**:612

Transverse dural venous sinuses, **2**:594

Transverse ligament; *see* Transverse atlantal ligament

Transverse plane, **1**:38

Transverse processes
of lumbar vertebrae, **1**:320
of thoracic vertebrae, **1**:318

Trapezium, **1**:60, **1**:61; *see also* Wrist
Clements-Nakayama method for fractures of, **1**:92-93
PA axial oblique projection for, **1**:92-93
tubercle of, **1**:63

Trapezius muscle, sectional anatomy of, **2**:596, **2**:602, **2**:605

Trapezoid, **1**:60, **1**:61; *see also* Wrist

Trauma
central nervous system and, **2**:499
cervical vertebrae, **1**:350-351
guidelines for, **1**:519-528
radiographs in, **1**:522, **1**:523-528
reversing/modifying position in, **1**:520, **1**:521
mandibular and temporomandibular joint, **2**:369
rib cage, **1**:405
sphenoid sinus effusion and, **2**:240
Towne method in, **2**:249, **2**:250

Treitz ligament, **2**:119

Trendelenburg position, **2**:93, **2**:115
modification of, **2**:112-113
in myelography, **2**:501
for urography, **2**:164

Triangular; *see* Triquetrum

Triangular bone, **1**:60

Tricuspid valve, **2**:516

Trigone, **2**:155

Triiodothyronine, **3**:265

Triquetral, **1**:60; *see also* Wrist

Triquetrum, **1**:60; *see also* Wrist

Trochanter, **1**:48; *see also* Greater trochanter
anatomy of, **1**:273

Trochlea, **1**:62, **1**:181; *see also* Humerus

Trochlear notch, **1**:61; *see also* Forearm

Trochlear surface, **1**:181

Trochoidal joint, **1**:46

True vocal folds, **2**:14; *see also* Neck

TSH; *see* Thyroid stimulating hormone

T-tube operative cholangiography, **2**:76, **2**:77

Tube
cathode ray; *see* Cathode ray tube
photomultiplier, **3**:272

Tubercle, **1**:48
of humerus, **1**:124; *see also* Humerus
of trapezium, **1**:63

Tuberculum sellae, **2**:222

Tuberosity, **1**:48
of metatarsals, **1**:181; *see also* Foot
of multangular; *see* Tubercle, of trapezium

Tumor volume, defined, **3**:296, **3**:304

Tumors
classification of, **3**:295
by radiosensitivity, **3**:294
metastasis of, positron emission tomography in, **3**:288
nuclear medicine and, **3**:271
radiation response of cells of, **3**:294
spinal cord, magnetic resonance imaging in, **3**:195

Turbinates, **2**:216, **2**:220; *see also* Nasal conchae

Turner, Burns, and Previtte method for intercondylar fossa, **1**:251

Twining method
for cervicothoracic region, **1**:352-353
for trachea and pulmonary apex, **1**:450-451

Twins, **2**:204

Tympanic antrum; *see* Mastoid antrum

Tympanic attic; *see* Epitympanic recess

Tympanic cavity, **2**:228

Tympanic membrane, **2**:228

Tympanum, **2**:226

U

Ulcerative colitis, **2**:130, **2**:131

Ulna, **1**:61; *see also* Forearm
styloid process of, **1**:61
trauma to, **1**:527

Ultrasound, **3**:205-247
advantages of, **3**:206
anatomical relationships and landmarks in, **3**:213, **3**:214-226
biologic effects of, **3**:212
clinical applications of, **3**:227-245
abdominal and retroperitoneal, **3**:227-231
of breast, **3**:237
cardiology, **3**:239-245
endorectal transducers in, **3**:237
neonatal neurosonography in, **3**:237, **3**:238
pelvic and obstetric, **3**:232-237, **3**:238
of penis, **3**:237
peripheral vascular, **3**:239-245
of prostate gland, **3**:237
of scrotum, **3**:237
of thyroid, **3**:237
continuous-wave, **3**:206, **3**:246
defined, **3**:247
diagnostic; *see* Diagnostic ultrasound
display modes in, **3**:210-212, **3**:246
Doppler, **3**:206, **3**:212
historical development of, **3**:207
physical principles of, **3**:208-213, **3**:214-226
acoustic impedance in, **3**:209
biological effects in, **3**:212
display modes in, **3**:210-212
longitudinal anatomic sections in, **3**:221-226, **3**:229-230, **3**:231
longitudinal waves in, **3**:208
sound wave properties in, **3**:208-209
transducers in, **3**:206, **3**:210
transverse anatomic sections in, **3**:215-220, **3**:227-228, **3**:229
pulsed-wave, **3**:206, **3**:210
transducers in, **3**:206, **3**:210

Unciform, **1**:60; *see also* Hamate

Undifferentiation, defined, **3**:293, **3**:304

Unidirectional tomographic motion, **3**:48-49
defined, **3**:73

Universal blood and body fluid precautions, **3**:8, **3**:9

Unstable nuclide, defined, **3**:304

Upper extremity; *see* Upper limb

Upper femur, **1**:276-279; *see also* Femoral neck and hip; Pelvis and upper femora

Upper gastrointestinal series, **2**:98-101

Upper limb, **1**:59-119
anatomy of, **1**:60-64
arteriography of, **2**:539
radial artery, in iatrogenic occlusion, **2**:539
articulations of, **1**:63-64
carpal bridge in, **1**:96-97
carpal canal in, **1**:94-95
digits in
first, **1**:72-73
second through fifth, **1**:70-71
elbow in, **1**:101-111
first carpometacarpal joint in, **1**:82
forearm in, **1**:98-100
general procedures for, **1**:65
hand in, **1**:74-81
humerus in, **1**:114-117
distal, **1**:106, **1**:108, **1**:112
proximal, **1**:118-119
lymphography for, **2**:580
thumb in, **1**:72-73
venogram of, **2**:540
wrist in, **1**:82-97; *see also* Wrist

Ureter, **2**:152, **2**:154-155; *see also* Urinary system
compression of, **2**:166
obstruction of, nuclear medicine and, **3**:270
retrograde urography and, **2**:179-182
sectional anatomy of, **2**:614
stent in, **2**:569

Ureteric compression, **2**:166

Ureterocystoscope, **2**:179

Urethra, **2**:152; *see also* Urinary system
female, **2**:155
male, **2**:155
retrograde urography and, **2**:181-182
sectional anatomy of, **2**:616, **2**:617, **2**:618

Urinary bladder, **2**:152, **2**:154-155
projections for
AP, **2**:184-185, **2**:190-192
AP oblique, **2**:186-187, **2**:189
lateral, **2**:188
PA, **2**:184-185
in R or L positions, **2**:188
in RPO and LPO positions, **2**:186-187, **2**:189
retrograde urography and, **2**:181-182
sectional anatomy of, **2**:616, **2**:618
and ureters, Chassard-Lapiné method for, **2**:183

Urinary incontinence, female, **2**:191-192

Urinary system, **2**:151-192
anatomy of, **2**:152-155
Barnes technique for, **2**:191-192
bladder in; *see* Urinary bladder
contrast media for, **2**:160, **2**:161
Cook, Keats, and Scale technique for, **2**:174
cystography of, **2**:158, **2**:181-182
retrograde; *see* Urinary system, retrograde cystography of
cystourethrography of, **2**:190-192
equipment for radiography of, **2**:164-165
Evans, Dubilier, and Monteith technique for, **2**:175

Index

Index